18 Update in Intensive Care and Emergency Medicine

Edited by J.-L. Vincent

K. Reinhart K. Eyrich
C. Sprung (Eds.)

Sepsis

Current Perspectives in Pathophysiology and Therapy

With 109 Figures and 56 Tables

Springer-Verlag
Berlin Heidelberg New York
London Paris Tokyo
Hong Kong Barcelona
Budapest

Series Editor

Prof. Dr. Jean-Louis Vincent
Clinical Director, Department of Intensive Care
Erasme University Hospital
Route de Lennik 808, 1070 Brussels, Belgium

Volume Editors

Prof. Dr. Konrad Reinhart
Direktor der Klinik für Anästhesiologie und Intensivtherapie
Klinikum der Friedrich Schiller-Universität Jena
Bachstraße 18, 07740 Jena, FRG

Prof. Dr. Klaus Eyrich
Klinik für Anästhesiologie und operative Intensivmedizin
Universitätsklinikum Steglitz der FU Berlin
Hindenburgdamm 30, 12200 Berlin, FRG

Prof. Dr. Charles Sprung
Department of Anesthesiology and Critical Care Medicine
Hadassah Hebrew University, Medical Center
P. O. Box 12000, 91120 Jerusalem, Israel

ISBN-13: 978-3-642-85038-7 e-ISBN-13: 978-3-642-85036-3
DOI: 10.1007/ 978-3-642-85036-3

Softcover reprint of the hardcover 1st edition 1994

Typesetting: Zechnersche Buchdruckerei, Speyer

19/3130-5 4 3 2 1 0 – Printed on acid-free paper

Preface

Sepsis is still the leading cause of death in surgical and general intensive care units. Although our knowledge of this complex syndrome has increased in recent years, it is still far from complete. New therapeutic approaches have been developed. Some did not fullfill the high expectations for their use in clinical practice; others are still under clinical evaluation.
It is the aim of this monograph to offer basic information on the etiology, definition, pathophysiology, prevention and therapy of sepsis and septic shock to both the clinician and the scientist. We believe that it presents an extensive overview that may help the clinician to better understand and treat sepsis and septic shock. We also hope that this work will give some directions for future research both in the clinical field as well as the laboratory.

Jena, Berlin, Jerusalem,
February 1994

K. Reinhart
K. Eyrich
C. Sprung

Table of Contents

I. Definition/Prognosis

II. Pathogenesis

III. Pathophysiology

IV. Monitoring

V. Therapy

List of Contributors

Prof. Dr. med. Dr. rer. nat. D. Adam
Vorstand der Abteilung
für Antimikrobielle Therapie
und Infektionsimmunologie
Dr. von Haunersches Kinderspital
der Universität
Lindwurmstraße 4
80337 München, FRG

Prof. G. R. Bernard, MD
Division of Pulmonary and Critical
Care Medicine
Center for Lung Research
Vanderbilt University
Nashville, TN 37232-2650, USA

Prof. B. Beutler, MD
Research Laboratories
Howard Hughes Medical Institute
5353 Harry Hines Boulevard
Dallas, TX 75235-9050, USA

Dr. med. F. Bloos
The Richard Ivey Critical Care
Trauma Centre
Victoria Hospital Corporation
375 South Street
London, Ontario NGA 4G5,
Canada

Dr. med. P. Boekstegers
Medizinische Klinik I
Ludwig-Maximilians-Universität
München
Klinikum Großhadern
Marchionistr. 15
81377 München, FRG

Prof. R. C. Bone, MD
The Medical College of Ohio,
Toledo
3000 Arlington Avenue
Toledo, OH 43699-0008, USA

Prof. K. L. Brigham, MD
Center for Lung Research
Department of Medicine
Vanderbilt University School
of Medicine
Nashville, TN 37232, USA

K. F. Bruin
Department of Inflammation
Research, AMC Hospital
University of Amsterdam
Medical Center
Meibergdreef 9
1105 AZ Amsterdam,
The Netherlands

Prof. S. M. Cain, MD, PhD
Department of Physiology
and Biophysics
University of Alabama
at Birmingham
Birmingham, AL 35294-0005, USA

Prof. F. B. Cerra, MD
Department of Surgery
University of Minnesota
406 Harvard Street Southeast
Minneapolis, MN 55455, USA

Prof. Dr. med. J. Cohen
Director of the Department of
Infectious Diseases & Bacteriology
Hammersmith Hospital
Du Cane Road
London W12 ONN, UK

Prof. J.F. Dhainaut, MD, PhD
Chef de Service de Réanimation
Cochin Port-Royal University
Hospital
27, Rue du Faubourg Saint-Jacques
75014 Paris, France

W.D. Döcke
Institut für Medizinische
Immunologie
Universitätsklinikum Charité
Humboldt-Universität
Schumannstr. 20/21
10098 Berlin, FRG

L. Eidelman, MD
Department of Anesthesiology
and Critical Care/Medicine
Hadassah Hebrew University,
Medical Center
PO Box 12000
91120 Jerusalem, Israel

Dr. med. B. Eisele
SGE Therapeutika
Klinische Forschung
Thrombose & Intensivmedizin
Behringwerke AG
Postfach 1140
35001 Marburg/Lahn, FRG

Priv.-Doz. Dr. med. E. Faist
Chirurgische Klinik und Poliklinik
Ludwig-Maximilians-Universität
München
Klinikum Großhadern
Postfach 701260
81337 München, FRG

Prof. Dr. med. K.J. Falke
Direktor der Klinik für
Anästhesiologie und operative
Intensivmedizin
Klinikum Rudolf Virchow
der Freien Universität Berlin
Augustenburger Platz 1
13344 Berlin, FRG

Prof. Dr. med. M. Georgieff
Geschäftsführender Direktor
der Universitätsklinik für
Anästhesiologie
Klinikum der Universität Ulm
Postfach 3830
89070 Ulm, FRG

Prof. G. Guiterrez, MD, PhD
Pulmonary and Critical Care
Medicine Division
The University of Texas Medical
School
6431 Fannin, MSMB 1.274
Houston, TX 77030, USA

J.A. Hazelzet, MD
Dr. Molewaterplein 60
3015 GJ Rotterdam,
The Netherlands

Dr. med. M. Kaul
Knoll AG
Oncology/Immunology
Postfach 210805
67008 Ludwigshafen, FRG

Dr. med. M. Kluge
Knoll AG
Oncology/Immunology
Postfach 210805
67008 Ludwigshafen, FRG

Prof. W.A. Knaus, MD
Director, ICU Research Unit
The George Washington University
2300 K Street, N.W.
Washington DC 20037, USA

Prof. Dr. med. H.G. Kress
Department of Anaesthesiology
and Intensive Care Medicine
University of Vienna (AKH)
Währinger Gürtel 18–20
1090 Vienna, Austria

Priv.-Doz. Dr. med. habil.
M. Kretzschmar
Klinik für Anästhesiologie
und Intensivtheraphie
Klinikum der
Friedrich-Schiller-Universität Jena
Bachstraße 18
07740 Jena, FRG

Prof. Dr. med. B. Lachmann
Department of Anesthesiology
Erasmus University Rotterdam
Postbox 1738
3000 DR Rotterdam,
The Netherlands

Dr. med. K. Lewandowski
Klinik für Anästhesiologie und
operative Intensivmedizin
Klinikum Rudolf Virchow
der Freien Universität Berlin
Augustenburger Platz 1
13344 Berlin, FRG

Prof. Dr. med. H. Lode
Pneumologie I – Infektiologie
und Immunologie
Krankenhaus Zehlendorf-Berlin
Zum Heckeshorn 33
14109 Berlin, FRG

J. C. Marshall, MD, FRCS(C), FACS
General and Critical Care Surgery
Toronto General Hospital
200 Elizabeth Street
Eaton North 9-234
Toronto, Ontario M5G 2C4,
Canada

Dr. med. A. Meier-Hellmann
Klinik für Anästhesiologie und
operative Intensivmedizin
Klinikum Steglitz der Freien
Universität Berlin
Hindenburgdamm 30
12200 Berlin, FRG

Priv.-Doz. Dr. med. M. D. Menger
Direktor des Instituts für
Chirurgische Forschung
Ludwig-Maximilians-Universität
München
Klinikum Großhadern
Marchioninistraße 15
81377 München, FRG

C. Natanson, MD
Critical Care Medicine Department
National Institutes of Health
9000 Rockville Pike
Bethesda, MD 20892, USA

S. M. Opal, MD
Infectious Disease Division
Memorial Hospital of Rhode Island
111 Brewster Street
Pawtucket, RI 02860, USA

M. D. Pasquale, MD
Department of Surgery
University of Minnesota
406 Harvard Street Southeast
Minneapolis, MN 55455, USA

Dr. med. M. Petri
Pneumologie I – Infektiologie
und Immunologie
Krankenhaus Zehlendorf-Berlin
Zum Heckeshorn 33
14109 Berlin, FRG

Z. M. N. Quezado, MD
Critical Care Medicine Department
National Institutes of Health
9000 Rockville Pike
Bethesda, MD 20892, USA

Prof. Dr. med. K. Reinhart
Direktor der Klinik
für Anästhesiologie
und Intensivtherapie
Klinikum der
Friedrich-Schiller-Universität Jena
Bachstraße 18
07740 Jena, FRG

Priv.-Doz. Dr. med. F. U. Schade
Institut für Experimentelle Biologie
und Medizin
Forschungsinstitut Borstel
Parkallee 1–40
23845 Borstel, FRG

Dr. med. R. R. Schumann
Max-Delbrück-Centrum
für molekulare Medizin
Robert-Rössle-Straße 10
13122 Berlin, FRG

Prof. Dr. med. W. Seeger
Medizinische Klinik I
Medizinisches Zentrum
für Innere Medizin
Klinikum der
Justus-Liebig-Universität Gießen
Klinikstraße 29
35385 Gießen, FRG

Prof. W. J. Sibbald, MD, FRCPC, FACP
Coordinator, The Richard Ivey
Critical Care Trauma Centre
Victoria Hospital Corporation
375 South Street
London, Ontario NGA 4G5,
Canada

Dr. med. C. Spies
Klinik für Anästhesiologie
und operative Intensivmedizin
Klinikum Steglitz der Freien
Universität Berlin
Hindenburgdamm 30
12200 Berlin, FRG

Ch. L. Sprung, MD, JD, FCCM
Department of Anesthesiology
and Critical Care/Medicine
Hadassah Hebrew University,
Medical Center
PO Box 12000
91120 Jerusalem, Israel

S. Sriskandan, MD
Department of Infectious
Diseases & Bacteriology
Hammersmith Hospital
Du Cane Road
London W12 ONN, UK

Prof. Dr. med. W. Teichmann
Chefarzt der 1. Chirurg. Abteilung
des Allgemeinen Krankenhauses
Altona
Paul-Ehrlich-Straße 1
22763 Hamburg, FRG

A. S. Tütüncü, MD
Department of Anesthesiology
Erasmus University Rotterdam
Postbox 1738
3000 DR Rotterdam,
The Netherlands

S. J. H. van Deventer, MD
Department of Inflammation
Research, AMC Hospital
University of Amsterdam
Medical Center
Meibergdreef 9
1105 AZ Amsterdam,
The Netherlands

Prof. Dr. J.-L. Vincent
Clinical Director, Department
of Intensive Care
Erasme University Hospital
Route de Lennik 808
1070 Brussels, Belgium

Prof. Dr. med. R. von Baehr
Geschäftsführender Direktor
des Instituts für Medizinische
Immunologie
Universitätsklinikum Charité
Humboldt-Universität
Schumannstr. 20/21
10098 Berlin, FRG

Prof. Dr. med. K. Werdan
Medizinische Klinik I
Ludwig-Maximilians-Universität
München
Klinikum Großhadern
Marchionistr. 15
81377 München, FRG

J. J. Zimmermann, MD, PhD
University of Wisconsin Children's
Hospital
600 Highland Avenue
Madison, WI 53792-4108, USA

I. Definition/Prognosis

Sepsis and Septic Shock: Update on Definitions

J.-L. Vincent

Introduction

Sepsis remains one of the most common causes of death in critically ill patients. Coming from a very old Greek term referring to "putrefaction," sepsis refers to the systemic response to infection and is recognized by a constellation of clinical, hemodynamic, hematologic, biochemical, and inflammatory signs which are all part of a whole body response (Table 1).

Although for many years, the terms "sepsis" and "infection" have been used alternatively, recent investigations have indicated that sepsis is related

Table 1. Signs of sepsis and septic shock

Sepsis

- Fever
- Tachycardia
- Tachypnea, respiratory alkalosis
- Elevated cardiac output, low systemic vascular resistance
- Hyperleukocytosis (with "left shift") or leukopenia
- Increased cellular metabolism, elevated oxygen consumption
- Increased insulin requirements
- Inflammatory signs: increased sedimentation rate, elevated C-reactive protein and fibrinogen levels
- Elevated cytokine levels: tumor necrosis factor, interleukin-6 etc.
- Cutaneous manifestations
- Ophthalmic manifestations
- Organ dysfunction: renal failure, ARDS, mental obtundation etc.

Septic shock[a]

- Arterial hypotension (systolic arterial pressure below 90 mm Hg or mean arterial pressure below 60 mm Hg) associated with signs of tissue hypoperfusion:
  - Increased blood lactate levels (>2 mEq/l)
  - Altered organ perfusion: oliguria, altered mentation etc.

[a] Abnormal $\dot{V}O_2/DO_2$ dependency, decreased gastric intramucosal pH can also be used to document tissue hypoperfusion. Cardiac output can be elevated, normal or low. Hypothermia, when present is a strong clue in favor of the diagnosis of septic shock

ARDS, adult respiratory distress syndrome; $\dot{V}O_2$, oxygen consumption; DO_2, oxygen delivery

to the immunological response of the host rather than to the invading organism itself. Sepsis involves the release of a wide array of mediators, including tumor necrosis factor (TNF), various interleukins, platelet activating factor (PAF), arachidonic acid metabolites, and many others. The release of the same mediators has been demonstrated in association with a variety of other disease processes such as trauma, pancreatitis, ischemia and reperfusion, and even heart failure [1]. Hence, although sepsis is the typical clinical syndrome recognized in association with infection, it must be borne in mind that infection is not always demonstrated in these conditions. Accordingly, the presence of positive blood cultures or an obvious source of infection is necessary to confirm that an infectious process is involved in genuine "sepsis." In some clinical conditions, sepsis could be of presumed, but unproven, infectious origin. In some of these patients, resorption could be of presumed, but unproven, infectious origin. In some of these patients, resorption of bacterial products from the gut may be implicated [2]. The prognosis may not be better in these patients without treatable infection. Marshall and Sweeny [3] found a similar degree of sepsis in patients dying without infection and those dying with uncontrolled infection.

Undoubtedly, these recent developments have created a problem of definition (Fig. 1). Yet, it is important for the members of the medical community to agree on definitions to describe patients. It is also important for clinical studies to have identifiable groups of patients so that the findings of these studies may result in their appropriate application.

Accordingly, there are basically two problems related to these definitions: The first is an immediate clinical one, that is the recognition of infection. It is essential to recognize infection early to find a possible source and to eradicate the responsible microorganisms. Overlooking an infectious process can

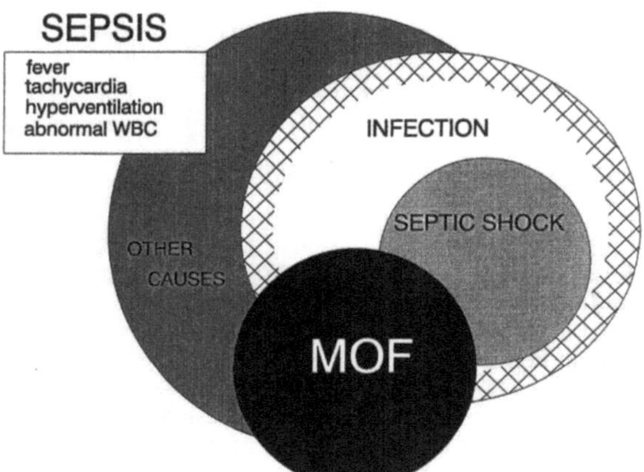

Fig. 1. Relation between sepsis, infection, septic shock and multiple organ failure (*MOF*). Infection is surrounded by a *hatched zone* corresponding to uncertainty about the presence of an infectious process. WBC, white blood count

prove fatal to the patient. The second problem is related to a possible influence of the immune response to infection. There is a wide range of possible therapeutic interventions, ranging from antibodies to TNF to the nonsteroidal anti-inflammatory agents. The basis for these forms of immunotherapy is that severe injury may result in an overreaction of the host, resulting in tissue damage from an excessive release of mediators. As the same cascade of septic mediators can be activated by several mechanisms, these forms of therapy may find a place in the prevention of multiple organ failure even in the absence of infection.

Does Infection Matter?

Clearly, the presence of infection is important for clinical purposes, such as in deciding upon an appropriate antibiotic strategy. When it comes to immunotherapy, if the same septic response is involved in severe infections and in other disease states, one may wonder if the documentation of an infection is of any importance. Although we do not have a precise answer to this important question, it is clear that mixing together septic patients with and without documented infections in clinical trials should be avoided, as it may confound some important issues. There can be important qualitative and quantitative differences in the activation of the immune/inflammatory cascade of mediators. For instance, the role of oxygen free radicals may be more important in the presence of trauma with ischemia-reperfusion and the role of proteases may be more important in the presence of severe pancreatitis. Hence, the effects of immunotherapy should be evaluated separately in infected and noninfected patients. As the septic reaction is more likely to be severe in infected patients, clinical trials should initially focus on these patients. Infections may also have a different pattern after trauma and in other forms of critical illnesses [4].

To refer to "suspected infection" is too vague and potentially misleading. Obviously, the difficulty resides in early identification of the infection, as the culture results cannot be immediately obtained. Nevertheless, in many patients, an infectious process can be documented. The various procedures and tests that can be performed to evaluate the presence and the source of infection in critically ill patients have been reviewed elsewhere [5].

Is Bacteremia Important?

Clearly, the presence of demonstrable bacteria in the blood is not a requirement for the diagnosis of sepsis. About 50% of patients with severe sepsis have documented bacteremia [6]. Despite the fact that the incidence of circulatory shock is higher when bacteremia is present [6, 7], recent studies found little significant difference between patients with and without positive blood cultures [8]. This lack of significance is probably in part due to the fact that many patients develop severe infections while treated by antibiotic therapy. It is also difficult to predict the presence of bacteremia from the patient's evaluation. Analyzing the data obtained on 2568 septic patients included in the Veterans Administration (VA) trial of corticosteroid therapy, Peduzzi et al. [9] found three factors to be independently predicitve of bacteremia: elevated temperature, low systemic blood pressure, and low platelet count. Nevertheless, none of these criteria had sufficient accuracy to be clinically useful.

The term "septicemia" refers to the association of sepsis with documented bacteremia. It is probably not very helpful, but the term exists and there is nothing wrong in using it.

Is the Type of Microorganism Important?

The type of bacteria involved is probably of little importance. Even though endotoxin is a potent trigger of the septic response, severe infections due to gram-negative and gram-positive bacteria have a similar pattern. Early studies on patients with septic shock described a different hemodynamic pattern in patients with infections due to gram-negative and gram-positive infections [10], but more recent studies did not confirm these findings [11, 12]. Another study reported a higher mortality rate in septicemia due to gram-positive than to gram-negative bacteria [13].

However, the presence of bacteria versus other forms of microorganisms is very important. Bacteria are usually more virulent and more likely to induce septic shock while fungal infections are more likely to develop in more debilitated, immunocompromised patients, whose prognosis is very poor.

Is the Source of Infection Important?

It is probably not warranted to mix patients with various sources of infection in clinical trials. In particular, it is well recognized that patients with infections due to urosepsis have a much lower mortality rate than those with other types of infection [14]. Hence, it is important to separate the different sources of infection.

How Important Is the Underlying Clinical Status?

The underlying status of the patient is probably the most important prognostic factor in severe sepsis. There is little doubt about the fact that a debilitated patient admitted for the third time to the intensive care unit for a fifth episode of septic shock has a much lower chance of survival than an otherwise healthy patient with urosepsis who comes from the emergency room. In a recent report on 448 episodes of gram-negative bacteremia [15], the underlying disease was found to represent the most important prognostic factor. The immune response, including nonspecific and specific factors, can be influenced by a number of elements [16].

Is the "Sepsis Syndrome" a Valid Clinical Entity?

Roger Bone must be commended for his essential contributions to this field. He introduced the term "sepsis syndrome," which is supposed to represent a severe form of sepsis, refering to the association of sepsis with altered organ perfusion and/or altered organ function. This entity has been used to establish a series of criteria applicable to multicenter studies [8].

Several important problems have emerged with the use of the term "sepsis syndrome", the most important being its inhomogeneity. This experience revealed that a total of 36% of patients had the criteria of septic shock on admission, and another 23% developed septic shock after study admission. The mortality rate for the entire group was around 25%, but only 13% in the absence of shock and 43% when shock developed after study admission [6]. A major problem is that patients with minor degrees of severity can meet the criteria, because some of these criteria are easily met (Table 2).

Do We Need the "Systemic Inflammatory Response Syndrome"?

Recently, an expert panel of North American colleagues proposed to reserve the term "sepsis" for the host response to invading microorganisms and to introduce the acronym "SIRS" (systemic inflammatory response syndrome) to define a generalized inflammatory response in a broader sense. The introduction of this neologism is not warranted for several reasons. First, the existing confusion is not likely to resolve with the introduction of yet another definition. Second, the term "SIRS" is conceptually a very sensitive entity so as to encompass a large number of critically ill patients with possible infection. In our experience, most intensive care unit (ICU) patients do meet the SIRS criteria [17]. Clinical studies using these very broad criteria should then rely heavily on the use of a severity index to stratify the degree of severity of illness of the patients. These indexes, however, have been usually validated for the prognosis 24 h after admission in the ICU but not for repeated eval-

Table 2. Potential problems with the common criteria used to define the sepsis syndrome

- Heterogenous group of underlying pathologies.
- Fever, tachycardia, tachypnea sometimes absent.
- Altered mental status cannot be quantified.
- Low systemic vascular resistance is related to: a reduced arterial pressure (included in the primary criteria) and/or an elevated cardiac output (not necessarily a sign of complication).

Table 3. Potential problems with the use of severity indexes in clinical trials

- There are several systems that could be used.
- Not all severity indexes are in the public domain.
- Some severity indexes are relatively complex.
- Severity indexes are not applicable to all groups of patients with the same degree of accuracy.
- Severity indexes have been usually validated
  - for evaluation after 24 h in the ICU
  - but not for repeated use in the ICU.
- The influence of therapy is not taken into account.

uation of individual patients during their ICU stay. Some of these indexes have become quite sophisticated, so that their use may require a computer program. Access to some programs is even protected (Table 3). Although progress made in prognostic assessment of the critically ill is certainly encouraging, it should not prevent us from basing our evaluation and our treatment on relatively simple criteria easily obtained at the bedside. Third, as expressed above, the primary diagnosis remains essential. It is not warranted to lump together a number of acutely ill patients with different disease states under the same SIRS label. Finally, for clinical purposes, placing a number of patients under the same diagnosis may reduce the incentive for searching for a source of infection.

Are the Signs of Sepsis Reliable?

There is a long list of signs of sepsis, which will not be summarized here [18]. Table 1 presents a few of the most important signs of sepsis. One must admit that none of these is either sensitive or specific, especially in the critically ill patient.

Fever is an important sign of infection, but it can be absent in a number of cases. This has been a common source of frustation for investigators in recent clinical trials in which patients with obviously severe infection did not reach the temperature criteria needed to enter the trial. Failure to develop fever has been related to increased fatality rates [19]. In the presence of acute circulatory failure, hypothermia can even occur, probably because of an impairment in the thermogenic mechanisms. Such hypothermia is actually an ominous sign, associated with higher mortality rates [20].

However, fever is often present in conditions other than infection, such as trauma or myocardial infarction.

After fever, tachycardia is the most important systemic sign of infection [13, 17]. It is usually present in relation to a sympathetic response to sepsis and sometimes hypovolemia. The degree of tachycardia has been related to mortality in septic shock [21, 22]. Sometimes, tachycardia is remarkably absent, especially in elderly patients or those treated with anti-arrhythmic agents.

Hyperventilation associated with respiratory alkalosis was identified many years ago as a sign of infection [23–25]. However, this clinical sign is often lost in critically ill patients, particularly since many patients with severe sepsis are mechanically ventilated.

Similarly, although an increased white blood count (WBC) is a valuable sign of infection, hyperleukocytosis is commonly found in critically ill patients in relation to a stress response to other stimuli.

Are There Important Differences in Clinical Management?

Obviously, treatment is a major determinant of survival. In the study by Kreger et al. [19] including 612 patients with gram-negative bacteremia, appropriate antibiotic therapy was associated with a 50% reduction in both circulatory shock and mortality rate. The management of underlying factors is also important. For instance, early stabilization of the traumatized patient can have a significant influence on morbidity and mortality [26, 27].

In any case, it may be difficult to assess the appropriateness of each form of therapy. There may be important differences in clinical management from one institution to another [28]. It should be kept in mind that these factors are not included in any severity index.

Is Septic Shock a Valid Clinical Entity?

Septic shock describes the clinical syndrome corresponding to acute circulatory failure. Septic shock is virtually always associated with a bacterial infection, even though the presence of bacteria is not always demonstrated. Septic shock is equally attributed to gram-negative and gram-positive infections [29]. It is difficult to objectively identify the patients who may develop septic shock. In a recent study on 331 patients with bacteremia, Aube et al. [29] identified the following to be risk factors for septic shock: male gender or age older than 75 years, creatinine level greater than 2 mg/dl, a prothrombin time less than 60% and the presence of an interstitial pattern on the chest roentgenogram.

Arterial hypotension is an important clinical sign, but it is neither specific nor very sensitive. Hypotension can be associated with other forms af acute circulatory failure. In particular, the differential diagnosis between hypovolemic and septic shock is not always evident, and it is generally the confirmation (or exclusion) of the infectious process that determines the eventual diagnosis. Transient hypotension can also occur in relation to a vagal reaction or to some reduction in venous return associated with some degree of hypovolemia, particularly when intrathoracic pressures are increased. These forms of transient hypotension are usually not associated with signs of organ failure. It is also evident that tissue hypoperfusion can sometimes occur in the absence of significant hypotension. The presence of tissue hypoxia can be reflected by an increase in blood lactate levels. Whenever possible, increased blood lactate levels should confirm the presence of tissue hypoxia.

Some investigators attempted to include some therapeutic aspects in the definition, such as "not responding to fluid therapy" or "requiring the use of vasopressor agents." These additions are probably not useful because they are nonspecific and largely dependent on the treatment protocols. How much fluid is required to state that there is no satisfactory response? Sometimes severely hypovolemic patients do not develop signs of hemodynamic instability. Similarly, the usage of vasopressors can differ substantially in the various centers. This is illustrated by some recent studies on the use of vasopressors in septic shock. Some investigators started the administration of epinephrine in patients with a mean pulmonary artery occlusion pressure (PAOP) of 19 mm Hg [30] while others started the administration of either norepinephrine [31] or epinephrine [32] in patients with a mean PAOP of only 9 mm Hg. Clearly, other clinicians would have started the vasopressor therapy earlier or later than in these studies. Could we then define a level of cardiac filling pressures? Unfortunately, in view of large variation in the optimal cardiac filling pressure in septic shock, it is also difficult to base the definition on such criteria. Thus, exactly as one would not define pneumonia by a requirement for penicillin, one should avoid the introduction of a therapeutic element in a definition of a disease state.

The use of "refractory shock" has been sometimes proposed to characterize the most severe form of circulatory shock. It usually refers to a situation in which prolonged adrenergic support is required [33]. The term is not helpful because it is too imprecise and too dependent on therapy. It could even have a negative connotation, implying that the situation has become hopeless. We think it important to consider that even the severest form of shock is potentially reversible. The degree of severity of shock can be assessed by other means, such as the degree of concurrent organ dysfunction or the degree of lactic acidosis.

In summary, the definition of shock must include several elements. The best definition of septic shock remains the development of arterial hypotension associated with signs of altered tissue perfusion (Table 1). This definition should not include a therapeutic variable. Although some assessment of the degree of severity of septic shock may be helpful, the use of the term "refractory shock" should be avoided.

Can Organ Failure Be Quantitated?

In septic patients, alterations in organ function can go from some degree of organ dysfunction (e.g., moderate elevation in creatinine or bilirubin levels) to severe organ failure (e.g., severe acute respiratory failure or coma). The most severe form leads to multiple organ failure (MOF), which often follows an episode of acute circulatory failure, although it sometimes arises in the absence of documented hemodynamic instability. It may also develop in the absence of infection. The translocation of bacteria and the resorption of endotoxin from the gut may be involved in these conditions.

The degree of failure of four organs can be quantitated in the following manner:

1. **Respiratory failure:** The degree of respiratory failure is best assessed by the evaluation of gas exchange, and the PaO_2/FiO_2 ratio is most commonly used for this purpose. As the degree of hypoxemia is influenced by the use of mechanical ventilation and positive end-expiratory pressure (PEEP) in particular, this form of therapy is often taken into account. In the assessment of the severity of the adult respiratory distress syndrome (ARDS), the score proposed by Murray et al. [34], including the PaO_2/FiO_2 ratio, the degree of PEEP used and the degree of alteration of the chest roentgenogram is commonly used, because it is relatively simple and yet reliable.
2. **Renal function:** The urea (or BUN) and creatinine concentrations are usually used to assess the degree of renal dysfunction. Oliguria is another objective parameter that can be included.
3. **Hematologic failure:** The degree of coagulation abnormalities is the most important component of this organ failure response to severe sepsis. It is best assessed by the platelet count combined with the prothrombin time (PT) and the activated partial thromboplastin time (APTT). A low hematocrit or a low white blood count (WBC) may be included in the definition of hematologic failure [35].
4. **Liver dysfunction:** The degree of hyperbilirubinemia is the most reliable and helpful parameter [36]. Elevated liver enzymes (SGOT and SGPT) can represent additional criteria.

In an attempt to be more complete, some investigators tried to include other criteria: It is evident that MOF often includes some degree of altered mentation. To assess neurological function, the Glasgow coma scale has been found most useful. However, there are two major problems. One is that since many patients are treated by sedative agents, evaluation in the presence of sedation is often difficult. The other is that many patients are treated with mechanical ventilation so that the assessment of speech capabilities becomes very subjective.

Some investigators also included the degree of cardiovascular dysfunction in the assessment of organ dysfunction [37]. Various criteria have been proposed, including the degree of adrenergic support, the cardiac output value, the presence of arrhythmias or the arterial pH. None of these criteria is very reliable. The degree of adrenergic support depends on the usual management in each particular unit. The cardiac output value is not clearly related to prognosis in severe sepsis. The development of arrhythmias can be associated with underlying cardiac disease or some electrolyte abnormalities rather than to the degree of MOF as a global consequence of an overwhelming septic process.

As expressed above, septic shock is a very important entity as such, because it can be a direct cause of failure of the various organs. Therefore, it should be considered as a source of complications rather than a complication.

Finally, some investigators listed some diagnoses, such as cholecystitis or stress ulcer, in the definition of MOF [38]. This can be hazardous, as these diagnoses are more often subjective.

In conclusion, it is advisable to include only objective, undisputable parameters in the assessment of organ failure. These, in turn, should be based on measurable parameters and not on clinical signs or symptoms. Unfortunately, the objective assessment of neurological complications is impossible today. Although the diagnosis of circulatory shock is of paramount importance, it should be considered as a major source rather than a part of the MOF syndrome.

Implications

A patient may appear septic in the absence of documented infection. In the presence of another recognized cause of inflammatory response, it is important to refer to this primary diagnosis and not to lump this disease state together with many others. Specifically, a patient with polytrauma or a patient with pancreatitis who develops a "sepsis-like" syndrome in the absence of demonstrable infection remains a patient with polytrauma or pancreatitis. These definitions, which are in agreement with our common clinical intuition, always raise the possibility that infection might be present. In any patient who appears septic, an infectious process should be actively sought.

What Is the Future of Clinical Studies on Immunotherapy?

Taken together, the clinical trials which have been recently completed or which are still under way are likely to show an overall moderate beneficial effect, characterized by a moderate reduction in morbidity and mortality rates. None of the tested substances will represent a "magic bullet" that will dramatically influence outcome. A major problem remains the identification of a group of patients most likely to benefit from these interventions.

In the future, there will basically be two types of approaches to this complex problem (Fig. 2).

The first is to include a very large number of patients into clinical trials so that confounding factors will be eventually eliminated. If a molecule is found effective, a subgroup analysis may then help to identify the patients who ben-

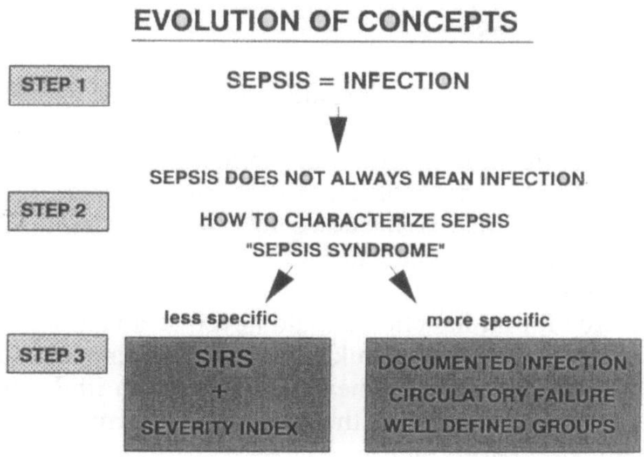

Fig. 2. Evolution of concepts related to severe sepsis

efit the most. These large trials must have relatively broad criteria for entry, except that a severity index must be used to stratify the patients. These trials must also be relatively simple to be practically feasible. They will be relatively expensive for the particular pharmaceutical industry, but the potential use of a therapeutic agent in large numbers of patients may be rewarding. A foreseeable problem is the availability of centers that will be ready to participate, in view of the multiplicity of the trials dealing with the same type of patients!

The second approach is to focus any new therapeutic intervention on a specific group of patients with an identifiable disease process. Rather than mixing traumatized with nontraumatized patients, urosepsis with other sources of infections, patients with early and advanced organ failure, these trials would include well defined groups of patients. Although the criteria need to be defined for each therapeutic intervention, it is likely that circulatory shock will represent a useful basis. A number of experimental studies have indicated that immunotherapeutic interventions are effective only in the most severe forms of overwhelming sepsis.

In any case, the clinical trials will need to stratify the patients according to the severity of the disease process and thus the chances of survival. Those patients with high chances of survival will be eliminated, because they are likely to do well in the absence of additional therapy. Furthermore, immunotherapy may even have deleterious effects by blocking the physiological septic response. At the other end of the spectrum, patients who are very debilitated and at the end of a long disease process should be also eliminated, because any form of investigational therapy is not likely to benefit those patients who are likely to die.

Conclusions

Sepsis is a clinical syndrome typically found in association with severe infections. However, one must recognize that an infection is not always found in the septic patient. The same immunological mediators can be released in a variety of other disorders. In any circumstance, it is important to consider a number of factors, including the type of patient, the severity of the underlying disease, and the cause of sepsis.

Clinically, it remains vital to search for infection in all conditions. The search for an infection should never be abandoned, and whenever a possible source is found, it should be eradicated to avoid the development of MOF.

Studies in immunotherapy are likely to find a therapeutic effect of some forms of treatment in the most severe forms of sepsis, i.e., those associated with circulatory failure.

References

1. Levine B, Kalman J, Mayer L, Fillit HM, Packer M (1990) Elevated circulating levels of tumor necrosis factor in severe chronic heart failure. N Engl J Med 323:236–241
2. Meakins JL (1990) Etiology of multiple organ failure. J Trauma 30:S165–S168
3. Marshall J, Sweeny D (1990) Microbial infection and the septic response in critical surgical illness. Arch Surg 125:17–23
4. Polk HC (1993) Factors influencing the risk of infection after trauma. Am J Surg 165:2S–7S
5. Norwood SH, Civetta JM (1987) Evaluating sepsis in critically ill patients. Chest 92:137–144
6. Bone RC, Fisher CJ, Clemmer TP, Slotman GJ, Metz CA, Balk RA (1989) Sepsis syndrome: a valid clinical entity. Crit Care Med 17:389–393
7. Mc Cabe WR, Treadwell TL, de Maria A (1983) Pathophysiology of bacteremia. Am J Med 75:7–18
8. Bone RC, Fisher CJ, Clemmer TP et al (1987) The methylprednisolone severe sepsis study group: a controlled clinical trial of high-dose methylprednisolone in the treatment of severe sepsis and septic shock. N Engl J Med 317:353
9. Peduzzi P, Shatney C, Sheagren J, Sprung C (1992) Predictors of bacteremia and gram-negative bacteremia in patients with sepsis. Arch Intern Med 152:529–535
10. Blain CM, Anderson TO, Pietras RJ, Gunnar RM (1970) Immediate hemodynamic effects of gram-negative vs gram-positive bacteremia in man. Arch Intern Med 126:260–265
11. Wiles JB, Cerra FB, Siegel JH, Border JR (1980) The systemic septic response: does the organism matter? Crit Care Med 8:55–60
12. Ahmed AJ, Kruse JA, Haupt MT, Chandrasekar PH, Carlson RW (1991) Hemodynamic responses to gram-positive versus gram-negative sepsis in critically ill patients with and without circulatory shock. Crit Care Med 19:1520–1525
13. Geerdes HF, Ziegler D, Lode H et al (1992) Septicemia in 980 patients at a university hospital in Berlin: prospective studies during 4 selected years between 1979 and 1989. Clin Infect Dis 15:991–1002
14. Wong DT, Wagner DP, Knaus WA (1992) Lower ICU mortality in septic shock due to urosepsis compared to non-urosepsis. Anesthesiology 77:A318 (abstract)
15. Uzun O, Akalin HE, Hayran M, Unal S (1992) Factors influencing prognosis in bacteremia due to gram-negative organisms: evaluation of 448 episodes in a Turkish university hospital. Clin Infect Dis 15:866–873

16. Cates L (1983) Host factors in bacteremia. Am J Med 75:19–25
17. Metrangolo L, Fiorillo M, Friedman G et al (1993) Hemodynamic profile in the first 24 hours of septic shock. Med Intens 17:S53 (abstract)
18. Harris RL, Musher DM, Bloom K et al (1987) Manifestations of sepsis. Arch Intern Med 147:1895–1906
19. Kreger BE, Craven DE, McCabe WR (1980) Gram-negative bacteremia. Am J Med 68:344–355
20. Clemmer TP, Fisher CJ, Bone RC, Slotman GJ, Metz GA, Thomas FO (1992) Hyperthermia in the sepsis syndrome and clinical outcome. Crit Care Med 20:1395–1401
21. Azimi G, Vincent JL (1986) Ultimate survival from septic shock. Resuscitation 14:245–253
22. Parker MM, Shelhamer JH, Natanson C (1987) Serial cardiovascular variables in survivors and nonsurvivors of human septic shock: heart rate as an early predictor of prognosis. Crit Care Med 15:923–929
23. Simmons DH, Nicoloff J, Guze LB (1960) Hyperventilation and respiratory alkalosis as signs of gram-negative bacteremia. JAMA 174:196–199
24. Blair E (1969) Hypocapnia and gram-negative bacteremic shock. Am J Surg 117:433–439
25. MacLean LD, Mulligan GW, McLean AP, Duff JH (1967) Alkalosis in septic shock. Surgery 62:655–662
26. Livingston DH (1993) Management of the surgical patient with multiple system organ failure. Am J Surg 165:8S–13S
27. Goris RJA, Gimbrere JSF, Van Niekerk JLM, Schoots FJ, Booy LHD (1982) Early osteosynthesis and prophylactic mechanical ventilation in the multitrauma patient. J Trauma 22:895–903
28. Vincent JL (1991) Diagnostic and medical management/supportive care of patients with gram-negative bacteremia and septic shock. Infect Dis Clin North Am 5:807–816
29. Aube H, Milan C, Blettery B (1992) Risk factors for septic shock in the early management of bacteremia. Am J Med 93:283–288
30. Moran JL, O'Fathartaigh MS, Peisach AR, Chapman MJ, Leppard P (1993) Epinephrine as an inotropic agent in septic shock: a dose-profile analysis. Crit Care Med 21:70–77
31. Desjars P, Pinaud M, Bugnon D, Taseau F (1989) Norepinephrine therapy has no deleterious renal effects in human septic shock. Crit Care Med 17:426–429
32. Bollaert PE, Bauer Ph, Audibert G, Lambert H, Larcan A (1990) Effects of epinephrine on hemodynamics and oxygen metabolism in dopamine resitant shock. Chest 98:949–953
33. Bone RC (1991) Sepsis, the sepsis syndrome, multi-organ failure: a plea for comparable definitions. Ann Intern Med 114:332–333
34. Murray JF, Matthay MA, Luce JM, Flick MR (1988) An expanded definition of the adult respiratory distress syndrome. Am Rev Respir Dis 138:720–723
35. Knaus WA, Draper EA, Wagner DP, Zimmermann JE (1985) Prognosis in acute organ-system failure. Ann Surg 202:685–693
36. Bone RC, Balk R, Slotman G et al (1992) Adult respiratory distress syndrome. Sequence and importance of development of multiple organ failure. Chest 101:320–326
37. Knaus WA, Draper EA, Wagner DP, Zimmermann JE (1985) APACHE II: a severity of disease classification system. Crit Care Med 13:818–829
38. Goris RJA, Boekhorst TPA (1985) Multiple organ failure. Arch Surg 120:1109–1115

Clinical Manifestations and Prognostic Indicators in Sepsis

R. C. Bone

Introduction

Sepsis can be defined as the systemic response to the presence in the body of microorganisms of their toxic products. Previous clinical studies have required *in vitro* laboratory growth of the organisms to confirm the diagnosis of sepsis. The septic syndrome is defined by specific clinical criteria and has a significant mortality rate in addition to other sequelae commonly associated with sepsis.

The criteria for the sepsis syndrome identify a population of patients at imminent risk for development of septic shock and adult respiratory distress syndrome (ARDS). The sepsis syndrome itself carries a clinically significant mortality rate. Identification and definition of this syndrome may allow for earlier detection and treatment of patients with sepsis and could potentially result in improved survival through prevention of shock and multiple system organ failure. Since the septic syndrome has the potential for earlier identification of septic patients, it may:

1. allow for earlier therapeutic intervention
2. aid in the search to uncover pathophysiologic mechanisms, and
3. provide a useful clinical point at which to evaluate new therapeutic modalities.

The high frequency and often devastating consequences of sepsis make it a major cause of death from infection in the United States today [1]. Although bacteremia may be asymptomatic, it too often comes to clinical attention as an acute catastrophic event recognized by a characteristic constellation of signs and symptoms. Indeed, the term "sepsis" implies bacteremia coupled with a host response to the circulating microorganisms. Factors that determine the presence or absence of clinical symptoms are largely unknown, though they are of obvious importance in the therapy of bacteremic patients. Conversely, several clinical and laboratory features of bacteremic patients mitigate for or against survival and the development of a particularly devastating manifestation of sepsis, ARDS.

This review will discuss risk factors, incidence, and prognostic indicators of sepsis and septic ARDS.

Clinical Manifestations of Sepsis

Manifestations of bacteremia are diverse in their range and representation in individual patients (Table 1). Skin lesions such as septic bullae, Janeway lesions, Roth spots, and others may be observed [2]. Fever and chills, thought to be pathophysiologically dependent upon the production of endogenous pyrogen (interleukin 1), frequently are present. Altered mental status may be observed and may, in fact, be the first manifestation of sepsis in elderly patients. Decreasing urine output, which may be associated with peripheral edema, is a reflection of inadequate perfusion and, more ominously, early renal failure [2]. Also, the gastrointestinal, pulmonary, and cardiovascular systems frequently show evidence of dysfunction in the presence of bacteremia [3]. Dysfunction of each of these organ systems is prognostically important, since mortality rate is well correlated to the number of organ systems injured [4]. Early dysfunction involving the cardiovascular system, however, is the single most reliable predictor of early death in endotoxemia [5] and is the most frequent immediate cause of death in septic patients in the first 24 h.

Laboratory abnormalities may be helpful in the evaluation of bacteremic patients (Table 2). Arterial blood gases obtained early in the course of bacteremia are likely to reflect respiratory alkalosis secondary to stimulation of central respiratory centers. If cardiovascular compensation is inadequate to maintain vital organ perfusion, lactic acidosis will supervene. Hypoxemia may be present, though abnormal arterial-alveolar oxygen ratios or gradients

Table 1. Clinical manifestations of bacteremia

- Fever or hypothermia
- Chills
- Skin lesions
- Altered mental status
- Organ dysfunction
  - Kidney
  - Gastrointestinal
  - Lung
  - Cardiovascular

Table 2. Laboratory abnormalities associated with bacteremia

- Arterial blood gases
  - Respiratory alkalosis → metabolic (lactic) acidosis
  - Increased alveolar-arterial oxygen gradient
- Coagulation abnormalities
- Granulocytosis/granulocytopenia
- Complement system activation

are earlier indicators of pulmonary dysfunction. Coagulation abnormalities, most commonly thrombocytopenia with or without other evidence of disseminated intravascular coagulation, are frequently observed [6]. Granulocytosis with predominance of immature forms, or granulocytopenia and falling white blood cell counts are suggestive of bacteremia. Patients with gram-negative bacteremia may have evidence of complement system activation [7].

Many investigators find it helpful to define a subset of bacteremic patients whose clinical features portend poorer prognosis. The term "sepsis" or "septic syndrome" implies that a patient has good evidence of a serious infection and a systemic response to that infection (Table 3). Criteria for definition of a serious infection include such factors as hyperthermia or hypothermia, granulocytosis or granulocytopenia, positive blood culture for a recognized pathogen, or gross pus in an enclosed space. Systemic response to infection is implied by the presence of clinical manifestations, such as otherwise unexplained arterial hypotension, low systemic vascular resistance, or metabolic acidosis. While most patients who are bacteremic and febrile but lack other manifestations of sepsis do well, the mortality rate for patients with cardiovascular collapse, even when the site of infection is known and appropriate antibiotics are given, is between 50% and 70% [6, 8]. Interestingly, treatment in an intensive care unit does not appear to alter the outcome of pneumococcal bacteremia once shock is established [9]. Thus, a more specific definition of sepsis may guide us toward the features of sepsis that can be used to predict outcome.

Sepsis Syndrome

The sepsis syndrome can be defined in terms of the systemic response to sepsis expressed as fever or hypothermia, tachycardia, tachypnea, and evidence of inadequate organ perfusion or organ dysfunction. More specifically,

Table 3. Definition of sepsis

Serious infection is evidenced by two or more of the following:
Core temperature $>39\,°C$ or $<35\,°C$
Neutrophil count $>12\,000/\mu l$ or $<3000/\mu l$ or $>20\%$ immature forms
One positive blood culture for a commonly accepted pathogen
A known or suspected source for systemic infection (such as the urinary tract) from which a recognized pathogen has been cultured
Gross pus in an enclosed space
Systemic response is evidenced by one of the following:
Unexplained arterial hypotension
Systemic vascular resistance <800 dynes/s cm^{-5}
Unexplained metabolic acidosis (base deficit >5 mEq/l)

it can be defined as hypothermia (<96 °F/35 °C), fever (>101 °F/39 °C), tachycardia (>90 bpm), tachypnea (>20 respirations/min), clinical suspicion of infection, and evidence of inadequate organ perfusion or function expressed as poor or altered cerebral function, hypoxemia (P_aO_2<75 mm Hg), elevated plasma lactate, or oliguria (urine output <30 ml/h or <0.5 ml/kg body weight per hour) [10]. When sepsis syndrome is accompanied by hypotension unresponsive to fluid therapy it is referred to as septic shock. Although the exact incidence is not known, 70000–300000 cases of sepsis are estimated to occur in the United States each year [11]. Shock develops in approximately 40% of these patients and adversely affects survival [6]. A number of recent innovations in medical practice may have actually increased the likelihood of sepsis and septic shock [11]. These innovations include: aggressive oncologic chemotherapy, corticosteroid or immunosuppressive therapy for organ transplantation or inflammatory diseases, increasing survival of patients predisposed to sepsis, and more frequent use of invasive medical procedures [11, 12].

Patients with the sepsis syndrome ($n=191$) were prospectively evaluated and comprised the placebo group of a multicenter trial of methylprednisolone in sepsis syndrome and septic shock [10]. Some 45% of the patients were found to be bacteremic; 31% were in septic shock (sepsis syndrome plus systolic blood pressure <90 mm Hg or decreased from baseline systolic blood pressure >40 mm Hg) at study entry. An additional 24% of the patients developed shock after admission, with 70% doing so within 24 h of study entry; shock reversal occurred with a frequency of 73%. Some 25% of the patients developed ARDS. Mortality for patients with sepsis syndrome who did not develop shock was 13%. Mortality for the groups of patients with shock at admission and shock subsequent to admission was 27.5% and 43.2%, respectively. A total of 47% of bacteremic patients developed shock after study admission compared to 29.6% of nonbacteremic patients ($p<0.05$). Other than development of shock, there were no significant differences between the bacteremic and nonbacteremic patients. Also, the outcomes for patients with gram-negative and gram-positive bacteremias did not differ significantly.

Prognostic Indicators in Sepsis

A large series of bacteremic patients reported by Kreger and McCabe detailed the clinical features and effects of antibiotic therapy in 612 patients with gram-negative bacteremia over a 10 year period [6]. For purposes of evaluation, patients were classified according to their underlying illness as being rapidly fatal, ultimately fatal, or nonfatal. Historical features that were associated with increased mortality in patients in any of the underlying disease categories are listed in Table 4. Factors that also were examined but did not materially affect the outcome of bacteremia included race, gender, and the coexistence of neoplastic diseases. The majority of factors listed in Ta-

Table 4. Preexisting factors that adversely influence the outcome of sepsis. Adapted from Kreger et al. [6]

- Antecedent antibiotics
- Antecedent antimetabolites
- Antecedent corticosteroids
- Azotemia
- Congestive heart failure
- Diabetes mellitus
- Nosocomial infection

ble 4 impair the immune response of the host and may be postulated to influence survival by this mechanism.

The single best clinical indicator of sepsis and poor outcome was the presence of shock. Shock occurred in 44% of the patients evaluated in this study; fatality in patients with shock was 47%, in contrast to mortality of 7% in patients who did not manifest shock. These data are in close accordance with those of Winslow et al. [8], who noted that 64% of patients with septic shock from gram-positive or gram-negative bacteremia died. Additional clinical factors in Kreger's patients that were associated with the development of shock were age 65 > years; antecedent corticosteroid, antimetabolite, or antibiotic therapy; azotemia; and congestive heart failure [6]. In a prospective study of serial cardiopulmonary variables in patients with septic shock, Abraham et al. reported that arterial hypotension was precipitated by a drop of the cardiac index from the high levels classically described in "warm" sepsis to normal ranges [13]. These data suggested to the investigators that loss of cardiac compensation for low systemic vascular resistance was the immediate cause of the hypotensive crisis.

Winslow et al. have reported that arterial lactic acid levels are higher in septic patients who died than in those who survived, though the overlap was too great to make this a test of prognostic significance in any individual patient [8]. The clinical and laboratory features associated with increased mortality in sepsis are listed in Table 5.

Additional laboratory tests that are reported to be abnormal in patients with sepsis are the levels of cyclooxygenase metabolites thromboxane B2 and 6-keto-prostaglandin (PG) $F_{1\alpha}$ [14, 15], plasma fibronectin, and angiotensin-converting enzyme. Thromboxane B2 is a metabolite of thromboxane A2, a vasoconstrictive and platelet aggregatory lipid. Similarly, 6-keto-$PGF_{1\alpha}$

Table 5. Clinical and laboratory features that adversely influence survival in sepsis

- Shock
- Lactic acidosis
- Elevated blood levels of cyclooxygenase metabolites
- Subtherapeutic levels of antibiotics
- Low levels of circulating antibodies to a common core lipopolysaccharide antigen of gram-negative bacteria

is a stable metabolite of prostacyclin, a vasodilatory and antiaggregatory metabolite of arachidonic acid metabolism. Although the mean levels of these metabolites were higher in nonsurviving than in surviving patients, the separation of values was insufficient to allow this test to be applied prognostically. Angiotensin-converting enzyme (ACE) is a carboxypeptidase that converts angiotensin 1 to angiotensin 2 and is found in highest concentrations in lung capillary endothelial cells. Endothelial cell injury causes release of ACE into the blood, the level of which is reported to be correlated to severity of lung injury [16]. Severe sepsis is associated with a decrease in plasma fibronectin, a nonimmunologic opsonin that facilitates removal of degradation products by the reticuloendothelial cell system [17]. Plasma fibronectin levels are touted as a prognostic indicator in sepsis. Each of these tests is of limited value in an individual patient, since the overlap with control patient populations remains significant.

For nearly 10 years, it has been recognized that high titers of antibody to a core lipopolysaccharide shared by most gram-negative bacteria protects patients against the development of shock and death [18]. More recently, levels of circulating antibodies to *Escherichia coli* endotoxin core were shown to correlate well to enhanced survival in patients with *Pseudomonas aeruginosa* septicemia [19]. These observations suggested that immunization against this common core antigen may be protective against cardiovascular changes associated with septicemia. Active immunization of sheep using the core glycolipid fraction of a J5 *E. coli* mutant is effective in reducing the pulmonary hypertension and the decrease in cardiac output and alveolar-arterial oxygen gradient that is secondary to gram-negative endotoxemia [20]. Passive immunization is also effective in this model, though protection is incomplete. Passive administration of antiserum raised in normal human volunteers against a mutant *E. coli* is reported to reduce mortality and death due to gram-negative bacteremia [21]. These results were reinforced by the observation that administration of plasma rich in antilipopolysaccharide immunoglobulin B provided a survival advantage to gynecologic patients with septic shock [22]. Since these two studies were unblinded and suboptimally controlled, however, verification of these results will be critically important.

Kreger's study [6] clearly demonstrated that early and appropriate antibiotic therapy is highly effective in reducing mortality secondary to gram-negative bacteremia. In all categories of patients, initial selection of appropriate antibiotic therapy improved outcome. Furthermore, this advantage extended to patients who had already entered into a shock state. These results have been extended by Moore et al., who found that administration of sufficient doses of aminoglycosides to achieve therapeutic levels reduced the mortality rate relative to patients similarly treated but in whom subtherapeutic levels of aminoglycosides were detected [23]. These data underscore the importance of delivering to patients judiciously chosen antibiotics in adequate doses as early as sepsis is suspected.

New treatments are now being defined and evaluated in animal models and multicenter studies.

References

1. McCabe WR (1973) Gram negative bacteremia: disease-a-month. Year Book Medical Publishers, Chicago
2. Sheagren JH (1986) Shock syndromes related to sepsis. Cecil textbook of medicine. Saunders, Philadelphia, pp 1473–1477
3. McCabe WR, Treadwell TL, Maria AD (1983) Pathophysiology of bacteremia. Am J Med 75:7–18
4. National Heart, Lung, and Blood Institute (1979) Extracorporeal support for respiratory insufficiency: Collaborative study. National Heart, Lung, and Blood Institute, Washington DC
5. Goldfarb RD, Tambolini W, Wiener SM et al (1983) Canine left ventricular performance during LD50 endotoxemia. Am J Physiol 244:H370–H377
6. Kreger BEW, Craven DE, McCabe WR (1980) Gram-negative bacteremia: IV. Reevaluation of clinical features and treatment in 612 patients. Am J Med 68:344–355
7. McCabe WR (1973) Serum complement levels in bacteremia due to gram negative organisms. N Engl J Med 288:21–23
8. Winslow EJ, Loeb HS, Rahimtoola SH et al (1973) Hemodynamic studies and results of therapy in 50 patients with bacteremic shock. Am J Med 54:421–432
9. Hook EW, Horton CA, Schaberg DR (1983) Failure of intensive care unit support to influence mortality from pneumococcal bacteremia. J Am Med Assoc 249:1055–1057
10. Bone RC, Fisher CJ, Clemmer TP et al (1989) The sepsis syndrome: a valid clinical entity. Crit Care Med 17:389–393
11. Parker MM, Parillo JE(1983) Hemodynamics and pathogenesis. J Am Med Assoc 250:3324–3327
12. Shubin H, Weil MH (1976) Bacterial shock. J Am Med Assoc 235:421–424
13. Abraham E, Shoemaker WC, Bland RD et al (1983) Plasma fibronectin in medical ICU patients. Crit Care Med 11:799–803
14. Halushka PV, Reines HD, Barrow SE et al (1985) Elevated 6-keto-prostaglandin F1a in patients in septic shock. Crit Care Med 13:451–453
15. Reines HD, Cook JA, Halushka PV et al (1982) Plasma thromboxane concentrations are raised in patients dying with septic shock. Lancet 2:174–175
16. Fourrier F, Chopin C, Wallaert B et al (1985) Compared evolution of plasma fibronectin and angio-converting enzye levels in septic ARDS. Chest 87:191–195
17. O'Connell MT, Becker DM, Steele BW et al (1984) Plasma fibronectin in medical ICU patients. Crit CareMed 12:479–482
18. Zinner SH, McCabe WR (1976) Effects of IgM and IgG antibody in patients with bacteremia due to gram-negative bacilli. J Infect Dis 133:37–45
19. Pollack M, Huang AI, Prescott PK et al (1984) Enhanced survival in pseudomonas aeruginosa septicemia associated with high levels of circulating antibody to E. coli endotoxin core. J Clin Invest 72:1874–1881
20. Girotti MJ, Menkes E, MacDonald JWD et al (1984) Effects of immunization on cardiopulmonary alterations of gram-negative endotoxemia. J Appl Physiol 56:582–589
21. Ziegler EJ, McCutchan JA, Fierer J et al (1982) Treatment of gram-negative bacteremia and shock with human antiserum to a mutant E. coli. N Engl J Med 307:1225–1230
22. Lachman E, Pitsoe SB, Gaffin SL (1984) Anti-lipopolysaccharide immunotherapy in management of septic shock of obstetric and gynecological origin. Lancet 1:981–983
23. Moore RD, Smith CR, Lietman PS (1984) The association of aminoglycoside plasma levels with mortality in patients with gram-negative bacteremia. J Infect Dis 149:443–448

What Determines Prognosis in Sepsis? Evidence for a Comprehensive Individual Patient Risk Assessment Approach to the Design and Analysis of Clinical Trials

W. A. Knaus, D. P. Wagner, F. E. Harrell and E. A. Draper

Proposition

In order to properly evaluate new therapeutic approaches to sepsis, we will have to provide a baseline estimate of a patient's short-term mortality risk based on patient characteristics available and reliably measured prior to treatment. This estimate should be uniform in regard in risk assessment and clinical definitions, but specific to the particular inclusion and exclusion criteria used in the clinical evaluations, and should be updated as new information becomes available regarding prognostic factors or the efficacy of specific new compounds.

Background and Rationale

No "Typical" Septic Patient

One of the major reasons infection and sepsis have increased as a cause of morbidity and mortality in hospitalized patients is that we are treating more severely ill patients at more advanced stages of disease [1]. The majority of patients who develop sepsis in our acute care hospitals have chronic illnesses such as cancer, cirrhosis, or other conditions that decrease their immunologic function and leave them vulnerable to infection. We are also providing more intensive care services to severely ill patients in the initial stages of illness, such as trauma and shock, and after complex operations, making it possible to survive previously fatal conditions. This progress comes at the cost of prolonged invasive life support that also increases the risk of acquiring infection.

As a result of these changes, there really is not any "typical" patient with sepsis. Potential candidates range from a young previously healthy individual with the sudden onset of urinary tract infection to a patient with cirrhosis, suffering from multiple organ system failure on prolonged ventilatory support in an intensive care unit (ICU) following emergency surgery for a leaking abdominal aneurysm who develops a sudden episode of septic shock. The term "sepsis" is not sufficient to describe either patient, and reliance on such terms alone is unlikely to assist in the value and indications of new therapeutic approaches.

Categorical Definitions and Patient Risk

Recognizing this problem, new categorical definitions such as "sepsis syndrome" or "sepsis syndrome with shock" were developed [2] that improved patient identification and refined entry criteria for clinical investigations. More recently, these categorical definitions have been refined to acknowledge that it is not only infection but systemic inflammation that is the underlying disorder, hence the new term "systemic inflammatory response syndrome" (SIRS) and "severe sepsis" to replace the former septic syndrome [3].

It has also been recently discovered that these categorical definitions, both new and old, have three important limitations [4]. First, they identify patients at a wide variety of baseline or pretreatment risk. This can be seen in Figs. 1–3, which provide the risk distributions for 519 ICU patients admitted with a primary diagnosis of sepsis and classified according to the categorical definitions for sepsis syndrome (severe sepsis) (Fig. 1), sepsis syndrome with shock (Fig. 2), and the new definition SIRS (Fig. 3). Regardless of the definition chosen, there is a wide distribution of patient risks for hospital mortality from less than 10% to over 90%. The risk predictions used in these analyses were based on the general APACHE III hospital mortality equation [4], and the relative advantages of this approach, compared to a disease-specific assessment, will be discussed shortly.

Second, depending on the manner in which these screening definitions are applied, the group mortality risk can also vary widely. This can be seen in Figs. 1–3. The overall group mortality risk will be a function of the proportion of patients selected for inclusion in the trial who fall at a specific risk level.

Third, it has been recognized that many patients with clinical evidence of sepsis may not fulfill the exact criteria for a categorical definition like sepsis syndrome, and yet have risks similar to those patients included. This can be

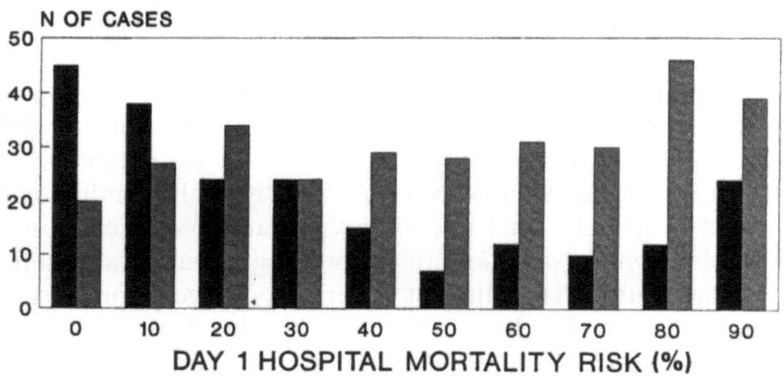

Fig. 1. Risk distribution of 519 ICU admissions with a primary clinical diagnosis of sepsis, divided into patients who met categorical criteria for septic syndrome ($n=308$; hatched) and those who did not ($n=211$; black). Risk predictions are calculated from the APACHE III first day hospital mortality risk equation. (From [4])

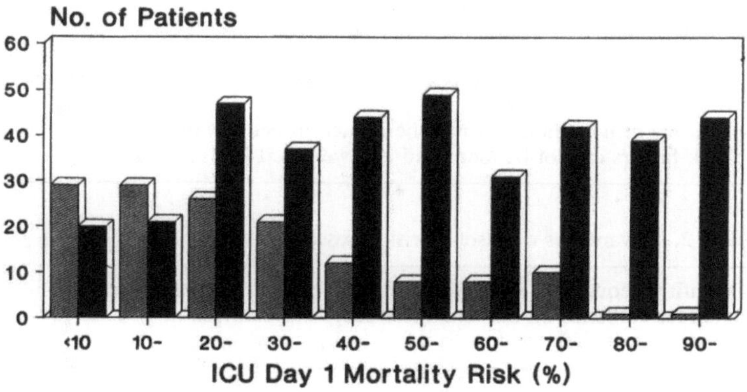

Fig. 2. Risk distribution of 519 ICU admissions with a primary clinical diagnosis of sepsis, divided into patients who met categorical criteria for shock ($n=374$; black) and those who did not ($n=145$; hatched). Risk predictions are calculated from the APACHE III first day hospital mortality risk equation [44].

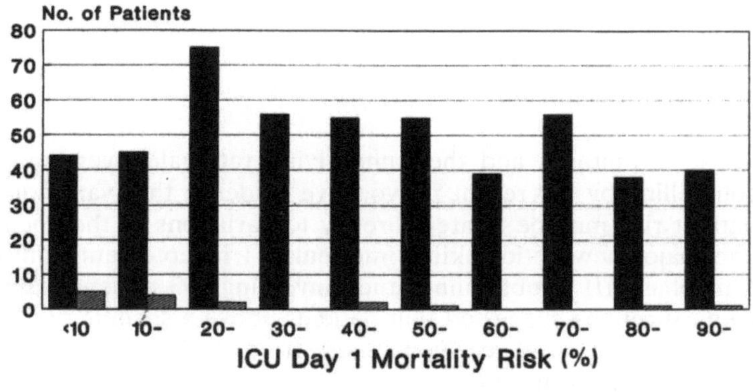

Fig. 3. Risk distribution of 519 ICU admissions with a primary clinical diagnosis of sepsis, divided into patients who met categorical criteria for systemic inflammatory response syndrome (SIRS) ($n=503$; black) and those who did not ($n=16$; hatched). Risk predictions are calculated from the APACHE III first day hospital mortality risk equation [44]. (From [3])

seen in Fig. 1 in which of the 519 patients admitted to an ICU with a primary diagnosis of sepsis, only 308 fulfill the definition for sepsis syndrome, and in Fig. 2 in which only 374 of 519 met criteria for another categorical definition, septic shock.

Recognition of these limitations, in part, encouraged the development of more general and inclusive definitions for the inflammatory cascade, e.g., SIRS. For example, in Fig. 3, it can be seen that virtually all (503) of the 519 patients with a clinical diagnosis of sepsis meet SIRS criteria. This is substantially more than the 308 who qualified for the more restrictive definition,

Table 1. Rationale for baseline risk assessment

– Using categorical definitions, e.g., severe sepsis, sepsis with shock, patients have a wide range of mortality risks.
– Efficacy of new therapies may be related directly to mortality risk.
– Risk factors cannot be identified and weighted from trial data.

Table 2. Advantages of baseline risk assessment

– Confirms equal risk distribution in placebo and treatment groups
– Reduces reliance on and enhances subgroup analyses
– Quantifies benefit relative to individual patient's risk

sepsis syndrome. Regardless of the definition chosen, however, it is now recognized that, in all future clinical trials, these definitions should be combined with appropriate risk stratification or risk prediction methods [3]. The rationale behind this recommendation are summarized in Table 1. The overall advantages for risk assessment are summarized in Table 2.

Risk Assessment and Drug Efficacy?

These advantages and their underlying rationales were made even more compelling by the recent provocative evidence that variations in estimated patient risk may be related directly to variations in therapeutic efficacy of one major new anticytokine, interleukin-1 receptor antagonist (IL-1ra) [5]. This phase III double-blind study involving 893 patients randomized at 63 medical centers suggested that patients above a specific risk level (24% risk of 28 day mortality) received benefit from IL-1ra, while patients whose risk was below 24% did not.

These results suggesting a relationship between patient risk and efficacy of IL-1ra are consistent with animal and recent clinical trial data evaluating the efficacy of another anticytokine, tumor necrosis factor (TNF) antagonists. A 1989 study of mice unable to produce TNF in response to infection demonstrated a 1000-fold greater susceptibility to lethal infection with *Escherichia coli* than TNF-responsive mice [6]. This suggested that certain levels of TNF may be involved in host protection, presumably patients with low risk may have low levels of TNF. A recent clinical trial of the influence of anti-TNF monoclonal antibody on cytokine levels also demonstrated a positive relationship between the efficacy of a murine anti-TNF and serum levels of TNF in a limited sample of 20 patients receiving a 10 mg/kg dose [7].

In that study, patients with a pretreatment TNF level less than 50 pg/ml had a 62% 28 day mortality (8/13), while patients with high pretreatment TNF levels (>50 pg/ml) appeared to benefit from blocking TNF, having a 14% (1/7) 28 day mortality ($p = 0.07$). The findings from these evaluations relate directly to one of the major rationales for a comprehensive approach to risk assessment, the possibility that a patient's pretreatment risk may be directly related to drug efficacy (Table 1).

By the mid-1980s, it was widely recognized that a lack of efficacy of traditional antimicrobial therapy against infection was not the primary reason for therapeutic failure [1]. Rather there was concern that prolonged life support was creating the opportunity for normally protective biologic responses to be magnified and to create irreversible organ system damage. Basic investigation turned to agents that might modify these responses. This lead to the development of compounds aimed at antagonizing components of the inflammatory cascade, e.g., IL-1, TNF, that are stimulated when infection occurs [8].

Each of these new therapeutic compounds varies widely in its presumed mechanism of action. One aspect common to all, however, is the presumption that the normal biologic responses designed to create a defense against infection can create untoward effects if they persist because of failure to entirely eliminate the infectious focus, and the continued application of life support. For example, the ability of IL-1 to mediate neutrophil emigration can also produce distant organ system damage if the mediator persists at high levels following the initial inflammatory cascade. The optimal role of new compounds, therefore, would be to allow the protective aspects of the inflammatory cascade to continue while blocking its potentially damaging influences. Such an action assumes that blocking the inflammatory response may be a life-saving strategy but total or premature blockade may leave the patient with a less than optimal response [9]. Presumably, this is the reason the preliminary results from the phase III evaluation of IL-1ra suggested a relationship between efficacy and patient severity or risk of death [5]. If we accept this hypothesis, the question then becomes whether predicted risk is the best way to measure the level or stage of the inflammatory response so that compounds may be appropriately targeted to block its persistent untoward effects while permitting its benefit.

One response would be to use the actual levels of the mediators, for example IL-1, to determine the appropriateness of therapy. Several investigators have attempted to correlate serum concentrations of mediators, including key mediators such as IL-1 and TNF, with patient outcome and risk, but the results have been disappointing [7, 10–21]. The frequency of detection is generally less than 50%. A short circulating half-life is partially responsible for these results, along with the compartmentalization of these mediators within tissues. This can result in a significant amount of cytokine activity but low to absent circulatory concentrations [16]. It is unlikely that these measurement problems will be resolved without substantial additional investigation.

Physiology as Major Risk Factor

Anticipating that the complex biologic and measurement challenges involved in cytokine assays will not be easily or shortly resolved, attention has focused on identifying other more reliable and accurate identifiers of patient risk that could be linked to the therapeutic activity of new anticytokine and other therapies. For example, Calandra et al. performed a logistic regression analysis of various risk factors for mortality from sepsis. While serum levels of IL-1 and TNF were independently associated with a poor outcome, stepwise regression analysis failed to confirm the associations. Instead, the severity of the patient's underlying disease, their age, urine output and arterial pH were found to be the major determinants of outcome [21].

These extremely important findings confirm numerous studies published during the past two decades that have pointed toward the importance of physiology and patient characteristics in determining outcome from sepsis. Some of these efforts have been designed at predicting mortality for ICU admissions while others have been specifically designed for outcome prediction in sepsis. A comprehensive review of these efforts is beyond the scope of this article, but an overview summarized in Table 3 suggests that a combination of patient factors, most importantly the acute severity of the patient's condition, were influential in determining outcome. What was not resolved from these efforts, however, was the exact weighting and optimal combination of these various risk factors and the relative influence of the type of infection or nature of infecting organism when compared to patient factors. The latter is a critical point. While type of organism has been linked in many studies to risk and patient outcome [22–30], exact identification of type of organism is not widely available when treatment decisions are being considered making this a problematic risk factor at this time.

More important, however, than the question of whether a particular prognostic variable should be included is how should the multiple risk factors in Table 3 be combined? It is not possible for every clinical trial to identify and determine the appropriate weight for each risk factor. First, the placebo arms of these clinical trials are not large enough to identify stable, reliable weighting schemes for each factor. Second, the data search or multiple comparisons inherent in such model-building are not appropriate when evaluating the po-

Table 3. Major current pretreatment prognostic variables in sepsis

- Severity of sepsis
  - General physiologic abnormalities [4, 21, 37–41, 44–46]
  - Shock [22–25, 28–30, 36, 42, 43]
  - Organ system failure [22–24, 27, 28, 30]
  - Neutropenia [25, 27, 29]
- Underlying acute disease [4, 22, 23, 25, 26, 28–30, 34–36, 40, 41, 44]
- Patient's chronic health condition [4, 41, 44]
- Timing of onset of sepsis [4, 41, 44, 46]

tential efficacy of new compounds. Third, the patients selected for these trials may not be representative of the larger population of patients with sepsis.

Furthermore, what previous efforts at evaluation have taught us, however, and what the items in Table 3 confirm is that there are *multiple* risk factors for death from sepsis, and unless we recognize and account for this complexity, we may continue to be limited in our ability to properly evaluate new therapeutic approaches. Relying on one or two risk factors, e.g., shock or a combination of these factors in categorical definitions, may also not improve our ability to discriminate because, as illustrated in Figs. 1–3, categorical definitions contain patients at multiple levels of risk.

In view of these findings, we are proposing the development of a comprehensive individual patient baseline risk assessment that would take into consideration all the key variables listed in Table 3 that have been demonstrated to influence the risk of any seriously ill patient with sepsis [1]. Such assessments and analyses are now possible using large clinical databases and multivariate statistical techniques [31]. These capabilities can be used to create an estimate for short-term mortality that would reduce the ambiguity of current attempts at case mix control and risk prediction. Such an effort might not only lead to a better understanding of risk in sepsis, but could also lead to indications of the potential value of these new drugs for individual patients. Since our knowledge in this field is expanding rapidly and many new compounds are undergoing clinical evaluation it will be important to create a uniform approach to risk assessment, so the results of such analyses can be combined for comparative purposes. It is also important that this be a dynamic process that can incorporate new insights rapidly.

Methods for a Comprehensive Baseline Risk Assessment in Sepsis

Recent advances in the storage and retrieval of clinically accurate patient data have resulted in the development of large contemporary databases. Simultaneous advances in the ability to analyze and model risk factors for outcome from an acute illness, like sepsis, have created a new technical and intellectual basis for risk adjustment in clinical evaluations of new therapeutic compounds. Using the steps outlined in Table 4, these databases can be used as large contemporary "control" groups. The groups can be used to investigate, confirm, and compile risk factors for outcome. As the size and representativeness of these databases expand, these efforts at risk prediction can be revisited and improved. If similar data collection procedures are followed then, as indicated in Table 4, the risk prediction may also involve comparisons of the efficacy of combinations of new therapeutic compounds. For our current purposes, however, we will begin with the development of an initial sepsis-specific risk model.

While there have been many candidates for prognostic factors in sepsis, the overwhelming evidence is that because of their reliability and availabili-

Table 4. Methods for developing a comprehensive risk assessment approach for patients with sepsis

Step 1. Apply exact study selection criteria, e.g., sepsis syndrome, severe sepsis, SIRS, to large clinically accurate database of severely ill hospitalized patients to select cohort of patients for risk assessment.
Step 2. Analyze cohort of patients meeting exact study entry criteria to create comprehensive risk assessment model. Investigate various approaches to modeling and risk assessment.
Step 3. Develop and validate risk model prior to analysis of clinical trial data.
Step 4. Apply independent risk prediction on patients at time of study qualification. Use risk assessment to check for imbalances in risk between treatment and control groups and to investigate relationship between risk and drug efficacy.
Step 5. Use results from clinical trial to refine entry criteria for next trial, or to develop indications for use.

As clinical trials are performed and the clinical databases described in step 1 expand, steps 2–4 can be repeated in improve risk prediction, and to investigate indications for specific compounds or combinations of compounds

ty, a combination of physiologic and other patient related risk variables, offer the most promising current approach. Each of the specific components in Table 3 is supported by studies that have examined its relationship with outcome, usually hospital or other short-term mortality outcomes. For example, a number of studies (see specific references in Table 3) have linked the development of physiologic changes such as shock and multiorgan system failure to mortality. As previously emphasized, what has not been done is to combine these factors into a single comprehensive model.

A preliminary step in this regard, however, was begun with the risk predictions used in Figs. 1–3 [44]. These risk predictions were produced using most of the components listed in Table 3 and represent an early attempt to provide a comprehensive risk adjustment. Specifically, a logistic regression equation was developed on 519 patients with sepsis as their primary reason for admission to the ICU. Hospital mortality was the dependent variable. The predictive variables were the first ICU day APACHE III score (the acute physiology score along with age and chronic health points), the etiology of sepsis defined as urosepsis or other sources, and the patient's treatment location prior to ICU admission (ward, emergency department, operating room, etc.) [44]. All three of these independent variables were significantly related to the hospital mortality risk. The APACHE III score was the most important with a partial Wald chi-square of 100 compared to 16 for etiology and 12 for prior treatment location. This supports the many studies listed in Table 3 that have associated physiologic abnormalities with outcome in sepsis. The model also acknowledges, however, that the etiology of the sepsis and the state of the patient prior to development of the septic episode are also important prognostically.

The overall explanatory power of the predictive system was good, with the receiver-operator-characteristics (ROC) curve=0.82. The accuracy of this approach to risk prediction can be seen in Fig. 4 in which the model is applied to the 503 patients from the original 519 who were admitted to an ICU with the primary diagnosis of sepsis and who also met criteria for SIRS.

In a more recent study and in keeping with the objective of constantly improving the risk adjustment, we have taken this approach the next logical step and created a sepsis-specific comprehensive risk predictive model [32]. This was done by analyzing a larger group of 1195 patients with a variety of indications of sepsis. Each of these patients had to meet entry criteria for clinical evaluations of septic drugs, e.g., sepsis syndrome or severe sepsis to use the more recently proposed definition.

Using this database, we refined our predictive model for sepsis by discovering that in addition to the acute physiologic abnormalities as measured by the acute physiology score of APACHE III, additional weight provided to two physiologic variables, white blood cell count and serum pH, improved explanatory power. These findings are compatible with previous investigations suggesting the importance of very low white counts and metabolic acidosis in sepsis. We also were able to take this opportunity to further refine two of the other constructs listed in Table 3, acute disease and timing of onset of sepsis. This was done by refining the use of diagnoses and by incorporating as predictive variables the number of days the patient was in the hospital and the ICU prior to meeting the criteria for sepsis syndrome. All of these factors were combined in a comprehensive model that would provide an estimate of the patient's risk of 28 day mortality at the time they were entered into a clinical trial (Table 4). The exact details of this modeling effort can be found in the manuscript [32], but the results support the conclusions

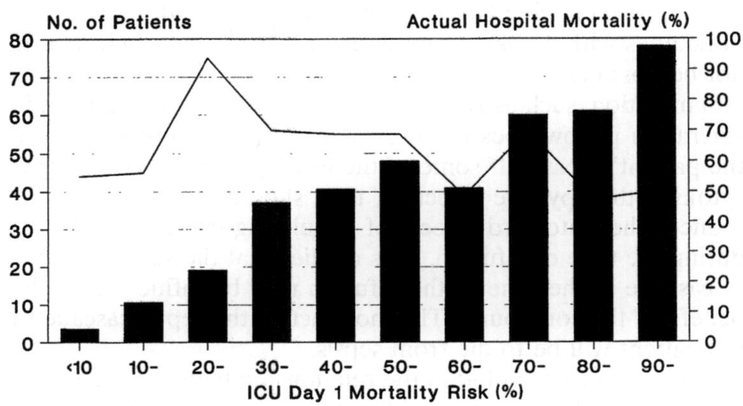

Fig. 4. Risk distribution of 503 patients with a primary clinical diagnosis of sepsis who met the criteria for SIRS, demonstrating the relationship between risk of hospital mortality, calculated on the first of the ICU day, and actual hospital mortality rates. Risk prediction are calculated from the APACHE III first day hospital mortality risk equation [44]. (From [3])

of previous efforts that the severity of the illness, etiology of the septic episode, prior health of the patient, and duration of illness prior to treatment are all independent and complimentary risk factors for mortality by 28 days. Evidence from validation efforts within the original 1195 patient database, an independent validation sample of 295 [32], and recent application to a large scale clinical evaluation all support the accuracy of this approach in predicting 28 day mortality risk [5].

But demonstrating that a comprehensive risk model based on the constructs listed in Table 3 can accurately predict risk in sepsis does not entirely address the question of whether this is the optimal approach to determining outcome. Ideally, one would also want to know that the approach was superior to other efforts and that it corresponded to the underlying severity of the septic or inflammatory cascade.

In regard to previous risk prediction efforts in sepsis, the comprehensive approach we have taken using a sepsis specific modification of a general prognostic scoring system, APACHE III, can be demonstrated to be superior to the use of the scoring system alone or earlier approaches to sepsis scoring [32].

It can also be demonstrated that, once a comprehensive measure of patient is available, it is superior in identifying patients who may benefit from new therapy than a variety of categorical definitions of infection or specific organ system failures such as shock or the adult respiratory distress syndrome. The latter finding is most likely because, as seen in Fig. 3, patients with the septic syndrome and shock still have a wide variety of baseline predicted risk.

But what evidence do we have that this comprehensive risk estimate is related to the underlying severity of the inflammatory cascade? One potential source of evidence would be to relate the risk predictions produced by this approach to circulating cytokine levels. Considering the afore mentioned difficulties with cytokine measurements, however, such determinations may not be possible or may only be possible with less specific determinations of inflammation, such as IL-6 [13, 17]. Another still indirect but important consideration is how does the pretreatment risk estimate relate to the time of the patient's death? If some of the new approaches to therapy, such as anticytokine therapy, are effective, they should be reducing deaths because it reduces the untoward effects of circulating cytokines. This can only occur during the time of infusion. This implies that the severity of the inflammatory cascade at the time of the infusion may be influential in determining the benefit of the compound. The more active the septic cascade the more likely the patient will be to die from sepsis.

In Fig. 5, we have plotted the relationship between the predicted risk of 28 day mortality from sepsis and the mean time to death. The risk prediction is drawn from the above mentioned comprehensive individual risk assessment [32], and the time to death is the mean time to death of all deaths (424) within the original 1195 patients upon which the risk prediction was based.

In Fig. 5, it can be seen that patients at low predicted risk of death take

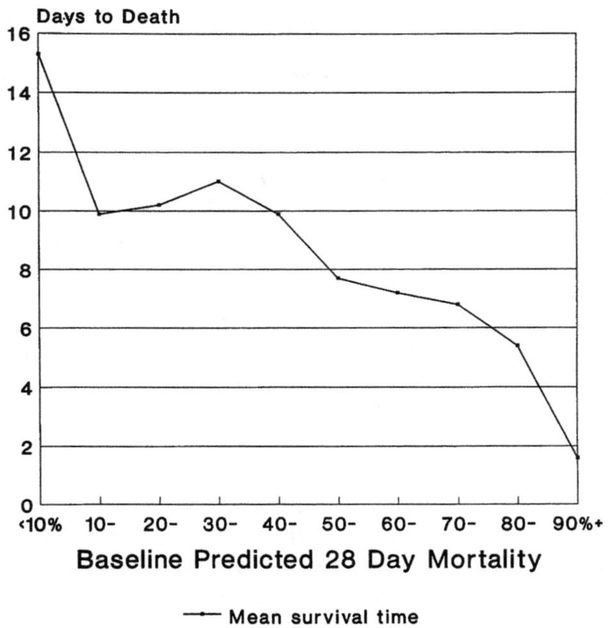

Fig. 5. Distribution of mean time to death of all 424 patients who died by 28 days within cohort of 1195 patients according to baseline predicted risk at the time they met criteria for septic syndrome (severe sepsis). Patients at low baseline risk of death demonstrate longer survival time. Baseline predicted risk of 28 day mortality calculated from a sepsis-specific risk model [32].

almost twice as long to die as those at high risk. Among the 95 patients with a baseline predicted mortality risk, less than 30% – mean survival time was 10.3 days. For the 245 patients in the 30%–70% predicted mortality range, mean survival time was 9.4 days, but for the 84 patients who died and had a predicted risk over 70%, mean survival time was only 5.2 days. This suggests that patient at a predicted high risk are not only at high risk of dying but at high risk of dying in the next few days. If this high risk of death in the short-term is from the effects of biologic mediators creating unstable hemodynamic and other acute end organ damage, then the association between the risk estimate and drug efficacy would be further established. It would suggest that the patients for whom anticytokine therapy is most useful are those patients with sepsis that are at substantial risk of short-term death.

Future Investigations

The sepsis-specific risk model referred to above must be considered dynamic. If a uniform data collection strategy encompassing the data elements included in Table 3 is adopted in most clinical evaluations, we will have larger and more comprehensive databases from which to build and refine predictive models. Included in Table 5 for future consideration is the nature of the infecting organism and the level of the circulating mediators. If our current measurement difficulties with these variables are overcome, they could be incorporated into future predictive efforts.

As we learn more about the contribution of various pretreatment patient elements we can refine the model to incorporate this new knowledge. For example, the risk model referred to above did not, because of data availability, contain information on platelet count or coagulation abnormalities. Since these elements have been related to patient risk in sepsis, they may contribute incrementally to the model's accuracy. As databases expand, we will also be able to explore the most appropriate statistical techniques for combining the predictive elements. In our recent sepsis-specific model, we found that an accelerated failure time statistical model log-normal provided the best fit between the predictive elements and patient outcome [32]. Specifically, we found that patients who were severely ill with substantial acute physiologic abnormalities die within a few days. The relative influence of these same acute physiologic abnormalities was substantially less 2 or 3 weeks later. This relationship is in violation of the Cox proportional hazards model and other commonly used statistical approaches to recent larger scale clinical trial evaluations [47, 48]. It is also becoming apparent from these and other recent trials [5] that determining the incremental value of new therapies, the magnitude of their mortality reduction, and their indications for use is a complex process. Large, independent data files and risk prediction can assist in this effort.

The risk prediction can be useful, for example, to investigate the influence of other treatment factors, such as the adequacy of antibiotic therapy, and the type of affecting organism on outcome. Both of these factors have been demonstrated to relate to outcome, but the exact role each plays, when considered along with a comprehensive measure of patient risk, requires further investigation. It is possible, for example, that the prognostic influence of infection with particular organisms, such as pseudomonas [25, 26, 27], is related to the type of patients that acquire such infections or the organism itself may have independent value. Likewise, the important influence of the adequacy

Table 5. Future possible prognostic factors in sepsis (assuming accurate pretreatment measurement)

– Cytokine levels
e.g., TNF, IL-1, IL-6
– Type of organism
e.g., Gram-negative/pseudomonas
– Factors related to efficacy of specific compounds
e.g., Low platelet counts: IL-1ra; myocardial depression: TNF

TNF, tumor necrosis factor; IL, interleukin; IL-1ra, interleukin-1 receptor antagonist

of antibiotic therapy must be continually scrutinized as a potential confounding factor [33, 34].

The availability of a comprehensive pretreatment risk assessment will also be useful in investigating the potential efficacy of new therapeutic compounds in regard to their most appropriate use. While current preliminary evidence suggests that a comprehensive physiologic based risk assessment may be a valid indicator of the incremental benefit of new compounds, additional work is needed to reinforce and refine that assessment. These efforts must await the availabilty of larger databases containing substantial number of patients treated with these new compounds. When such databases are available we can examine the interaction among the risk estimate, use of the new compound, and patient benefit taking into consideration other potentially useful patient descriptors such as type of organ system failure or individual physiologic measures. These efforts could then lead not only to improve clinical evaluations, but to refinements in development of exact indications for use.

Summary

Current evidence suggests that the most reliable and accurate method for determining prognosis from sepsis is a comprehensive risk model consisting of the patient risk factors of physiologic severity, disease etiology, a patient's chronic health condition, and the time point during hospitalization that sepsis occurs. These factors can be used to describe patients by their estimated risk of death at the time they are entered into clinical trials or at the time new drug administration is being considered.

The use of this risk estimate will be helpful in ensuring that distribution of patient risk is equivalent across treatment groups. It can also be used to investigate the relationship between risk and the therapeutic efficacy of new compounds. If this risk estimate can be demonstrated to correctly and prospectively identify those patients who can benefit from new therapy, it could also assist in investigating and developing indications for use for these potentially life-saving compounds.

Acknowledgement. Supported by The Agency for Health Care Policy and Research (HSO 7137).

References

1. Bone RC (1991) The pathogenesis of sepsis. Ann Intern Med 115:457–469
2. Bone RC et al (1989) Sepsis syndrome: a valid clinical entity. Crit Care Med 17:389–394
3. Bone RC, Balk RA, Cerra FB et al (1992) Definitions of sepsis and organ failure and guidelines for the use of innovative therapies in sepsis. Chest 101:1644–1655
4. Knaus WA, Sun X, Nystrom PO, Wagner DP (1992) Evaluation of definitions for sepsis. Chest 101:1656–1662

5. Fisher CJ Jr, Dhainaut J-F, Pribble JP, Knaus WA, IL-1 Receptor Antagonist Study Group (1993) A study evaluating the safety and efficacy of human recombinant interleukin-1 receptor antagonist in the treatment of patients with sepsis syndrome. Presented at the 13th international symposium on intensive care and emergency medicine, Brussels, Belgium
6. Cross AS, Sadoff JC, Kelly N, Bernton E, Gemski P (1989) Pretreatment with recombinant murine tumor necrosis factor α/cachectin and murine interleukin 1 α protects mice from lethal bacterial infection. J Exp Med 169:2021–2027
7. Fisher CJ, Opal SM, Dhainaut JF et al (1993) Influence of an anti-tumor necrosis factor monoclonal antibody on cytokine levels in patients with sepsis. Crit Care Med 21:318–327
8. Dinarello CA, Gelfand JA, Wolff SM (1993) Anticytokine strategies in the treatment of the systemic inflammatory response syndrome. JAMA 269:1829–1835
9. Dinarello CA (1992) Role of interleukin-1 in infectious diseases. Immunol Rev 127:119–146
10. Wortel CH, von der Mohlen MAM, van Deventer SJH et al (1992) Effectiveness of a human monoclonal antiendotoxin antibody (HA-1A) in gram-negative sepsis: relationship to endotoxin and cytokine levels. J Infect Dis 166:1367–1374
11. Tracey KJ (1992) Tumor necrosis factor in the biology of septic shock syndrome. Circ Shock 35:123–128
12. Waage A, Halstensen A, Espevik T (1987) Association between tumour necrosis factor in serum and fatal outcome in patients with meningococcal disease. Lancet 1:355–357
13. Calandra T, Gerain J, Heumann D, Baumgartner JD, Glauser MP (1991) High circulating levels in interleukin-6 in patients with septic shock: evolution during sepsis, prognostic value, and interplay with other cytokines. Am J Med 91:23–29
14. Debets JMH, Kampmeijer R, van der Linden MPMH, Buurman WA (1989) Plasma tumor necrosis factor and mortality in critically ill septic patients. Crit Care Med 17:489–494
15. Girardin E, Grau GE, Dayer JM, Roux-Lombard P, J5 Study Group (1988) Tumor necrosis factor and interleukin-1 in the serum of children with severe infectious purpura. N Engl J Med 319:397–400
16. Lowry SF (1993) Anticytokine therapies in sepsis. New Horizons 1:120–126
17. Hack CE, DeGroot ER, Felt-Bersma RJF et al (1989) Increased plasma levels of interleukin-6 in sepsis. Blood 74:1704–1710
18. Waage A, Brandtzaeg P, Halstensen A, Kierulf P, Espevik T (1989) The complex pattern of cytokines in serum from patients with meningococcal septic shock. J Exp Med 169:333–338
19. Hamilton G, Hofbauer S, Hamilton B (1992) Endotoxin, TNF-alpha, interleukin-6 and parameters of the cellular immune system in patients with intra-abdominal sepsis. Scand J Infect Dis 24:362–368
20. Dinarello CA, Wolff SM (1993) The role of interleukin-1 in disease. N Engl J Med 328:106–113
21. Calandra T, Baumgartner JD, Grau GE et al (1990) Prognostic values of tumor necrosis factor, interleukin-1, interferon-α, and interferon-γ in the serum of patients with septic shock. J Infect Dis 161:982–987
22. Uaun O, Akalin HE, Hayran M, Unal S (1992) Factors influencing prognosis in bacteremia due to gram-negative organisms: evaluation of 448 episodes in a Turkish university hospital. Clin Infect Dis 15:866–873
23. Gracia de la Torre M, Romero-Vivas T, Martinez-Beltran J, Guerrero J, Meseguer M, Bouza E (1985) Klebsiella bacteremia: an analysis of 100 episodes. Rev Infect Dis 7:143–150
24. Bouza E, Garcia de la Torre M, Erice A, Losa E, Diaz-Borrego JM, Buzon L (1985) Enterobacter bacteremia: an analysis of 50 episodes. Arch Intern Med 145:1024–1027
25. Bisbe J, Gatell JM, Puig J et al (1988) Pseudomonas aeruginosa bacteremia: univariate and multivariate analyses of factors influencing the prognosis in 133 episodes. Rev Infect Dis 10:629–635

26. Gallager PG, Watanakunakorn C (1989) Pseudomonas bacteremia in a community teaching hospital, 1980–84. Rev Infect Dis 11:846–852
27. Hilf M, Yu VL, Sharp J, Zuravleff JJ, Korvick JA, Muder RR (1989) Antibiotic therapy for pseudomonas aeruginosa bacteremia: outcome correlations in a prospective study of 200 patients. Am J Med 87:540–546
28. Gatell JM, Trilla A, LaTorre X et al (1988) Nosocomial bacteremia in a large Spanish teaching hospital: analysis of factors influencing prognosis. Rev Infect Dis 10:203–210
29. Ashkenazi S, Leibovici L, Samra Z, Konisberger H, Drucker M (1992) Risk factors for mortality due to bacteremia and fungemia in childhood. Clin Infect Dis 14:949–951
30. Cooper GS, Havlir DS, Shlaes DM, Salata RA (1991) Polymicrobial bacteremia in the late 1980's: predictors of outcome and review of the literature. Medicine (Baltimore) 69:114–123
31. Knaus WA, Wagner DP, Lynn J (1991) Short-term mortality predictions for critically ill hospitalized adults: science and ethics. Science 254:389–394
32. Knaus WA, Harrell FE, Fisher CJ, Wagner DP, Opal SM, Sadoff JC (1993) The clinical evaluation of new drugs for sepsis: a prospective study design based on survival analysis. JAMA 270:1233–1241
33. Graninger W, Ragette R (1992) Nosocomial bacteremia due to enterococcus fecalis without endocarditis. Clin Infect Dis 15:49–57
34. Hoge CW, Adams J, Buchanan B, Sears SD (1991) Enterococcal bacteremia, to treat or not to treat, a reappraisal. Rev Infect Dis 13:600–605
35. Malone DA, Wagner RA, Myers JP, Watanakunakorn C (1986) Enterococcal bacteremia in two large community teaching hospitals. Am J Med 81:601–606
36. Fidalgo S, Vazquez F, Mendoza MC, Perez F, Mendez FJ (1990) Bacteremia due to staphylococcus epidermidis: microbiologic, epidemiologic, clinical, and prognostic features. Rev Infect Dis 12:520–528
37. Elebute EA, Stoner HB (1983) The grading of sepsis. Br J Surg 70:29–31
38. Stevens LE (1983) Grading the severity of surgical sepsis. Arch Surg 118:1190–1192
39. Knaus WA, Zimmerman JE, Wagner DP, Draper EA, Lawrence DE (1981) APACHE – acute physiology and chronic health evaluation: a physiologically based classification system. Crit Care Med 9:591–597
40. Dellinger EP, Wertz MJ, Meakins JL et al (1985) Surgical infection stratification system for intra-abdominal infection. Arch Surg 120:21–29
41. Knaus WA, Draper EA, Wagner DP, Zimmerman JE (1985) APACHE II: a severity of disease classification system. Crit Care Med 13:818–829
42. Goris RJA, te BoeDherst TPA, Nuytinek JKS et al (1985) Multiple organ failure: generalized autodestructive inflammation. Arch Surg 120:1109–1115
43. Knaus WA, Draper EA, Wagner DP, Zimmerman JE (1985) Prognosis of acute organ-system failure. Ann Surg 202:685–693
44. Knaus WA, Wagner DP, Wagner DP et al (1991) The APACHE III prognostic system: risk prediction of hospital mortality for critically ill hospitalized adults. Chest 100:1619–1636
45. Meck M, Munster AM, Winchurch RA, Dickerson C (1991) The Baltimore sepsis scale: measurement of sepsis in patients with burns using a new scoring system. J Burn Care Rehabil 12:564–568
46. Baumgartner JD, Bula C, Vaney C, Wu M, Eggiman P, Perret C (1992) A novel score for predicting the mortality of septic shock patients. Crit Care Med 20:953–960
47. Ziegler EJ, Fisher CJ, Sprung CL et al (1991) Treatment of gram-negative bacteremia and septic shock with HA-1A human monoclonal antibody against endotoxin. N Engl J Med 324:429–436
48. Greenman RL, Schein RMH, Martin MA, Wenzel RP, MacIntyre NR, Emmanuel G (1991) A controlled clinical trial of E5 murine monoclonal IgM antibody to endotoxin in the treatment of gram-negative sepsis. JAMA 266:1097–1102

A Scoring System for Multiple Organ Dysfunction Syndrome

J. C. Marshall

Introduction

Critically ill patients admitted to a contemporary intensive care unit (ICU) rarely die as a consequence of the progression of the disease process which resulted in their admission to hospital. Instead, and despite the widely heterogeneous processes which precipitate ICU admission, the most common cause of mortality in the ICU is a syndrome variously known as multiple system failure [1], multiple organ failure [2], multiple systems organ failure [3], or, more recently, the multiple organ dysfunction syndrome (MODS) [4]. Moreover death from MODS usually results not so much from failure of vital organ function refractory to support with existing technology, but from the conscious decision of the responsible intensivist that functional recovery is improbable, and that prolongation of exogenous life support is inappropriate. Expressed differently, critically ill patients rarely die because we are unable to ventilate them; they die because we decide to turn off the ventilator.

MODS can be defined as *a clinical syndrome characterized by the development of progressive, but potentially, reversible physiologic dysfunction developing in two or more organs or organ systems and arising in the wake of an acute threat to homeostasis*. MODS has been further classified as **primary** or **secondary** [4]. Primary MODS refers to organ dysfunction which arises immediately after an acute homeostatic insult and as a direct consequence of the process responsible for that insult, whereas secondary MODS develops later and arises as a result of the host response to the primary disease process. Examples of primary MODS include pulmonary contusion and coagulopathy following massive blood loss and transfusion; examples of secondary MODS include the adult respiratory distress syndrome (ARDS) and coagulopathy developing in association with peritonitis. The distinction between primary and secondary MODS is neither absolute nor always clinically obvious.

MODS is at once a paradigm and a syndrome. As a paradigm, it reflects the evolution of intensive care as a discipline centred around the support of organ system function during a period of acute physiologic insufficiency. Since the ICU exists as a geographic locale for the support and monitoring of respiratory, cardiovascular, and renal function, the need for this support is a compelling method of describing the acute disease process evolving in the ICU, and conversely, the prolonged failure of support to restore normal physiologic function justifies its discontinuation and the demise of the patient. From this perspective, MODS is a reflection of the severity of physiologic derangement over time and of the degree of therapeutic intervention required.

But MODS appears to be more than a simple inventory of ICU technology or the process of death in slow motion. Studies in both animal models and humans suggest that there are pathophysiologic processes common to the evolution of MODS in a heterogeneous group of patients. The syndrome can be initiated by a variety of stimuli including infection, ischemia, injury, and inflammation which are amenable to therapeutic manipulation; MODS is thus at least partially preventable. Moreover it is increasingly apparent that the events triggered by these disparate stimuli are mediated by common, endogenously derived cellular mediators including cytokines, prostanoids, and intermediates of oxygen and nitrogen. Thus the course of organ injury may be amenable to modulation, raising the exciting prospect of specific mediator-directed therapy in critical illness in addition to nonspecific organ system support. The goal of effective mediator-directed therapy has yet to be achieved.

If MODS is to be considered a syndrome with the implicit potential for therapeutic intervention, rather than simply a concept defining the limits of critical care technology, it is necessary that there be consensus on what constitutes the syndrome, so that its epidemiology can be properly defined and so that prophylactic or therapeutic interventions can be evaluated. There is as yet no consensus on the criteria necessary to define the syndrome – neither with respect to the organ systems which comprise it nor the degree of abnormality which defines failure. Studies to date have been largely retrospective in nature and have relied on arbitrary and variable criteria to define organ system failure or dysfunction. Despite this there is a striking degree of concordance between reports, and the consistent finding of these is that ICU mortality is a linear function of the number of failing systems, regardless of which systems are considered or what criteria are used to define failure.

This chapter describes an ongoing project to refine and validate a system of characterizing the severity of MODS using a numeric score and summarizes the rationale for such an approach and the current status of the score.

Multiple Organ Dysfunction Syndrome: How Do We Describe it? How Should We Describe it?

Review of Published Descriptions

A review of 19 published reports shows considerable variability in the descriptions of the syndrome – both in the systems whose dysfunction or failure defines the syndrome and in the variables used to define dysfunction or failure in a given system. Seven organ systems – the respiratory, renal, hepatic, cardiovascular, hematologic, gastrointestinal, and central nervous system – appear in more than half of these reports; other organs or systems occasionally mentioned include the endocrine/metabolic system, the pancreas, the immune system, and the skin. The spectrum of variables used to define dysfunction are summarized in Table 1.

Table 1. Published criteria for organ system failure

System	Number of citations	References	Variables used to define failure
Respiratory	19	[2, 3, 5–7, 9–11, 16–26]	Increased A-a gradient, reduced PO_2/FIO_2 ratio, requirement for mechanical ventilation, elevated FIO_2, X-ray evidence of ARDS, ventilation for longer than 72 h, pulmonary failure, use of PEEP, hypercarbia, abnormally low or high respiratory rate
Renal	19	[2, 3, 5–7, 9–11, 16–26]	Requirement for dialysis, elevated creatinine, reduced creatinine clearance, oliguria, elevated BUN
Hepatic	18	[2, 3, 5–7, 9–11, 16–22, 24–26]	Hyperbilirubinemia, jaundice, hypoalbuminemia, elevation SGOT, LDH, SGPT, or AP
Cardiovascular	16	[5–7, 9–11, 16–18, 20–26]	Requirement for inotropes, myocardial infarction, endocarditis, arrhythmia, cardiac arrest, congestive failure, tamponade, bradycardia, hypotension, acidosis, ventricular tachycardia
Hematologic	14	[2, 5–7, 9–11, 15–18, 21, 22–26]	Thrombocytopenia, elevation of PT, PTT, fibrin degradation products, need for clotting factors, leukopenia, leukocytosis, DIC, reduced hematocrit
Central nervous	13	[5, 6, 9–11, 17, 18, 20, 21, 23–26]	Lethargy, coma, failure to respond to other than painful stimuli, meningitis, intracranial hemorrhage, reduced Glasgow Coma Score
Gastrointestinal	13	[2, 3, 5–7, 9, 11, 17, 20–22, 25–26]	Bleeding stress ulcera, acalculous cholecystitis, ileus, bowel perforation, intolerance of enteral feeding
Endocrine/ metabolic	5	[5, 10, 11, 18, 19]	Diabetes, hypercortisolemia, persistent hypermetabolism, glucose intolerance
Pancreas	2	[5, 25]	Pancreatitis
Immune	2	[10, 17]	Impaired delayed hypersensitivity, ICU-acquired infection
Skin, wound healing	1	[17]	Decubitus ulcera, impaired formation of granulation tissue

The difficulty in defining MODS reflects a more basic divergence of views on the fundamental biology of the process. Many authors regard organ failure as a dichotomous event which is either present or absent and define the severity of MODS by the **number** of failing systems [3, 5–8]; for others, organ dysfunction is a continuous process with incremental degrees of dysfunction within each organ system [9–11]. Some authors consider discrete local pathologic processes such as myocardial infarction, endocarditis, and intracranial hemorrhage to be part of the spectrum of MODS; others restrict criteria for organ dysfunction to abnormalities which cannot be otherwise explained on the basis of local pathology. A number of descriptions include physiologic variables which reflect acute injury and incomplete resuscitation such as a reduced hematocrit or oliguria, while others incorporate only criteria which are not readily corrected in the process of resuscitation. Finally organ failure is variously defined by clinical and biochemical abnormalities or by the need for institution of specific ICU supportive measures.

The diversity of the criteria used to characterize MODS reflects the fact that organ dysfunction and its support or reversal is the dominant paradigm of intensive care. Characterization of MODS as a syndrome requires a more critical consideration of the choice of descriptors. There is, at present, no consensus on which variables best reflect the clinical process that the intensivist sees as MODS, but it would seem intuitively evident that the standard by which these variables would be judged is their correlation with ICU mortality.

Dysfunction or Failure?

Although MODS was originally described as organ failure, reflected in inadequate physiologic function to sustain the normal needs of the host without exogenous intervention [1], we believe that it is more appropriate to consider the syndrome as a continuum of deranged physiologic dysfunction, rather than as an ordinal event which is either present or absent. The demonstration that outcome with MODS occurs as a continuous function of increasing physiologic derangement, rather than at a definable threshold, permits description of the syndrome using a continuous organ dysfunction score.

If MODS is a continuum of severity, then it would follow that ICU mortality is a function not only of the **number** of failing systems, but also of the **degree** of dysfunction within any given system. Thus, ICU mortality would rise in a linear fashion with increasing dysfunction in any given system, rather than demonstrating an incremental rise at a discrete level separating failure from nonfailure. In a previous report, we showed this to be the case for variables reflecting dysfunction in eight separate organ systems [10].

Which Systems Comprise Multiple Organ Dysfunction Syndrome?

Although four organ systems – the lungs, kidneys, liver, and cardiovascular system – are included in more than 80% of published reports of MODS, it is apparent from Table 1 that abnormalities of physiologic function can be readily demonstrated for virtually any organ system whose function is assessed. Most authors describe MODS by considering at least four different organ systems. We have included six separate systems in our Multiple Organ Dysfunction (MOD) score, thus reflecting a process which is highly variable in its expression and minimizing the discrete contribution of dysfunction in any single system to the overall quantitation of severity. The six systems are included in the majority of published reports, and it is possible, with varying degrees of success, to define appropriate descriptors to reflect a spectrum of increasingly severe dysfunction for each system.

Criteria for Optimal Descriptors of Organ Dysfunction

The choice of variables to reflect altered function in a given organ system is critical. For some systems – the lungs or kidneys, for example – variables reflecting worsening function are readily identified. For other systems – the cardiovascular system, for example – the process is more difficult. Implicit in the majority of descriptions of MODS is the concept that dysfunction of any given organ system is mediated indirectly by some remote pathologic process, rather than directly as a result of local organ pathology. Thus we believe that processes such as meningitis or myocardial infarction should not be viewed as part of the organ dysfunction syndrome. Nonetheless, the distinction between the direct and indirect consequences of critical illness is not always readily evident.

The ideal variable to describe function in any given organ system is one which is:

1. Simple
2. Objective
3. Readily, regularly, and reliably measured
4. Reproducible in heterogeneous groups of critically ill patients
5. An accurate reflection of function in the given organ system
6. Specific for the function of that particular organ system
7. Unaffected by direct therapeutic intervention
8. A continuous, rather than a categorical variable
9. Abnormal in one direction only (i. e., only levels above or below normal are considered)
10. One for which increasingly abnormal function correlates independently with increasing ICU mortality

Our approach has been to use ICU mortality, rather than hospital mortality, as the endpoint to evaluate candidate variables, since intrinsic to the concept of MODS is the need for ICU support and the consequences of its success or failure.

The Multiple Organ Dysfunction Score

We have described a system for characterizing MODS as an organ dysfunction score using descriptors of deranged function in six separate organ systems [12]. The variables and intervals are summarized in Table 2. Organ dysfunction in each of the six systems is scored on a scale from 0 (normal function) to 4 (markedly impaired function), and the sum of the worst values for each of the six systems comprises the MOD score. The MOD score, therefore, represents a composite of the worst values over time and is an outcome measure rather than a predictor. Within each system, abnormal values are those present at a standard time of assessment (the morning in the present series), rather than the worst values over 24 h to minimize the impact of marked, but transient, functional abnormalities as might occur, for example, as consequence of a mucus plug in the airway. Missing values are assigned a score of 0.

The score was developed using prospectively collected data from 692 separate admissions to the surgical intensive care unit of the Victoria General

Table 2. The multiple organ dysfunction (MOD) score

System	0	1	2	3	4
Respiratory (PaO_2/FIO_2 ratio)	>250	151–250	101–150	61–100	≤60
Renal (Serum creatinine μmol/L)	≤100	101–200	201–350	351–500	>500
Hepatic (Serum bilirubin μmol/L)	≤20	21–60	61–120	121–240	>240
Cardio-vascular	Pulse rate ≤120	Pulse rate 121–140	Pulse rate >140	Need for inotropes to maintain mean BP>80	Lactate >5
Hematologic (Platelet Count per mm^3)	>120000	81–120000	41–80000	21–40000	≤20000
Central nervous (Glasgow Coma Score)	15	13–14	10–12	6–9	<6

Hospital, Halifax, Nova Scotia, Canada, over a 21 month period from May 1988 to February 1990. Comprehensive clinical, laboratory, radiographic, and microbiologic data were collected for all patients admitted for at least 2 days. Candidate variables in each of the selected systems were developed using the first 336 patients in the data base, then tested on the remaining patients to assess their reproducibility. For each system, intervals of abnormality were selected with the objective that the mortality associated with a

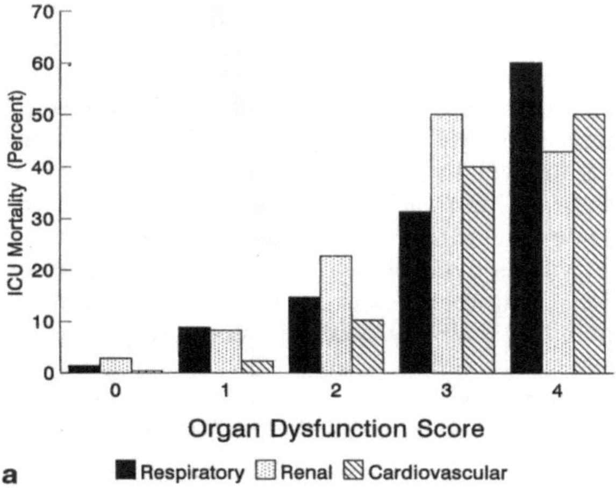

a

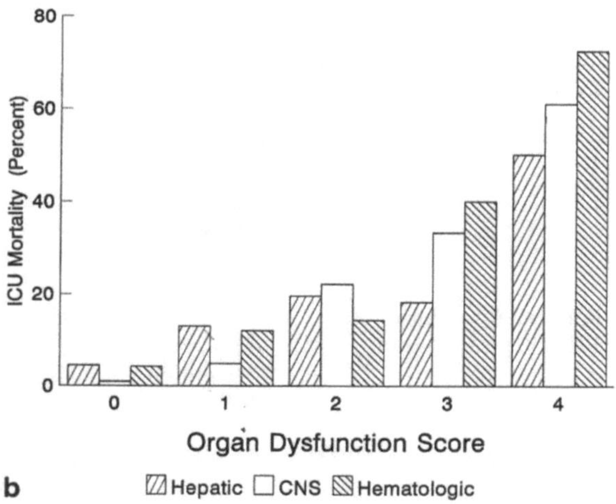

b

Fig. 1. For each of the six organ systems in the multiple organ dysfunction (MOD) score – the respiratory, renal, and cardiovascular system (**a**) and the hepatic, hematologic, and central nervous system (**b**) – increasing abnormality of the variables used to characterize organ system function correlated with ultimate ICU mortality

score of 0 in any given system would be less than 5%, while that associated with a score of 4 would be 50% or higher.

Fig. 1 demonstrates the correlation between incremental increases in individual organ dysfunction scores and ICU mortality and shows that for each system assessed it was possible to demonstrate a strong correlation between increasingly deranged function and the probability of death. Interestingly, only certain variables demonstrated a linear relationship between increasing abnormality and ICU mortality. The maximal level of positive end-expiratory pressure (PEEP), for example, showed a pattern similar to that seen for the oxygen tension/fraction of inspiled oxygen (PO_2/FIO_2) ratio; the maximal PCO_2 level did not differ between survivors and nonsurvivors.

When each of the six individual components of the score were totalled to produce the MOD score, it was evident that ICU mortality increased with increasing MOD scores (Fig. 2). A MOD score of 10 was associated with an ICU mortality of approximately 25%, whereas a score of 15 or greater carried a mortality of over 75%. The distribution of scores in the study population is shown in Fig. 3.

Stepwise logistic regression analysis using ICU mortality as the dependent variable showed an independent contribution to mortality for each organ system except the liver and generated an equation linking organ dysfunction with ICU mortality:

P|Death| = −0.104 + 0.078 (CNS) + 0.049 (Hematologic) + 0.036 (Cardiovascular) + 0.039 (Renal) + 0.027 (Respiratory)

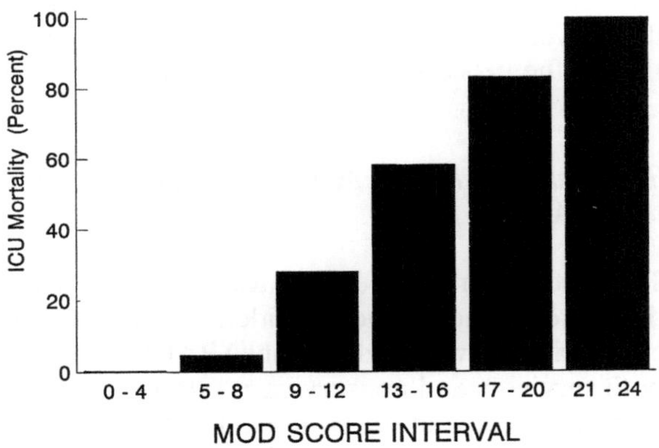

Fig. 2. ICU mortality rose progressively as multiple organ dsyfunction (MOD) scores increased. In the absence of organ dysfunction, survival was 100%; in the presence of marked dysfunction, it was 0%. A similar association was seen when the correlation of MOD score with hospital mortality was studied, although the additional influence of events happening after the ICU admission had the net effect of shifting the curve to the left

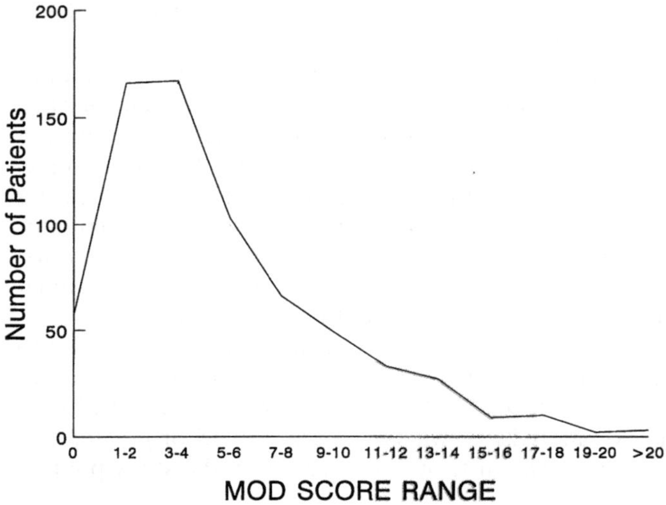

Fig. 3. Distributions of multiple organ dysfunction (MOD) scores among the 692 patients in the study population; significant organ dysfunction developed in a minority of patients

Do We Need Another Score?

The increasing complexity and volume of clinical data collected within the ICU and the ready accessibility of microcomputers has spawned an enormous number of prognostic scores designed to organize data to predict a particular outcome. The MOD score described here, however, is not primarily a predictor of an outcome, but a descriptor of an outcome. Although it has been developed using ICU mortality as the standard against which candidate variables are assessed, its utility lies in providing a numeric description of the process which ultimately led to that mortality.

The Relationship of Multiple Organ Dysfunction Score to APACHE II

The distinction between the use of a score as a predictor and its use as a descriptor is more readily evident from a review of Fig. 4, which shows the correlation between admission APACHE II scores [8] and MOD scores for both survivors and nonsurvivors. Global illness severity at the time of admission, as reflected in the admission APACHE II score, contributes to the subsequent severity of organ dysfunction, since mean MOD scores for survivors increase with incremental increase in APACHE II score. For all nonsurvivors, however, MOD scores are similar over the entire range of APACHE II scores. This observation suggests two conclusions: (1) that although APACHE II predicts ICU mortality, events occurring after ICU admission

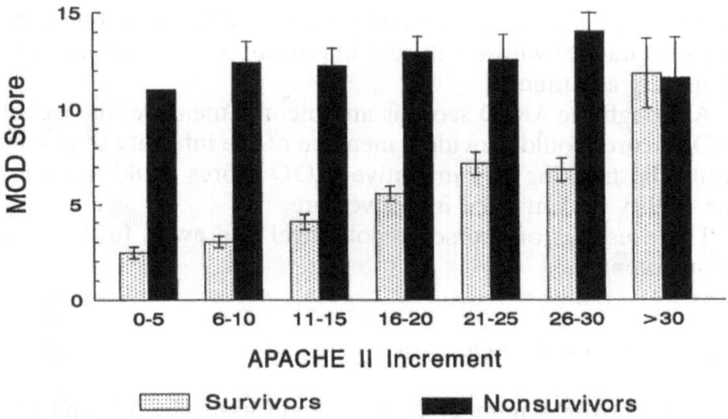

Fig. 4. The association between admission APACHE II and multiple organ dysfunction (MOD) scores over the duration of the ICU admission. That MOD scores for nonsurvivors are similar, regardless of admission APACHE II scores, suggests that the MOD score may be useful as a surrogate outcome for ICU mortality

make a significant contribution to outcome, and (2) perhaps more importantly, that the MOD score can be used as a surrogate for mortality as an outcome measure in critical care.

Applications of the Multiple Organ Dysfunction Score

A numeric descriptor for a complex process such as MODS has a number of potential applications. As an outcome measure, it can potentially substitute for mortality as an endpoint in clinical trials, with the result that more subtle biologic changes can be detected using smaller groups of patients than are required for mortality studies. In a matched cohort study, for example, we have shown that blood transfusion in the first 48 h following ICU admission has an adverse impact on ICU outcome, reflected in significantly higher MOD scores in transfused patients in the face of a slight, but statistically insignificant, increase in mortality [13]. Moreover the use of the MOD score provides insights into the biologic processes associated with this adverse outcome, showing that the increase in organ dysfunction is accounted for by changes in the central nervous system, hepatic, and hematologic components of the score, but not by changes in the respiratory or renal components.

Since the MOD score reflects morbidity over time, it may have a role to play as a measure of the intensity of resource utilization and as a quality assurance marker. It can be hypothesized, for example, that the mean MOD score for patients stratified by admission APACHE II score is a measure of the quality of care provided in a particular ICU. For similar admission APACHE II scores, differing units would be expected to show similar MOD scores, and discrepancies could be interpreted as reflecting differences in patterns of practice whose nature is important to ascertain as part of the process of quality assurance.

Although the MOD score is an outcome measure, the calculation of daily MOD scores could provide a measure of the intensity of resource utilization, while the tracking of cumulative MOD scores could assist in documenting the futility of continued intensive care.

The uses are, of course, hypothetical and await further studies to assess their potential.

Summary and Conclusions

It is clear from a number of recent editorials [14, 15] and from the recommendations emerging from consensus conferences [4] that there is a pressing need for clarity and consensus in describing the complex events which unfold in the critically ill patient. The work described here represents one attempt at trying to achieve greater clarity. It is by no means definitive and is better seen as an initial foray into what will inevitably be a long and challenging process. It does, however, establish the feasibility of using a numeric score based on incremental increases in the abnormal function of a number of organ systems as a descriptor of a common and important clinical process.

In the development of a score whose purposes are purely prognostic without particular reference to an underlying disease process (APACHE II is the prototype of such a score) it is sufficient for the investigator to show that a given abnormality predicts death to justify its incorporation into the score. The challenge in developing a descriptor of MODS is more difficult. Not only must the potential variables correlate with death, they must also reflect the clinical dimensions of a complex process which, like pornography, all can recognize but none can satisfactorily define. It is clear from a review of the literature that although there is considerable consensus on what MODS is and how best to describe it, there is also considerable variability from one author to another and from one centre to the next. The challenge is to develop a descriptive instrument which truly reflects a consensus of a clinical description and which applies equally well in a surgical ICU in Canada, a pediatric ICU in South America, and a medial ICU in Europe.

References

1. Baue AE (1975) Multiple, progressive, or sequential systems failure. A syndrome of the 1970's. Arch Surg 110:779–781
2. Eiseman B, Beart R, Norton L (1977) Multiple organ failure. Surg Gynecol Obstet 144:323–326
3. Fry DE, Pearlstein L, Fulton RL, Polk HC (1980) Multiple system organ failure. The role of uncontrolled infection. Arch Surg 115:136–140
4. ACCP/SCCM Consensus Conference (1992) Definitions of sepsis and multiple organ failure. Crit Care Med 20:864–874

5. Bell RC, Coalson JJ, Smith JD, Johanson WG (1983) Multiple organ system failure and infection in adult respiratory distress syndrome. Ann Intern Med. 99:293–298
6. Bihari D, Smithies M, Gimson A, Tinker J (1987) The effects of vasodilation with prostacyclin on oxygen delivery and uptake in critically ill patients. N Engl J Med 317:397–403
7. Henao FJ, Daes JE, Dennis RJ (1991) Risk factors for multiorgan failure: a case-control study. Trauma 31:74–80
8. Knaus WA, Draper EA, Wagner DP, Zimmermann JE (1985) APACHE II: a severity of disease classification system. Crit Care Med 13:818–829
9. Goris RJA, te Boekhurts TPA, Nuytinck JKS, Gimbrere JSF (1985) Multiple-organ failure. Generalized autodestructive inflammation? Arch Surg 120:1109–1115
10. Marshall JC, Christou NV, Horn H, Meakins JL (1988) The microbiology of multiple organ failure. The proximal GI tract as an occult reservoir of pathogens. Arch Surg 123:309–315
11. Moore FA, Moore EE, Poggetti R, McAnena OJ, Peterson VM, Abernathy CM, Parsons PE (1991) Gut bacterial translocation via the portal vein: a clinical perspective with major torso trauma. Trauma 31:629–638
12. Marshall JC, Cook DJ, Sibbald WJ, Roy PD, Christou NV (1992) The multiple organ dysfunction (MOD) score: a reliable descriptor of a complex clinical outcome. Crit Care Med 20:S80 (abstract)
13. Chiu P, Roy PD, Marshall JC (1993) Blood transfusion is a risk factor for ICU-acquired infection and the multiple organ dysfunction syndrome (MODS). Crit Care Med 21:S126 (abstract)
14. Bone RC (1991) Let's agree on terminology: definitions of sepsis. Crit Care Med 19:973–976
15. Sibbald WJ, Marshall J, Christou N, Girotti M, McCormack D, Rotstein O, Martin C, Meakins J (1991) "Sepsis" – clarity of existing terminology or more confusion? Crit Care Med 19:996–998
16. Bone RC, Balk R, Slotman G, Maunder R, Silverman H, Hyers TM, Kerstein MD, and the Prostaglandin E_1 Study Group (1992) Adult respiratory distress syndrome. Sequence and importance of development of multiple organ failure. Chest 101:320–326
17. Border JR, Chenier R, McMenamy RH, La Duca J, Seibel R, Birkhahn R, Yu L (1976) Multiple systems organ failure: muscle fuel deficit with visceral protein malnutrition. Surg Clin North Am 56:1147–1167
18. Carrico CJ, Meakins JL, Marshall JC, Fry D, Maier RV (1986) Multiple-organ-failure-syndrome. Arch Surg 121:196–208
19. Cerra FB, McPherson JP, Konstantinides FN, Konstantinides NN, Teasley KM (1988) Enteral nutrition does not prevent multiple organ failure syndrome (MOFS) after sepsis. Surgery 104:727–733
20. DeCamp MM, Demling RH (1988) Posttraumatic multisystem organ failure. JAMA 260:53–534
21. Deitch EA (1992) Multiple organ failure. Pathophysiology and potential future therapy. Ann Surg 216:117–134
22. Faist E, Baue AE, Dittmer H, Heberer G (1983) Multiple organ failure in polytrauma patients. J Trauma 23:775
23. Knaus WA, Draper EA, Wagner DP, Zimmerman JE (1985) Prognosis in acute organ system failure. Ann Surg 202:685–692
24. Pine RW, Wertz MJ, Lennard ES, Dellinger EP, Carrico CJ, Minshew BH (1983) Determinants of organ malfunction or death in patients with intra-abdominal sepsis. Arch Surg 118:242–249
25. Tilney NL, Bailey GL, Morgan AP (1973) Sequential system failure after rupture of abdominal aortic aneurysms: an unsolved problem in postoperative care. Ann Surg 178:117–122
26. Tran DD, Groeneveld ABJ, van der Meulen J, Nauta JJP, Strack van Schijndel RJM, Thijs LG (1990) Age, chronic disease, sepsis, organ system failure, and mortality in a medical intensive care unit. Crit Care Med 18:474–479

II. Pathogenesis

Endotoxemia and Sepsis: Important Roles for Lipopolysaccharide Binding Protein and CD14 in Endotoxin Signal Transduction

K. F. Bruin, M. A. M. von der Möhlen and S. J. H. van Deventer

Introduction

Septic shock associated with gram-negative septicemia is still a leading cause of death in the western world. In the last decade, it has become increasingly clear that endotoxin, a lipopolysaccharide (LPS) component of the outer membrane of gram-negative bacteria, is a pivotal trigger of gram-negative septic shock and that its biological effects are mediated by endogenous (glyco)proteins known as cytokines. Despite the considerable heterogeneity of endotoxins from different gram-negative bacteria, these molecules all have a similar molecular structure that underlies bioactivity. The lipid moiety of endotoxin, lipid A, is the biologically active component, and is also essential for binding of endotoxin to immunocompetent cells. Since in intact bacteria lipid A is completely embedded within the outer bacterial membrane, it is likely that endotoxins need to be released from bacteria in order to cause inflammation. The clinical importance of endotoxemia and the possible role of various antibiotics in the process of endotoxin liberation have been recently reviewed [1]. Once liberated from bacteria, endotoxin rapidly binds to various plasma proteins, and it has recently become clear that some of these interactions importantly alter the host response to endotoxin.

In this chapter we rewiev current knowledge of the endotoxin signal transduction pathway, with special emphasis on the role of plasma proteins in this process.

The Quest for the Endotoxin Receptor

Although several membrane-associated structures which can interact with endotoxin or lipid A have been identified, their distinct roles in the endotoxin signal transduction pathway remain to be identified. The CD 11b/CD 18 family of glycoproteins can bind endotoxin [2], but binding does not result in activation of monocytes or macrophages [3], and phagocytes express other lipid A binding sites [4]. One of these has been characterized as the scavenger receptor, a macrophage receptor that binds a large variety of known ligands. Binding of the lipid A analogue lipid IV_A to the scavenger receptor is followed by internalization of the ligand-receptor complex and subsequent degradation of the molecule [5]. Thus, the scavenger receptor may play a role in the detoxification of endotoxin. However, interaction of endotoxin and the scavenger receptor does not result in activation of macrophages, as reflected by an absence of tumor necrosis factor (TNF) production. A membrane-associated endotoxin binding protein of 73 kDa, originally detected on murine splenocytes, is now known to have an analogue which is expressed by human monocytes [6–8]. A monoclonal antibody generated against this receptor activated macrophages, as indicated by induction of cell-mediated cytotoxicity [9, 10]. Interestingly, this receptor not only recognizes endotoxin, but also peptidoglycan from *Staphylococcus aureus* [11] and pertussis toxin [12, 13], suggesting the possibility of a "final common pathway" for monocyte activation by gram-negative and gram-positive microorganisms.

Is CD14 the Endotoxin Receptor?

The latest endotoxin binding molecule to be characterized has been identified as CD14. CD14 is a 55 kDa cell membrane-associated glycoprotein originally classified as a differentiation antigen on cells of the myelomonocytic lineage. It is present on monocytes, macrophages and activated granulocytes, as well as on some mature tumor cell lines, but not on cells in earlier stages of differentiation or on immature tumor cell lines such as U937, HL60 or K562 [14–17]. The gene for CD14 has been cloned and mapped to the long arm of human chromosome 5, to a region encoding several growth factors and receptors such as interleukin-3 (IL-3), granulocyte-macrophage colony stimulating factor (GM-CSF), the platelet-derived growth factor (PDGF) receptor, the β2 adrenergic receptor and endothelial cell growth factor (ECGF) [18]. This localization prompted speculation regarding a possible role of CD14 as a receptor. From the predicted amino acid sequence of the protein it became clear that, although a characteristic leader peptide was present, the protein contained no membrane spanning hydrophobic domain [19]. It was then found that CD14 is attached to the cell membrane by a glycophosphatidylinositol (GPI) anchor [4, 20], which seemed to exclude a function as a cell signaling protein. It has been demonstrated recently, however, that even though GPI-anchored proteins do not have a transmembrane region, they may be involved in signal transduction (reviewed in [21]). In accordance with these data is the finding that cross-linking of CD14 on monocytes and granulocytes results in an increase in the intracellular calcium concentration, which is suggestive of involvement of CD14 in signal transduction [22]. One of the consequences of GPI anchoring of a protein is the relatively easy nonproteolytic cleavage from the cell membrane by GPI-specific phospholipases C or D (PI-PLC or PI-PLD) and a high mobility in the plane of the cell membrane. Indeed, shedding of CD14 has been observed *in vitro* [23], and does occur *in vivo* as well, since two soluble forms of CD14, respectively of molecular weights 53 and 48 kDa, have been detected in urine and in plasma [24, 25]. The 53 kDa form results from cleavage off the cell membrane by a specific phospholipase and still contains the GPI-anchor [26], whereas the 48 kDa form no longer does.

Monocytes rapidly internalized CD14 when incubated with a specific anti-CD14 monoclonal antibody, and CD14-antibody complexes could be demonstrated intracellularly [27]. The kinetics of this process strongly resembled those of receptor-mediated endocytosis, suggesting a function as a receptor, however a ligand was not yet identified. Interestingly, the antibody used in these experiments, ROMO 1, acted as a monocyte activating factor in mononuclear cell suspensions, as reflected by the production of O_2-, H_2O_2, and interleukin-1 (IL-1) [28]. It was shown later that endotoxin-induced IL-1, interleukin (IL-6), interleukin-8 (IL-8) and TNF release by human monocytes is mediated by CD14 and that this effect is strongly enhanced by, but not completely dependent on, the presence of serum [2, 29, 30].

Soluble Endotoxin Binding Factors

Soluble factors which bind endotoxin and modulate its biological effects, such as lipopolysaccharide binding protein (LBP) and bactericidal permeability increasing protein (BPI), have been recently characterized [31]. LBP is an approximately 60 kDa protein present in the acute phase serum of several species, including humans, mice, rats and rabbits. The primary structure of the protein was deduced from the cloned and sequenced LBP gene [32]. LBP shares 45% amino acid sequence identity at its NH_2-terminal end with a 60 kDa endotoxin-binding protein, BPI, that is present in the primary secretory granules of neutrophils [33, 34]. Both proteins specifically bind endotoxin at their NH_2-terminal and form high affinity complexes with lipid A, the biologically active moiety of endotoxin [35]. Recently, the genes of LBP and BPI were mapped to the same region of the long arm of human chromosome 20, suggesting that the proteins are members of a family of endotoxin binding proteins [36].

Lipopolysaccharide-Lipopolysaccharide Binding Protein-CD14 Interactions

Binding of endotoxin (LPS) to LBP facilitated its interaction with macrophages [37]. This interaction occurred through a receptor that was mobile in the plane of the cell membrane [5], later identified as CD 14 [38] (Fig. 1A). The binding of endotoxin to human monocytes was greatly enhanced in the presence of serum. This effect could be reversed by preincubation of the cells with an anti-CD14 monoclonal antibody (My4), by enzymatic removal of CD14 from the cell surface, or by depletion of LBP from the serum [39]. Macrophage responsiveness to endotoxin, lipid A or lipid A partial structures, as measured by TNF production *in vitro,* was a 1000-fold lower in the presence of LBP-depleted serum than in the presence of normal serum [40].

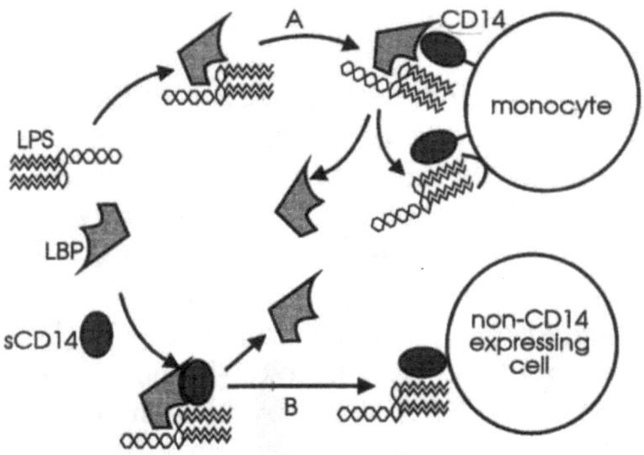

Fig. 1. Lipopolysaccharide (*LPS*)-lipopolysaccharide binding protein (*LBP*)-CD14 interactions. *sCD14*, soluble CD14

A similar effect was observed when monocytes from patients with paroxysmal nocturnal hemoglobinuria (PNH), which lack GPI-anchored proteins including CD14, were stimulated with endotoxin. These cells were able to react to endotoxin, but needed a 100-fold higher dose of endotoxin to do so. Since CD14 deficiency does not cause complete endotoxin unresponsiveness, it would appear that there is an additional, CD14-independent, pathway of endotoxin signal transduction. Alternatively, CD14 interacts with other endotoxin receptors to up-regulate the efficiency of signal transduction.

Regulation of CD14 Expression

CD14 expression on monocytes is modulated by a variety of substances including endotoxin itself. In whole blood *in vitro,* a dose-dependent increase in monocytic CD14 expression and a concurrent increase in binding of FITC-labeled endotoxin was observed rapidly (within 30 min) after stimulation with endotoxin [41]. This increase was not dependent on protein synthesis since it was not blocked by cycloheximide. Culture of monocytes in the presence of IL-6 also resulted in an increase of CD14 expression as quantitated by binding of ^{125}I-labeled anti-CD14 monoclonal antibodies [6]. Finally, TNFα induced the release of soluble CD14 from cultured monocytes [42]. Interleukin-4 (IL-4) down-regulated the expression of membrane-associated CD14 by monocytes after 2–3 days of culture [43]; this effect could be blocked by anti-IL-4 but not by anti-interferon(IFN)-γ [44]. A parallel decrease in the release of soluble CD14 was observed, suggesting that this down-regulation is not due to enhanced CD14 shedding, and it was demonstrated that transcription of CD14 mRNA was decreased [6]. IFN-γ also decreased membrane CD14 expression in a dose-dependent fashion within 3 h [6, 45], and in addition, IL-4 and IFN-γ decreased the release of soluble CD14 by monocytes and macrophages [46]. This effect of IFN-γ is remarkable, because this cytokine is known to increase endotoxin sensitivity *in vivo* [47, 48]. Interleukin-2 (IL-2) and IFN-γ decreased both membrane CD14 expression and soluble CD14 release in mononuclear cells, which is possibly mediated by IFN-γ. Other cytokines, such as IL-1, IL-2, IL-3, IL-5, TNFβ and GM-CSF, however, did not influence CD14 expression in human monocytes.

Soluble CD14

Soluble CD14 was first identified in plasma and urine as a 53 kDa glycoprotein [4]. It is present in normal serum at concentrations of 2–6 μg/ml. Serum CD14 levels may vary in the course of several disease processes. In polytraumatized patients and patients with severe burn injuries, serum CD14 levels were initially depressed, but increased and remained elevated for some time after admittance to the hospital [49]. In patients with a clinical diagnosis of gram-negative sepsis, levels of soluble CD14 were also elevated (von der Möhlen and van Deventer, unpublished results).

Since it was discovered that CD14 mediates the enhanced induction of the biological effects of endotoxin by complexes of endotoxin and LBP, the potential regulatory role of soluble CD14 has been the topic of much debate. Several possible functions for soluble CD14 have been postulated. Firstly, it has been suggested that soluble CD14 may function as a naturally occurring endotoxin antagonist by binding endotoxin-LBP complexes in the systemic circulation, thereby preventing activation of monocytes or macrophages [50]. There is some evidence that soluble CD14 can indeed reduce endotoxin-induced monocyte activation *in vitro* in the presence of serum [6]. However, *in vivo*, even in severe sepsis, the molar excess of soluble CD14 to lipopolysaccharide does not prevent endotoxin-induced biological effects, which suggests that this mechanism is not very important *in vivo.* Secondly, soluble CD14 may arise from cleavage of the CD14 molecule from the monocyte membrane as a way of preventing (further) activation of monocytes by endotoxin [4]. Thirdly, soluble CD14 has the exciting property to enable cells that do not express CD14 on their membranes to respond to endotoxin-LBP complexes in the systemic circulation [51, 52] (Fig. 1B).

Conclusions

No doubt endotoxin is a key bacterial pathogenic factor in sepsis. Its biological effects are in large part mediated by an inflammatory host response, which, if appropriately regulated, is necessary for succesful clearance of the invading bacteria. However, uncontrolled release of inflammatory mediators, in particular of cytokines such as TNF and IL-1, may cause extensive organ damage and death. The endotoxin-induced inflammatory response is normally tightly controlled at multiple levels. Here we have reviewed the complex and fine-tuned pathways that are involved in endotoxin signaling by immunocompetent cells. These data are not only of importance for our understanding of the pathogenesis of sepsis, but may also lead to novel intervention strategies.

References

1. Hurley JC (1992) Antibiotic-induced release of endotoxin: a preappraisal. Clin Infect Dis 15:840–854
2. Wright SD, Levin SM, Jong MTC, Chad Z, Kabbash LG (1989) CR3 (CD11b/CD18) expresses one binding site for Arg-Gly-Asp-containing peptides and a second site for bacterial lipopolysaccharide. J Exp Med 169:175–183
3. Couturier C, Jahns G, Kazatchkine MD, Haeffner-Cavaillon N (1992) Membrane molecules which trigger the production of interleukin-1 and tumor necrosis factor α by lipopolysaccharide-stimulated human monocytes. Eur J Immunol 22:1461–1466
4. Golenbock DT, Hampton RY, Raetz CRH, Wright SD (1990) Human phagocytes have multiple lipid A binding sites. Infect Immun 58:4069–4075
5. Hampton RY, Golenbock DT, Penman M, Krieger M, Raetz CRH (1991) Recognition and plasma clearance of endotoxin by scavenger receptors. Nature 352:342–344
6. Lei MG, Morrison DC (1989) Specific endotoxic lipopolysaccharide binding proteins on murine splenocytes. I. Detection of LPS binding sites on splenocytes and splenocyte subpopulations. J Immunol 141:996–1005
7. Lei MG, Morrison DC (1989) Specific endotoxic lipopolysaccharide binding proteins on murine splenocytes. II. Membrane localization and binding characteristics. J Immunol 141:1006–1011
8. Lei MG, Stimpson SA, Morrison DC (1991) Specific endotoxic lipopolysaccharide binding receptors on murine splenocytes. III. Binding specificity and characterization. J Immunol 147:1925–1932
9. Bright SW, Chen TY, Flebbe LM, Lei MG, Morrison DC (1990) Generation and characterization of hamster-mouse hybridomas secreting monoclonal antibodies with specificity for lipopolysaccharide receptor. J Immunol 145:1–7
10. Chen TY, Bright SW, Pace JL, Russel SW, Morrison DC (1990) Induction of macrophage-mediated tumor cytotoxicity by a hamster monoclonal antibody with specificity for lipopolysaccharide receptor. J Immunol 145:8–12
11. Dziarski R (1991) Peptidoglycan and lipopolysaccharide bind to the same binding site on lymphocytes. J Biol Chem 266:4719–4728
12. Clark CG, Amstrong GD (1990) Lymphocyte receptors for pertussis toxin. Infect Immun 58:3840–3846
13. Lei MG, Morrison DC (1992) Interrelationship of LPS, pertussis toxin and the p73 LPS receptor on lymphoreticular cells. In: Levin J, Alving CR, Munford RS, Stütz PL (eds) Bacterial endotoxin: recognition and effector mechanisms. Elsevier, Amsterdam, pp 143–150 (Endotoxin research series, vol 2)
14. Todd RF III, Nadler LM, Schlossman SF (1981) Antigens on human monocytes identified by monoclonal antibodies. J Immunol 126:1435–1442
15. Griffin JD, Ritz J, Nadler LM, Schlossman SF (1981) Expression of myeloid differentiation antigens on normal and malignant myeloid cells. J Clin Invest 68:932–941
16. Maliszewski CR, Ball ED, Graziano RF, Fanger MW (1985) Isolation and characterization of MY23, a myeloid cell-derived antigen reactive with the monoclonal antibody AML-2-23. J Immunol 135:1929–1936
17. Goyert SM, Ferrero EM, Seremetis SV, Winchester RJ, Silver J, Mattison AC (1986) Biochemistry and expression of myelomonocytic antigens. J Immunol 137:3909–3914
18. Goyert SM, Ferrero EM, Rettig WJ, Yenamandra AY, Obata F, Le Beau MM (1987)

The CD14 monocyte differentiation antigen maps to a region encoding groth factors and receptors. Science 239:497–500
19. Haziot A, Chen S, Ferrero E, Low MC, Silber R, Goyert SM (1988) The monocyte differentiation antigen, CD14, is anchored to the cell membrane by a phosphatidylinositol phosphate. J Immunol 141:547–552
20. Simmons DI, Tan S, Tenen DG, Nicholson-Weller, Seed B (1989) Monocyte antigen CD14 is a phospholipid anchored membrane protein. Blood 73:284–289
21. Robinson PJ (1991) Phosphatidylinositol membrane anchors and T-cell activation. Immunol Today 12:35–41
22. Lund-Johansen F, Olweus J, Aarli Å, Bjerknes R (1990) Signal transduction in human monocytes and granulocytes through the PI-linked antigen CD14. FEBS Lett 273:55–58
23. Bazil V, Strominger JL (1991) Shedding as a mechanism of downmodulation of CD14 on stimulated human monocytes. J Immunol 147:1567–1574
24. Bazil V, Horejsi V, Baudys M, Kristofova H, Strominger JL, Kostka W, Hilgert I (1986) Biochemical characterization of a soluble form of the 53-kDa monocyte surface antigen. Eur J Immunol 10:1583–1589
25. Goyert SM, Tesio L, Ashman LK et al (1989) Report on the CD14 cluster workshop. In: Knapp W et al (eds) Leucocyte typing IV. White cell differentiation antigens. Oxford University Press, Oxford, pp 789–794
26. Bazil V, Baudys M, Hilgert I, Stefanova I, Low MG, Zbrozek J, Horejsi V (1989) Structural relationship between the soluble and membrane-bound forms of human monocyte surface glycoprotein CD14. Mol Immunol 26:657–662
27. Jonas L, Schutt C, Neels P, Walzel H, Siegl E (1988) Electron microscopic visualization of receptor internalization induced by a monoclonal antibody recognizing the monocyte specific glycoprotein CD14. Acta Histochem (Jena) 85:167–173
28. Schutt C, Ringel B, Nausch M et al (1988) Human monocyte activation induced by an anti-CD14 antibody. Immunol Lett 19:321–328
29. Couturier C, Haeffner-Cavaillon N, Caroff M, Kazatchkine MD (1991) Binding sites for endotoxins (lipopolysaccharides) on human monocytes. J Immunol 147:1899–1904
30. Dentener MA, Bazil V, von Asmuth EJU, Ceska M, Buurman WA (1993) Involvement of CD14 in lipopolysaccharide-induced tumor necrosis factor α, IL-6 and IL-8 release by human monocytes and alveolar macrophages. J Immunol 150:2885–2891
31. Tobias PS, Mathison JC, Ulevitch RJ (1988) A family of lipopolysaccharide binding proteins involved in responses to gram-negative sepsis. J Biol Chem 263:13479–13481
32. Schumann, Leong SR, Flaggs GW et al (1990) Structure and function of lipopolysaccharide binding protein. Science 249:1429–1431
33. Marra MN, Wilde CG, Griffith JE, Snable JL, Scott RW (1990) Bactericidal/permeability-increasing protein has endotoxin-neutralizing activity. J Immunol 144:662–666
34. Gray PW, Flaggs G, Leong SR, Gumina RJ (1989) Cloning of the cDNA of a human neutrophil bactericidal protein. J Biol Chem 264:9505–9509
35. Tobias PS, Soldan K, Ulevitch RJ (1989) Identification of a lipid A binding site in the acute phase reactant lipopolysaccharide binding protein. J Biol Chem 264:10867–10871
36. Gray PW, Corcorran AE, Eddy RL, Byers MG, Shows TB (1993) The genes for lipopolysaccharide binding protein (LPS) and the bactericidal permeability increasing protein (BPI) are encoded in the same region of human chromosome 20. Genomics 15:188–190
37. Wright SD, Tobias PS, Ulevitch RJ, Ramos RA (1989) Lipopolysaccharide (LPS) binding protein opsonizes LPS bearing particles for recognition by a novel receptor on macrophages. J Exp Med 170:1231–1241
38. Wright SD, Ramos RA, Tobias PS, Ulevitch RJ, Mathison JC (1990) CD14, a receptor for complexes of lipopolysaccharide (LPS) and LPS binding protein. Science 249:1431–1433

39. Heumann D, Gallay P, Barras C et al (1992) Control of lipopolysaccharide (LPS) binding and LPS-induced tumor necrosis factor secretion in human peripheral blood monocytes. J Immunol 148:3505–3512
40. Mathison JC, Tobias PS, Wolfson E, Ulevitch RJ (1992) Plasma lipopolysaccharide binding protein. A key component in macrophage recognition of gram-negative LPS. J Immunol 149:200–206
41. Marchant A, Duchow J, Delville JP, Goldmann M (1992) Lipopolysaccharide induces up-regulation of CD14 molecule on monocytes in whole blood. Eur J Immunol 22:1663–1665
42. Schütt C, Schilling T, Grunwald U, Schönfeld W, Krüger C (1992) Endotoxin-neutralizing capacity of soluble CD14. Res Immunol 143:71–78
43. Lauener RP, Goyert SM, Geha RS, Vercelli D (1990) Interleukin 4 down-regulates the expression of CD14 in normal human monocytes. Eur J Immunol 20:2375–2381
44. Landmann R, Ludwig C, Ohrist R, Obrecht JP (1991) Effect of cytokines and lipopolysaccharide on CD14 antigen expression in human monocytes and macrophages. J Cell Biochem 47:317–329
45. Landmann R, Wesp M, Olbrecht JP (1991) Cytokine regulation of the myeloid glycoprotein CD14, Pathobiology 59:131–135
46. Landmann R, Fischer A, Olbrecht JP (1992) Interferon-γ and interleukin-4 down-regulate soluble CD14 release in human monocytes and macrophages. J Leukocyte Biol 52:323–330
47. Vogel SN, Moore RN, Sipe JD, Rosenstreich DL (1980) BCG-induced enhancement of endotoxin sensitivity in C3H/HeJ mice. I. In vivo studies. J Immunol 124:2004
48. Galanos C, Freudenberg MA, Katschinski T, Salomao R, Mossmann H, Kumazawa Y (1992) Tumor necrosis factor and host response to endotoxin. In: Ryan JL, Morrison DC (eds) Immunopharmacology and pathophysiology. CRC, Ann Arbor, pp 75–104 (Bacterial endotoxic lipopolysaccharides, vol 2)
49. Krüger C, Schütt C, Obertacke U et al (1991) Serum CD14 levels in polytraumatized and severely burned patients. Clin Exp Immunol 85:297–301
50. Maliszewski CR (1991) CD14 and the immune response to lipopolysaccharide (Comment). Science 252:1321–1322
51. Patrick D, Betts J, Frey EA, Prameya R, Doroviv-Zis K, Finlay BB (1992) Haemophilus influenzae lipopolysaccharide disrupts confluent monolayers of bovine brain endothelial cells via a serum-dependent cytotoxic pathway. J Infect Dis 165:865–872
52. Frey EA, Miller DS, Gullstein Jahr T et al (1992) Soluble CD14 participates in the response of cells to lipopolysaccharide. J Exp Med 176:1665–1671

Bacterial Exotoxins and Sepsis

W. Seeger, H. Schütte, F. Grimminger,
N. Suttorp, and S. Bhakdi

Introduction

Researchers engaged in the study of septic shock pathogenesis generally regard this syndrome to be the consequence of detrimental endotoxin effects in the host organism. This is understandable since causal relationships are firmly established between the action of endotoxin on various inflammatory competent cells. Surprisingly, proteinaceous microbial toxins have received only little attention as potentially important instigators of systemic inflammation and multiorgan dysfunction. Our present discussion will focus on some of these widespread, yet less well known, bacterial exotoxins that exert direct effects on target cells.

When considering the modes of action of bacterial protein toxins, it is useful to distinguish between toxins that enter the cell, as opposed to those that act primarily at the level of the cell plasma membrane. Examples of the former group are the ADP-ribosylating toxins and the neurotoxins. Although several are of cardinal medical importance, they are not generally associated with septic organ failure. In contrast, recent evidence has accumulated indicating that membrane-perturbating toxins may directly evoke pathophysiological reactions leading to vascular damage and shock.

Basically, a protein toxin may attack the plasma membrane either via enzymatic action or via physical perturbation of bilayer integrity. Phospholipase C ist the best known representative of a medically important, membrane-damaging bacterial enzyme. This toxin is elaborated by several bacterial species and it is established as an important pathogenic factor of *Clostridium perfringens.* Massive release of phospholipase C probably contributes to pathological processes seen in *Cl. perfringens* infections due to its combined effects on blood and tissue cells. The second mechanism of membrane damage by bacterial toxins is via physical perturbation of bilayer integrity evoked in the main through the formation of transmembrane pores. Evidence has accumulated over the past decade that the majority of medically relevant pathogens produce toxins belonging to the category of pore formers. Amongst the pathogens that are frequently associated with septic shock, *Escherichia coli* and several members of the family of Enterobacteriaceae, and *Staphylococcus aureus* deserve special mention. These and other producers of pore forming toxins are listed in Table 1. In the following, basic properties of pore forming proteins and the functional consequences of membrane damage will be discussed. The potential importance of pore forming toxins for the induction of septic organ failure will be illustrated for the lung vasculature.

Table 1. Prototypes of pore forming bacterial exotoxins

Producing organism	Designation	Salient features
Gram-positive bacteria[a]		
Staphylococcus aureus	α-Toxin (-hemolysin)	Binds to unidentified specific sites on target cells; forms voltage-independent hexameric pores of 1.5 nm diameter; identified susceptible human cells: platelets, monocytes, lymphocytes, endothelial cells
Streptococcus pyogenes A	Streptolysin-O	Prototype of polymerizing toxin that forms large pores (up to 30 nm diameter and more); probably binds to cholesterol; all examined mammalian cells susceptible
Gram-negative bacteria[b,d]		
Escherichia coli	*E. coli* hemolysin (HlyA, α-hemolysin)	"Receptor" problem unclarified, may bind nonspecifically to lipid bilayers; forms voltage-dependent, cation-selective pores of 2 nm diameter possibly through membrane insertion of toxin monomers; potent cytocidal effects on all white blood and endothelial cells
Serratia marcescens[c]	*Serratia* hemolysin	Forms voltage-independent pores of 1 nm diameter
Aeromonas hydrophilia[d]	Aerolysin	Forms heptameric pores of 1 nm diameter; glycophorin serves as binding site

[a] At least 14 other related and probably functionally similar toxins are produced by gram-positive organisms including *Listeria monocytogenes, Streptococcus pneumoniae, Bacillus cereus*)

[b] At least 10 other related toxins are produced by gram-negative organisms including *Proteus* sp., *Morganella morganii, Pasteurella hemolytica, Actinobacillus pleuropneumoniae* and *Bordetella pertussis*

[c] Related toxin is also produced by certain strains of *Proteus vulgaris*

[d] Other poreforming toxins are produced by *Vibrio cholerae* and *Vibrio parahemolyticus* and *Klebsiella*

General Features of Transmembrane Pore Formation

All pore forming toxins are produced and released by bacteria initially as water soluble proteins, but are able to undergo a unique and possibly always irreversible transition from a hydrophilic to an amphiphilic state upon interaction with a target lipid bilayer [1, 2]. Primary binding to a target membrane may require the presence of specific binder molecules. A well documented example for this type of interaction is represented by the sulfhydryl-activated cytolysins (e.g., streptolysin-O) which probably initially bind to membrane cholesterol. Often, however, cytolysins will be of the "receptorless" type that binds indiscriminately to lipid bilayers. E. *coli* hemolysin and related toxins are considered representatives of this second group. Staphylococcal α-toxin can interact both with specific binding sites and, at high concentrations, via nonspecific absorption to lipid bilayers.

Insertion into the lipid bilayer follows as a second and sometimes temporally dissociated step after toxin molecules have bound to the membrane surface. In some instances, pores are probably generated by insertion of protein monomers into the bilayer (e.g., *E. coli* hemolysin). Alternatively, some pore formers need to aggregate to form oligomers before pores can be generated; this is the case with α-toxin and streptolysin-O [1, 2]. Monomeric pores are too small to be visualized by electron microscopy, whereas several oligomeric pores are generally seen as partially or fully circularized structures. Oligomeric pores are sometimes heterogeneous in size due to variations in the number of protomers that constitute the individual channels [1–3]. *S. aureus* α-toxin oligomers tend to be more homogenous (Fig. 1). The effective functional diameters of pores span a very large range, from approximately 1.5 nm (α-toxin) to over 35 nm (streptolysin-O). Even the smallest pores are, however, large enough to permit rapid transmembrane flux of ions and small molecules. Generally, oligomeric pores have been found to display little ion selectivity and no dependence on membrane potential. In contrast, monomeric pores created by *E. coli* hemolysin require a distinct transmembrane potential and display a strong selectivity for cations over anions.

Although the primary structures of α-toxin, *E. coli* hemolysin and several sulfhydryl-activated toxins are known, the domains that are membrane-embedded have yet to be identified. No details are available on the polypeptide conformation and three-dimensional structure of any protein pore, and the fate of pores after their formation in membranes of nucleated cells has not been analyzed.

Susceptibility of Target Cells

Two main categories of factors, cellular and humoral, influence the overall susceptibility of cells towards a given toxin under physiological conditions.

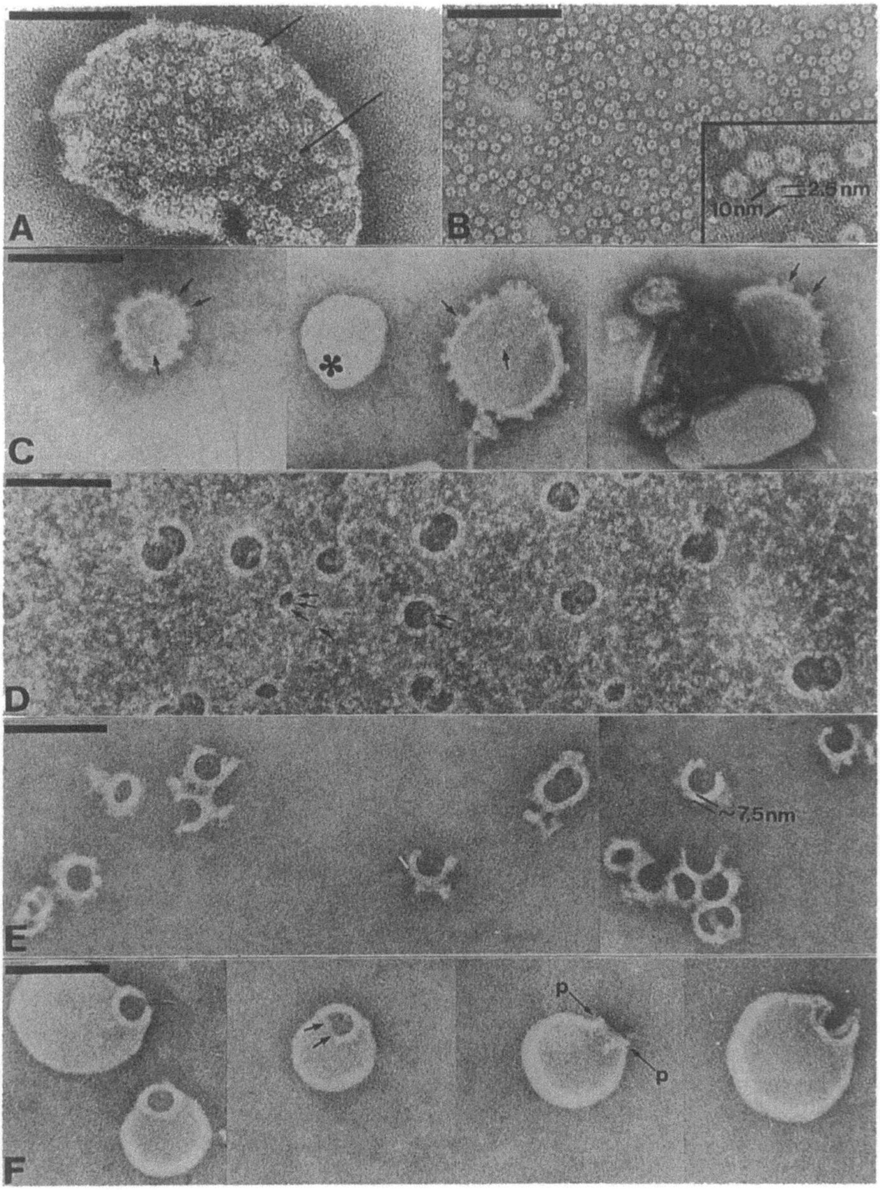

Fig. 1. A Negatively stained fragment of rabbit erythrocyte lysed with staphylococcal α-toxin. Numerous 10 nm ring-shaped structures are seen over the membrane (*arrows*). **B** Isolated toxin hexamer in detergent solution. **C** Lecithin liposomes carrying reincorporated α-toxin hexamers. The hexamers are seen as stubs along the edge of the liposomal membrane and as rings over the membrane (*arrows*). Characteristically, liposomes that escape incorporation of the toxin are impermeable to the stain. **D** Negatively stained erythro-

Cellular factors

1. *Specific high-affinity binding sites* will direct attack of a toxin to the respective cell target.
2. *Nonspecific cell surface characteristics* such as the surface organization of charged molecules can probably affect the efficiency and speed at which diffusion of a toxin to a membrane bilayer occurs. Slow binding may imply that a toxin will not be able to efficiently attack a cell under physiological conditions.
3. *Intrinsic resistance* towards a toxin is exemplified by human leukocytes and their resistance to *S. aureus* α-toxin (unpublished data). The term implies that a toxin can bind to a cell without inflicting functional membrane damage.
4. *Limited repair* for damaged membrane sites of nucleated cells is theoretically conceivable. However, membrane repair has not been clearly documented for any bacterial pore former to date. Notably, however, in hemolysin-perfused intact lungs reversibility of toxin effects was noted after washout of the bacterial agent, which might be compatible with repair mechanisms.

Humoral factors

Pore forming bacterial toxins are generally potent immunogens, and their respective antibodies are therefore normally present in healthy individuals. Moreover, many pore formers are bound and inactivated by plasma lipoproteins. When liberated into the host environment, the attack of a given toxin will thus be counteracted by several inhibitory humoral factors. For example, *E. coli* hemolysin binds extremely rapidly to leukocytes, but relatively slowly to erythrocytes (unpublished data). Whenever present, humoral components hence will be able to prevent *E. coli* hemolysin from attacking erythrocytes, but their action may often be too slow to similarly protect leukocytes. As a consequence, addition of low amounts of *E. coli* hemolysin to whole human blood results in its selective attack on leukocytes and monocytes [4, 5]. Another example for selective attack of a pore forming cytolysin is the action of α-toxin on human blood platelets [6]. Upon addition of this toxin to whole human blood, the cytolysin binds rapidly to specific sites on blood platelets

---

cyte membrane lysed by streptolysin-O (SLO) showing numerous 25–100 nm long and approximately 7.5 nm broad, curved rods of 13–16 nm inner radius of curvature. Most rods are approximately semicircular, often joined in pairs at their ends. Dense accumulation of strain is seen at the concave side of the rods. When these do not form closed profiles, the stain deposit is partly bordered by a "free" edge of the erythrocyte membrane (*arrows*). **E** Negative staining of isolated SLO oligomers showing numerous curved rod structures identical to those found on toxin-treated membranes. **F** Purified SLO complexes reincorporated into cholesterol-free lecithin liposomes. The toxin oligomers form holes in the liposomes (*unlabeled arrows*); *p* indicates a lesion seen in profile. Scale *bars* indicate 100 nm in all frames. Sodium silicotungstate was used as negative stain in **B–F**. Uranylacetate was used in *A*. (From [3])

and leukocytes, less efficiently to lymphocytes, and not at all to erythrocytes. Leukocytes can intrinsically withstand toxin attack, but platelets and monocytes are highly susceptible. As a consequence, selective activation/injury of the latter blood cells ensues [6, 7]. In addition to such toxin attack on circulating cells, sessile inflammatory cells (such as macrophages), endothelial cells and parenchymal cells may be highly susceptible to the membrane-perturbating activities of the various bacterial agents. An impressive example is the staphylococcal α-toxin-induced severe injury of capillary endothelial cells in intact rabbit lungs, concomitant with the demonstration of main pulmonary artery endothelial cell activation by this agent *in vitro* (see below).

Theoretically, it should be possible to augment the neutralizing capacity of antibodies to pore forming bacterial exotoxins by increasing antibody titers. In a model study, high-titered human hyperimmune globulins against *S. aureus* α-toxin were prepared by immunization of volunteers. It was found that these hyperimmune globulins, but not any of the commercially available intravenous immunoglobulin preparations, were able to suppress deleterious actions of α-toxin [8]. Clinical trials with these hyperimmune globulins are currently being planned.

Secondary Cellular Reactions

Cell death is the most obvious and inevitable consequence of transmembrane pore formation, if a lesion cannot be removed or repaired. Death ensues because the cell is rapidly depleted of ATP (via efflux through the pores [4]), and because it is unable to counteract the deleterious effects of ionic disequilibrium and loss of its "milieu intérieur" that are essential for sustainment of metabolic processes. Killing of leukocytes and monocytes by hemolysin [4, 5] cripples the local phagocytic defense system and probably fosters the invasion of other pathogens that colonize the lesions. Damage to endothelial cells by *S. aureus* α-toxin causes massive derangements in lung vasculature and loss of endothelial cell lining leads to rapid development of pulmonary edema [9]. Renal tubular epithelia are highly susceptible to hemolysin, and this may partially explain disturbances in tubular function that commonly develop during renal infections with toxin-producing bacterial strains [10]. Until recently, awareness that perturbation of the plasma membrane permeability barrier might trigger various cellular reactions was generally lacking. Today, it is apparent that such reactions are inevitable, and that they contribute substantially to the progression of tissue lesions. Passive flux of extracellular calcium ions into the damaged cells represents a major trigger for such secondary reactions, and further triggering mechanisms of intracellular signal transduction events may be involved. Depending on the cell target, a variety of responses may ensue, of which the following have been studied in some detail.

1. Secretion. Exocytotic liberation of vesicular components has been demonstrated in leukocytes, platelets and neurological cells. Leukocytes succumbing to attack by hemolysin release large amounts of vesicular components. The release of elastase (Fig. 2) is noteworthy since this enzyme has been discussed as a factor that may contribute towards development of diffuse vascular leakage and multiple organ injury. Platelets attacked by α-toxin secrete large quantities of granule constituents including platelet factor 4 and factor 5. Release of the latter leads to assembly of platelet-bound prothrom-

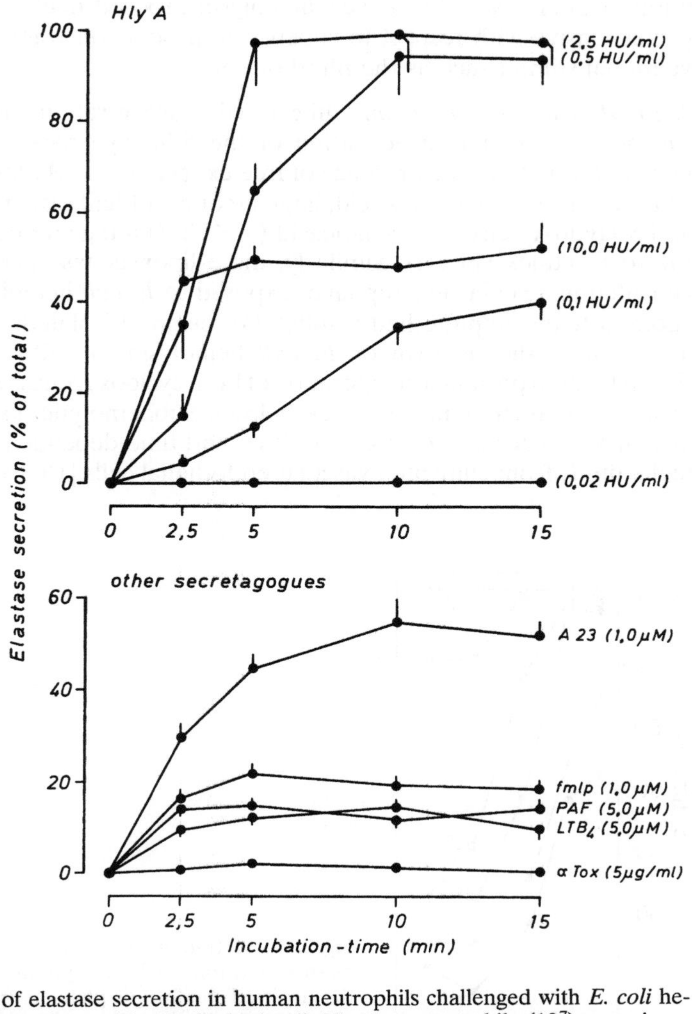

Fig. 2. Time course of elastase secretion in human neutrophils challenged with *E. coli* hemolysin (*HlyA*): comparison with standard stimuli. Human neutrophils (10^7) were incubated with different concentrations of the hemolysin (*upper panel*; concentrations given in hemolytics units (HU)/ml) or with standard stimuli used at their optimum doses (*lower panel*). Elastase secretion is given in percent of total neutrophil enzyme content. Mean ± SEM of 4–5 independent experiments is depicted. The strong potency of subcytolytic hemolysin concentrations to induce PMN degranulation is evident. (From [13])

binase complexes that generate thrombin [6]. *S. aureus* α-toxin thus activates human platelets and promotes coagulation (Fig. 3), processes that bear high potential relevance in staphylococcal infections [11].

2. Generation of reactive oxygen species. Leukocytes attacked by very low doses of *E. coli* hemolysin produce large amounts of oxygen radicals [12, 13]. At optimum toxin concentrations in the subcytolytic range, maximum responses are elicited, comparable to those in response to optimum FMLP or phorbol ester doses. Moreover, hemolysin-exposed neutrophils become hyperresponsive with respect to superoxide production when exposed to conventional stimuli such as the phorbol esters.

3. Lipid mediator generation. Subcytolytic concentrations of *E. coli* hemolysin induce pronounced activation of the 5-lipoxygenase system in human neutrophils [14]. In the presence of free exogenous arachidonic acid or donor cells of this precursor fatty acid, large amounts of leukotrienes (LTA_4, LTB_4) and 5-Hydroxy-eicosatetraenoicacid (5-HETE) are generated in response to the toxin attack (Fig. 4). Similarly, the 5-lipoxygenase pathway is strongly activated in alveolar macrophages exposed to *E. coli* hemolysin or staphylococcal α-toxin (unpublished results). Perfusion of isolated, blood-free rabbit lungs with either α-toxin or *E. coli* hemolysin, or with viable hemolytic *E. coli* leads to pronounced liberation of both cyclooxygenase and lipoxygenase products of arachidonic acid (see below). Subhemolytic doses of hemolysin and staphylococcal α-toxin evoke dose- and time-dependent release of prostaglandin I_2 from cultivated vascular endothelial cells [15, 16]. Marked gener-

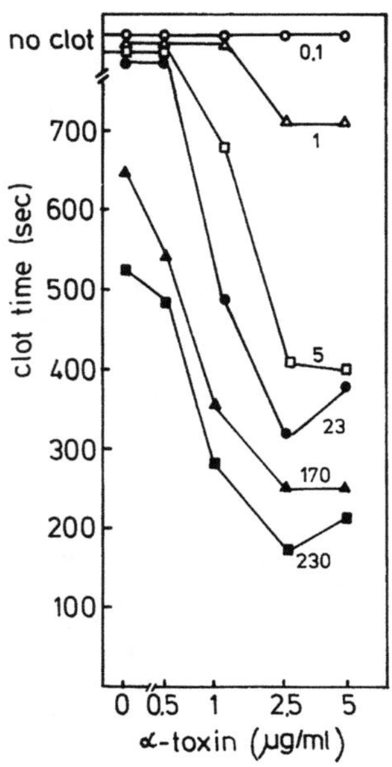

Fig. 3. Reduction in clot times of recalcified human plasma by α-toxin. Citrated plasma samples containing the depicted number of platelets (per nanoliter) were given 12 m*M* Ca^{2+} and α-toxin at the given final concentrations. Marked reductions in clot times were noted at α-toxin concentrations of 1–2.5 μg/ml, dependent on the presence of platelets in the plasma sample. No clot indicates lack of clot formation within 900 s. (From [6])

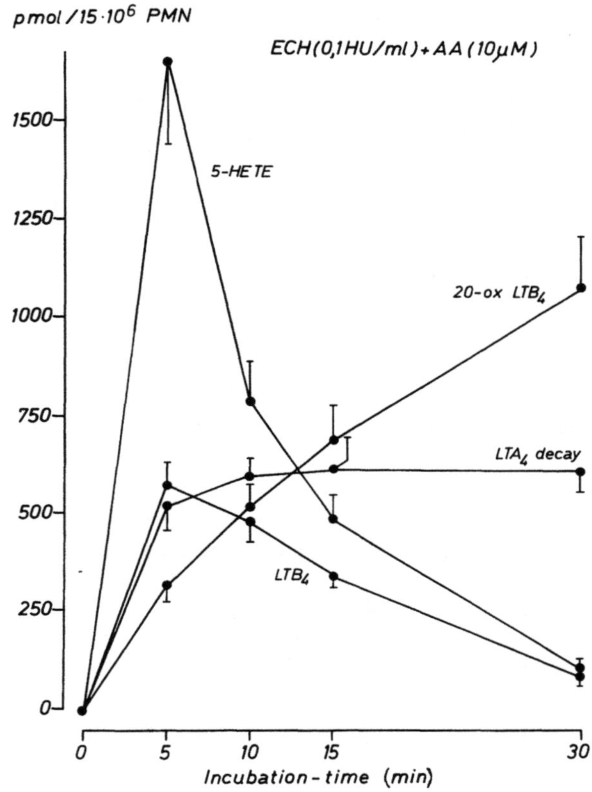

Fig. 4. Time course of leukotriene generation in human neutrophils challenged with *E. coli* hemolysin (*ECH*) in the presence of free exogenous arachidonic acid (*AA*). Human neutrophils (1.5×10^7) were incubated with the hemolysin (0.1 HU/ml) and free AA (10 μM) for different time periods. Supernatants were extracted and 5-lipoxygenase products were separated by HPLC techniques and quantified by UV detection. 20-OH-LTB_4 and 20-COOH-LTB_4 compromised as *20-ox-LTB_4*; nonenzymatic hydrolysis products of LTA_4 (6-trans-diastereomeric pair of LTB_4 and 5,6-DiHETEs) are summarized as *LTA_4 decay*. Mean ±SEM of six independent experiments is depicted. The strong activation of the 5-lipoxygenase pathway is evident. The decrease in the LTB_4 level after 5–10 min is caused by its enzymatic conversion to the 20-ox products; the decline in 5-HETE is due to membrane incorporation of this hydroxy fatty acid. (From [14])

ation of platelet activating factor (PAF) and lyso-PAF is elicited in *E. coli* hemolysin-challenged human neutrophils [13].

4. Derangement of cytoskeleton organization and function. In cultured pulmonary artery endothelial cells, staphylococcal α-toxin and *E. coli* hemolysin induce intercellular gap formation, which permits enhanced passage of fluids and macromolecules across the originally intact monolayer (see below). Evidence was obtained that this derived from contraction and rounding up of the adherent cells, probably because of rearrangement of the endothelial cytoskeleton.

5. Other processes. Attack on monocytes by *S. aureus* α-toxin and *E. coli* hemolysin causes liberation of large amounts of interleukin-1β [5, 7]. In addition, release of tumor necrosis factor-α was observed in α-toxin-activated monocytes. A prerequisite for the interleukin-1β liberation appears to be the prior intracellular accumulation of the interleukin-1β precursor. Thus, unstimulated monocytes do not release interleukin-1β in response to toxin attack, but large amounts of cytokine are liberated from cells that have been in short-term culture or that have been costimulated with very low amounts of lipopolysaccharide (LPS). Pore forming toxins may therefore synergize with LPS and with other substances that induce interleukin-1β synthesis. This concept is supported by the finding that incubation of freshly isolated monocytes with toxin-producing *E. coli* causes production and release of interleu-

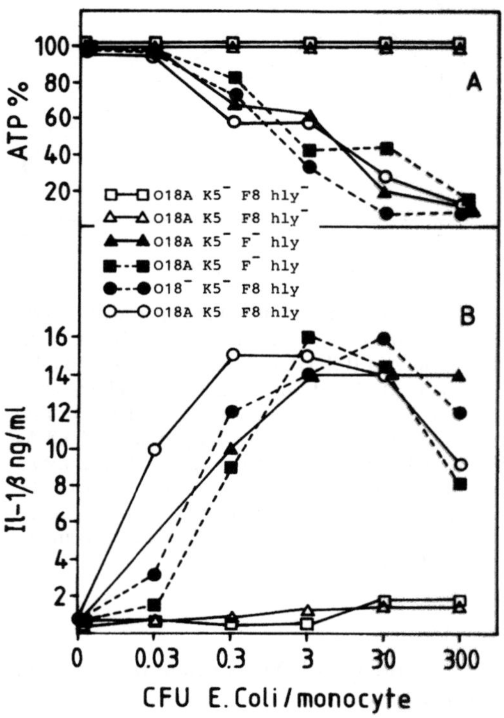

Fig. 5 A, B. Effects of incubation of viable *E. coli* with freshly isolated human monocytes. Six strains were used with the given characteristics and at the given approximate bacteria to cell ratios. Measurements of cellular ATP (**A**) and of interleukin-1β (IL-1β) (**B**) in the cell supernatants were performed after 70 min incubation at 37°C. All strains of toxin-producers (*hly*) evoked ATP depletion and IL-β production. The 100% ATP content corresponded to 140 pmol ATP per well. (From [5])

kin-1β within a few hours (Fig. 5). Such a dramatic and rapid effect was not observed when cells were incubated with genetically related, nonhemolytic *E. coli*. Taken together, these results demonstrate that Interleukin-1β, tumor necrosis factor and possibly a variety of further cytokines not yet experimentally addressed belong to the battery of inflammatory mediators which can be elicited by pore forming bacterial exotoxins.

Signal Transduction Events in E. coli Hemolysin-Challenged Target Cells: More Than Pore Formation

Two concepts have hitherto emerged to explain the different cell activation phenomena which are observed in different target cells exposed to subcytolytic toxin concentrations. The first of these is calcium flux through toxin-created nonphysiological bypass gates. Prostanoid generation and vasoconstriction in cell-free perfused rabbit lungs as well as prostacyclin generation and cell retraction phenomena in cultured endothelial cells in response to both staphylococcal α-toxin and *E. coli* hemolysin are strictly dependent on extracellular calcium [15–18]. An enhanced passive influx of ^{45}Ca into the toxin-treated cells was directly demonstrated. These data suggest that the toxin-created pores may act as nonphysiological calcium gates, allowing extra- to intracellular calcium flux along the steep gradient of this bivalent cation and thereby initiating different calcium-dependent cellular processes. These processes include stimulation of phospholipolytic activities in the endothelial cells and putatively in toxin-exposed thromboxane-generating lung macrophages, calcium-dependent cell retraction phenomena with generation of intercellular gaps in the endothelial cells and, possibly, processing of intracellular interleukin-1β precursor in monocytes. Such toxin-related calcium gating [19] is thus distinctly different from the action of a calcium ionophore such as A23187, or from calcium shifts following receptor occupancy and activation of receptor-operated events. The second concept is that of induction of phosphoinositide hydrolysis and related metabolic responses. A different signal transduction pathway in response to *E. coli* hemolysin challenge was recently noted in human granulocytes [13]. In these cells, the toxin provoked rapid secretion of elastase and myeloperoxidase, generation of superoxide and synthesis of PAF and lyso-PAF. Concomitantly, marked phosphatidylinositol hydrolysis with sequential appearance of the inositol phosphates IP_3, IP_2 and IP_1 and formation of diacylglycerol occurred [13]. The metabolic responses displayed distinct cell-shaped dose dependencies, with maximum events noted at subcytolytic toxin concentrations ranging between 0.1–0.5 HU/ml (Fig. 6). Phosphatidylinositol hydrolysis and metabolic responses elicited by the hemolysin exceeded those evoked by optimum concentrations of FMLP, PAF, LTB_4, A23187 and staphylococcal α-toxin. The toxin-induced effects were sensitive to pertussis toxin, thus indicating involvement of G proteins. These data suggest that the marked capacity of low doses of hemo-

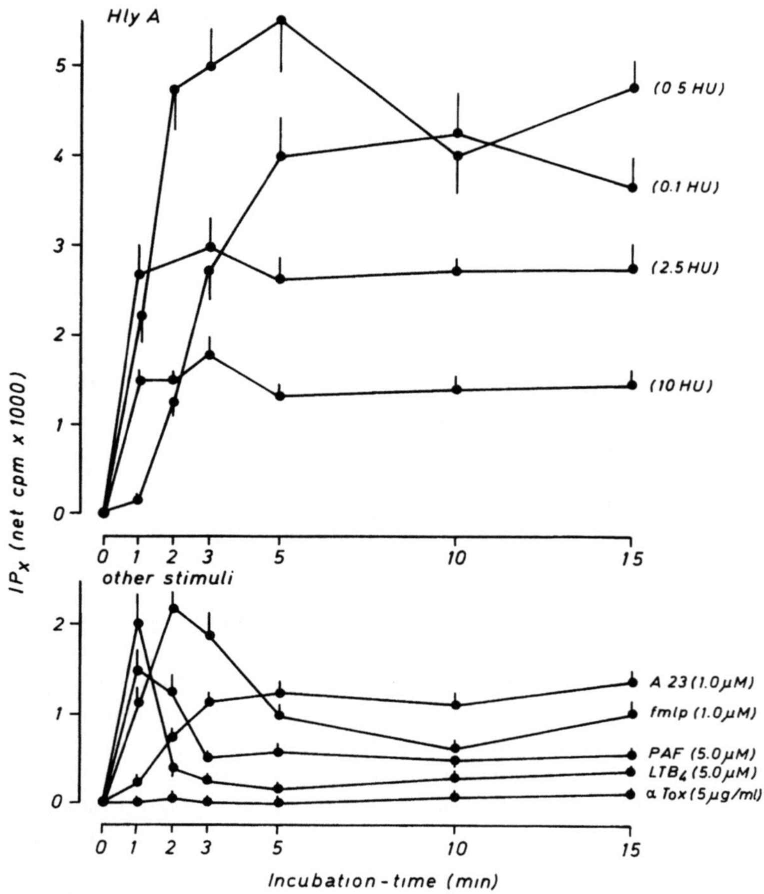

Fig. 6. Sum of inositol phosphates (*IP_x*) generated in human neutrophils in response to *E. coli* hemolysin (*Hly A*) stimulation: comparison with standard stimuli. Human neutrophils (10^7) preincubated with [^{3}H]Insotol were stimulated with different concentrations of the hemolysin (upper panel; concentrations given in hemolytic units (HU)/ml) or with standard stimuli used at their optimum doses (*lower panel*). The sum of extracted inositol phosphates (IP_3, IP_2, IP_1) is given (mean ± SEM of at least four independent experiments). Background activity of nonhemolysin challenged control cells was subtracted. The strong potency of subcytolytic hemolysin concentrations to induce inositol phosphate liberation is evident. (From [13])

lysin to elicit degranulation, respiratory burst and lipid mediator generation in human neutrophils probably proceeds via the preformed phosphatidylinositol hydrolysis signal transduction pathway.

Intercellular Cooperation Underlying Hemolysin-Induced Leukotriene Generation

E. coli hemolysin is a potent inductor of the 5-lipoxygenase metabolism in neutrophils. In the absence of exogenous arachidonic acid supply, the toxin induced the generation of minor amounts of leukotriene B_4 and its Ω-oxidation products in human polymorphonuclear neutrophils (PMNS) [14]. Simultaneous disposal of free arachidonic acid during hemolysin challenge did, however, result in a severalfold increase in mediator generation (Fig. 4). This feature corresponds to the effect of the chemotactic agents FMLP and PAF, which similarly activate the PMN 5-lipoxygenase complex without major mobilization of endogenous arachidonate pools. The dependence of PMN lipoxygenase metabolism on exogenous precursor fatty acid supply suggests intercellular cooperativity in eicosanoid synthesis under *in vivo* conditions (depicted in Fig. 7). Vascular endothelial cells "feed" the adjacent PMN with free arachidonic acid, thereby promoting ongoing leukotriene synthesis. Countercurrently, the labile leukotriene intermediate LTA_4 is transferred from the PMN to the vascular acceptor cell, where it is further processed to cysteinyl leukotrienes by the endothelial glutathione-S-transferase. The complementary enzymatic equipments of LTA_4 "donor" and LTA_4 "acceptor" cell thus cooperate to generate cysteinyl leukotrienes, which are not generated by each cell type alone. Extracellular decay of PMN-derived LTA_4 is avoided in such system of intercellular cooperativity. Accordingly, *E. coli* hemolysin challenge of cocultures of human neutrophils and endothelial cells results in marked generation of the vasoactive cysteinyl leukotrienes; and a severalfold amplification of the overall 5-lipoxygenase product formation takes place.

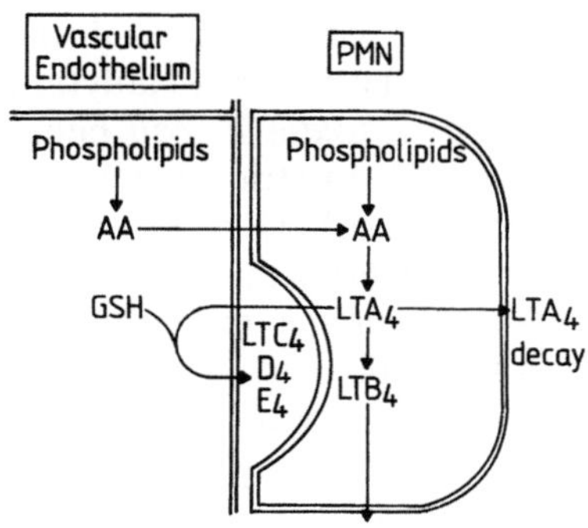

Fig. 7. Cooperativity of endothelial cells and adhering neutrophils in leukotriene synthesis. For details see text

Hemolysin-Induced Neutrophil Activation: Impact on Host Defense Mechanisms

Neutrophils represent the first line of defense against bacterial infections. These leukocytes sense, migrate toward and engulf distant microorganisms, killing them by release of microbicidal compounds from granules and by the generation of reactive oxygen metabolites. These responses are initiated by the interaction of inflammatory mediators with specific neutrophil cell surface receptors, directing locomotion to the inflammatory focus. Hemolysin reduces both the chemotactic motility and the phagocytotic capacity of neutrophils. At the same time, the toxin induces liberation of all granule constituents into the extracellular environment and onset of respiratory burst, physiologically restricted to the phagosomal compartment of the PMN in order to destroy ingested organisms. These events are elicited by subcytolytic hemolysin concentrations; they must thus be assumed to take place at some distance from the toxin-liberating microorganisms. Thereby, the destructive capacity of attracted leukocytes is mislead against the host itself, and neutrophils are completely depleted of their defense arsenal before reaching the site of infection, or they may even be paralyzed distant from this location. Overall, the toxin-induced neutrophil activation may be operative as an effective principle to counteract the antimicrobial capacity of these cells.

Endothelial Cell Function

Exotoxin-Induced Synthesis of Endothelium-Derived Vasodilators

A hallmark of the hyperdynamic phase of septic shock is a substantial decrease of the total peripheral vascular resistance, which barely responds to vasoconstricting agents. The underlying mechanisms are not fully elucidated, but may include an increased synthesis of and/or an increased reactivity to endothelium-derived vasodilating mediators. A putative role of bacterial exotoxins in such loss of systemic vascular resistance in sepsis has hitherto not been directly addressed. Interestingly, however, cultured endothelial cells responded with a marked increase in vasodilating mediator generation after stimulation with sublytic subcytolytic concentrations of the exotoxins *S. aureus* α-toxin, *E. coli* hemolysin or *Pseudomonas aeruginosa* cytotoxin [15, 16, 20]. In strict dependence on the exotoxin dose, large quantities of prostaglandin I_2 (Fig. 8) and nitric oxide (NO) (manuscript in preparation) were liberated within 5–30 min. In perfused rabbit lungs, the mentioned exotoxins all induce marked prostaglandin (PG) I_2 generation, concomitant with thromboxane (Tx) formation (see below). In that model, the vasoconstrictive potency of the latter agent surpasses the vasodilating properties of PGI_2, thus resulting in a net vasoconstrictor response in the pulmonary vasculature. It is, however, conceivable that the slightly longer half-time of PGI_2 as compared to TxA_2, and/or differential sensitivities to PGI_2 (and NO) vs

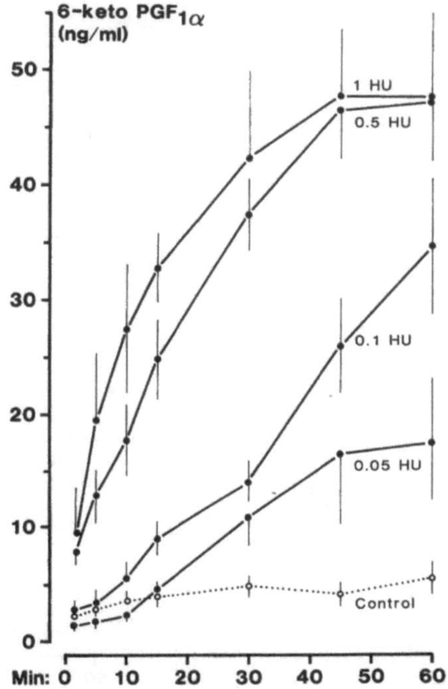

Fig. 8. Time- and dose-dependent prostacyclin (PGI_2) synthesis in porcine pulmonary artery endothelial cells by *E. coli* hemolysin. Cells were incubated with increasing toxin concentrations for 1–60 min. The cell supernatant was taken for determination of PGI_2 levels (measured radioimmunologically as 6-keto-$PGF_{1\alpha}$). (From [15])

TxA_2 of vascular smooth muscles in various systemic perfusion areas may result in a net decrease in the overall peripheral vasomotor tone in response to exotoxin challenge.

Exotoxin-Induced Loss of Endothelial Barrier Function

A major feature of septic shock and septic organ failure is the general vascular leakage syndrome. The underlying mechanism is a loss of endothelial barrier function including both increased permeability for water and small solutes and decreased sieving properties with respect to macromolecules. Such altered endothelial function results in protein-rich edema formation in various perfusion areas [21]. In order to address the influence of bacterial exotoxins on endothelial barrier function, we developed an *in vitro* model of pulmonary endothelial cells grown on polycarbonate filter membranes [15, 22–24]. In this model, addition of staphylococcal α-toxin resulted in a rapid, severe loss of endothelial barrier function. This included both increased hydraulic conductivity and decreased albumin-reflecting properties [22, 23] (Fig. 9). Corresponding profound alterations of endothelial permeability characteristics were noted upon monolayer challenge with *E. coli* hemolysin and *P. aeruginosa* cytotoxin [15]. Washout of the exotoxins after induction of

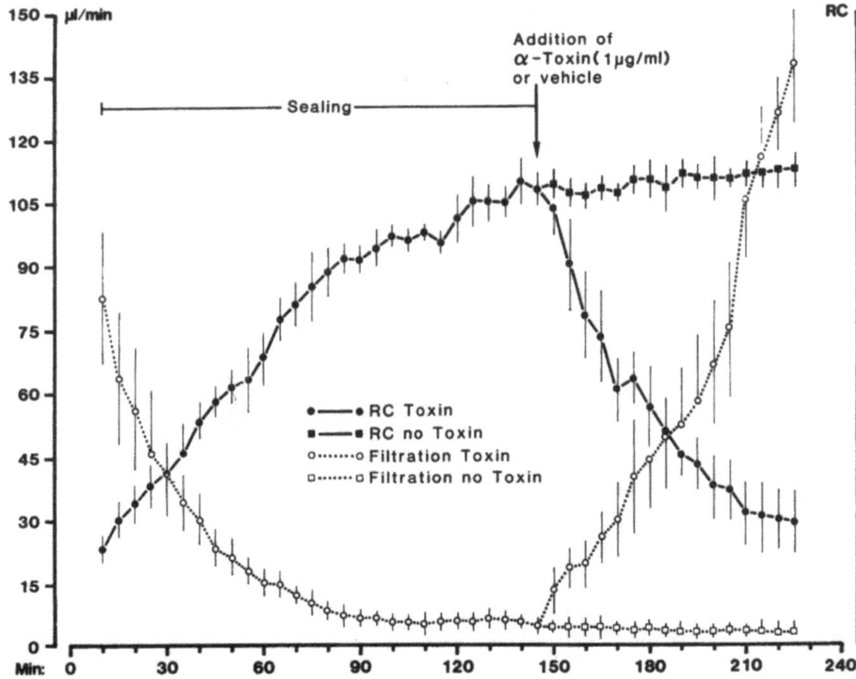

Fig. 9. Filtration rate across endothelial cell monolayer (in µl/min) and reflection coefficient (*RC*) for albumin during sealing period and after addition of 1 µg/ml staphylococcal α-toxin. Initial filtration rate (≈80 µl/min) was high, and RC (≈0.2) was low. Application of a transendothelial pressure gradient of 10 cm H_2O resulted in marked "sealing" of the monolayer system during a 2 h control period; the filtration rate slowly decreased to ≈4 µl/min (hydraulic conductivity of 2×10^{-6} cm × s^{-1} × cm H_2O^{-1}), and the RC slowly increased and stabilized at 0.73. Addition of staphylococcal α-toxin to this sealed monolayer resulted in a sharp increase in filtration rate and in a dramatic collapse of albumin-reflecting properties. Control monolayers were stable throughout the entire experimental time. (From [23])

leakage was not capable of reversing the loss of barrier function. Preincubation of the toxins with specific antibodies did, however, suppress their permeability increasing properties.

Light and scanning electron microscopic studies of the cultured pulmonary artery endothelial cells demonstrated typical tight monolayer packing under baseline conditions (Fig. 10 A, B). Following administration of staphylococcal α-toxin (Fig. 10 C, D), *P. aeruginosa* cytotoxin or *E. coli* hemolysin, inter-endothelial gap formation occurred, allowing enhanced paracellular fluid exchange [15, 23]. Moreover, morphological studies with cytoskeleton staining suggested endothelial cell "contraction" as an underlying event [22, 23].

These data are compatible with the notion that an exotoxin-triggered sharp increase in intracellular free Ca^{2+} concentrations may be responsible

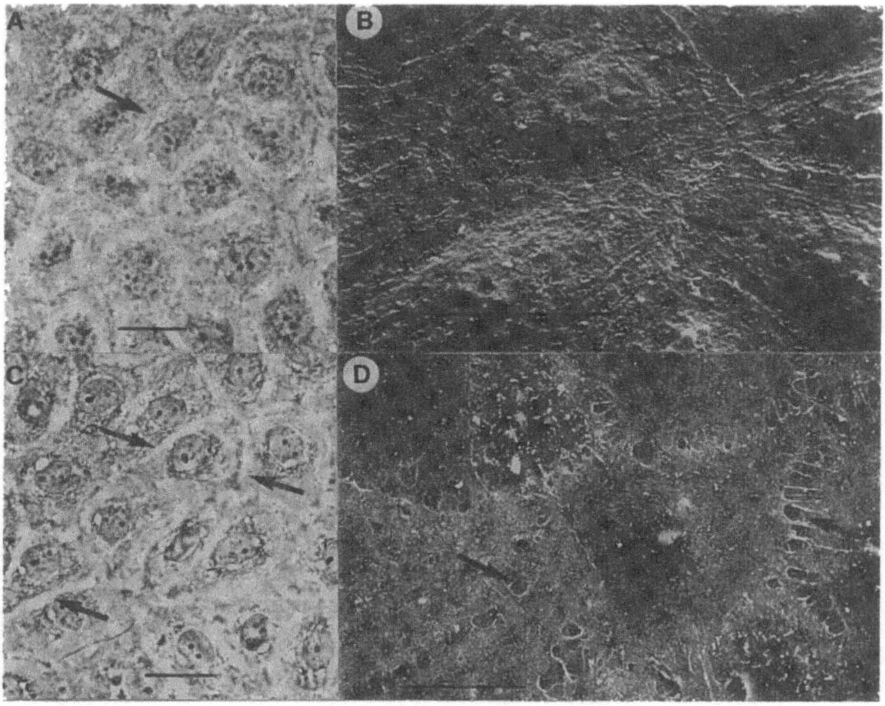

Fig. 10. A, B Sealed endothelial cell monolayer of pig pulmonary artery grown on gelatine-coated cover slips and exposed for 90 min to a hydrostatic pressure of 10 cm H_2O. Examination by phase contrast (**A**) and scanning electron microscopy (**B**) shows that virtually all interendothelial junctions (intercellular space, *arrows*) are closed. **C, D** Endothelial cell monolayer exposed for 90 min to staphylococcal α-toxin. Note large interendothelial gaps (*arrows*) that are seen both by phase contrast (**C**) and scanning electron microscopy (**D**). Bars indicate 20 μm. (From [23])

for altered cytoskeleton function and gap formation. Ca^{2+}/calmodulin-dependent activation of myosin-light chain kinase is known to cause phosphorylation of the myosin light chains, thereby triggering myosin-actin interaction and onset of contraction phenomena. Such endothelial cell contraction is assumed to result in a widening of the intercellular junctions with subsequently increased water- and protein filtration properties (vascular leakage).

The presumably Ca^{2+} flux-related interaction of pore forming bacterial exotoxins with the endothelial microfilament system may allow the development of new pharmacological strategies designed to interfere with vascular leakage under conditions of sepsis.

Sequential Pathogenetic Events in a Model of Exotoxin-Induced Lung Injury

Bacterial sepsis is the most consistent factor associated with the development of adult respiratory distress syndrome (ARDS) [25–27]. Moreover, acute diffuse lung injury of different etiology is often complicated by nosocomial pneumonia [28, 29]. In experimental models, septic lung failure is mimicked by administration of lipopolysaccharide components of gram-negative bacteria (endotoxins), and plenty of detailed information is available on the mechanisms of lung injury by these agents. However, only very little information is available on abnormalities inflicted by "nonendotoxin toxins" in the pulmonary circulation. We hypothesized that these toxins might induce marked inflammatory mediator generation, thereby eliciting pulmonary circulatory disorders and disturbances of gas exchange.

Vasoconstrictor Potency of E. coli Hemolysin in the Pulmonary Circulation: The Role of Prostanoid Generation

To assess this issue, isolated hemolysin and hemolysin liberating viable *E. coli* bacteria were infused in a model of isolated, perfused and ventilated rabbit lungs.

In the first study [18], direct intravascular administration of the toxin was performed. Low concentrations of the toxin in the perfusate caused a dose- and time-dependent release of potassium, TxA_2 and PGI_2, but not of lactate dehydrogenase, into the recirculating medium (Fig. 11). Concomitantly, a dose-dependent liberation of the prostanoids into the bronchoalveolar space was noted. These events were paralleled by pulmonary hypertension, and studies with different inhibitors collectively indicated that the vasoconstrictor response was mediated predominantly by pulmonary Tx generation. In addition, hemolysin elicited a protracted, dose-dependent increase in the lung capillary filtration coefficient, which was independent of the prostanoid-mediated pressor response and resulted in severe pulmonary edema formation.

In the second study [30], viable hemolysin-forming *E. coli* bacteria were infused in the model of isolated rabbit lungs. Control experiments used an *E. coli* strain which releases an inactive form of the hemolysin (lack of the hemolysin C gene). A concentration of 10^4–10^7 hemolysin-forming *E. coli*/ml perfusate caused a dose- and time-dependent appearance of the toxin in the recirculating buffer fluid, again accompanied by the release of potassium, TxA_2 and PGI_2 into the buffer fluid. Concomitantly, marked pulmonary hypertension developed (Fig. 12). Inhibitor studies with use of cyclooxygenase inhibitors, Tx synthetase inhibitors and a Tx receptor antagonist again indicated that the pressor response was predominantly mediated via pulmonary Tx generation. Administration of hemolysin-forming *E. coli* additionally caused a protracted, dose-dependent increase in the lung capillary filtration

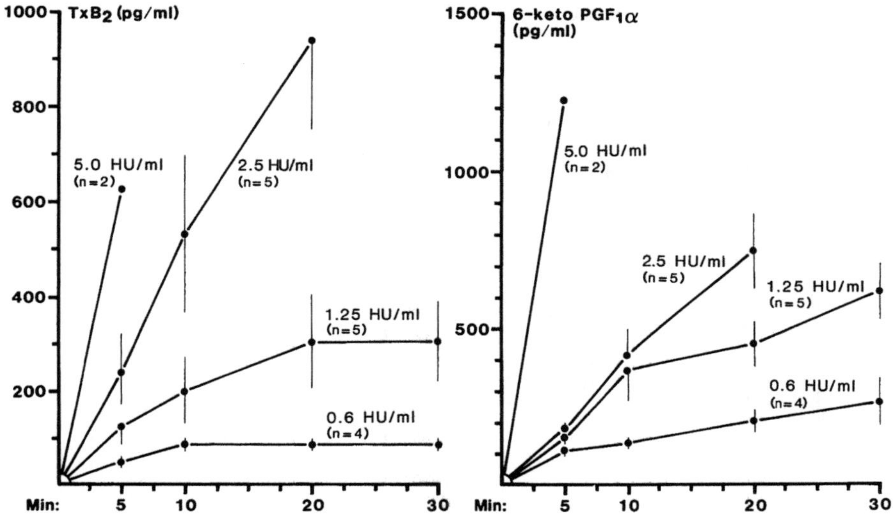

Fig. 11. Dose dependency and time course of *E. coli* hemolysin-induced prostanoid release into the buffer fluid of perfused rabbit lungs. Concentrations of thromboxane B_2 (*TxB_2*; *left*) and 6-keto-$PGF_{1\alpha}$ (*right*) are given measured in aliquots of the recirculating medium at different times after administration of the various doses of *E. coli* hemolysin to Krebs-Henseleit buffer-perfused rabbit lungs. In the studies with administration of 2.5 and 5.0 HU/ml, the experiments had to be stopped before termination of the 30 min period because of excessive edema formation. (From [18])

coefficient, followed by severe edema formation (Fig. 13). The hemolysin C lacking *E. coli* strain completely failed to provoke the described biophysical and biochemical responses.

These two studies strongly suggest that *E. coli* hemolysin is a potent vasoconstrictor in the pulmonary vascular bed. Dose-dependent release of potassium in the absence of significant LDH liberation indicates toxin-induced membrane permeabilization as a primary exotoxin effect also in this intact organ model. Secondary generation of the potent vasoconstrictive agent TxA_2 occurs, which surpasses the vasodilatory effect of the simultaneously generated PGI_2 and which is predominantly responsible for the toxin-evoked pulmonary hypertension. In addition, prostanoid-independent vascular leakage ensues, which results in the formation of protein-rich interstitial and alveolar edèma. The high sensitivity of the pulmonary vasculature towards hemolysin was true even in the presence of plasma with putative hemolysin inactivating capacity (antibodies, lipoproteins). This finding supports the notion that rapid exotoxin binding to target cells competes with toxin neutralization. Furthermore, it is conceivable that a direct transfer of the exotoxin from target cell-adherent bacteria occurs. In such a "hidden microenvironment," plasma inactivators may be virtually ineffective. The pulmonary target cells responsible for the predominant Tx generation in the intact rabbit

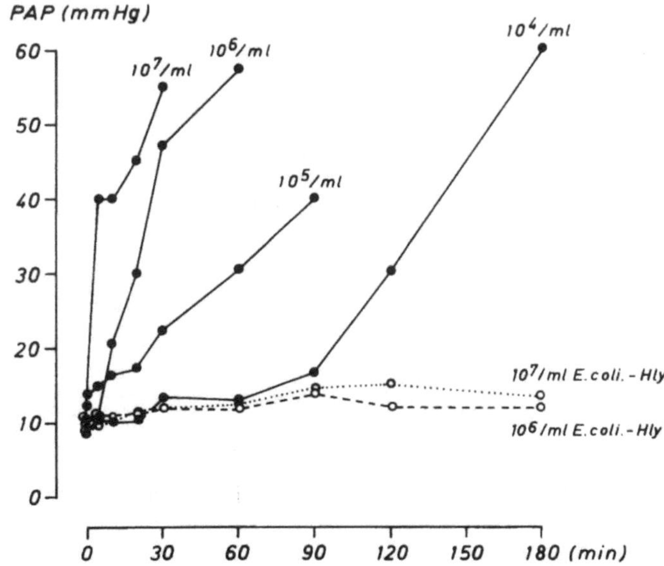

Fig. 12. Dose dependency and time course of pulmonary artery pressure (*PAP*) rise evoked by hemolysin-forming viable *E. coli* in buffer-perfused lungs. The experiments were performed in Krebs Henseleit albumin buffer-perfused rabbit lungs. Time was set zero when the hemolysin-forming *E. coli* were administered to the buffer medium at the given final concentrations. Mean values of two to three experiments at each concentration are given. As controls, 10^6/ml and 10^7/ml bacteria of a genetically related *E. coli* strain, which secretes an inactive toxin (Hly^-) were used. (From [30])

vasculature have not yet been conclusively identified. Intravascular resident, interstitial and intra-alveolar macrophages are likely candidates. Additional cell types such as alveolar epithelial cells type II and interstitial FibroBlast may, however, also be involved. The lung microvascular endothelium is the most likely candidate for the hemolysin-evoked PGI_2 generation.

Exotoxin-Induced Ventilation/Perfusion Mismatch

The hemolysin-elicited vasoconstriction results in an inhomogenous narrowing of the pulmonary vascular bed [31]. As a consequence, the profile of perfusion distribution is markedly affected, resulting in severe ventilation/perfusion mismatch in otherwise healthy lungs. This marked effect on perfusion distribution is exemplified in Fig. 14. Such mismatch results in severe gas exchange disturbances even in the absence of lung edema formation and atelectasis.

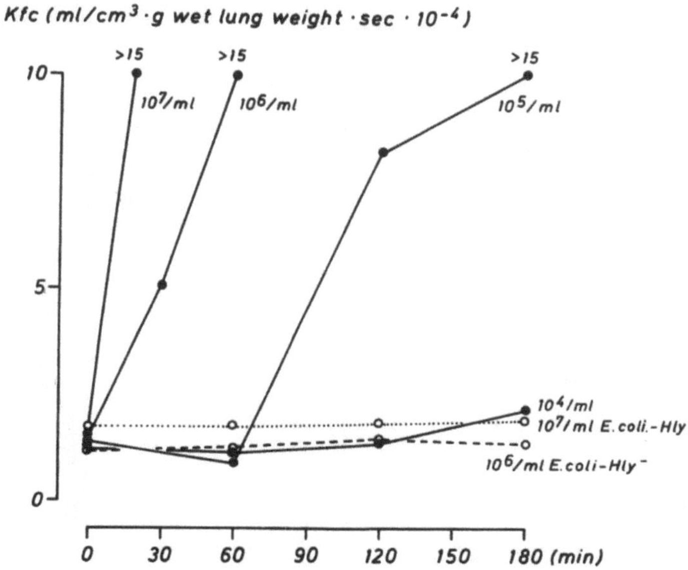

Fig. 13. Dose dependency and time course of capillary filtration coefficient (*Kfc*) increase evoked by hemolysin-forming viable *E. coli* in buffer-perfused lungs. The experiments were performed in Krebs Henseleit albumin buffer-perfused rabbit lungs in the presence of 500 μM acetylsalicylic acid, in order to block any major hemolysin-induced pressor response. Baseline Kfc data (O') were determined directly before administration of the hemolysin-forming *E. coli* to the buffer medium at the given final concentrations. Mean values of two to three experiments at each concentration are given. As controls, 10^6/ml and 10^7/ml *E. coli* of a nonhemolysin-forming strain (Hly^-) were used. (From [30])

Hemolysin as a Potent Inductor of Arachidonic Acid Lipoxygenase Metabolism in Perfused Rabbit Lungs

In addition to its induction of prostanoid generation in the isolated rabbit lungs and in cultured pulmonary artery endothelial cells, hemolysin was noted to be a potent inductor of arachidonic acid lipoxygenase metabolism. In perfused lungs, subcytolytic concentrations of the exotoxin caused a rapid release of large quantities of cysteinyl leukotrienes and leukotriene B_4 into the intravascular space [32]. Moreover, a marked liberation of 5-HETE into the buffer medium occurred, whereas LTB_4 represented the predominant compound in the bronchoalveolar lavage fluid. The hemolysin-induced burst of leukotriene and HETE generation preceded the onset of vascular leakage in this model. Similarly, large amounts of arachidonic acid lipoxygenase products were elicited by infusion of viable hemolysin-liberating *E. coli* bacteria in the perfused lung model [33]. In accordance with the physiological measurements, nonhemolysin-forming *E. coli* bacteria again failed to induce substantial arachidonic acid lipoxygenase metabolism. The leukotriene in-

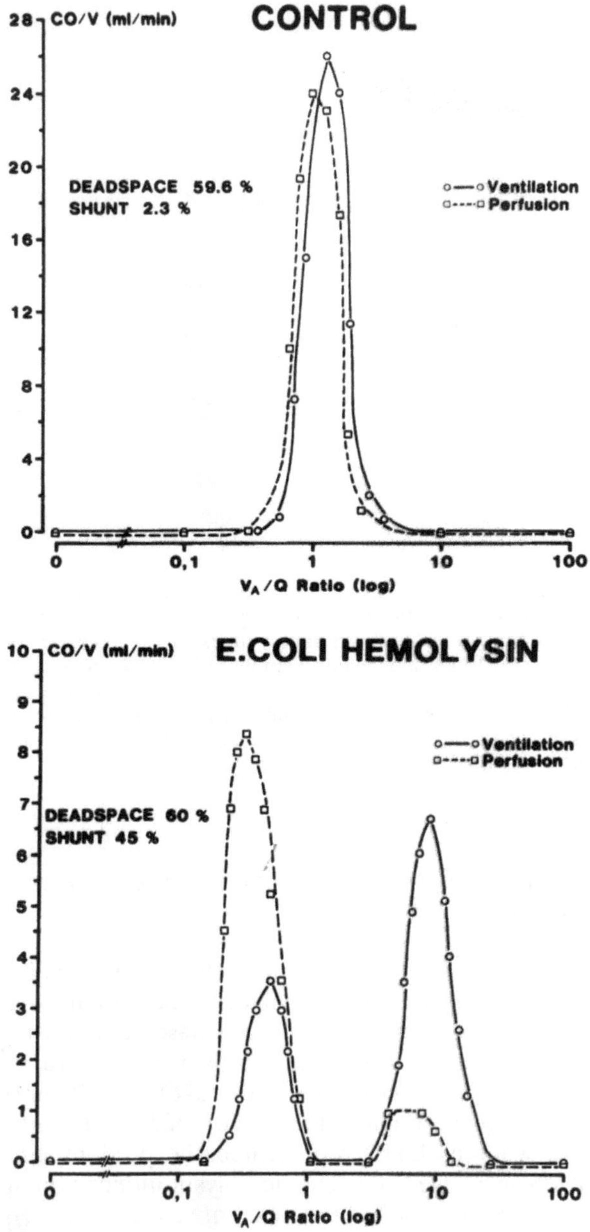

Fig. 14. Hemolysin-induced ventilation/perfusion mismatch. Ventilation (V_A)/perfusion (Q) ratios of the different lung compartments were assessed by the multiple inert gas elimination technique, detailed in [31]. Under baseline conditions, both ventilation and perfusion ("cardiac output," *CO*) are distributed nearly quantitatively to areas with V_A/Q ratios approximating 1. In the presence of *E. coli* hemolysin, mismatch of ventilation and perfusion occurs and shuntflow dramatically increases

duction by in situ liberation of hemolysin was not inhibited in the presence of plasma with toxin neutralizing capacity.

Preadministration of human granulocytes, which sequestered in the lung microvasculature, caused a severalfold increase in leukotriene generation upon subsequent challenge with hemolysin-forming *E. coli* bacteria. This finding deserves special attention, since granulocytes have been noted to be preferred hemolysin targets within the circulating blood cells (see above), and the toxin-induced strong activation of the PMN 5-lipoxygenase pathway predisposes these cells for cooperative leukotriene synthesis, as depicted in Fig. 7. This amplification of 5-lipoxygenase metabolism is predominantly caused by increased generation of cysteinyl leukotrienes and, to a minor extent, LTB_4. Concomitantly, 5-HETE- and LTA_4-hydrolysis product release decreases as compared to hemolysin neutrophil stimulation *in vitro*. This pattern of metabolite generation is in accordance with previous studies, in which selective stimulation of sequestered neutrophils in the lung vasculature [34, 35] and direct intravascular administration of freshly prepared LTA_4 demonstrated neutrophil-endothelial cell cooperativity in leukotriene metabolism. Moreover, toxin-induced interaction of neutrophils with alveolar macrophages and alveolar epithelial cells type II within the alveolar space results in marked LTB_4 generation. This potent chemotactic agent must be assumed to cause further neutrophil influx into the alveolar compartment, and to perpetuate inflammatory events due to its autocrine/paracrine activation of neutrophils and sessile alveolar cells (macrophages, pneumocytes type II).

Morphological Examination of Hemolysin-Exposed Rabbit Lungs

In a preceding electron microscopical examination of staphylococcal α-toxin-exposed rabbit lungs, pulmonary hypertension and vascular leakage were found to be paralleled by severe structural changes. In particular, increasing electron density of microvascular endothelial cell nuclei and subsequently of their cytoplasm was noted, followed by detachment of these cells from their mutual endoepithelial basal lamina [9]. Edema was localized in the blood-gas exchange area, in contrast to hydrostatically induced lung fluid accumulation. A recent electron microscopical examination of perfusion-fixed lungs after hemolysin incubation did, however, display a different morphological picture [36]. Interstitial edema formation was again noted, but this was predominantly located in areas remote from the blood-gas exchange barrier. The endothelial cells displayed normal electron density and were not detached from the fused basal lamina. These findings suggest alterations of functional endothelial sieving properties in hemolysin-treated lungs, rather than gross endothelial cell damage. There were, however, markedly increased numbers of endothelial plasmalemmal vesicles, which may suggest intercompartimental fluid shifts. Such transport processes, when directed from the abluminal to the luminal side of the microvessels, have been suggested as second line defense against pulmonary edema formation in lungs with hydrostatically induced edema.

References

1. Bhakdi S, Tranum-Jensen J (1987) Damage to mammalian cells by proteins that form transmembrane pores. Rev Physiol Biochem Pharmacol 107:147
2. Bhakdi S, Tranum-Jensen J (1991) Damage to cell membranes by pore-forming bacterial cytolysins. Prog Allergy 40:1
3. Bhakdi S, Tranum-Jensen J (1984) Mechanism of complement cytolysis and the concept of channel-forming proteins. Philos Trans R Soc Lond [Biol] 306:311
4. Bhakdi S, Greulich S, Muhly M, Eberspächer F, Becker H, Thiele A, Hugo F (1989) Potent leukocidal action of Escherichia coli hemolysin mediated by permeabilization of target cell membranes. J Exp Med 169:737
5. Bhakdi S, Muhly M, Korom S, Schmidt G (1990) Effects of Escherichia coli hemolysin on human monocytes. Cytocidal action and stimulation of interleukin-1 release. J Clin Invest 85:1746
6. Bhakdi S, Muhly M, Mannhardt U, Hugo F, Klapettek K, Mueller Eckhardt C, Roka L (1988) Staphylococcal alpha toxin promotes blood coagulation via attack on human platelets. J Exp Med 168:527
7. Bhakdi S, Muhly M, Korom S, Hugo F (1989) Release of interleukin-1β associated with potent cytocidal action of staphylococcal alpha-toxin on human monocytes. Infect Immun 57:3512
8. Bhakdi S, Mannhardt H, Ronneberger R, Hungerer KD (1989) Human hyperimmune globulin protects against the cytotoxic action staphylococcal alpha-toxin in vitro and in vivo. Infect Immun 57:3214
9. Seeger W, Birkemeyer RG, Ermert L, Suttorp N, Bhakdi S, Duncker HR (1990) Staphylococcal alpha-toxin induced vascular leakage in rabbit lungs. Lab Invest 63:341
10. Keane WF, Welch R, Gekker G, Peterson PK (1987) Mechanism of Escherichia coli alpha-hemolysin induced injury to isolated renal tubular cells. Am J Pathol 126:350
11. Arvand M, Bhakdi S, Dahlback B, Preissner KT (1990) Staphylococcus aureus alpha-toxin attack on human platelets promotes assembly of the prothrombinase complex. J Biol Chem 265:14377
12. Bhakdi S, Martin E (1991) Superoxide generation by human neutrophils induced by low doses of Escherichia coli hemolysin. Infect Immun 59:2955
13. Grimminger F, Sibelius U, Bhakdi S, Suttorp N, Seeger W (1991) Escherichia coli hemolysin is a potent inductor of phosphoinositide hydrolysis and related metabolic responses in human neutrophils. J Clin Invest 88:1531
14. Grimminger F, Scholz C, Bhakdi S, Seeger W (1991) Subhemolytic doses of Escherichia coli hemolysin evoke large quantities of lipoxygenase products in human neutrophils. J Biol Chem 266:14262
15. Suttorp N, Flöer B, Seeger W, Schnittler H, Bhakdi S (1990) Effects of E. coli hemolysin on endothelial cell function. Infect Immun 58:3796
16. Suttorp N, Seeger W, Dewein E, Bhakdi S, Roka L (1985) Staphylococcal alpha-toxin-induced PGI_2 production in endothelial cells: role of calcium. Am J Physiol 248:C127
17. Seeger W, Bauer M, Bhakdi S (1984) Staphylococcal alpha-toxin elicits hypertension in isolated rabbit lungs. Evidence for thromboxane formation and the role of extracellular calcium. J Clin Invest 74:849
18. Seeger W, Walter H, Suttorp N, Bhakdi S (1989) Thromboxane-mediated hypertension and vascular leakage evoked by low doses of Escherichia coli hemolysin in rabbit lungs. J Clin Invest 84:220

19. Suttorp N, Habben E (1988) Effect of staphyococcal alpha-toxin on intracellular Ca^{2+} in polymorphonuclear leukocytes. Infect Immun 56:2228
20. Suttorp N, Seeger W, Uhl J, Lutz F, Roka L (1985) Pseudomonas aeruginosa cytotoxin stimulates prostacyclin production in cultured pulmonary artery endothelial cells: membrane attack and calcium influx. J Cell Physiol 123:64
21. Glauser MP, Zanetti G, Baumgartner J-D, Cohen J (1991) Septic shock: pathogenesis. Lancet 338:732
22. Suttorp N, Fuchs T, Seeger W, Wilke A, Drenckhahn D (1989) Role of Ca^{2+} and Mg^{2+} for endothelial permeability of water and albumin in vitro. Lab Invest 61:183
23. Suttorp N, Hessz T, Seeger W, Wilke A, Koob R, Lutz F, Drenckhahn D (1988) Bacterial exotoxins and endothelial permeability for water and albumin. Am J Physiol 255:C369
24. Suttorp N, Polley M, Seybold J, Schnittler H, Seeger W, Grimminger F, Aktories K (1991) ADP-ribosylation of G-actin by botulinum C2 toxin increases endothelial permeability in vitro. J Clin Invest 87:1575
25. Fowler AA, Hamman RF, Zerbe GO, Benson KN, Hyers TM (1985) Adult respiratory distress syndrome. Prognosis after onset. Am Rev Respir Dis 132:472
26. Montgomery AB, Stager MA, Carrico CJ, Hudson LD (1985) Causes of mortality in patients with the adult respiratory distress syndrome. Am Rev Respir Dis 132:485
27. Petty TL (1985) Indicators of risk, course, and prognosis in adult respiratory distress syndrome (ARDS). Am Rev Respir Dis 132:471
28. Andrews CP, Coalson JJ, Smith JD, Johanson WG (1981) Diagnosis of nosocomial pneumonia in acute, diffuse lung injury. Chest 80:254
29. Bodey GP, Jadea L, Elting I (1985) Pseudomonas bacteremia. Arch Intern Med 145:1621
30. Seeger W, Obernitz R, Thomas M et al. (1991) Lung vascular injury after administration of viable hemolysin-forming Escherichia coli in isolated rabbit lungs. Am Rev Respir Dis 143:797
31. Walmrath D, König R, Ernst C, Brückner H, Grimminger F, Seeger W (1992) Ventilation-perfusion relationships in isolated bloodfree perfused rabbit lungs. J Appl Physiol 72(1):374
32. Grimminger F, Walmrath D, Birkemeyer RG, Bhakdi S, Seeger W (1990) Burst of leukotriene- and HETE-generation elicited by low dose Escherichia coli hemolysin in rabbit lungs. Infect Immun 58:2659
33. Grimminger F, Thomas M, Obernitz R, Walmrath D, Bhakdi S, Seeger W (1990) Inflammatory lipid mediator generation elicited by viable hemolysin-forming Escherichia coli in lung vasculature. J Exp Med 172:1115
34. Grimminger F, Kreusler B, Schneider U, Becker G, Seeger W (1990) Influence of microvascular adherence on neutrophil leukotriene generation – evidence for cooperative eicosanoid synthesis. J Immunol 144:1866
35. Grimminger F, Menger M, Becker G, Seeger W (1988) Potentiation of leukotriene generation following sequestration of neutrophils in isolated lungs. Blood 72:1687
36. Ermert L, Rousseau S, Schütte H et al. (1992) Induction of severe vascular leakage by low doses of Escherichia coli hemolysin in perfused rabbit lungs. Lab Invest 66:362

Bacterial Translocation: Myth versus Reality

M.D. Pasquale, M.D. Cipolle and F.B. Cerra

Introduction

Bacterial translocation has been defined as the passage of viable bacteria through the epithelial mucosa and lamina propria of the gastrointestinal (GI) tract to extraintestinal sites such as the mesenteric lymph nodes (MLN), spleen, liver, peritoneum, and blood [1]. More recently, however, Alexander et al. [2] have suggested a refinement of this definition to include all microbial translocation (viable and nonviable) as well as microbial products, e.g., endotoxin, across an anatomically intact intestinal barrier. It should be noted that neither definition describes the host or bacterial mechanisms responsible for such movement. Currently, it is felt that indigenous bacteria translocate continuously from the GI tract. The numbers of bacteria that translocate are low and the host immune system is able to destroy them prior to systemic spread. This process may very well be a major mechanism of immune sampling to maintain "natural immunity" to a variety of pathogens. Thus, in the presence of normal GI ecology and a well-functioning immune system, the relative impermeability of the GI mucosa, "gut barrier function", prevents invasion of bacteria into extraintestinal sites [3].

The gut barrier has both extrinsic and intrinsic components [4]. The extrinsic barrier, located within the intestinal lumen, stabilizes the microenvironment at the intestinal epithelial surface and consists of mucus, secretory IgA, the "unstirred layer" overlying the epithelium, and the luminal flora and microflora themselves [4]. The intrinsic barrier has two components, the epithelial cells (transcellular) and the spaces around them (paracellular) [4]. Some investigators have called translocation a transcellular process. Others feel that gut barrier disruption involves primarily the paracellular route that may or may not be associated with bacterial movement from gut lumen to lymph nodes [1]. The major pathway for passive permeation of luminal contents (and perhaps bacteria) through the intestinal epithelium is paracellular, with the tight junction being the primary rate-limiting structure. Intercellular tight junctions or zonulae occludentes (ZO) form a narrow band encircling the apical pole of epithelial cells. Within this band, the lateral cytoplasmic membranes of adjacent cells are fused at multiple points called "kisses". It is felt that although kisses are generally impermeable, there are areas of discontinuity (pores) which permit passive transepithelial permeation.

A variety of immunologic mechanisms support this barrier system. The intestinal wall is rich in lymphocytes, macrophages, and Peyer's patches, and the mesentery is filled with regional lymph nodes. The specialized mucosal lymph nodes have antigen sampling and processing systems thought to maintain an optimal state of natural immunity. The intraluminal secretion of IgA provides a specialized defense system and aids recognition of appropriate antigens for gut absorption [5]. Finally, Kupffer cells of the liver and the spleen serve as a backup barrier to trap and detoxify bacteria and their products if they penetrate beyond the epithelium and the regional lymphatic tissue.

Translocation per se is currently viewed as a normal physiologic occurrence, probably primarily occurring by the transcellular mechanism. Disruption of the paracellular barrier provides another possible port for bacterial movement through the lamina propria. This intestinal epithelial barrier can be abnormal in disease states, even when the epithelium remains confluent and there is no discernible biochemical or morphological alteration [4]. Fine initially proposed that in hemorrhagic shock the gut became the source of endotoxin and invasive gram-negative bacteria and in the presence of a defective reticuloendothelial system (RES) led to systemic bacteremia. Schimpff [7] later demonstrated that the GI tract acts as a source of pathogens in granulocytopenic patients. Other authors [8–11] have demonstrated the ability of intestinal gram-negative bacterias enterococci, clostridia and *Candida* to cause bacteremia. This invasion of bacteria, into extraintestinal sites has led to the description of the gut as the motor of multiple organ dysfunction, the so-called "gut hypothesis" [12].

Factors known to lead to increased bacterial translocation and a concomitant increase in bacteremia are disruption of the intestinal mucosal barrier, suppression of the immune system, and alteration of the normal GI ecology [2, 3].

Disruption of the Gut Barrier Function

Conditions which lead to mesenteric hypoperfusion such as those seen in hemorrhagic shock, multiple trauma, burns, and sepsis have been shown to cause breakdown of the intestinal mucosal barrier [13]. This breakdown is most likely the end result of inadequate oxygen delivery (DO_2) to the intestinal tissues. When DO_2 is unable to meet tissue requirements, the rate of ATP hydrolysis exceeds the rate of ATP synthesis, resulting in a net production of hydrogen ions and mucosal acidosis [14]. Mucosal acidosis leads to sloughing of cells along with loss of cellular membrane integrity and tight cellular junctions. The overall result is a breakdown in the "gut barrier."

Studies looking at the effect of decreased mesenteric flow and its relationship to breakdown of the GI barrier function have centered on animal models of hemorrhagic shock, thermal injury, and sepsis. In humans, clinical evaluations of polytrauma patients have provided useful insight into this problem.

Hemorrhagic Shock

In a rat model where intestinal blood flow was reduced to one-third of the resting control level, increased mucosal permeability to macromolecules and morphological injury to small intestinal villi was noted within 2 h [15]. The colonic mucosa appeared to be more resistant in that a longer period of ischemia was required to give such changes [15]. Deitch et al. [16, 17] have shown in a rat model of hemorrhagic shock that increasing periods of hypotension are associated with mucosal injury and subsequent translocation of bacteria into extraintestinal sites. Histologically, early (2 h) changes consisted of subepithelial edema in the cecum and ileum which progressed to focal sloughing and necrosis in the mucosa at 24 h [17]. Intestinal permeability to horseradish peroxidase was increased at 2 h [17]. Note that horseradish peroxidase is a macromolecular histochemical tracer that typically penetrates the epithelium via both the paracellular and transcellular pathways [18]. In a canine model of mesenteric hypoperfusion, Chiu et al. [19] demonstrated early subepithelial edema starting at the apex of the intestinal villus and progressing down the sides, resulting in the lifting of the epithelial layer from the lamina propria. The later progressed to disintegration of the lamina propria, hemorrhage, ulceration, and transmural necrosis [19]. Further evidence of mucosal injury resulting from decreased visceral flow has been demonstrated in a swine model by Saydjari et al. [20]. In this model, mechanical occlusion of the celiac and superior mesenteric arteries caused a significant increase in ornithine decarboxylase (ODC) activity in the colon [20]. The increase in ODC activity suggests a regenerative response to injury of the bowel [20]. It is this physical disruption of the gut barrier that then leads to invasion of the MLN and/or portal circulation by the luminal contents [21].

Thermal Injury

In sheep undergoing a 40% total body surface burn, mesenteric blood flow was noted to be significantly decreased from baseline 1–2 h post-burn, despite maintenance of normal cardiac output with rigorous fluid resuscitation [22]. Despite a return to normal flow by 20 h post-burn, these animals were noted to have a significant increase in bacterial counts in the MLN, liver, and lungs at 48 h when compared to sham controls [22]. The decrease in mesenteric blood flow that occurs post-burn is felt to be due to an increase in mesenteric vascular resistance. Navaratnam et al. [23] have shown that by maintaining mesenteric blood flow with selective sodium nitroprusside infusion, the decrease in intestinal blood flow and the increased bacterial translocation could be prevented. These authors conclude that post-burn, a decrease in mesenteric blood flow promotes bacterial translocation by disrupting the gut barrier [22, 23]. The role of ischemia in this situation is further supported by the fact that pretreatment with xanthine oxidase inhibitors (allopurinol or tungsten) will reduce the incidence of bacterial translocation [24]. Evidence also suggests that reperfusion after an episode of intestinal ischemia releases oxygen free radicals generated by xanthine oxidase [25]. The free radicals are then capable of augmenting the ischemic mucosal injury. Reperfusion of ischemic intestine results in the influx and extravasation of large numbers of neutrophils and the reactive oxygen species (ROS) generated by these cells [26].

Endotoxin

It appears as though endotoxin can induce bacterial translocation from the gut, as well as induce hemodynamic, metabolic, and immunologic disturbances [27]. The primary mechanism by which endotoxin promotes bacterial translocation is by physical disruption of the gut barrier [28]. The subepithelial edema once felt to be characteristic of lipopolysaccharide (LPS), however, is probably best considered a nonspecific response to a number of types of injury. Morphological studies in mice have shown that this increase in bacterial translocation is due to selective damage to the ileal and cecal mucosa [28]. The endotoxin-induced damage appears to be mediated, at least in part, by xanthine oxidase-generated oxygen free radicals and is evidenced by an increase in the enzyme's activity in the ileal and cecal mucosa and the fact that translocation can be reduced by inhibiton of xanthine oxidase with allopurinol [29]. Allopurinol's protective effect appears to be related to its action as an xanthine oxidase inhibitor rather than as an antioxidant [29, 30]. The effect of endotoxin on ileal mucosal permeability was tested by comparing the ratio of clearance of EDTA to the clearance of urea in two groups of pigs [31]. EDTA is a more specific marker of paracellular permeability [32]. In the experimental group, mesenteric hypoperfusion was induced by infusion of LPS, while in a second group comparable decreases in perfusion were obtained with a mechanical occluder [31]. There was an approximate six-fold increase in permeability noted in the LPS group while there was no significant effect on permeability in the mechanically occluded group [31]. In a canine model, Bulkley et al. [33] showed that intestinal permeability was not affected by ischemic reperfusion unless the decrement in oxygen consumption ($\dot{V}O_2$) across the gut was decreased by more than 50% during the period of low flow. This further supports the fact that the adverse effect of endotoxin on mucosal permeability cannot be accounted for by mesenteric hypoperfusion alone. Additional support for the role of the xanthine oxidase-mediated disruption of the gut mucosal barrier comes from Deitch et al. [34] in a study of zymosan-induced bacterial translocation. Zymosan, a component of the cell wall of the yeast *S. cerevisiae* was used as the inflammatory agent since it is nonbacterial and nonendotoxic [34]. Zymosan reportedly exerts its inflammatory and hemodynamic effects by activating complement, macrophages, and neutrophils [35]. Prior work by Deitch et al. [36] indicated that zymosan promoted bacterial translocation by damaging the intestinal mucosa. Deitch et al. [34] were able to demonstrate in mice that zymosan-induced mucosal injury and subsequent bacterial translocation were not complement-, macrophage- or mast cell-dependent. This group also demonstrated that zymosan's effect on the intestinal barrier was most likely mediated through the activation of xanthine oxidase and could be largely prevented by pretreatment with allopurinol [34]. Walker and Porvaznik [37], examining the morphological integrity of ZO using a freeze-fracture technique, have shown that the ileal mucosal tight junctions are disrupted by endotoxin. O'Dwyer et al. [38] have demonstrated that a single dose of endotoxin will increase the intestinal permeability in humans.

Mechanism of Translocation

Models of hemorrhagic shock, thermal injury, and endotoxemia have been shown to result in physical disruption of the gut mucosal barrier. The injury induced by these various etiologies is similar and probably involves similar mechanisms. In vivo studies have shown that parenteral LPS induces intestinal pathology similar to that seen in mild to moderate mesenteric ischemia, i.e., subepithelial edema and cellular degeneration of the lamina propria [19]. This disruption provides the luminal contents of the intestine ready access to extraintestinal sites. Other factors which lead to physical disruption of the intestinal mucosa should also lead to increased bacterial translocation. It is known that the physical integrity of the gut mucosa depends on an adequate nutritional state. In starved rats excessive small bowel weight loss and reduced proliferation of intestinal epithelial cells has been demonstrated [39]. Mucosal atrophy occurs after prolonged periods of parenteral feeding most likely due to the lack of access to nutrients in the gut lumen. A number of nutrients provided in the gut lumen have mucosotrophic properties. Glutamine is one fuel used by the intestinal tract, and in animals subjected to an acute stress, such as operative trauma, transmesenteric uptake of this amino acid increased dramatically [40]. Interestingly, glutamine can support the gut mucosa when supplied parenterally [12]. Barton et al. [41] have suggested that essential fatty acid deficiency may result in structural changes within the intestinal epithelium that lead to failure of the mechanical barrier function. In rats fed a diet deficient in essential fatty acids the incidence of bacterial translocation to the MLN was increased compared to those fed an essential fatty acid-replete diet [41].

With disruption of the gut barrier, one would expect that translocation would primarily be of a paracellular nature due to breakdown in the tight cellular junctions. The exact mechanism of translocation, however, is not well understood. Whether or not bacteria translocate via a transcellular or paracellular route remains to be elucidated. Wells et al. [42, 43] have reported that intestinal macrophages can phagocytize inert latex particles and live bacteria from the gut and then transport them to the MLN. It was felt by this group that during the transport there was a failure of the normal intracellular killing by the macrophage and thus viable bacteria can be delivered to the MLN [42, 43]. In their murine model, the degree of translocation was greatly decreased in macrophage-defective mice which had been decontaminated and colonized with *E. coli* [42, 43]. Mainous et al. [44] demonstrated that in rats, the physiologic response to zymosan and zymosan-induced bacterial translocation was dose-dependent. At a zymosan dose of 0.1 mg/g body weight, bacterial translocation was limited to the MLN and the animals manifested no signs of systemic toxicity [44]. At a dose of 0.5 mg/g, however, there was systemic bacterial translocation and sepsis with a mortality of 40% [44]. The authors note that at this higher dose both mesenteric lymph flow and intestinal blood flow were increased, either of which could promote systemic spread [44]. It has been hypothesized that once the bacteria reach the MLN they may gain access to the systemic circulation via the thoracic duct [42, 45]. In Thiry-Vella loops of thermally burned guinea pigs and rats, Alexander et al. [46] noted that both large (*C. albicans*) and small (*E. coli*) intact microbes and endotoxin translocated directly through morphologically intact enterocytes. This type of transcellular translocation is consistent with reports by Cole et al. [47] who demonstrated direct internalization of *Candida* by enterocytes after intragastric inoculation. Likewise, Wells et al. [48] have shown that enterococci translocated through rather than between enterocytes in mice. These findings suggest that endotoxin and intact organisms once in the lamina propria may pass between cells and through the muscular layer of the bowel wall to the serosa. This would explain the transmural migration of endotoxin through ischemic colons in dogs described by Papa et al. [49] and the translocation of enteric bacteria through the intestinal wall into intraperitoneal abscesses described by Wells et al. [50]. Thus, the gut barrier function of the host is important in preventing the initial translocation of bacteria; however, as mentioned earlier, indigenous bacteria are continuously translocating across the mucosa in small numbers. Normally these are killed by the host immune defense system either during transport to or in the MLN and other organs of the RES. If for some reason the host is immunosuppressed, then bacteria may multiply and spread to extraintestinal sites without being destroyed. Thus, organisms could theoretically become invasive at normal translocation rates in the presence of compromised immune function of either the specific or the nonspecific immune system. Similarly, more organisms may be found in lymph nodes resulting from decreased cytotoxic activity without a change in the real translocation rate.

Immunosuppression

Virtually all drugs used to treat malignancies and prevent rejection will also reduce the number and effectiveness of immune cells. Depression of bone marrow is well known and several chemotherapeutic agents also depress delayed-type hypersensitivity, secondary antibody responses, and immunoglobulin levels. Corticosteroids are also known to cause lymphopenia and depress lymphocyte activation in mixed lymphocyte culture [51]. Intraperitoneal injection of methotrexate, 5-fluorouracil, cytarabine hydrochloride, cyclophosphamide, or prednisone appear to promote bacterial translocation in mice from the GI tract to the MLN, spleen, liver, and kidneys [52]. In a separate study by Berg and Itoh [53], 50% of the MLN, spleens, livers, and kidneys of congenitally athymic (nu/nu) mice contained viable indigenous GI bacteria, compared to only 5.2% positive organ cultures from heterozygous (nu/+) mice. The authors concluded that T-cell-dependent mechanisms are important in the inhibition of bacterial translocation [53]. Other more complicated models in which host immunosuppression appears to play a role in allowing bacterial translocation include hemorrhagic shock, thermal injury, endotoxemia, and diabetes. It is important to understand that in most of these studies, translocation rates are determined by the number of bacterial colonies counted on culture of the lymph nodes. This methodology is probably not able to discriminate between an absolute increase in the number of bacteria and/or a reduction in the lymphocyte cytotoxicity rate.

Trauma and Hemorrhagic Shock

Within 2 h of trauma or hemorrhagic shock, there is decreased neutrophil chemotaxis and phagocytosis which can persist for several days [54]. Twenty-four hours after a traumatic insult, a reversal of the T-cell helper-to-suppressor ratio, decreased opsonin levels, and inhibition of the RES result [55–57]. The immune system is further compromised by the catabolism that occurs after severe trauma. Bacterial invasion leading to post-traumatic sepsis is believed to be secondary to trauma-induced immune suppression. The ability of the RES to clear endotoxin from the blood in hemorrhagic shock is impaired, promoting increased circulating endotoxin levels [58]. Hemorrhagic shock also inhibits the peritoneal inflammatory response in rats and decreases the ability of the animal to clear bacteria from the bloodstream [59]. Severe trauma has also been noted to result in a generalized suppression of T-cell-mediated immunity, which, as mentioned previously, appears to be important in the suppression of bacterial translocation [60]. Trauma patients are also noted to have suppression of the secretory IgA system and an excess release of prostaglandin E_2 (PGE_2) [61, 62]. It should be noted that secretory IgA does not kill bacteria but rather binds to it, and thus prevents the binding of the bacteria to cells of the mucous surface. PGE_2, on the other hand, suppresses immune function by inhibiting the production of interleukin-2 (IL-2) and thus the generation of helper T-cells – phenomena that can suppress the cytotoxic T-cell response [62].

Thermal Injury and Sepsis

Burn injury alone results in multiple alterations in the host, including hypermetabolism, counterregulatory hormone changes, alterations in neutrophil function and lymphocyte subpopulations, and impaired immune responses [63–66]. Patients with sepsis have multiple immune problems and are particularly prone to develop additional infections [67]. Decreased blood lymphocyte counts have been noted along with a predominance of immature polymorphonuclear leukocytes [67]. There is also a decrease in several of the complement factors [67]. The hepatic Kupffer cells which usually clear the portal blood of gut-derived endotoxin and microorganisms exhibit depressed function in the presence of hepatic ischemia [68]. Two to 3 h following the administration of zymosan or in a septic state, there is a marked reduction in hepatic blood flow [69, 70]. The end result of portal bacteremia and hepatic ischemia, then, could overwhelm the hepatic RES and allow viable bacteria to gain access to the systemic circulation. In a study by Jones et al. [71], rats undergoing 30% scald burn followed by immediate inoculation of the burn wound with 1×10^8 colony forming units (CFU) of *Pseudomonas aeruginosa* were used to study the effects of ongoing infection after thermal injury on bacterial translocation. The addition of infection after thermal injury produced marked cachexia with peripheral protein wasting [71]. There was also an associated increase in hepatic mRNA for tumor necrosis factor (TNF) that was not seen with burn injury alone [71, 72]. Although it is unclear whether or not the organisms from the burn wound, or from an enteric source, or both induced the increased hepatic mRNA for TNF, the presence of bacterial translocation appears to have an impact on hepatic immunologic function [71]. Bacterial translocation can be reduced by specific or nonspecific vaccination. A heat-killed *E. coli* vaccine injected intraperitoneally weekly for 4 weeks reduced translocation of *E. coli* from the GI tract to the MLN in mice decontaminated by antibiotics or germ-free mice challenged orally with this *E. coli* strain [53]. Vaccination with a nonspecific immunomodulator, formalin-killed *Propionibacterium acnes,* also decreased translocation of *E. coli* [53].

Diabetes

Patients with diabetes are generally considered to have a five to ten times greater risk of infection after trauma or surgery than the general population [67]. The exact reason for this is unknown, but it is known that there is impaired killing of engulfed bacteria [67]. In mice with streptozocin-induced diabetes, the incidence of bacterial translocation to the MLN decreased from 49% to 17% when their hyperglycemia was controlled with daily insulin injections [53].

Nutrition

Malnutrition is known to impair host immune defenses as well as to lead to gut mucosal atrophy [73]. In patients with essential fatty acid deficiency, Barton et al. [41] proposed that depressed levels of arachidonic acid and its metabolites impair the cellular immune response to invading bacteria within the intestinal epithelium. They further proposed that depressed levels of these metabolites alter monokine production and/or superoxide generation leading to a failure of intracellular killing of ingested bacteria [41]. Impaired neutrophil migration and superoxide generation in the setting of essential fatty acid deficiency may also contribute to the deterioration in immune barrier function [41]. Lastly, it has been shown that parenteral nutrition causes a marked reduction in the amount of secretory IgA, the immunoglobulin that prevents attachment of luminal bacteria to the mucosal cells [74].

In summary, it appears that there is ample evidence to suggest that immune suppression exists to varying degrees in stressed states. Theoretically, this may lead to spread of viable bacteria and bacterial products from the intestinal lumen to extraintestinal sites, even without an increase in the rate of bacterial translocation per se. One further point should be made regarding the host immune defenses, and that is that the indigenous GI flora itself provides a defense against bacterial translocation. Thus, alterations in the relationships among the gut flora and/or enteric bacterial overgrowth can result in increased bacterial translocation [75].

Bacterial Overgrowth

Certain enteric bacteria (*E. coli, K. pneumoniae, P. mirabilis* and *P. aeruginosa*) readily translocate from the GI tract when they reach a high level, e.g., 10^8/g intestinal contents [3]. Normally, bacterial antagonisms by other indigenous microflora control the GI population level of these enterics to 10^3–10^5/g intestinal contents [3]. This inhibitory process, termed "colonization resistance," also prevents more pathogenic exogenous bacteria from colonizing the GI tract. In germ-free and antibiotic-decontaminated mice the cecal populations of gram-negative enteric bacteria have been found to be directly related to the rate of translocation from the GI tract to the MLN in otherwise healthy animals [3]. In mice who underwent ligation of their common bile ducts, cecal levels of gram-negative enteric bacteria were 100-fold higher and the incidence of bacterial translocation was significantly higher than controls (33% vs. 7%) [76, 77]. The authors believed that intestinal bacterial overgrowth was the major factor responsible for bacterial translocation [76, 77]. Mucosal injury was also noted with these patients, i.e., subepithelial edema [76, 77]. Other studies involving rats and mice have shown that certain liquid diets promoted cecal bacterial overgrowth, and this resulted in an increased incidence of bacterial translocation from the intestinal tract to the draining MLN [78, 79]. It is also known that when the ecological balance in the GI tract is disrupted with oral antibiotics (penicillin, clindamycin, metronidazole), enteric bacilli can increase in numbers and result in increased translocation [3].

Review of the data to this point would suggest that although bacteria may translocate from the intestinal lumen to extraintestinal sites, the number of bacteria that do so is usually small and controlled by the host immune defense system. Conditions which lead to either physical disruption of the gut mucosal barrier, immune suppression, and/or intestinal bacterial overgrowth can lead to an increase in the effective bacterial translocation and spread to the MLN and other organs of the RES. The questions that remain to be answered are whether or not this process is truly a pathogenetic mechanism that is clinically relevant; whether or not it can lead to multiple organ dysfunction syndrome (MODS); and whether or not therapy directed to suppress translocation can improve relevant clinical outcomes.

Gut as Motor for MODS

It indeed, the gut can be considered as a cause of MODS rather than just another target, bacteria must escape from the intestine, spread systematically, and cause subsequent morbidity and mortality. It remains to be determined whether or not bacteria pass into the circulation at the intestinal level, via the lymphatic system, or neither. The first line of defense against bacteria passing from the GI tract to the portal venous system is the hepatic RES, namely, the Kupffer cells. Teleologically, the important role played by the RES is suggested by the fact that the liver and the lungs, two large RES organs, are in series and can therefore filter particulate matter from the blood draining the GI tract, thereby preventing passage to the systemic circulation [80]. Kupffer cells normally clear translocating bacteria and endotoxin from the portal blood, and thus factors which lead to hepatic dysfunction would be expected to impair this function of the Kupffer cells and thereby allow the systemic passage of bacteria and endotoxin. Endotoxin from the gut has been shown to cause hepatic dysfunction along with activation of Kupffer cells in the absence of a demonstrable focus of infection of bacteremia [81, 82]. Ultimately, this may lead, at least in part, to the development of MODS [81, 82]. Keller et al. [83] have shown in a rat cell culture preparation that LPS-activated Kupffer cells are capable of modulating adjacent hepatocyte protein synthesis. Kupffer cell blockade in an animal model of hemorrhagic shock has been shown to be associated with diminished hepatic phagocytosis and a concomitant increase in pulmonary localization of viable *E. coli* [84, 85]. Saba and Jaffe [86] have shown that hepatic reticuloendothelial function is depressed as a result of depletion of the reticuloendothelial opsonin and fibronectin while the presence of bacteria and endotoxin in the portal circulation promotes Kupffer cell secretion of cytokines, i.e., TNF, interleukin-1 (IL-1), and PGE_2 [87]. These findings suggest a potential role for the Kupffer cell population in the pathogenesis of both the metabolic and immunologic aberrations of MODS. This has led to the "gut hypothesis" whereby the gut, via translocation and subsequent hepatic dysfunction, leads to MODS. Supporting this concept are studies by Marshall et al. [88] and Kahky et al. [89], which show that *E. coli* and TNF infusion into the portal vein result in a significant increase in toxicity and mortality when compared to infusion of these agents into the inferior vena cava. If this is the case, then, as Marshall et al. [90] concluded, the gut must serve as an occult reservoir of bacteria which can translocate to the liver as well as the systemic circulation.

In a rat hemorrhagic shock model, Baker et al. [91] showed that 30–60 min shock resulted in one-half of the MLN having positive cultures while there was less than 20% spread to the liver and spleen and a mortality rate of only 15%–20%. After 90 min shock, however, all MLN had positive cultures and grew greater numbers of enteric bacteria (*E. coli, Enterococcus, Pseudomonas, Proteus*) [91]. Spread to systemic organs was 60% and mortality was 40% [91].

Sori et al. [92], in rats who were fed carbon-14-labeled *E. coli* and underwent subsequent hemorrhagic shock, demonstrated a greater incidence of positive cultures in portal blood than in arterial blood. The authors felt that this represented entrance of bacteria into the bloodstream at the intestinal level rather than via the lymphatic system. Of the 14 animals subjected to hemorrhagic shock, 7 had elevated plasma radioactivity levels and all were dead within 84 h of shock [92]. In contrast, 83% of animals without plasma carbon-14 activity survived [92]. The authors conclude from this study that the degree of bacterial translocation from the intestine correlated with mortality [92].

In a prolonged hemorrhagic shock model, Koziol et al. [93] noted that blood cultures became positive within 30 min of the initiation of shock and bacteremia continued to be present throughout the ensuing 48 h [93]. *Pseudomonas* and *Enterococcus* predominated early, while cultures became polymicrobial over time [93]. The authors noted that germ-free rats subjected to the same shock had significantly better survival [93]. In this model, the authors have also shown correlation between bacteremia and the degree of endotoxemia [94]. The detrimental effect of endotoxin on hepatic function has been mentioned earlier.

Goris et al. [95], in a study of rats undergoing intraperitoneal instillation of zymosan, showed that although $\dot{V}O_2$ decreased, serum lactate increased, multiple organs deteriorated in function several days post-instillation, and blood cultures remained sterile. The authors concluded that a severe inflammatory response in itself was capable of inducing multiple organ failure [95]. In contrast, Deitch et al. [96] demonstrated a dose-dependent translocation of bacteria from the intestine to other organs in pathogen-free mice injected intraperitoneally with zymosan. While saline-injected controls had sterile organ cultures, 85% of mice receiving zymosan 0.1 mg/g body weight had documented translocation to MLN [96]. When the zymosan dosage was increased to 0.5 mg/g, bacterial translocation passed the MLN and could be recovered from liver, spleens, and blood of the mice [96]. Animals receiving zymosan were randomized into saline control or cefoxitin-treated groups to study whether or not the lethal effects of zymosan were related to bacterial translocation [96]. At a dosage of zymosan 0.5 mg/g there were no deaths in either group, while at a dosage of zymosan 0.75 mg/g cefoxitin significantly improved 7-day survival [96]. Cefoxitin also improved short- and long-term survival in mice receiving zymosan 1 mg/g; however, it did not prevent mortality in a group receiving zymosan 2 mg/g [96]. In the cefoxitin-treated survivors, translocating bacteria were cleared and cecal populations returned to normal [96]. Since antibiotic treatment reduced mortality from 100% to 20% in mice challenged with zymosan (1 mg/g), the authors concluded that gut-derived sepsis plays a causal role in the morbidity/mortality associated with zymosan [96]. Fukushima et al. [97] investigated the effect of bacterial translocation on mortality after a thermal injury. Previously transfused BALB/c mice were gavaged with carbon-14-labeled *E. coli* prior to inflicting a 20% full-thickness flame burn [97]. Radionuclide counts in the blood (obtained by retroorbital puncture 4 h post-burn) correlated well with both radionuclide counts and numbers of viable bacteria in the tissue [97]. Survivors had significantly less bacterial translocation as evidenced by blood radionuclide counts compared with nonsurvivors, and there was a significant inverse correlation between the degree of translocation and the length of survival [97].

Important in consideration of the concept of bacterial translocation as a promoter of MODS is the fact that translocation is not an all-or-nothing concept, and independent stresses can have additional effects on it. This is nicely demonstrated by models looking at thermal injury with and without concomitant infection. Jones et al. [71] compared control rats with a group undergoing a 30% scald burn and a third group undergoing a 30% scald burn followed by immediate inoculation of the burn wound wit 1×10^8 CFU *Pseudomonas aeruginosa.* The authors noted that the lymph nodes, organs, and blood of control animals remained sterile at essentially all time points, while burn injury resulted in significant bacterial translocation of enteric organisms to MLN [71]. The abdominal organs and blood remained free of translocating organisms and by day 4 translocation was not evident in the MLN [71]. Burn-infected animals failed to clear the initial translocation after thermal injury and had evidence of continued bacterial translocation to MLN, liver, spleen, and blood [71]. These cultures were polymicrobial with a predominance of *E. coli* [71].

This data would suggest that bacterial translocation plays a significant role in the development of MODS. There is, however, an increasing amount of evidence that translocation per se may not be the major mechanism of the gut origin of sepsis, organ dysfunction, and adverse clinical outcomes.

In porcine models of hemorrhagic shock, Morales et al. [98] could not demonstrate significant bacterial translocation to the liver, spleen, and portal blood in ischemica/reperfusion despite profound shock and significant evidence of lipid peroxidation after resuscitation. The authors concluded that although translocation to MLN does occur, its importance in the development of MODS remains to be proven [98]. Likewise, Wells et al., in a murine model of gut injury and translocation, observed that multiple agents can disrupt the mucosal barrier and alter translocation rates, but that there was a very poor correlation between the translocation rate and subsequent mortality.

Moore et al. [99] inserted portal vein catheters for sequential blood sampling in 20 injured patients requiring emergent laparotomy and who were at known risk of MODS. Eight of 212 portal blood cultures were positive and 7 were presumed contaminated [99]. The only positive systemic culture (1/212) was of *S. aureus* on day 5 in one patient with a concurrent staphylococcal pneumonia [99]. Endotoxin could not be detected in portal or systemic blood at 48 h [99]. This prospective clinical trial could not confirm portal or systemic bacteremia within the first 5 days after injury, despite an eventual 30% incidence of MODS [99].

If the gut is indeed the motor of MODS, then therapy directed at preservation of barrier function and/or elimination of potentially pathogenic microbacteria (PPM) would be expected to decrease the incidence of organ dysfunction and subsequent mortality. It is important to understand, however, that even if efficacy were demonstrated with such therapy it would not necessarily confirm or deny the translocation hypothesis [1]. Other mechanisms effected by these same therapies may account for the outcome effects, such mechanisms including: enhanced immune function in the gut; enhanced systemic immune function; reduced or altered systemic endothelial injury and/or macrophage activation; more effective gut hormone signalling and more effective nutrient regulation of the systemic metabolism.

Therapy Directed at Bacterial Translocation

Nutritional Support

The presence of food in the lumen of the gut appears to be the most important stimulus of mucosal growth. Enteral feeding stimulates the mechanical desquamation of cells at the villus tip, provides nutrients, and stimulates trophic hormone production [12]. When the gut cannot be fed via the enteric route, atrophy of the intestinal mucosa can be expected to occur [12, 100]. Enteral feeding will also stimulate bile flow, increasing the luminal supply of epidermal growth factor, IgA and bile salts, promote peristalsis and bacterial clearance, and supply substrates not available by the parenteral route. Enteral feeding could be expected to maintain gut barrier function during critical illness. Mochizuki et al. [101] studied the hormonal and gut epithelial responses in guinea pigs that had been subjected to a 30% burn injury. When enteral feedings were instituted shortly after the time of injury, the mucosa was preserved and the catabolic response to injury was attenuated [101]. Animals receiving fixed doses of 5-fluorouracil were given isocaloric, isonitrogenous diets that contained either 2% glutamine or other nonessential amino acids [102]. Animals receiving the glutamine-containing diet had improved nitrogen balance, increased mucosal cellularity, and decreased mortality compared to animals receiving standard nutrient formulas [102].

Nutritional support in trauma and burn patients has been associated with improvements in patient outcome [103, 104]. These improvements appear to result from the prevention of nutrient deficiencies and starvation. In patients who have advanced into persistent hypermetabolism, however, the current data would indicate that standard enteral nutritional support does not alter the course of the disease process [105]. In a randomized, prospective study, Daly et al. [106] examined the effects of enteral nutrition with supplemental arginine, RNA, and omega-3 fatty acids on clinical outcome in a group of postoperative critically ill patients. In critically ill and injured patients, the use of these omega-3 fatty acids along with arginine and nucleic acids has been associated with restoration of immune reactivity in *in vitro* tests of immune function, while recent clinical trials have documented improvement in patient outcome [107]. Daly's group [106] documented a significant decrease in infectious and wound complications along with a significantly shorter mean length of hospital stay in the group of patients given nutritional supplementation with arginine, RNA, and omega-3 fatty acids.

Selective Gut Decontamination

It has been hypothesized that oral antibiotics designed to suppress the luminal aerobic, but not anaerobic flora, i.e., selective gut decontamination (SGD), will reduce the incidence of nosocomial infections and subsequent mortality. Presumably, such an effect would be mediated by the limitation of movement of gut bacteria up or through the gut lumen. Trials of SGD which utilized oral application of antimicrobials along with gut and systemic administration of antimicrobials have shown a reduction in nosocomial infections and mortality [108–110]. Others, however, have not been able to document any significant improvement in morbidity and mortality with the use of SGD [111, 112]. In a prospective, randomized, double-blind, placebo-controlled clinical trial in patients in a surgical intensive care unit who had persistent hypermetabolism, Cerra et al. [113] showed that SGD (norfloxin 500 mg suspension every 8 h, nystatin one million units every 6 h) significantly reduced the incidence of nonsocomial infections and the mean length of hospital stay. There was, however, no concomitant decrease in progressive MODS, ARDS, or mortality [113].

From the available data it appears that SGD does reduce the rate of colonization of the upper GI tract and airway by potentially pathogenic microorganisms. This is accompanied by a reduction in infection rates, most notably pneumonia [114]. SGD also prevents the selection of multiply resistant strains of gram-negative enterics [114]. Unproven effects of SGD remain the reduction of infection-related mortality and the prevention and treatment of MODS [114]. Interpreted another way, it would appear that in patients with disruption of the gut barrier or in those with profound immune suppression, control of the gut microflora is unlikely to be fully effective in preventing gut-origin septic states.

Restoration of Adequate Oxygen Delivery

As mentioned earlier in this chapter, conditions which lead to mesenteric hypoperfusion can lead to disruption of the gut barrier function. Consistent with this is the fact that xanthine oxidase inhibitors (allopurinol) have been shown to decrease the amount of disruption and the amount of translocation in animal models. Another area of investigation has been to attempt to protect the intestinal mucosa by the intraluminal instillation of protease inhibitors, nutritional supplements, or oxygen. Intraluminal infusion of 10% glucose minimized morphological mucosal damage and increased ATP concentration in a canine model of small bowel ischemia [115]. Other studies have suggested that oxygen delivered by an intraluminal route may provide protection to the intestinal mucosa during ischemia [116, 117]. Salzman et al. [118] likewise have documented preservation of the barrier function of ischemic gut mucosa when oxygen is delivered by an intraluminal route dissolved in a buffer in a guinea pig model. A clear benefit of intraluminal oxygenation was evident during the reperfusion phase of injury, at both the functional and histologic levels [118]. The amelioration of injury during reperfusion may have resulted from a protective effect of intraluminal oxygenation on cellular function during the period of ischemia [118]. Complete recovery of mucosal levels of ATP after reperfusion occurred only in oxygenated segments of bowel [118]. Findings of subnormal levels of ATP in nitrogenated bowel segments after reperfusion suggest a supply-demand mismatch in the mucosa (oxygen debt) during the ischemic phase [118].

Growth Factors

A number of studies have now evaluated the effects of several growth factors on the gut mucosal barrier function after injury. The gut mucosal cells contain receptors for insulin-like growth factor 1. In a rat model of burn injury, the administration of insulin-like growth factor 1 was associated with decreased mucosal atrophy and reduced bacterial translocation to the MLN [119]. In a murine model of burn injury, fibroblast growth factor in combination with sucralfate was associated with a major reduction in bacterial translocation to MLN, liver, spleen, and blood [120].

Summary

The movement of bacteria from the gut lumen through the gut wall and into the regional lymph and blood drainage systems has been termed "translocation." In normal man, it is a normal physiologic occurrence and may have a survival advantage in promoting natural immunity that results from the frequent sampling of the bacterial flora by the gut immune system. The mechanisms of translocation in health and disease remain to be precisely clarified. In general, the two major routes available would be transcellular or paracellular. Three primary classes of variables promote an increase in effective translocation. These classes are variables that affect the normal gastrointestinal bacterial ecology, suppression of the immune system, and ischemic, physical, and pharmacological variables that disrupt gut permeability.

Whether the gut is the "motor" of the multiple organ dysfunction syndrome remains controversial. Whether translocation is a pathogenic mechanism in this context also remains hypothetical. It may also be that the translocation rate remains relatively constant and that the increase in positive node cultures after injury reflects a suppression of the cytotoxicity function of that system. A number of therapies directed at improving the gut barrier function have undergone testing; therapies such as nutritional support, selective gut decontamination, optimization of oxygen transport and the administration of various growth factors into the gut lumen. Improved barrier function and patient outcomes have been observed with these techniques. The component of the barrier function that was affected to achieve these improved outcomes, however, remains unknown. Possibilities would include improved balance of the intestinal flora, decreased bacterial translocation, or improved gut immune function. Continued experimental and human investigations are necessary in order to clarify these issues and to develop more effective treatments.

References

1. Berg RD, Garlington AN (1979) Translocation of certain indigenous bacteria from the gastrointestinal tract to the mesenteric lymph nodes and other organs in a gnotobioic mouse model. Infect Immun 23:403
2. Alexander JW, Boyce ST, Babcock GF et al (1990) The process of microbial translocation. Ann Surg 212:496
3. Berg RD: Conspectus: bacterial translocation from the gastrointestinal tract
4. Madera JL (1990) Pathobiology of the intestinal epithelial barrier. Am J Pathol 137:1273
5. Dobbins WO (1982) Gut immunophysiology: a gastroenterologist's view with emphasis on pathophysiology. Am J Physiol 242:G1
6. Fine J (1965) Current status of the problem of traumatic shock. Surg Gynecol Obstet 120:537
7. Schimpff SC (1980) Infection prevention during profound granulocytopenia. Ann Intern Med 93:358

8. Kreger BE, Craven DE, Carling PC et al (1980) Gram negative bacteremia. III. Reassessment of etiology, epidemiology, and ecology in G12 patients. Am J Med 68:332
9. Garrison RN, Fry DE, Beberich S et al (1982) Enterococcal bacteremia: clinical implications and determinants of death. Ann Surg 196:43
10. Fry DE, Klamer TW, Garrison RN et al (1981) Atypical clostridial bacteremia. Surg Gynecol Obstet 153:28
11. Stone HH, Kolb LD, Carrie CA et al (1974) Candida sepsis: pathogenesis and principles of treatment. Ann Surg 179:697
12. Wilmore DW, Smith RJ, O'Dwyer ST et al (1988) The gut: a central organ after surgical stress. Surgery 104:917
13. Saadia R, Schein M, MacFarlane C et al (1990) Gut barrier function and the surgeon. Br J Surg 77:487
14. Fink MP (1993) Adequacy of gut oxygenation in endotoxemia and sepsis. Crit Care Med 21:54
15. Haglund U (1993) Systemic mediators released from the gut in critical illness. Crit Care Med 21:515
16. Deitch EA, Bridges W, Baker J et al (1988) Hemorrhagic shock-induced bacterial translocation is reduced by xanthine-oxidase inhibition or inactivation. Surgery 104:191
17. Deitch EA Morrison J, Berg RD et al (1990) Effect of hemorrhagic shock on permeability in conventional and antibiotic-decontaminated rats. Crit Care Med 18:529
18. Hidalgo IJ, Raub TJ, Barchardt RT (1989) Characterization of the human colon carcinoma cell line (Caco-2) as a model system for intestinal epithelial cell permeability. Gastroenterology 96:736
19. Chiu CJ, McArdle AH, Brown R et al (1970) Intestinal mucosal lesion in low-flow states. Arch Surg 101:478
20. Saydjari R, Beerthuizen GIJM, Townsend CM et al (1991) Bacterial translocation and its relationship to visceral blood flow, gut mucosal ornithine decarboxylase activity, and DNA in pigs. J Trauma 31:639
21. Baker JW, Deitch EA, Li M et al (1988) Hemorrhagic shock induced bacterial translocation from the gut. J Trauma 28:896
22. Morris SE, Navaratnam N, Herndon DN (1990) A comparison of effects of thermal injury and smoke inhalation on bacterial translocation. J Trauma 30:639
23. Navaratnam N, Morris SE, Townsend CM et al (1989) Bacterial translocation and selective mesenteric artery perfusion in an ovine model. Proc Am Burn Assoc 21:240
24. Ma L, Ma JW, Deitch EA et al (1989) General susceptibility to mucosal damage leads to bacterial translocation in a murine burn model. J Trauma 29:1245
25. Parks DA, Bulkley GB, Granger DN et al (1982) Ischemic injury in the cat small intestine: role of superoxide radicals. Gastroenterology 82:9
26. Grisham MB, Hernandez LA, Granger DN (1986) Xanthine oxidase and neutrophil infiltration in intestinal ischemia. Am J Physiol 251:567
27. Deitch EA, Berg RD, Specian RD (1987) Endotoxin promotes the translocation of bacteria from the gut. Arch Surg 122:185
28. Deitch EA, Taylor M, Grisham MB et al (1989) Endotoxin induces bacterial translocation and increases xanthine oxidase activity. J Trauma 29:1679
29. Deitch EA, Specian RD, Berg RD (1991) Endotoxin-induced bacterial translocation and mucosal permeability: role of xanthine oxidase complement activation and macrophage products. Crit Care Med 19:78
30. Zimmermann BT, Parks DA, Grisham MB et al (1988) Allopurinol does not enhance antioxidant properties of extracellular fluid. Am J Physiol 255:H202
31. Fink MP, Antorrsson JB, Wang H et al (1991) Increased intestinal permeability in endotoxic pigs: mesenteric hypoperfusion as an etiologic factor. Arch Surg 126:211
32. Menzies IS (1987) Transmucosal passage of inert molecules in health and disease. In: Skadhauge E, Heintze K (eds) Falk Symposium 36. MTP Press, Lancaster, p 527
33. Bulkley GB, Kuietys PR, Parks DA et al (1985) Relationship of blood flow and oxygen consumption to ischemic injury in a canine small intestine. Gastroenterology 89:852

34. Deitch EA, Specian RD, Grisham MB et al (1992) Zymosan-induced bacterial translocation: a study of mechanisms. Crit Care Med 20:782
35. Schirmer WJ, Schirmer JM, Neff GB et al (1988) Systemic complement activation produces thermodynamic changes characteristic of sepsis. Arch Surg 123:316
36. Deitch EA, Ma W, Ma L et al (1990) Protein malnutrition predisposes the inflammatory-induced gut-origin septic states. Ann Surg 211:560
37. Walker RI, Porvaznik MJ (1978) Disruption of the permeability barrier (zonula occludens) between intestinal epithelial cells by lethal doses of endotoxin. Infect Immun 21:655
38. O'Dwyer ST, Michie HR, Ziegler TR et al (1988) A single dose of endotoxin increases intestinal permeability in humans. Arch Surg 123:1459
39. Steiner M, Bourges HR, Freedman LS et al (1968) Effect of starvation on the tissue composition of the small intestine in the rat. Am J Physiol 215:75
40. Souba WW, Klimberg VS, Plumley DA et al (1990) Current research review: the role of glutamine in maintaining a healthy gut and supporting metabolic response to injury and infection. J Surg Res 48:383
41. Barton RG, Cerra FB, Wells CL (1992) Effect of a diet deficient in essential fatty acids on the translocation of intestinal bacteria. JPEN 16:122
42. Wells CL, Maddaus MA, Simmons RL (1987) Role of the macrophage in the translocation of intestinal bacteria. Arch Surg 122:48
43. Wells CL, Maddaus MA, Simmons RL (1987) Role of the macrophage in the translocation of intestinal bacteria. Arch Surg 122:48
44. Mainous MR, Rso P, Berg RD et al (1991) Studies of the route, magnitude, and time course of bacterial translocation in a model of systemic inflammation. Arch Surg 126:33
45. Wells CL, Maddaus MA, Simmons RL (1988) Proposed mechanisms for the translocation of intestinal bacteria. Rev Infect Dis 10:858
46. Alexander JW, Boyce ST, Babcock GF et al (1990) The process of microbial translocation. Ann Surg 212:496
47. Cole GT, Sesham KR, Pope LM et al (1988) Morphologic aspects of gastrointestinal tract invasion by Candida albicans in the infant mouse. J Med Vet Mycol 26:173
48. Wells CL, Jechorek RP, Erlandson SL (1990) Evidence for the translocation of Enterococcus faecalis across the mouse intestinal tract. J Infect Dis 162:82
49. Papa M, Halperin Z, Rubinstein E et al (1983) The effect of ischemia of the dog's colon on transmural migration of bacteria and endotoxin. J Surg Res 35:264
50. Wells CL, Rotstein OD, Pruett TL et al (1986) Intestinal bacteria translocate into experimental intra-abdominal abscesses. Arch Surg 121:102
51. Rosenberg JC, Kaplan MP, Lyse K (1980) Mechanisms of steroid suppression of immune function: effect of methylprednisolone on lymphocyte activation and proliferation. Surgery 88:193
52. Berg RD (1983) Bacterial translocation from the gastrointestinal tract of mice receiving immunosuppressive chemotherapeutic agents. Curr Microbiol 8:285
53. Berg RD, Itoh K (1986) Bacterial translocation from the gastrointestinal tract — immunologic aspects. Microecol Ther 16:131
54. Christan NV, McLean RPH, Meakins JL (1980) Host defense in blunt trauma: interrelationships of kinetics of energy and depressed neutrophil function, neutrophil status and sepsis. J Trauma 20:833
55. O'Mahorrey JB, Palder S, Roderick M et al (1983) Depression of cellular immunity after multiple trauma in the absence of sepsis. J Trauma 23:654 (abstract)
56. Sab T, Blumernstock FA, Scoville WA (1978) Cryoprecipitate reversal of opsenic alpha-2 surface binding glycoprotein deficiency in septic surgical and traumatic patients. Science 20:622
57. Altura BM, Hershey SG (1973) Reticuloendothelial function in experimental injury and tolerance to shock. Adv Exp Med Biol 33:545
58. Ravin HA, Fine J (1962) Biological implications of intestinal endotoxins. Fed Proc 21:65

59. Fink MP, Gardiner M, Macvittie JJ (1985) Sublethal hemorrhage impairs the acute peritoneal inflammatory response in rats. J Trauma 25:334
60. Owens WE, Barg RD (1980) Bacterial translocation from the gastrointestinal tract of athymic (nu/nu) mice. Infect Immun 27:461
61. Border JR, Hassett J, LaDuce J et al (1987) The gut origin septic states in blunt multiple trauma (ISS=40) in the ICU. Ann Surg 206:427
62. Faist E, Riedel A, Riebu H et al (1986) Prostaglandin E_2 dependent suppression of interleukin 2 production in patients with major trauma. Conference Program American Association for the Surgery of Trauma, Honolulu, p 56
63. Wilmore DW, Lang JM, Mason AD et al (1974) Catecholamines: mediators of the hypermetabolic response to thermal injury. Ann Surg 180:653
64. Bjerson AB, Bjorson HS, Altemeier WA (1981) Serum mediated inhibition of polymorphonuclear leukocyte function following burn injury. Ann Surg 194:568
65. Antonacci AC, Good RA, Gupten S (1982) T-cell subpopulations following thermal injury. Surg Gynecol Obstet 155:1
66. Alexander JW, Moncrief JA (1986) Alterations of the immune response following severe thermal injury. Arch Surg 93:75
67. Wilson RF (1986) Sepsis prophylaxis in the surgical patient at risk. In: Sibbald WJ, Sprung CL (eds) New Horizons, p 301
68. Holper K, Olcay I, Kitahama A et al (1974) Effect of ischemia on hepatic parenchymal and reticuloendothelial function in the baboon. Surgery 76:423
69. Schirmer WJ, Schirmer JM, Naff GB et al (1987) Alternate pathway complement activation induces reductions in effective hepatic blood flow. Ann Surg 44:304
70. Machiedo GN, Hurd T, Rush BF Jr et al (1988) Temporal relationship of hepatocellular dysfunction and ischemia in sepsis. Arch Surg 123:42
71. Jones WF II, Minei JP, Barber AE et al (1990) Bacterial translocation and intestinal atrophy after thermal injury and burn wound sepsis. Ann Surg 211:399
72. Marano MA, Moldawer LL, Fong Y et al (1988) Cachectin/TNF production in experimental burns and Pseudomonas infection. Arch Surg 123:1383
73. Chandra RK (1983) Nutrition, infection and immunity: present knowledge and future directions. Lancet i:688
74. Meyer J, Yurt RN, Dubancy R et al (1988) Differential neutrophil activation before and after endotoxin infusion in enterally versus parenterally fed volunteers. Surg Gynecol Obstet 167:501
75. Berg RD, Owens WE (1979) Inhibition of translocation of viable E. coli from the gastrointestinal tract of mice by bacterial antagonism. Infect Immun 25:820
76. Deitch EA, Sittig K, Li M, Berg R (1990) Obstructive jaundice promotes bacterial translocation from the gut. Am J Surg 159:79
77. Slocum MM, Sittig KM, Specian RD et al (1992) Absence of intestinal bile promotes bacterial translocation. Am Surg 58:305
78. Alverdy JC, Aoys E, Moss GS (1988) Total parenteral nutrition promotes bacterial translocation from the gut. Surgery 104:185
79. Spaeth G, Specian RD, Berg RD et al (1990) Bulk prevents bacterial translocation induced by the oral administration of total parenteral nutrition solution. JPEN 14:442
80. Carrico CY, Meakins JL, Marchall JC et al (1986) Multiple-organ failure syndrome. Arch Surg 121:196
81. Billiar TR, Maddaus MA, West MA et al (1988) Intestinal gram negative bacterial overgrowth in vivo augments in the in vitro response of Kupffer cells to endotoxin. Ann Surg 208:532
82. Cerra FB (1987) Hypermetabolism, organ failure, and metabolic support. Surgery 101:1
83. Keller GA, West MA, Cerra FB et al (1985) Multiple systems organ failure: modulation of hepatocyte protein synthesis by endotoxin activated Kupffer cells. Ann Surg 201:87

84. Pardy BJ, Spencer RC, Dudley HAF (1977) Hepatic reticuloendothelial protection against bacteremia in experimental hemorrhagic shock. Surgery 81:193
85. Katz S, Grosfield JL, Gross K et al (1984) Impaired bacterial clearance and trapping in obstructive jaundice. Ann Surg 199:14
86. Sabe TM, Jaffe E (1980) Plasma fibronectin (opsonic glyceprotein): its synthesis by vascular endothelial cells and role in cardiopulmonary integrity following trauma as related to reticuloendothelial function. Am J Med 68:577
87. Cerra FB, Holman RT, Bankey PE et al (1990) Nutritional pharmacology: its role in the hypermetabolism-organ failure syndrome. Crit Care Med 18:S154
88. Marshall JC, Lee C, Meakins JV et al (1987) Kupffer cell modulation of the systemic immune response. Arch Surg 122:191
89. Kahky MP, Daniel CO, Cricz AB et al (1990) Portal infusion of tumor necrosis factor increases mortality in rats. J Surg Res 49:138
90. Marshall JC, Christou NV, Horn R et al (1988) The microbiology of multiple organ failure: the proximal gastrointestinal tract as an occult reservoir of pathogens. Arch Surg 123:309
91. Baker JN, Deitch EA, Berg RD et al (1988) Hemorrhagic shock induces bacterial translocation from the gut. J Trauma 28:896
92. Sori AJ, Rush BF Jr, Lyse TW et al (1988) The gut as source of sepsis after hemorrhagic shock. Am J Surg 155:187
93. Koziol JM, Rush BF Jr, Smith SM et al (1988) Occurrence of bacteremia during and after hemorrhagic shock. J Trauma 28:10
94. Rush BF Jr, Sori AJ, Murphy TF et al (1988) Endotoxemia and bacteremia during hemorrhagic shock. Ann Surg 207:549
95. Goris RJA, Boekholtz WKF, van Bebber IPT et al (1986) Multiple organ failure and sepsis without bacteremia: an experimental model. Arch Surg 121:897
96. Deitch EA, Kemper AC, Specian RD et al (1992) A study of the relationship among survival, gut origin sepsis, and bacterial translocation in a model of systemic inflammation. J Trauma 32:141
97. Fukushima R, Gianotti L, Alexander JW et al (1992) The degree of bacterial translocation is a determinant factor for mortality after burn injury and is improved by prostaglandin analogs. Ann Surg 216:438
98. Morales J, Kibsey P, Thomas PD et al (1992) The effects of ischemia and ischemia-reperfusion on bacterial translocation, lipid peroxidation and gut histology: studies on hemorrhagic shock in pigs. J Trauma 33:221
99. Moore FA, Moore EE, Poggetti R et al (1991) Gut bacterial translocation via the portal vein: a clinical perspective with major torso trauma. J Trauma 31:629
100. Levine GM, Deren JJ, Steiger E et al (1974) Role of intake in maintenance of gut mass and disaccharide activity. Gastroenterology 67:975
101. Mochizuki H, Trocki O, Dominioni L et al (1984) Mechanism of prevention postburn hypermetabolism and catabolism by early enteral feeding. Ann Surg 200:297
102. O'Dwyer ST, Scott T, Smith RJ et al (1987) 5-fluorouracil toxicity on small intestinal mucosa but not white blood cells is decreased by glutamine. Clin Res 35:369 (abstract)
103. Alexander JW (1986) Nutrition and infection: new perspectives for an old problem. Arch Surg 121:966
104. Moore FA et al (1989) TEN versus TPN following major abdominal-reduced septic morbidity. J Trauma 29:916
105. Cerra FB et al (1991) Nutrient modulation of inflammatory and immune function. Ann J Surg 161:230
106. Daly JM, Lieberman MD, Goldfine J et al. (1992) Enteral nutrition with supplemental arginine, RNA and omega-3 fatty acids in patients after operation: immunologic, metabolic, and clinical outcome. Surgery 112:56
107. Cerra FB et al (1990) Effects of enteral nutrient on in vitro tests of immune function in ICU patients: a preliminary report. Nutrition 56:84

108. Stowtenbeek CP, Seane HFK, Miranda DR et al (1984) The effect of SDD on colonization and infection rate in multiple trauma patients. Intensive Care Med 10:185
109. Ledingham IM, Eastaway AT, McKay IC et al (1988) Triple regimen of SDD, systemic cefotaxime, and microbiological surveillance for prevention and acquired infection in ICU. Lancet i:785
110. Kerver AIH, Rommes JA, Meuisseu-Verhage EAE et al (1988) Prevention of colonization and infection in critically ill patients: a prospective randomized study. Intensive Care Med 16:1087
111. Brun-Buissen C, Legrande P, Rauss A et al (1989) Intestinal decontamination for control of nosocomial multi-resistant and gram negative bacilli. Study of an outbreak in an intensive care unit. Ann Intern Med 110:873
112. Hartenauer U, Muney AE, Williams PS et al (1990) Infection surveillance and selective decontamination of the digestive tract (SDD) in critically ill patients: results of a controlled study. Infection 18:522
113. Cerra FB, Maddaus MA, Dunn DL et al (1992) Selective gut decontamination reduces nosocomial infections and length of stay but not mortality or organ failure in surgical intensive care unit patients. Arch Surg 127:163
114. Koruda MJ (1993) Gut sterilization to prevent nosocomial infection. In: Solonkin JS (ed) New Horizons, p 1994
115. Chin C, Scott W, Gurd F (1970) Intestinal mucosal lesion in low-flow states. II: the protective effect of intraluminal glucose as energy substrate. Arch Surg 101:484
116. Shute K (1976) Effect of intraluminal oxygen on experimental ischemia of the intestine. Gut 17:1001
117. Oldham K, Guice K, Gore D et al (1987) Treatment of intestinal ischemia with oxygenated intraluminal perfluorocarbons. Am J Surg 153:291
118. Salzman A, Wallert S, Warre H et al (1993) Intraluminal oxygenation ameliorates ischemia/reperfusion-induced gut mucosal hypermeability in pigs. Circ Shock 40:37
119. Hyuang KF, Chung DH, Herndon DN (1993) Insulinlike growth factor reduces gut atrophy and bacterial translocation after severe burn injury. Arch Surg 128:47
120. Gianotti L, Alexander W, Jukushima R, Pyles T (1993) Reduction of bacterial translocation with oral fibroblast growth factor and sucralfate. Am J Surg 165:195

Tumor Necrosis Factor and Other Cytokines in Septic Syndrome

B. Beutler

Introduction

Historically, interventions in the septic syndrome have consisted of attemps to deal with the infection that causes it. In some respects, a great deal of sophistication has been acquired, since antimicrobial therapy has remained effective despite the evolving resistance of pathogenic organisms. Even in patients who lack immune mechanisms necessary for protection against microbes, an *"artificial immune system"* may be rendered pharmacologically through the use of antibiotics.

Beyond this, the major focus of therapy is no more than supportive care: the assurance of adequate blood pressure, tissue perfusion, ventilation, electrolyte balance, and organ function. Each of these aspects of host physiology is threatened during sepsis. Remarkably, many different types of invasive organism are able to cause the septic syndrome. Certain viruses (e.g., dengue and yellow fever), parasites (e.g., malaria), and eubacteria (both gram-negative and gram-positive organisms) can provoke such a response, although they have little or no structural similarity to one another. This fact, in itself, bespeaks a final common pathway leading to demise of the host.

Why should such a pathway exist, and what are its molecular components? It might be expected that a precise understanding of the sequence of events would allow specific interventions to be used in protecting the host. The recognition that infection initiates sepsis, but that treatment of infection is not sufficient to terminate the septic syndrome, is not new. However, the elucidation of events leading to widespread organ failure is new and remains an unfinished story.

Herein, an attempt will be made to follow the sequence of reactions that transpire in sepsis, with emphasis given to possible (and actual) interventional strategies.

Microbial Inducers and the Host Sensing Mechanism

Teleologically speaking, the immune system represents the imperfect product of an attempt by higher organisms to deal with an overwhelming assembly of hostile organisms that attempt to colonize and kill them. Due to their short generation time, viruses, bacteria and other microbial invaders are capable of defeating their metazoan hosts in an evolutionary "footrace;" if it is to their advantage to develop and sustain a high level of pathogenicity, they will invariably do so. Yet the host is shaped by the presence of pathogens in its environment and, correspondingly, evolves an array of broadly active protective devices that may have an anticipatory quality about them. Hence, the immune system features a humoral and cell-bound system of proteins that are capable of binding virtually any antigen that might arise in nature. The cytokine system is a second, and probably more primitive, immune mechanism, whereby a subset of cells may signal the presence of disease so as to allow the mobilization of host defenses at a distance.

The release of cytokines, which serve to protect the host but which also may injure it, entails recognition of microbial products by receptors which have been but partly characterized. Perhaps the most studied recognition system is that which initiates the response to the lipopolysaccharides (LPSs) released by gram-negative bacteria. LPS, or endotoxins, have been known for nearly a century as heat-stable toxins derived from bacteria which eventuate shock in experimental animals and humans (for reviews, see [1, 2]). LPS are of variable structure, but feature a disaccharide backbone containing two phosphate groups and a number of acyl chains attached to still other acyl chains by acyloxyacyl linkages. A polysaccharide moiety of variable size confers antigenicity to the LPS molecule, but does not seem to mediate toxicity. Rather, toxicity is a function of the lipid moiety, which engages specific receptors on cells.

LPS is not toxic to most cells, which, indeed, are quite indifferent to its presence. The indirect nature of endotoxin action was revealed by transplantation studies involving the endotoxin-resistant C3H/HeJ mouse [3]. Animals of this strain were shown to be homozygous for a mutation, mapped to chromosome 4 [4, 5], which renders them unresponsive to all of the biological effects of LPS. Originally considered a potential LPS receptor, the protein encoded by this gene remains obscure and may actually represent an early component of the LPS signaling pathway. In any case, it was shown that mice of the C3H/HeJ strain were rendered sensitive to the lethal effect of LPS by transplantation of hematopoietic precursors derived from LPS-sensitive animals. Conversely, LPS-sensitive mice could be rendered resistant to LPS by transplantation with stem cells from C3H/HeJ mice.

Additional studies, involving the adoptive transfer of macrophages, indicated that macrophages were the principal cellular mediator of endotoxic shock [6].

The best characterized receptor for LPS is that molecule known as CD14 [7]. CD14 resides on a number of cell types including macrophages. It is a glycerolphosphoinositol-linked component of the plasma membrane, and may also exist in a secreted form [8–14]. By directly engaging LPS, or LPS linked to LPS-binding protein (LBP), CD14 effectively concentrates the agonist and allows the sensing of minute concentrations of LPS in plasma or in tissues.

However, CD14 is not the product of the *Lps* gene, which is required for biological responses to endotoxin. CD14 does not transmit a signal to the cytoplasm and, indeed, may be bypassed by administration of high concentrations of LPS to cells. Hence, 70Z/3 cells, which lack CD14, are LPS-responsive provided that high concentrations of LPS are added to the culture.

Certain monoclonal antibodies against CD14 do not impair LPS binding, yet block further transduction of the LPS signal [15]. Such studies suggest the direct interaction between CD14 and more distal components of the LPS signaling pathway. Interestingly, modified forms of LPS, such as lipid IVa (a form which lacks acyloxyacyl side groups), are capable of directly activating mouse cells, but antagonize the response of human cells to LPS [16–18]. Since there appears to be no difference in the binding of lipid IVa to human and mouse CD14 (P. Tobias, personal communication), a direct interaction between LPS and later components of the signaling pathway reasonably be suspected.

In many ways the identification of the product of the *Lps* gene would represent a breakthrough in understanding of LPS signal transduction. This protein is, in fact, the gateway to LPS response. It is to be hoped that novel approaches to the cloning of this gene may soon shed light on its function.

Of course, other components of eubacteria and other microorganisms are capable of activating macrophages to produce cytokines. For example, lipopeptides drived from *Treponema pallidum* and from *Borrelia burgdorferi* stimulate macrophages to secrete tumor necrosis factor (TNF) [19], apparently through a pathway distinct from that utilized by LPS. The TNF gene is also activated by gram-positive organisms, perhaps through interaction with lipoteichoic acid (B. Beutler, unpublished observation). Lipoarabinomannan (LAM) and other products of mycobacteria also may act as an inducer of TNF synthesis [20–22]. Plasmodium species [23–26] and trypanosomes [27–29] also are capable of activating TNF synthesis, presumably through the action of lipid-bearing inducing molecules.

The molecular targets of these toxins are obscure. Aside from CD14, no biologically relevant receptors for these nonprotein toxins have been identified. It is noteworthy that many of the inducing agents are lipids; however, this observation does not, in itself, provide much information as to the nature of the receptors.

Certain proteins of microbial origin also activate TNF and/or interleukin-1 (IL-1) synthesis. Bacterial exotoxins, including Shiga toxin (SLT-I) [30, 31], toxic shock toxin (TSST-1) [32–34], and staphylococcal enterotoxin B (SEB) [35] have each been reported to stimulate TNF production by cultured monocytes or macrophages, or *in vivo*. In mice, SLT-I appears to induce TNF reporter gene expression specifically in renal tissue [31]. This is of interest, since the kidney is the principal target of SLT-I action when this exotoxin induces the hemolytic uremic syndrome. It is possible that site-specific expression of the TNF gene, determined by exotoxin receptor specificity, may lead to many different clinical presentations wrought by a single cytokine.

Pivotal Cytokines and Their Control

Many cytokines are synthesized in response to an activator such as LPS. Which of these are most relevant to the development of shock? The *inflammatory character, tissue origins, temporal pattern of production, effect of passive immunization,* and *direct toxicity* of each cytokine must be considered in assessing its relative contribution to the septic syndrome. In Table 1, a number of cytokines are examined according to these criteria.

Since septic shock represents an uncontrolled, disseminated inflammatory process, the cytokines that initiate it likely exert an inflammatory effect, normally operating at a local level. IL-1α, IL-1β, TNF, interleukin-8 (IL-8), macrophage inflammatory protein (MIP)-1α, MIP-1β, and interferon-γ each qualify in this respect. The first six cytokines are involved in the recruitment and activation of neutrophils, whereas the last cytokine plays a prominent role in the activation of mononuclear phagocytes IL-8 and the MIPs belong to a large and growing family of small inflammatory polypeptide hormones. Other members of the group include monocyte chemotaxis activating factor (MCAF), gro-α, gro-β, RANTES, and platelet factor IV (for a review, see [36, 37]). While structural homology is rather vague among members of the so-called "intercrine" family, which is split into two major divisions, the overlap of function is large, and it is not clear that any one member dominates in the pathogenesis of sepsis. IL-1α and IL-1β share common receptors and have numerous proinflammatory effects [38–43], overlapping in many of their activities with TNF. Sensitization to the effects of IL-1 and TNF and augmentation of their production are rendered by interferon-γ, which also is known to have certain inflammatory characteristics, such as pyrogenicity [44]. Other cytokines, such as interleukin-6 (IL-6), play an uncertain role in the inflammatory response. IL-6 is known to abet certain features of the acute phase response, such as thrombocytosis [45–49], and the production of

Table 1. Properties of cytokines released during sepsis, with bearing on their pathogenetic importance

Cytokine	Propensity to cause inflammation	Hematopoietic origin	Early production	Protection by passive immunization	Direct toxicity
TNF-α	++++	+++	++++	+++	++++
TNF-β	++++	++++	++	?	++++
IL-1α/β	+++	++	++	+++	++
Interferon-γ	++	++++	++	++	+++
IL-6	+	−	+	−	−
IL-8	++	++++	+	−	−
MIP	++	+++	++	−	−

TNF, tumor necrosis factor; IL-interleukin; MIP, macrophage inflammatory protein

acute phase reactants [50], but cannot be described as a major organizer of the inflammatory response.

The lethal factor(s) in sepsis is(are) derived from cells of hematopoietic origin, as noted above [3]. The secondary participation of cytokines derived from nonhematopoietic cells may not be discounted; however, the initiation of the syndrome must depend upon mediators produced by cells that originate in the marrow. TNF is such a protein, as it seems to be produced chiefly by monocyte/macrophages [51–56]. IL-1 might also qualify, although it is also produced by extrahematopoietic cells such as keratinocytes, which are said to contain enormous quantities of the protein [57, 58]. Other candidate mediators include interferon-γ (principally a product of T cells), the MIPs (produced chiefly by macrophages) and IL-8 (also derived from macrophages).

If a cytokine plays a central or initiating role in the pathogenesis of septic shock, one would expect that it must be produced very early in the process. To some extent, this feature supercedes that of direct toxicity or inflammatory potential. While many toxic and inflammatory factors might be produced in the course of shock, there is no escape from the conclusion that the initiating factor(s) must be produced early and must be hematopoietically derived. TNF is made earlier than all of the other candidate mediators listed in Table 1. Its production is followed by "waves" of other cytokines (including IL-1 and IL-6) [59]. This finding constitutes a strong argument favoring its role as an initiating mediator.

It is to be expected that selective blockade of important mediators of the septic syndrome, whether by antagonists, antibodies, or soluble receptors, ought to prevent or at least diminish the consequences of challenge with LPS, or any relevant infectious agent. Passive immunization against TNF [60–64] or neutralization of TNF [65] has been shown to attenuate the lethal effect of LPS. Similar studies have confirmed the participation of IL-I [66, 67] and interferon-γ [68] in the septic syndrome. These observations may be interpreted to indicate the involvement of all three factors, although the results say nothing about the order of involvement, or about which (if any) of the factors are the primary mediators of shock. For example, it is clear that interference with production or action of terminal mediators of shock (e.g., leukotrienes, or platelet activating factor) also has a protective effect in animal models [69–74]. Very little work has been done to test the effect of combined blockade of multiple cytokines. It is very likely, as pointed out below, that such an approach would lead to vastly more effective protection against shock than the use of a single agent.

A final test of cytokine involvement in shock is that of direct toxicity. Administered alone or in combination with other cytokines, a given agent should be able to reproduce the derangements that characterize sepsis in the absence of a true infectious stimulus. Of course, attempts to recreate the septic syndrome may be unsuccessful, because it may not be possible to reproduce the temporal pattern of cytokine production and because systemic administration of a cytokine may not mimic its site-specific production *in vivo*. However, such an approach can give considerable insight into the individual and coordinated effects of different cytokines.

On the basis of studies carried out to date, TNF may be assigned the earliest and most fundamental role among cytokines that mediate septic shock. It is clear that TNF can induce the synthesis of IL-1 [75] as well as IL-6 [75–78] and that blockade of TNF activity will prevent the induction of IL-1 as well as IL-6 by the infusion of an invasive stimulus such as live *E. coli* [59]. IL-1, while oddly lacking in toxicity if administered as an isolated preparation, clearly contributes to the septic syndrome, since antagonism of its action in the context of sepsis sharply diminishes the incidence of lethal outcome [66, 67]. Interferon-γ blockade also prevents lethality [68], and it may be assumed that it, like IL-1, plays a contributory role in shock. In part, this role may depend upon its ability to sensitize to the toxic effects of other cytokines and encourage their production.

Signaling Events in the Production of Tumor Necrosis Factor and Related Cytokines

Expression of the TNF gene has been thoroughly studied, and at least some of the mechanisms that control TNF biosynthesis apply in the regulation of other cytokines. In studying expression of cytokine genes, the nature of the signaling pathway that activates these genes is examined de facto. It has become apparent, for example, that most cytokine genes are dependent upon nuclear factor (NF)-κB [79–82] or the related factor NF-GMα [79] for activation. NF-κB is a positively acting transcription factor that, in quiescent cells, exists as a cytoplasmic complex with a second protein that functions as an inhibitor of NF-κB action (IκB) [81]. IκB is modified, perhaps by phosphorylation, so as to release NF-κB following cell activation. The NF-κB then translocates to the nucleus, binding to a recognition motif within the promoter of diverse cytokines and facilitating initiation of transcription.

Other transcription factors, such as AP1 (often consisting of a dimer composed of the proteins fos and jun) may also contribute to activation of many cytokine genes at a transcriptional level. Still other factors may act to negatively influence expression. Thus, the response to LPS induction is, in at least some cases, short-lived [83]. Indeed, cells become refractory to LPS activation after an initial exposure, a phenomenon which may to some extent be exercised at the level of cytokine gene transcription.

Transcriptional activation may be blocked by certain drugs, such as dexamethasone [84], pentoxifylline [85, 86], and 2-aminopurine [87], each of which acts through a distinct mechanism to interfere with signal transduction. Although the precise mechanism of action by which each of these agents acts remains obscure, dexamethasone (like other glucocorticoid hormones) appears to act at very early stage in the signaling pathway, since its administration to cells blocks translational activation (see below) and transcriptional activation of TNF synthesis within macrophages. Pentoxifylline exerts a specific effect on TNF synthesis (to the exclusion of effects on IL-1 or IL-6 synthesis, for example) [88–90]. It is known to inhibit phosphodiesterase, thereby increasing cytoplasmic cAMP levels, and may conceivably exert its action through other effects as well. Elevation of cAMP, whether caused by inhibition of phosphodiesterase or by other mechanisms, strongly inhibits TNF gene transcription [86]. Finally, 2-aminopurine acts as a protein kinase inhibitor and as such appears capable of abrogating signals that initiate transcription as well [87].

Transcriptional activation is but one process by which cytokine release is effected. At least some cytokines, and perhaps most of them, are also translationally repressed by virtue of their content of a (U + A)-rich element within the 3′-untranslated region of their respective mRNAs [91, 92]. Translational repression is overcome by cell activation in the case of the TNF mRNA, which is more efficiently translated following stimulation by LPS [93] or ultraviolet light [94]. The molecular events that cause translational repression or favor its release remain to be deciphered, although certain RNA binding proteins may very well be involved [95].

Clearly, within a common cellular environment, some cytokine genes respond to a given activating signal more strongly than others. Moreover, temporal differences in response exist, suggesting that the state of cell activation evolves over time, favoring the activation of one set of genes, then another, and then still others. Certain drugs may interrupt cell activation and arrest the progressive release of cytokines; however, commitment to activation also occurs [84] so that some agents (notably glucocorticoids) become ineffectual, and it is necessary to halt the activation process by a different approach at later and later stages.

The Posttranslational Processing and Secretion of Cytokines

Most cytokines are expressed as prohormones, bearing a classical signal sequence that dictates their efficient secretion. There are exceptions, however, and with time the distinction between cytokines and cell surface proteins has become blurred, since many bioactive proteins, capable of engaging specific cell surface receptors, can exist in both soluble and cell bound forms.

TNF, for example, has a hydrophobic signal peptide sequence and is, for the most part, efficiently secreted after proteolytic cleavage of the prohormone to yield a mature product, through the action of an elastase-like enzyme that has two potential cleavage sites within the murine protein sequence [96]. However, a fraction of the TNF that is synthesized fails to undergo cleavage and therefore is diverted to the plasma membrane, where it may retain weak biological activity [97, 98]. The function of this membrane-associated TNF remains to be determined. It has been observed on both macrophages and on lymphocytes, and certain noncleavable mutants have been produced so as to assure membrane localization [98]. The physical state of the membrane-associated TNF has yet to be determined. Specifically, given that secreted TNF is a trimeric protein [99], it is not clear whether the major form of membrane-associated TNF is a homotrimer consisting of three prohormone subunits, or whether a single prohormone anchors two processed subunits to the membrane.

Some cytokines, such as the IL-1 molecules, are secreted through a different and poorly understood mechanism, which may in fact be lysis of the cell [100]. The IL-1 molecules are also produced as prohormones which undergo cleavage by IL-1 converting enzyme (ICE), the cDNA for which has now been cloned [101–104]. ICE is the object of considerable interest, since specific ICE antagonists may effectively prevent the formation of biologically active IL-1 [105].

Many cytokines are glycosylated; however, aside from influencing the stability of the protein in circulation, it is unclear that glycosylation functionally alters any of the cytokines, which can effectively engage their receptors whether or not a glycosyl moiety is present.

The Immediate Consequences of Cytokine Release

The receptors for different cytokines transmit distinct signals but often are activated by aggregation on the cell surface. This appears to be the case with the TNF and lymphotoxin receptors, the receptor for interferon-γ and the receptors for hemopoietins such as erythropoietin. In aggregating, it seems probable that an active site is generated, yielding a specific but yet to be identified enzymatic activity. Few details of the signaling pathway triggered by any cytokine have been elucidated. Therefore, it may be said that neither the pathways leading to cytokine biosynthesis nor the pathways leading to cytokine effect are clearly understood and that a great many therapeutic opportunities await their determination.

Once cytokine release has occurred, a second series of events transpire within the target cell population. A part of the action of cytokines may be of an autocrine nature. Many cytokines (among them, TNF) exert part of their influence through NF-κB activation [78, 79, 106–108]. Thus, the same signal that leads to cytokine release in the first instance may also lead to a second wave of release and/or perpetuation of the primary response.

Endothelial Cells and Neutrophils as Important Targets of the Cytokine Cascade

In septic syndrome, margination of neutrophils with resulting microvascular occlusion and transudation of fluid and cells from the intravascular space may lead to generalized hypotension and tissue injury. These events transpire as the result of a cytokine-driven interaction between the neutrophils and the endothelium, the molecular components of which have now been partially deciphered.

TNF is the cytokine best studied in this respect. On the endothelial surface, TNF induces the production of intercellular adhesion molecule-1 (ICAM-1) and endothelial leukocyte adhesion molecule-1 (ELAM-1) which bind to corresponding receptors on the neutrophil, among them the antigens lymphocyte function antigen (LFA)-1 and Mac-1 (which is also up-regulated by TNF). LFA-1 and Mac-1 are members of the β_2-integrin family. They are heterodimers consisting of a CD18 chain combined with a CD11 or CD11b chain, respectively. The importance of these and other heterodimers bearing the CD18 chain has been established from the fact that severe immunodeficiency results from mutational deletion of CD18 [109].

The endothelial surface is normally anticoagulant in character, but on exposure to TNF, IL-1, and perhaps other cytokines acquires procoagulant characteristics. These cytokines stimulate the production of tissue factor and diminish the expression of cell surface thrombomodulin, leading to the accretion of thrombus [110]. Possibly, the development of disseminated intravascular coagulation depends upon this process.

What Can Be Done To Halt Development of the Septic Syndrome?

Despite the complexity of shock, it is now clear that the syndrome begins in a rather simple fashion. Mutation of a single gene, for example, can abolish the toxicity of LPS. Many other agents that trigger the septic syndrome may similarly confront a "bottleneck," either at the level of signal transduction or at the level of cytokines that they induce. Such points of activation represent targets for pharmacotherapy.

It will be noted that many opportunities to intervene in sepsis have already presented themselves. Agents which:

1) disrupt signaling so as to prevent activation of cytokine synthesis,
2) selectively destroy cytokines [111],
3) prevent interaction between cytokines and their cell membrane receptors,
4) impede signaling events in the target cell population, or
5) prevent the secondary effects of cytokines (e.g., the functioning of molecules that cause adhesive interaction) are likely to interrupt the septic syndrome.

Some of these approaches have already been reduced to practice and are the subject of ongoing investigation at a clinical level. There is reason for optimism that the once baffling constellation of problems that occurs in shock may yield to our understanding of the molecules that cause it.

References

1. Morrison DC, Ryan JL (1979) Bacterial endotoxins and host immune responses. Adv Immunol 28:293–450
2. Morrison DC, Ulevitch RJ (1978) The effects of bacterial endotoxins on host mediation systems. Am J Pathol 93:526–617
3. Michalek SM, Moore RN, McGhee JR, Rosenstreich DL, Mergenhagen SE (1980) The primary role of lymphoreticular cells in the mediation of host responses to bacterial endotoxin. J Infect Dis 141:55–63
4. Watson J, Riblet R, Taylor BA (1977) The response of recombinant inbred strains of mice to bacterial lipopolysaccharides. J Immunol 118:2088–2093
5. Watson J, Kelly K, Largen M, Taylor BA (1978) The genetic mapping of a defective LPS response gene in C3H/HeJ mice. J Immunol 120:422–424
6. Freudenberg MA, Keppler D, Galanos C (1986) Requirement for lipopolysaccharide-responsive macrophages in galactosamine-induced sensitization to endotoxin. Infect Immun 51:891–895
7. Beck G, Benach JL, Habicht GS (1989) Isolation of interleukin 1 from joint fluids of patients with lyme disease. J Rheumatol 16:800–806
8. Wright SD, Jong MTC (1986) Adhesion-promoting receptors on human macrophages recognize Escherichia coli by binding to lipopolysaccharide. J Exp Med 164:1876–1888
9. Wright SD, Tobias PS, Ulevitch RJ, Ramos RA (1989) Lipopolysaccharide (LPS) binding protein opsonizes LPS-bearing particle for recognition by a novel receptor on macrophages. J Exp Med 170:1231–1241
10. Schumann RR, Leong SR, Flaggs GW et al (1990) Structure and function of lipopolysaccharide binding protein. Science 249:1429–1431
11. Wright SD, Ramos RA, Tobias PS, Ulevitch RJ, Mathison JC (1990) CD14, a receptor for complexes of lipopolysaccharide (LPS) and LPS binding protein. Science 249:1431–1433
12. Ferrero E, Goyert SM (1988) Nucleotide sequence of the gene encoding the monocyte differentiation antigen, CD14. Nucleic Acids Res 16:4173
13. Tobias PS, Ulevitch RJ (1993) Lipopolysaccharide binding protein and CD14 in LPS dependent macrophage activation. Immunobiology 187:227–232
14. Tobias PS, Soldau K, Kline L, Lee J-D, Kato K, Martin TP, Ulevitch RJ (1993) Cross-linking of lipopolysaccharide (LPS) to CD14 on THP-1 cells mediated by LPS-binding protein. J Immunol 150:3011–3021
15. Lee JD, Kravchenko V, Kirkland TN et al (1993) Glycosylphosphatidylinositol anchored or integral membrane forms of CD14 mediate identical cellular responses to endotoxin. Proc Natl Acad Sci USA (in press)
16. Birkland TP, Cornwell RD, Golenbock DT, Proctor RA (1990) Comparative study of lipopolysaccharide-, lipid IVa-, and lipid X-induced tumor necrosis factor production in murine macrophage-like cell lines. Adv Exp Med Biol 256:399–402
17. Riedo FX, Munford RS, Campbell WB, Reisch JS, Chien KR, Gerard RD (1990) Deacylated lipopolysaccharide inhibits plasminogen activator inhibitor-1, prostacyclin, and prostaglandin E_2 induction by lipopolysaccharide but not by tumor necrosis factor-α. J Immunol 144:3506–3512
18. Munford RS, Hall CL (1986) Detoxification of bacterial lipopolysaccharides (endotoxins) by a human neutrophil enzyme. Science 234:203–205
19. Radolf JD, Norgard MV, Brandt ME, Isaacs RD, Thompson PA, Beutler B (1991) Lipoproteins of Borrelia Burgdorferi and Treponema Pallidum activate cachectin/TNF synthesis: analysis using a CAT reporter construct. J Immunol 147:1968–1974
20. Wallis RS, Amir-Tahmasseb M, Ellner JJ (1990) Induction of interleukin 1 and tumor necrosis factor by mycobacterial proteins: the monocyte western blot. Proc Natl Acad Sci USA 87:3348–3352
21. Valone SE, Rich EA, Wallis RS, Ellner JJ (1988) Expression of tumor necrosis factor

in vitro by human mononuclear phagocytes stimulated with whole Mycobacterium bovis BCG and myobacterial antigens. Infect Immun 56:3313–3315
22. Grau GE, Parida SK, Pointaire P, Barnes PF, Modlin RL (1992) TNF and mycobacteria. In: Beutler B (ed) Tumor necrosis factors: The molecules and their emerging role in medicine. Raven, New York, pp 329–340
23. Taverne J, Bate CAW, Sarkar DA, Meager A, Rook GAW, Playfair JHL (1990) Human and murine macrophages produce TNF in response to soluble antigens of Plasmodium falciparum. Parasite Immunol 12:33–43
24. Kwiatkowski D, Cannon JG, Manogue KR, Cerami A, Dinarello CA, Greenwood BM (1989) Tumour necrosis factor production in Falciparum malaria and its association with schizont rupture. Clin Exp Immunol 77:361–366
25. Taverne J, Bate CAW, Playfair JHL (1989) Induction of TNF in vitro as a model for the identification of toxic malaria antigens. Lymphokine Res 8:317–322
26. Bate CAW, Taverne J, Playfair JHL (1988) Malarial parasites induce TNF production by macrophages. Immunology 64:227–231
27. Hotez PJ, Le Trang N, Fairlamb AH, Cerami A (1984) Lipoprotein lipase suppression in 3T3-L1 cells by a haematoprotozoan-induced mediator from peritoneal exudate cells. Parasite Immunol 6:203–209
28. Goldberg SS, Cordeiro MN, Silva Pereira AA, Mares-Guia ML (1983) Release of lipopolysaccharide (LPS) from cell surface of Trypanosoma cruzi by EDTA. Int J Parasitol 13:11–18
29. Ketteridge DS (1978) Lipopolysaccharide from Trypanosoma cruzi. Trans R Soc Trop Med Hyg 72:101–102
30. Barrett TJ, Potter ME, Strockbine NA (1990) Evidence for participation of the macrophage in Shiga-like toxin II-induced lethality in mice. Microb Pathog 9:95–103
31. Harel Y, Weinberg A, Silva M, Giroir B, Beutler B (submitted 1993) A reporter transgene indicates renal-specific induction of TNF by Shiga-like toxin: possible involvement of TNF in hemolytic-uremic syndrome (abstract)
32. Fast DJ, Schlievert PM, Nelson RD (1989) Toxic shock syndrome-associated staphylococcal and streptococcal pyrogenic toxins are potent inducers of tumor necrosis factor production. Infect Immun 57:291–294
33. Ikejima T, Dinarello CA, Gill DM, Wolff SM (1984) Induction of human interleukin-1 by a product of Staphylococcus aureus associated with toxic shock syndrome. J Clin Invest 73:1312–1320
34. Hirose A, Ikejima T, Gill DM (1985) Established macrophaselike cell lines synthesize interleukin-1 in response to toxic shock syndrome toxin. Infection Immunity 50:765–770
35. Nedwin GE, Svedersky LP, Bringman TS, Palladino MA, Goeddel DV (1985) Effect of interleukin 2, interferon-γ and mitogens on the production of tumor necrosis factors α and β. J Immunol 135:2492–2497
36. Mukaida N, Hishinuma A, Zachariae CO, Oppenheim JJ, Matsushima K (1991) Regulation of human interleukin 8 gene expression and binding of several other members of the intercrine family to receptors for interleukin-8. Adv Exp Med Biol 305:31–38
37. Oppenheim JJ, Zachariae CO, Mukaida N, Matsushima K (1991) Properties of the novel proinflammatory supergene "intercrine" cytokine family. Annu Rev Immunol 9:617–648
38. Dinarello CA (1984) Interleukin-1. Rev Infect Dis 6:51–95
39. Duff G (1985) Many roles for interleukin-1. Nature 313:352–353
40. Allison AC (1985) The interleukin-1 family of molecules. BioEssays 3:260–262
41. Oppenheim JJ, Kovacs EJ, Matsushima K, Durum SK (1986) There is more than one interleukin 1. Immunol Today 7:45–56
42. Unanue ER, Allen PM (1987) The basis for the immunoregulatory role of macrophages and other accessory cells. Science 236:551–557
43. Martin M, Resch K (1988) Interleukin 1: more than a mediator between leukocytes. TIPS 9:171–177
44. Von Hoff DD, Fleming TR, Macdonald JS et al (1990) Phase II evaluation of recom-

binant gamma-interferon in patients with advanced pancreatic carcinoma: a Southwest Oncology Group study. J Biol Response Mod 9:584–587
45. Williams N, Bertoncello I, Jackson H, Arnold J, Kavnoudias H (1992) The role of interleukin 6 in megakaryocyte formation, megakaryocyte development and platelet production. Ciba Found Symp 167:160–170
46. Zeidler C, Kanz L, Hurkuck F et al (1992) In vivo effects of interleukin-6 on thrombopoiesis in healthy and irradiated primates. Blood 80:2740–2745
47. Hill RJ, Warren MK, Stenberg P et al (1991) Stimulation of megakaryocytopoiesis in mice by human recombinant interleukin-6. Blood 77:42–48
48. Imai T, Koike K, Kubo T et al (1991) Interleukin-6 supports human megakaryocytic proliferation and differentiation in vitro. Blood 78:1969–1974
49. Stahl CP, Zucker-Franklin D, Evatt BL, Winton EF (1991) Effects of human interleukin-6 on megakaryocyte development and thrombocytopoiesis in primates. Blood 78:1467–1475
50. Andus T, Geiger T, Hirano T, Kishimoto T, Heinrich PC (1988) Action of recombinant human interleukin 6, interleukin 1β and tumor necrosis factor α on the mRNA induction of acute-phase proteins. Eur J Immunol 18:739–746
51. Matthews N (1978) Tumour-necrosis factor from the rabbit. II. Production by monocytes. Br J Cancer 38:310–315
52. Matthews N (1981) Production of an anti-tumour cytotoxin by human monocytes. Immunology 44:135–142
53. Matthews N (1981) Tumour-necrosis factor from the rabbit. V. Synthesis in vitro by mononuclear phagocytes from various tissues of normal and BCG-injected rabbits. Br J Cancer 44:418–424
54. Satomi N, Haranaka K, Kunii O (1981) Research on the production site of tumor necrosis factor (TNF). Jpn J Exp Med 51:317–322
55. Fisch H, Gifford GE (1983) In vitro production of rabbit macrophage tumor cell cytotoxin. Int J Cancer 32:105–112
56. Beutler B, Greenwald D, Hulmes JD et al (1985) Identity of tumour necrosis factor and the macrophage-secreted factor cachectin. Nature 316:552–554
57. Sauder DN (1984) Epidermal cytokines: properties of epidermal cell thymocyte-activating factor (ETAF). Lymphokine Res 3:145–151
58. Kupper TS, Ballard DW, Chua AO et al (1986) Human keratinocytes contain mRNA indistinguishable from monocyte interleukin 1 alpha and beta mRNA. J Exp Med 164:2095–2100
59. Fong Y, Tracey KJ, Moldawer LL et al (1989) Antibodies to cachectin/tumor necrosis factor reduce interleukin 1β and interleukin 6 appearance during lethal bacteremia. J Exp Med 170:1627–1633
60. Beutler B, Milsark IW, Cerami A (1985) Passive immunization against cachectin/tumor necrosis factor (TNF) protects mice from the lethal effect of endotoxin. Science 229:869–871
61. Tracey KJ, Fong Y, Hesse DG et al (1987) Anti-cachectin/TNF monoclonal antibodies prevent septic shock during lethal bacteremia. Nature 330:662–666
62. Mathison JC, Wolfson E, Ulevitch RJ (1988) Participation of tumor necrosis factor in the mediation of gram negative bacterial lipopolysaccharide-induced injury in rabbits. J Clin Invest 81:1925–1937
63. Exley AR, Cohen J, Buurman W et al (1990) Monoclonal antibody to TNF in severe septic shock. Lancet 335:1275–1277
64. Opal SM, Cross AS, Kelly NM, Sadoff JC, Bodmer MW, Palardy JE, Victor GH (1990) Efficacy of a monoclonal antibody directed against tumor necrosis factor in protecting neutropenic rats from lethal infection with Pseudomonas aeruginosa. J Infect Dis 161:1148–1152
65. Ashkenazi A, Marsters SA, Capon DJ et al (1991) Protection against endotoxic shock by a tumor necrosis factor receptor immunoadhesin. Proc Natl Acad Sci USA 88:10535–10539

66. Ohlsson K, Bjork P, Bergenfeldt M, Hageman R, Thompson RC (1990) Interleukin-1 receptor antagonist reduces mortality from endotoxin shock. Nature 348:550–552
67. Wakabayashi G, Gelfand JA, Burke JF, Thompson RC, Dinarello CA (1991) A specific receptor antagonist for interleukin 1 prevents Escherichia coli-induced shock in rabbits. FASEB J 5:338–343
68. Redmond HP, Chavin KD, Bromberg JS, Daly JM (1991) Inhibition of macrophage-activating cytokines is beneficial in the acute septic response. Ann Surg 214:502–508
69. Hagmann W, Keppler D (1982) Leukotriene antagonists prevent endotoxin lethality. Naturwissenschaften 69:594–595
70. Doebber TW, Wu MS, Robbins JC, Choy BM, Chang MN, Shen TY (1985) Platelet activating factor (PAF) involvement in endotoxin-induced hypotension in rats. Studies with PAF-receptor antagonist kadsurenone. Biochem Biophys Res Commun 127:799–808
71. Fleisch JH, Rinkema LE, Haisch KD et al (1985) LY171883,1-<2-hydroxy-3-propyl-4-<4-(1H-tetrazol-5-yl)butoxy>phene, an orally active leukotriene D4 antagonist. J Pharmacol Exp Ther 233:148–157
72. Braquet P, Etienne A, Mencia-Huerta J-M, Clostre F (1988) Effects of the specific platelet-activating factor antagonists, BN 52021 and BN 52063, on various experimental gastrointestinal ulcerations. Eur J Pharmacol 150:269–276
73. Terashita Z-I, Stahl GL, Lefer AM (1988) Protective effects of a platelet activating factor (PAF) antagonist and its combined treatment with prostaglandin (PG) E1 in traumatic shock. J Cardiovas Pharmacol 12:505–511
74. Heuer H (1989) Effect of a new and specific paf-antagonist, WEB 2086, on paf and endotoxin/tumor necrosis factor induced changes in mortality and intestinal transit velocity. Prog Clin Biol Res 308:919–924
75. Dinarello CA, Cannon JG, Wolff SM et al (1986) Tumor necrosis factor (cachectin) is an endogenous pyrogen and induces production of interleukin-1. J Exp Med 163:1433–1450
76. Shalaby MR, Waage A, Aarden L, Espevik T (1989) Endotoxin, tumor necrosis factor-α and interleukin 1 induce interleukin 6 production in vivo. Clin Immunol Immunopathol 53:488–498
77. Cicco NA, Lindemann A, Content J et al (1990) Inducible production of interleukin-6 by human polymorphonuclear neutrophils: role of granulocyte-macrophage colony-stimulating factor and tumor necrosis factor-alpha. Blood 75:2049–2052
78. Zhang Y, Lin J-X, Vilcek J (1990) Interleukin-6 induction by tumor necrosis factor and interleukin-1 in human fibroblasts involves activation of a nuclear factor binding to a kappaB-like sequence. Mol Cell Biol 10:3818–3823
79. Shannon MF, Pell LM, Lenardo MJ, Kuczek ES, Occhiodoro FS, Dunn SM, Vadas MA (1990) A novel tumor necrosis factor-responsive transcription factor which recognizes a regulatory element in hemopoietic growth factor genes. Mol Cell Biol 10:2950–2959
80. Baeverle PA, Baltimore D (1991) The physiology of the NF-kB transcription factor. In: Cohen P, Foulkes JG (eds) Hormonal control regulation of gene expression. Biomedical Press, Elsevier/North Holland, pp 409–432
81. Lenardo MJ, Baltimore D (1989) NF-KB: A pleiotropic mediator of inducible and tissue-specific gene control. Cell 58:227–229
82. Lenardo MJ, Fan C-M, Maniatis T, Baltimore D (1989) The involvement of NF-KB in β-interferon gene regulation reveals its role as widely inducible mediator of signal transduction. Cell 57:287–294
83. Mathison JC, Virca GD, Wolfson E, Tobias PS, Glaser K, Ulevitch RJ (1990) Adaptation to bacterial lipopolysaccharide controls lipopolysaccharide-induced tumor necrosis factor production in rabbit macrophages. J Clin Invest 85:1108–1118
84. Beutler B, Krochin N, Milsark IW, Luedke C, Cerami A (1986) Control of cachectin (tumor necrosis factor) synthesis: mechanisms of endotoxin resistance. Science 232:977–980

85. Han J, Huez G, Beutler B (1991) Interactive effects of the TNF promoter and 3′-untranslated regions. J Immunol 146:1843–1848
86. Han J, Thompson P, Beutler B (1990) Dexamethasone and pentoxifylline inhibit endotoxin-induced cachectin/TNF synthesis at separate points in the signalling pathway. J Exp Med 172:391–394
87. Goldfeld AE, Maniatis T (1989) Coordinate viral induction of tumor necrosis factor α and interferon β in human B cells and monocytes. Proc. Natl Acad Sci USA 86:1490–1494
88. Waage A, Sorensen M, Stordal B (1990) Differential effect of oxpentifylline on tumour necrosis factor and interleukin-6 production. Lancet 335:543
89. Semmler J, Wachtel H, Endres S (1993) The specific type IV phosphodiesterase inhibitor rolipram suppresses tumor necrosis factor-α production by human mononuclear cells. Int J Immunopharmacol 15:409–413
90. Prada J, Prager C, Neifer S, Bienzle U, Kremsner PG (1993) Production of interleukin-6 by human and murine mononuclear leukocytes stimulated with Plasmodium antigens is enhanced by pentoxifylline, and tumor necrosis factor secretion is reduced. Infect Immun 61:2737–2740
91. Caput D, Beutler B, Hartog K, Brown-Shimer S, Cerami A (1986) Identification of a common nucleotide sequence in the 3′-untranslated region of mRNA molecules specifying inflammatory mediators. Proc Natl Acad Sci USA 83:1670–1674
92. Shaw G, Kamen R (1986) A conserved AU sequence from the 3′ untranslated region of GM-CSF mRNA mediates selective mRNA degradation. Cell 46:659–667
93. Han J, Brown T, Beutler B (1990) Endotoxin-responsive sequences control cachectin/TNF biosynthesis at the translational level. J Exp Med 171:465–475
94. Bazzoni F, Jongeneel CV, Shakhov A, Beutler B (1993) Induction of the TNF gene by ultraviolet light. J Clin Invest (submitted)
95. Bohjanen PR, Petryniak B, June CH, Thompson CB, Lindsten T (1991) An inducible cytoplasmic factor (AU-B) binds selectively to AUUUA multimers in the 3′-untranslated region of lymphokine mRNA. Mol Cell Biol 11:3288–3295
96. Cseh K, Beutler B (1989) Alternative cleavage of the cachectin/TNF propeptide results in a larger, inactive form of secreted protein. J Biol Chem 264:16256–16260
97. Kriegler M, Perez C, DeFay K, Albert I, Lu SD (1988) A novel form of TNF/cachectin is a cell surface cytotoxic transmembrane protein: Ramifications for the complex physiology of TNF. Cell 53:45–53
98. Perez C, Albert I, DeFay K, Zachariades N, Gooding L, Kriegler M (1990) A nonsecretable cell surface mutant of tumor necrosis factor (TNF) kills by cell to cell contact. Cell (in press)
99. Eck MJ, Sprang SR (1989) The structure of tumor necrosis factor-alpha at 2.6A resolution: implications for receptor binding. J Biol Chem 264:17595–17605
100. Chaplin DD, Hogquist KA (1992) Interactions between TNF and interleukin-1. In: Beutler B (ed) Tumor necrosis factors: the molecules and their emerging role in medicine. Raven, New York, pp 197–220
101. Black R, Kronheim S, Sleath P, Greenstreet T, Virca GD, March C, Kupper T (1991) The proteolytic activation of interleukin1 β. Agents Actions [Suppl] 35:85–89
102. Molineaux SM, Casano FJ, Rolando AM et al (1993) Interleukin 1 β (IL1 β) processing in murine macrophages requires a structurally conserved homologue of human IL1 beta converting enzyme. Proc Natl Acad Sci USA 90:1809–1813
103. Howard AD, Chartrain N, Ding GF, Kostura MJ, Limjuco G, Schmidt JA, Tocci MJ (1991) Probing the role of interleukin-1 β convertase in interleukin-1 beta secretion. Agents Actions [Suppl] 35:77–83
104. Thornberry NA, Bull HG, Calaycay JR et al (1992) A novel heterodimeric cysteine protease is required for interleukin-1 β processing in monocytes. Nature 356:768–774
105. Reiter LA, Martin JJ (1993) Interleukin-1β converting enzyme. Synthesis of hydroxyethyl dipeptide surrogate-containing compounds as potential ICE inhibitors. Int J Pept Protein Res 41:476–483

106. Meichle A, Schütze S, Hensel G, Brunsing D, Krönke M (1990) Protein kinase C-independent activation of nuclear factor kappaB by tumor necrosis factor. J Biol Chem 265:8339–8343
107. Hohmann H-P, Remy R, Poschl B, van Loon APGM (1990) Tumor necrosis factors-α and β bind to the same two types of tumor necrosis factor receptors and maximally activate the transcription factor NF-kB at low receptor occupancy and within minutes after receptor binding. J Biol Chem 265:15183–15188
108. Castigli E, Pahwa R, Good RA, Geha RS, Chatila TA (1993) Molecular basis of a multiple lymphokine deficiency in a patient with severe combined immunodeficiency. Proc Natl Acad Sci USA 90:4728–4732
109. Anderson DC, Springer TA (1987) Leukocyte adhesion deficiency on inherited defect in the MAC-1, LFA-1, and P150.95 glycoproteins. Annu Rev Med 38:175
110. Stern DM, Nawroth PP (1986) Modulation of endothelial hemostatic properties by tumor necrosis factor. J Exp Med 163:740–745
111. Alzani R, Corti A, Grazioli L, Cozzi E, Ghezzi P, Marcucci F (1993) Suramin induces deoligomerization of human tumor necrosis factor α. J Biol Chem 268:12526–12529

Role of Oxygen Free Radicals in the Pathophysiology of Sepsis

M. Kretzschmar

Introduction

Septic shock (SS) is a complex disease state characterized by significant hemodynamic, cardiovascular and metabolic disturbances which may result in multiple organ failure (MOF). Despite successful management of early complications in severely injured patients, i.e., polytraumatized patients in hemorrhagic shock, SS has an increasing incidence tendency [1–3]. Due to the high associated mortality rate, this disease is a major health concern. Although much research has been carried out to characterize the main pathophysiological changes that occur with SS, treatment has been ineffective in most cases.

Despite our limited understanding of the pathophysiology of SS, there is agreement regarding the initiating event [4], which is the presence of gram-negative bacteria or bacterial cell wall products (endotoxins) in the circulation. The endotoxins are lipopolysaccharides (LPS) found in the outer cell wall of gram-negative bacteria. There is some evidence that free radicals are responsible for the pathophysiological changes observed following exposure to LPS [5], and some experiments have demonstrated that tumor necrosis factor (TNF), believed to be a key mediator of tissue injury in SS [6, 7], amplifies the generation of these free radicals [8].

We shall now look at the role of oxygen-derived free radicals as mediators in the pathophysiology of SS.

Nature of Free Radicals

Chemistry of Free Radicals

Electrons in atoms occupy regions of space known as orbitals. Each orbital can hold a maximum of two electrons. A free radical is simply defined as any species that contains one or more unpaired electrons, an unpaired electron being one that is alone in an orbital [9, 10] and which is capable of independent existence. Examples of free radicals are superoxide ($O_2{}^{-\circ}$, an oxygen-centered radical), thiyl (RS°, a sulphur-centered radical), trichloromethyl ($CCl_3{}^\circ$, a carbon-centered radical), and nitric oxide (NO°), where the unpaired electron is delocalized between the two atoms.

According to Halliwell et al. [11], free radicals can react with other molecules. If two radicals meet, they can combine their unpaired electrons and form a covalent bond ($X^\circ + X^\circ \rightarrow X-X$). A radical may donate its unpaired electron to another molecule. It may pair with an electron from another molecule or it may simply join onto that molecule. When a radical donates an electron to, takes an electron from, or simply joins a nonradical (such as biological molecules), that nonradical becomes a radical. Thus, a feature of the reaction of free radicals with nonradicals is that they usually proceed as chain reactions: one radical begets another. Only when two radicals meet do they disappear (this is called termination reaction).

In principle, the hydrogen atom containing a single electron is a radical. Hence, removal of a hydrogen atom from a biological molecule leaves behind an unpaired electron on the atom to which the hydrogen was originally attached. Highly reactive radicals such as hydroxyl (OH°) frequently attack biological molecules by subtracting a hydrogen atom.

Free Radicals in Vivo

Many endogenous sources of radical generation *in vivo* have been found. For example, they are released within microsomal electron transport chains [12].

Activated phagocytes (polymorphonuclear leukocytes, PMN) and macrophages utilize oxygen radicals to kill phagocytosed bacteria and to clear necrotic tissue in synergism with their proteases. Activation of PMN by an activated complement cascade induces a respiratory burst in which the oxygen consumption of the PMN increases up to 80 times. This oxygen is almost exclusively utilized for the production of short-lived ($O_2{}^{-\circ}$, H_2O_2, OH°) and long-lived (HClO) toxic oxygen species (see below, The Early Phase: Activation of Leukocytes). This mechanism occurs in infectious diseases, in local infections, in inflammatory diseases (e. g., arthritis, adult respiratory distress syndrome) and in physiological wound healing, and is secondarily involved in ischemia-reperfusion syndrome [9, 13]. The latter is characterized by the paradoxical fact that reperfusion following ischemia and reoxidation after hypoxia may lead to tissue damage. If sufficient oxygen for aerobic metabolism is not provided, tissue energy stores are depleted of high-energy phosphorus compounds such as ATP. Upon reoxygenation, hypoxanthine is used to restore ATP. If, however, tissue hypoxia is prolonged, xanthine oxidase is formed, which on reoxidation forms xanthine and subsequently uric acid from hypoxanthine, a process producing $O_2{}^{-\circ}$. This phenomenon can be observed in patients with different forms of vascular occlusion (e. g., myocardial infarction) or impaired microcirculation (e.g., reflex sympathetic dystrophy), in all hypoxemic conditions [14], in shock states, in surgery involving the use of a bloodless field or the clamping of blood vessels, and in organ preservation and transplantation.

Important exogenous sources of oxygen radical formation are hyperoxia (leading to the activation of enzyme systems with a high K_m for oxygen, some of which produce oxygen radicals), ionizing radiation, cigarette smoke, and redox cycling of xenobiotics like the herbicide paraquat or the cytostatic doxorubicin. The toxic effects of free radicals in biological systems are manifold and include damage to all cell constituents that are prone to oxidative attack, e.g., lipids, carbohydrates, proteins, and nucleic acids. Oxidation of thiol groups of proteins may result in a loss of enzyme function (e.g., protease inhibitors such as α_1-antitrypsin are inactivated by oxygen radicals, leading to excessive activity of elastase), transmembrane ion and metabolite transport, and in contractile function [15]. Peroxidation of membrane phospholipids results in altered fluidity of membranes and altered membrane characteristics, leading to increased influx of Ca^{++} with resulting dysregulation of cell functions and uncoupling of oxidative phosphorylation. It has become apparent that the calcium ion is important for both physiological and destructive processes. A disturbance of Ca^{++} homeostasis, leading to a sustained increase in cytosolic Ca^{++} levels, has been associated with cytotoxicity in response to a variety of agents in different cells. Several biochemical mechanisms have been identified that appear to be generally involved in Ca^{++}-dependent cell injury and death. An increase in cystosolic Ca^{++} can result in a dissociation or proteolytic cleavage of actin microfilaments from vital anchoring proteins in the plasma membrane, leading to blebbing and increased membrane permeability. Activation of phospholipases or proteases can also cause structural or functional injury to other cell components leading to cell death [16, 17].

Peroxidation of lung surfactant results in atelectasis and pulmonary dysfunction (≙ adult respiratory distress syndrome, ARDS) [18].

The most extensively documented effect of oxygen-derived free radicals concerns the involvement in the oxidative breakdown of polyunsaturated fatty acids, known as lipid peroxidation (LPO). Whether LPO occurs *in vivo* is a difficult question to answer. HO° and HO_2°, but not $O_2^{-\circ}$ and H_2O_2 can abstract a hydrogen atom from a methylene bridge in a carbon chain, yielding a carbon-centered radical (R°), which after molecular rearrangement produces a conjugated diene due to a shift in the position of double bonds.

Initiation: $RH + initiator \rightarrow R^\circ$

The diene conjugate lipid radical combines rapidly with O_2 to produce a peroxyl radical (ROO°) capable of setting off propagation reactions.

Propagation: $R^\circ + O_2 \rightarrow ROO^\circ$

$ROO^\circ + RH \rightarrow ROOH + R^\circ$

The following steps are termination or amplification reactions.

Amplification: $ROOH + Fe^{2+} \rightarrow RO^\circ + OH^- + Fe^{3+}$

Termination: $R^\circ + R^\circ \rightarrow R\text{-}R$

$R^\circ + ROO^\circ \rightarrow ROOR$

In some cases free radical termination reactions could yield triplet carbonyl compounds, which are products of great toxicity:

$$ROO^{\circ}+ROO^{\circ}\rightarrow ROH+{}^{3}RO^{*}+O_2$$
$$ROO^{\circ}+ROO^{\circ}\rightarrow ROH+RO+{}^{1}O_2$$

The cain propagation, termination, and/or amplification reactions, however, will be determined by the character of the nearby lipid and the microenvironment of the cell compartment. Schaich and Borg [19] demonstrated that the intramembranous formation of HO° is feasible *in vivo* provided that appropriately complexed non-heme iron and suitable reducing equivalents are available. Fatty acid hydroperoxides formed during LPO can be further decomposed in a variety of fashions by hemoproteins, heme, ferritin, and transition metals, giving as molecular products a broad spectrum of volatile hydrocarbons and cytotoxic aldehydes suitable for the detection of chemical endpoints of *in vivo* radical reactions [20].

The consequences of cellular oxidative stress are not limited to lipid peroxidation. Proteins also undergo oxidative damage when exposed to $O_2^{\circ}-$, H_2O_2 and HO°. The oxidative modification of proteins varies with the nature of the oxidant and the protein under study: the oxidant must gain access to critical residues of the protein which are important for the maintenance of protein conformation and/or biological activity [21]. Oxidized proteins exhibit increased proteolytic susceptibility, probably sustained by denaturation and augmented hydrophobicity.

Principle of Multicausality in Injury Caused by Free Radicals

The generation of stable molecular products from lipid peroxidation (mainly the reactive toxic aldehydes) are generally referred too as the *diffusible products of LPO*. They form the basis of dissemination of toxigenic substances distant from lipid peroxidation *loci* over sizeable distances [22]. 4-hydroxy-alkenals (the main by-products of LPO) react with thiol groups in glutathione, cystine, proteins, and aminogroups of certain amino acids, inhibit enzyme activities, and have various other effects on cells and organs [23]. The broad target spectrum for these reactive aldehydes has further contributed to the concept that the principle of "unicausality" of the free radical-mediated damage is not longer tenable, and it is more realistic a sequence of events involving: *free radical attack→membrane damage→formation of toxic nonradical products.*

Rises in intracellular free Ca^{++}, protein damage, and DNA damage are often more important events in causing cell injury than the bulk peroxidation of membrane lipids [24]. LPO is often, but by no means always, a late event accompanying rather than causing final cell death. It therefore follows that a failure to protect against tissue damage by chain-breaking antioxidant inhibitors of lipid peroxidation does not rule out free radical damage as an injury mechanism. Of course, even if peroxidation is important, antioxidants may fail to protect if they do not reach the required site of action in sufficient concentrations [11].

Protection Against Injury Caused by Free Radicals

The first line of defense against injury caused by free radicals includes the factors that prohibit the formation of or primarily scavenge initiators of the lipid or protein peroxidation processes. These factors include metal-ion-binding proteins or the enzymes superoxide dismutase (SOD), catalase, and selenium-dependent glutathione peroxidase (GSHPx) [25]. There are several forms of the metalloprotein SOD: a Cu/Zn SOD (found mainly in the cytoplasm of cells), a Mn-dependent SOD (within the mitochondrial matrix), and an extracellular SOD. SOD catalyzes the transformation of two superoxide anion radicals to hydrogen peroxide (H_2O_2) and molecular oxygen:

$$2O_2{}^{-\circ} + 2H^+ \xrightarrow{SOD} H_2O_2 + O_2$$

Catalase is a heme (Fe^{3+})-containing enzyme able to catalyze the breakdown of H_2O_2 into water and oxygen. A low intracellular concentration of H_2O_2 is predominantly removed by GSHPx:

$$H_2O_2 + 2GSH \xrightarrow{GSHPx} GSSG + 2H_2O$$

This leads to the oxidation of GSH (the reduced form of glutathione) into its oxidized form GSSG. Adequate levels of GSH are maintained by the NADPH-dependent enzyme glutathione reductase (GSSG red) that generates GSH from GSSG.

GSH is important as a substrate for GSHPx, transferases, and several other enzymes, and as a general "radical quencher" in cells [26]. It could be the most important antioxidant in the aqueous phase of cells (cytosol). Two major GSHPx forms have been described: a selenium-dependent GSHPx which is able to reduce H_2O_2 and organic hydroperoxides and a selenium-independent GSHPx (similar to GSH-transferase) which preferentially utilizes organic hydroperoxides. Recently, a GSH-dependent α-tocopherol (vitamin E) free radical reductase was described indicating an interplay between the cytosolic antioxidant GSH and the membrane-bound (lipophilic) α-tocopherol antioxidant factor [27]. The vitamins E and C (ascorbic acid) as well as β-carotene may scavenge oxygen radicals and can therefore be classified as being part of the first line of defense. However, vitamin E (toc-OH) and vitamin C can be regarded as chain-breaking antioxidants [26, 28]. Toc-OH acts in the lipid phase by trapping peroxy radicals:

$$LOO^\circ + \mathit{toc}\text{-}OH \rightarrow LOOH + \mathit{toc}\text{-}O^\circ -$$

The resulting α-tocopherylchromanoxy radical is resonance-stabilized and relatively unreactive. It can react with a second peroxy radical:

$$Toc\text{-}O^{\circ} - + LOO^{\circ} \rightarrow \textit{nonradical products}$$

Vitamin E might also be regenerated by the membrane-bound toc-OH regeneration system which is dependent on ascorbic acid and GSH. The chain-breaking antioxidant effect circumvents the propagation of the LPO process. This constitutes the second line of defense.

The metabolism of LPO products forms the third line of defense. As mentioned above, the peroxidation products may initiate damage in general or may cause an LPO chain reaction. Aldehydes can be removed by GSH-transferases. Lipid hydroperoxides can be reduced to the respective alcohols by GSHPx.

Oxygen-Derived Free Radicals as Mediators in the Pathophysiology of Sepsis and Septic Shock

The Early Phase: Activation of Leukocytes

A primary hemorrhagic-traumatic insult with tissue necrosis and microbial invasion triggers "cascade systems" in the organism (Fig. 1). This includes complement, especially through the alternative pathway, coagulation and fibrinolysis. Increasing attention is now also directed to maintaining the nutritional integrity of gut mucosa. A continuous, adequate oxygen supply to the intestinal wall has been recognized as the prominent prerequisite for preserving barrier function [29]. Splanchnic and in particular mucosal ischemia seems to be the most common triggering event leading to increased permeability of the intestinal epithelium. Evidence has been accumulated in support of the notion that in such situations enterocytes not only undergo hypoxic

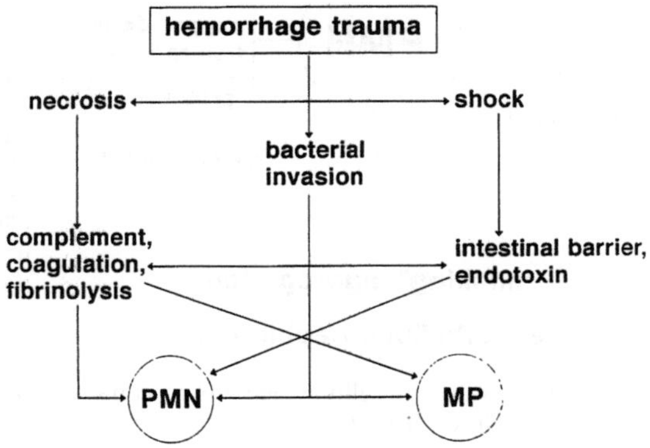

Fig. 1. Activation of the "fire brigades" and the "cascade system" following a hemorrhagic-traumatic insult with tissue necrosis, microbial invasion, and shock. PMN, polymorphonuclear leukocytes; MP, macrophages. (Modified from [40])

damage but are also affected by *reperfusion injury*. This stems from the local activation of xanthine oxidase and from respiratory bursts in granulocytes, which consequently release oxygen-derived free radicals [30, 31].

This process occurs rapidly. In rats, for instance, a 30-min episode of shock (mean arterial pressure 30 mmHg) was sufficient to enhance bacterial translocation through the epithelial layer of the gut mucosa [32]. Very early in the process of intestinal barrier failure one has to reckon with a marked influx of bacterial endotoxin released from dead, damaged, and/or proliferating gram-negative bacteria [33]. These events activate the cellular "fire brigades" of the organism, i.e., the PMN and the macrophages (Fig. 1). Within limits, this activation is a desirable part of natural defense mechanisms. The PMN are activated more quickly than the macrophages. The early stage is dominated by highly unstable and therefore "aggressive" oxygen-derived free radicals, proteases, and arachidonic acid derivatives or eicosanoids (Fig. 2).

The oxygen radicals released during the "respiratory burst" of the PMN can be monitored at the experimental level by the chemiluminescence of blood or tissue samples [34, 35], and comprise superoxide radical $O_2^{-\circ}$, hydrogen peroxide H_2O_2, and the hydroxyl radical OH°. Essentially all cellular membranes are susceptible to this attack (see above, Free Radicals *in Vivo*), but their potential for *direct* damage is strictly localized, because they desintegrate within seconds. In addition to causing tissue injury themselves, these radicals may also lead to the accumulation, adherence, and activation of PMN. Like the terminal "membrane attack sequence" C5–C9 of the complement system, the oxygen radicals facilitate the entry of extracellular calcium into cells, disturbing intracellular functions and structures (see above, ibid.). Furthermore, they activate a cellular membrane enzyme, phospholipase A_2, which liberates arachidonic acid from membranes [16]. Its free form is metabolized by two enzymes, cyclooxygenase and lipooxygenase, each initiating a multistep metabolic pathway leading to the generation of eicosanoids [36],

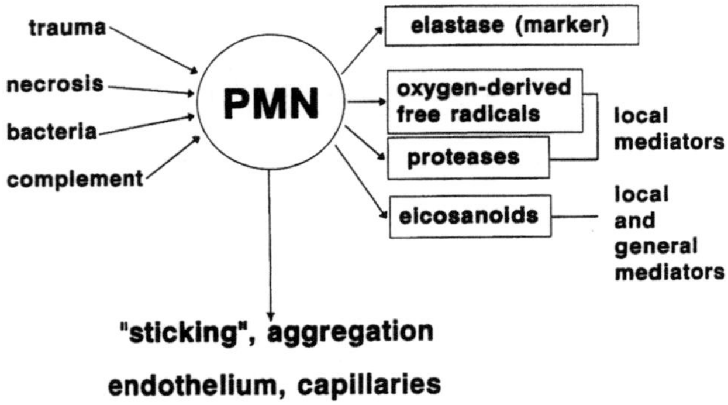

Fig. 2. Early stage of cellular activation, centering on the polymorphonuclear leukocytes (PMN). (Modified from [40])

showing biological activity at even low plasma concentration levels. It is now accepted that increased levels of such substances [e.g., thromboxane A_2 (TXA_2), the prostaglandin F (PGF) series, leukotrienes (LTB_4)] are associated with greater morbidity in states of SS [37]. Arachidonic acid products may influence PMN in reperfusion injury. Firstly, they may act as chemoattractants and induce PMN adhesion to the endothelium (e.g., LTB_4 and TXA_2). Secondly, arachidonic acid products may activate PMN to produce more oxygen radicals and also proteolytic enzymes. LTB_4 is a potent stimulus of H_2O_2 generation in PMN following ischemia [38]. Thirdly, leukotrienes and TXA_2 affect blood flow and therefore tissue perfusion by direct action on the microvasculature.

Figure 2 and the mediator effects discussed so far make it clear why the generalized damage arising during the early course of major trauma centers on the microcirculation. Apart from the resulting decreased perfusion, the activated PMN aggregate and adhere to the epithelium, releasing mediators capable of damaging the microvasculature. A characteristic example of this is the "lung-in-shock syndrome" (ARDS) [39, 40].

The effects of oxygen-derived free radicals are summarized in Fig. 3, which clearly indicates their role as mediators of the early stage of SS.

The Late Phase: Activation of Macrophages

The progressive activation of macrophages, which are capable of secreting a hundred different products, is a crucial development during the late phase of post-traumatic mediator release [41] (Fig. 4). The most important causes are persistent areas of tissue necrosis and/or bacterial invasion continuing the complement activation. At the same time, the risk of endotoxemia or bac-

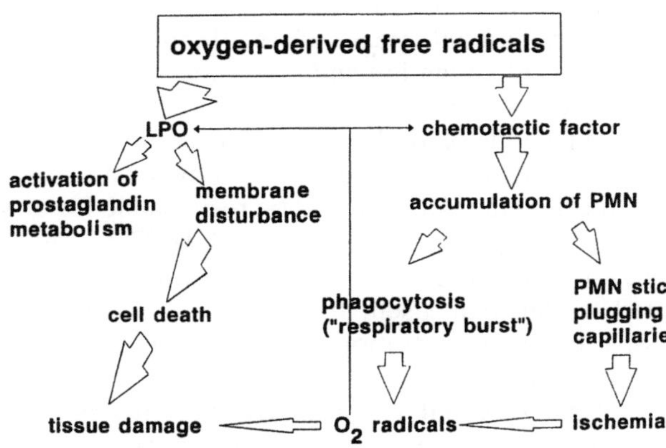

Fig. 3. Effects of oxygen-derived free radicals as mediators of the early stage of septic shock. LPO, lipid peroxidation; PMN, polymorphonuclear leukozytes

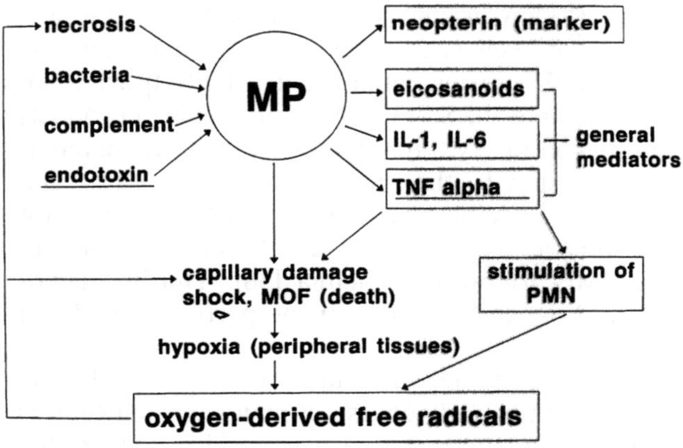

Fig. 4. Later stage of cellular activation, centering on the macrophages (MP) and the role of oxygen-derived free radicals in the triggering of the vicious circle leading to the generalized, often irreversible septic shock. IL, interleukin; TNF tumor necrosis factor; PMN polymorphonuclear leukozytes; MOF, multiple organ failure

teremia due to a progressive weakening of the intestinal barrier grows [40]. The marker of macrophage activation is neopterin. The principal mediators released comprise the eicosanoids, interleukins, and TNFα. TNFα (cachectin) is a mediator with potentially irreversible, lethal effects [42]. It is now known that the degree to which the macrophages are "primed" by ongoing, forced phagocytic labor largely determines their capacity to synthesize and release large quantities of TNF when "triggered" by endotoxin [43].

Among the several interleukins that can now be distinguished, interleukin-1 (IL-1) remains established as an activator of the arachidonic acid cascade. It leads to an additional release of free (lipid) radicals. IL-1 is a major factor responsible for inflammation and promotes a hyperdynamic circulatory state with increased cardiac output and decreased peripheral vascular resistance. High concentrations of IL-1 result in hyperdynamic shock [44] leading to a reduced O_2 supply and, consequently, to hypoxia and the generation of free radicals. Interleukin-6 (IL-6) could be responsible for a "switching on" of the "acute phase reaction" (for review see [45]). TNF, when released from macrophages after induction by endotoxin, produces most of the effects formerly attributed to the toxin itself. In general, TNF produces severe shock with progressive hemoconcentration, lactic acidosis, and hyperglycemia followed by subnormal serum glucose levels. Histological examination reveals the presence of patchy capillary thrombosis with pericapillary hemorrhage, edema, and cellular infiltration. In the lungs, liver, kidney, and gastrointestinal tract, the histological lesions are indistinguishable from those seen in MOF [40].

The later phase of cell activation is characterized by the function of oxygen-derived (and lipid) free radicals as local triggering substances in a vicious cycle:

1) TNFα stimulates the PMN and amplifies the generation of free radicals.
2) TNFα causes (usually with IL-1) a hyperdynamic shock state leading to hypoxia of peripheral tissues with liberation of free radicals.
3) The released free radicals are able to promote the capillary damage by destruction of endothelial cells, leading to an additional decrease in tissue perfusion.
4) Cell necrosis caused by the free radical action stimulates macrophages, LPO, and, additionally, the activation of the arachidonic acid cascade. Therefore, oxygen-derived free radicals could be the mediators responsible for the self-perpetuation of SS leading to irreversible MOF and death.

Experimental and Clinical Experiences

The only technique that allow us to "see" free radicals is electron spin resonance (ESR) spectroscopy. This measures the energy changes that occur as unpaired electrons align in response to an external magnetic field [46]. However, biologically important radicals do not accumulate to high enough concentrations to be directly observable by ESR. Therefore so called "spin-traps" (such as phenyl-tert-butyl nitrone) have been used in detecting certain free radicals and demonstrating the effects of antioxidants *in vivo*. Currently available "spin traps" do not appear to have convincingly succeeded in detecting $O_2^{-\circ}$ or OH° *in vivo*, nor can they be safely administered to humans [11].

First *in vivo* evidence for the role of free radicals in SS-associated tissue injury and the mechanisms underlying the generation of free radicals in sepsis was provided by Lloyd et al. [47] using a primate model. These authors combined ESR spectroscopy and spin-trapping techniques. Baboons were administered the "spin trap" DMPO during an infusion of *Escherichia coli* with or without TNF. ESR spectra suggesting the trapping of carbon-centered and oxygen-centered radicals detected in liver lipid extracts of *E. coli*-infused animals that exhibited pathophysiological changes indicative of sepsis. In animals demonstrating a toxic response to *E. coli*, TNF challenge appeared to intensify the ESR signal observed. These data provide evidence of free radical production during sepsis and suggest that TNFα plays a part in the production of free radicals.

For clinical purposes, "end-point measurements" should be useful for detecting free radical action and LPO *in vivo*. Most often the thiobarbituric acid test is used. This test is very simple but nonspecific and can offer, at best, an empirical view on the complex process of LPO [48]. The measurement of the consumption of antioxidants (mainly GSH) in plasma should be a more effective method to detect oxidative stress in intact biological systems (including man) using the plasma compartment [49–51]. Recently, we started a longitudinal study in polytraumatized patients to determine changes in cytokines immediately following trauma and their possible correlation to antioxidant consumption (GSH and its oxidized form GSSG) as well as changing serum concentrations of thiobarbituric acid-reacting material. Figures 5 and 6 demonstrate the typical course in a 31-year-old male patient who had suffered severe polytraumatic injury (57 points on the Hannover trauma score). The patient was monitored from early stage after the injury until his death from MOF on the 12th post-traumatic day. Initially, we observed peaks of endotoxin, TNFα, and endotoxin-binding capacity in serum. There were also increased TNFα levels from the 4th day after injury to the death of the patient, associated with an increase in serum endotoxin levels on days 8 and 11 after injury. We measured increasing GSSG plasma levels over the

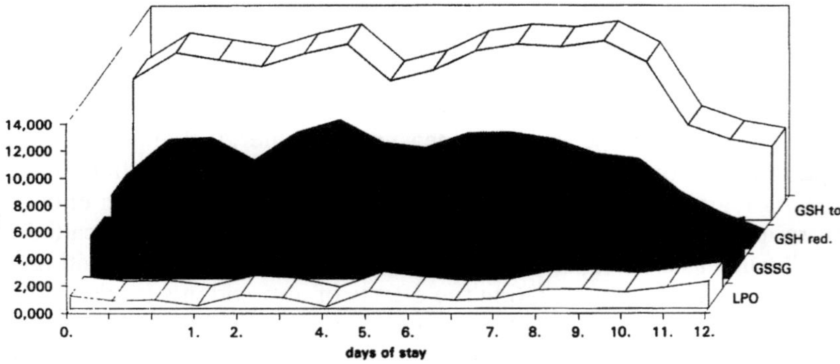

Fig. 5. Course of plasma levels of GSH, GSSG, and lipid peroxidation (LPO; expressed in terms of thiobarbituric acid-reacting substances) in a patient suffering from severe polytrauma leading to fatal systemic inflammatory response syndrome

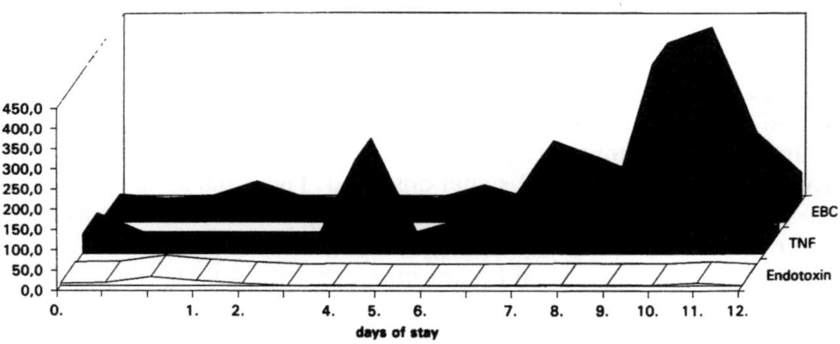

Fig. 6. Course of plasma levels of endotoxin, endotoxin binding capacity (EBC), and tumor necrosis factor (TNF) in the same patient

whole observation period. Serum lipid peroxides (expressed as thiobarbituric acid-reacting substances) were dramatically increased from the 6th day after injury until the patients death. In association with these results, we observed a continuous decrease in GSH after the 6th day following the injury. This decreased to zero, indicating a total loss of the GSH-dependent antioxidative defense system. These results correlate with the assumption that oxygen-derived free radicals are responsible for locally triggering the vicious cycle leading to MOF during sepsis or systemic inflammatory response syndrome (SIRS).

Conclusion

The initiating factor in MOF is frequently an episode of acute hemorrhage with resulting visceral ischemia. The syndrome of MOF manifests itself clinically by the onset of *enteric sepsis* and *ileus.* This suggests that altered splanchnic vascular flow may be an initiating event.

Oxygen-derived free radicals have been proposed as important mediators of tissue injury. They are released during reperfusion after hypovolemic shock, by leukotriene B_4, and during the peroxidase-catalyzed enzymatic reduction of hydroperoxy fatty acids. These radicals also take part in the triggering of SS and leading to MOF.

Acknowledgements. The author is grateful to Prof. W. Schirrmeister, Prof. W. Klinger, and Dr. F. Knebel for critically reading the manuscript. Many thanks to Mrs. Marina Wolf for typing the manuscript. The study discussed in this paper was supported by the Deutsche Forschungsgemeinschaft (DFG Kr 1220/1–2).

References

1. Goris RJA (1987) The adult respiratory distress syndrome and multi-organ failure. Intensive Care News 1:1–7
2. Luce JM (1987) Pathogenesis and management of septic shock. Chest 91:883–888
3. Mc Guise GP, Pearl GR (1990) Sepsis and the trauma patient. Crit Care Clin 6:121–146
4. Wendel A (1991) Reactive oxygen species, antiproteases, and cytokines in sepsis. Klin Wochenschr 69:969–974
5. Manson NH, Hess ML (1983) Interaction of oxygen free radicals and cardiac sarcoplasmic reticulum: proposed role in the pathogenesis of endotoxin shock. Circ Shock 10:205–213
6. Tracey KJ, Beutler B, Lowry SF et al (1986) Shock and tissue injury induced by recombinant human cachectin. Science 234:470–474
7. Tracey KJ, Fong Y, Hesse DG et al (1987) Anti-cachectin/TNF monoclonal antibodies prevent septic shock during lethal bacteraemia. Nature 330:662–664
8. Klebanoff SJ, Vadas MA, Harlan JM, Sparks LH, Gamble JR, Agosti JM, Waltersdorfph AM (1986) Stimulation of neutrophils by tumor necrosis factor. J Immunol 136:4220–4325

9. Bast A, Goris RJA (1989) Oxidative stress – biochemistry an human disease. Pharm Weekbl 11:199–206
10. Elstner EF (1991) Oxygen radicals – biochemical basis for their efficacy. Klin Wochenschr 69:949–956
11. Halliwell B, Gutteridge JMC, Cross CE (1992) Free radicals, antioxidants, and human disease: where are we now? J Lab Clin Med 119:598–620
12. Halliwell B, Gutteridge JMC (1989) Free radicals in biology and medicine, 2nd edn. Clarendon, Oxford
13. Menger MD, Lehr HA, Messmer K (1991) Role of oxygen radicals in the microcirculatory manifestations of postischemic injury. Klin Wochenschr 69:1050–1055
14. De Groot H, Littauer A (1989) Hypoxia, reactive oxygen, and cell injury. Free Radical Biol Med 6:541–551
15. Gilbert HF (1989) Catalysis of thiol/disulfide exchange: single-turnover reduction of protein disulfide-isomerase by glutathione and catalysis of peptide disulfide reduction. Biochemistry 28:7298–7305
16. Nicotera P, McConkey DJ, Dypbukt JM, Jones DP, Orrenius S (1989) Ca^{2+}-activated mechanisms in cell killing. Drug Metab Rev 20:193–201
17. Orrenius S, McConkey DJ, Bellomo G, Nicotera P (1989) Role of Ca^{2+} in toxic cell killing. Trends Pharmacol Sci 10:281–285
18. Cochrane C, Spragg RG, Revak SD (1983) The presence of neutrophil elastase and evidence of oxidation activity in bronchoalveolar lavage fluid of patients with adult respiratory distress syndrome. Am Rev Respir Dis 127:525–527
19. Schaich KM, Borg DC (1987) Fenton reactions in lipid phases: iron solubility, HO° production and initiation of lipid peroxidation. Fourth International Congress on Oxygen Radicals, La Jolla, Abstracts, pp 102–105
20. Saran M, Bors W (1991) Direct and indirect measurement of oxygen radicals. Klin Wochenschr 69:957–964
21. Davies KJA (1987) Protein damage and degradation by oxygen radicals: I. General aspects. J Biol Chem 262:9895–9901
22. Esterbauer H (1986) Lipid peroxidation products: formation, chemical properties and biological activities. In: Poli G, Cheeseman KH, Dianzini MU, Stater TF (eds) Free radicals in liver injury. IRL Press, Oxford, pp 29–47
23. Esterbauer H, Zollner H, Schaur RJ (1988) Hydroxyalkenals: cytotoxic products of lipid peroxidation. ISI Atlas of Science Biochem 1:311–317
24. Cochrane C (1991) Mechanisms of oxidant injury of cells. Mol Aspects Med 12:137–147
25. Sies H (1991) Oxidative stress: oxidants and antioxidants. Academic, New York
26. Meister A (1992) On the antioxidant effects of ascorbic acid and glutathione. Biochem Pharmacol 44:1905–1915
27. Chow CK (1991) Vitamin E and oxidative stress. Free Radic Biol Med 11:215–232
28. Wefers H, Sies H (1989) Antioxidant effects of ascorbate and glutathione in microsomal lipid peroxidation are dependent on vitamin E. In: Poli G, Cheeseman KH, Diansini MU, Stater TF (eds) Free radicals in liver injury. IRL Press, Oxford, pp 309–316
29. Deitch EA, Bridges W, Ma L, Berg R, Specian RD, Granger DN (1990) Hemorrhagic shock included bacterial translocation: the role of neurophils and hydroxyl radicals. J Trauma 30:942–951
30. Arndt H, Kubes P, Granger DN (1991) Involvement of neutrophils in ischemia-reperfusion injury of the small intestine. Klin Wochenschr 69:1056–1060
31. Siems W, Kowalewski J, Werner A, Schimke I, Gerber G (1989) Radical formation in the rat small intestine during and following ischemia. Free Radic Res Commun 7:347–353
32. Deitch EA, Morrison J, Berg R, Specian RD (1990) Effect of hemorrhagic shock on bacterial translocation, intestinal morphology, and intestinal permeability in conventional and antibiotic-decontaminated rats. Crit Care Med 18:529–536
33. Kraft R, Ruchti C, Burkhardt A, Cottier H (1992) Pathogenetic principles in the devel-

opment of gut derived infectious-toxic shock (GITS) and multi-organ failure. Curr Stud Hematol Blood Transfus 59:204–240
34. Pryor WA, Godber SS (1991) Noninvasive measures of oxidative stress status in humans. Free Radic Biol Med 10:177–184
35. Weber GF (1990) The measurement of oxygen-derived free radicals and related substances in medicine. J Clin Chem Clin Biochem 28:569–603
36. Welbourn CRB, Goldman G, Paterson IS, Valeri CR, Shepro D, Hechtman HB (1991) Pathophysiology of ischemia reperfusion injury: central role of the neutrophil. Br J Surg 78:651–655
37. Oettinger W, Berger HG (1989) How specific is eicosanoid release in the surgical sepsis syndrome? Current state of clinical evidence. Theor Surg 3:171–180
38. Paterson IS, Klausner JM, Goldman G (1989) Thromboxane mediates the ischemia induced neutrophil oxidative burst. Surgery 106:224–229
39. Brigham KL (1991) Oxygen radicals – an important mediator of sepsis and septic shock. Klin Wochenschr 69:1004–1008
40. Lundsgaard-Hansen P, Blauhut B (1992) Markers and mediators in enterogenic infectious-toxic shock. Curr Stud Hematol Blood Transfus 59:163–203
41. Nathan CF (1987) Secretory products of macrophages. J Clin Invest 79:319–326
42. Damas P, Reuter A, Gysen P, Demonty J, Lamy M, Franchimont P (1989) Tumor necrosis factor and interleukin-1 serum levels during severe sepsis in humans. Crit Care Med 17:975–978
43. Mitchie HR, Wilmore DW (1990) Sepsis, signals, and surgical sequelae (a hypothesis). Arch Surg 125:531–536
44. Cannon JG, Tompkins RG, Gelfond JA et al (1990) Circulating interleukin-1 and tumor necrosis factor, in septic shock and experimental endotoxin fever. J Infect Dis 61:982–987
45. Wise WC, Cook JA, Tempel GE, Reines HD, Halushba PV (1989) The rat in sepsis and endotoxin shock. Prog Clin Biol Res 299:243–252
46. Janzen EG (1990) Spin trapping and associated vocabulary. Free Radic Res Commun 10:63–68
47. Lloyd SS, Chang AK, Taylor FB, Janzen EG, McCay PB (1993) Free radicals and septic shock in primates: the role of tumor necrosis factor. Free Radic Biol Med 14:233–242
48. Yagi K (1987) Lipid peroxides and human diseases. Chem Phys Lipids 45:327–351
49. Kretzschmar M, Klinger W (1990) The hepatic glutathione system – influences of xenobiotics. Exp Pathol 38:145–164
50. Kretzschmar M, Müller D, Hübscher J, Marin E, Klinger W (1991) Influence of aging, training and acute physical exercise on plasma glutathione and lipid peroxides in man. Int J Sports Med 12:218–222
51. Kretzschmar M, Pfeifer U, Machnik G, Klinger W (1992) Glutathione homeostasis and turnover in the totally hepatectomized rat: evidence for a high glutathione export capacity of extrahepatic tissues. Exp Toxicol Pathol 44:273–281

III. Pathophysiology

Cardiocirculation in Sepsis

F. Bloos and W. J. Sibbald

Introduction

Sepsis is a syndrome in which organ dysfunction frequently determines outcome. Myocardial dysfunction is not only part of the process of organ dysfunction, but may contribute to its further propagation. For example, the myocardium needs to generate a high cardiac output in sepsis to support the elevated tissue O_2 needs typical of this syndrome. Failure to maintain a "supranormal" systemic O_2 delivery has been associated with organ dysfunction and death [45].

Cardiac dysfunction appears early in sepsis, but at this stage, can be restored by appropriate fluid resuscitation [46]. As sepsis progresses, myocardial performance declines further, as demonstrated by a depression in the ventricular ejection fractions, left ventricular dilatation [32, 47] and an alteration of the Frank-Starling mechanism [49]. Myocardial dysfunction at this time is not easily explained by intravascular fluid loss since this phenomenon persists in the resuscitated normotensive state of sepsis. Importantly, these changes are reversible when the patient recovers from this syndrome [47].

Measures of contractility (i.e., left ventricular pressure-volume curves), which are independent of changes in preload and afterload, are depressed in sepsis [26, 54]. This suggests a direct involvement of the myocardium's contractile apparatus. Indeed, data show that endotoxemia causes a derangement of Ca^{2+} metabolism in the cardiac sarcolemma [40]. This is accompanied by structural changes of the cardiac tissue in sepsis. In the healthy myocardium, collagen supports the orientation of myocytes. In sepsis, myocardial collagen content is depressed and collagen orientation is significantly reduced [57].

While these studies show that the myocardium is clearly affected by sepsis, controversy remains about the pathophysiology of myocardial depression in this syndrome. Two theories have been proposed to explain the development of myocardial dysfunction in sepsis:

1) *Myocardial depressant substances:* Studies have shown that serum from septic patients inhibited the contraction of beating heart cells *in vitro* [48] and that hemofiltration had a beneficial effect on cardiac performance in septic dogs [26]. Therefore, it was concluded that the serum of septic pa-

tients contains one or more substances which directly depress cardiac function [48].

2) *Myocardial ischemia:* This concept has been addressed by several studies which have assessed transmyocardial O_2 metabolism in different animal models of sepsis and in septic patients.

The objective of this chapter is to review studies investigating the adequacy of the coronary circulation in sepsis.

Regulation of Myocardial O_2 Availability in Health

Unlike skeletal muscle, the heart cannot accept an O_2 debt. Therefore, O_2 supply to the myocardium must always match the O_2 need of this organ and any failure to do so will cause myocardial dysfunction (even if no necrosis occurs) [38]. Two mechanisms regulate myocardial O_2 availability to ensure that oxygen is provided even under critical conditions of systemic O_2 supply: autoregulation and metabolic regulation (Fig. 1).

Autoregulation of Coronary Blood Flow

Autoregulation describes the ability of the coronary vasculature to maintain blood flow independent of arterial perfusion pressures [43]. At rest, the autoregulatory range of the heart includes coronary perfusion pressures from 70 mm Hg to 130 mm Hg [30, 43]. Thus, when outside these limits, coronary blood flow becomes dependent on coronary pressure.

The site of autoregulation is located mainly in arterioles with a diameter less than 100 μm [33]. Nevertheless, the mechanism that supports autoregu-

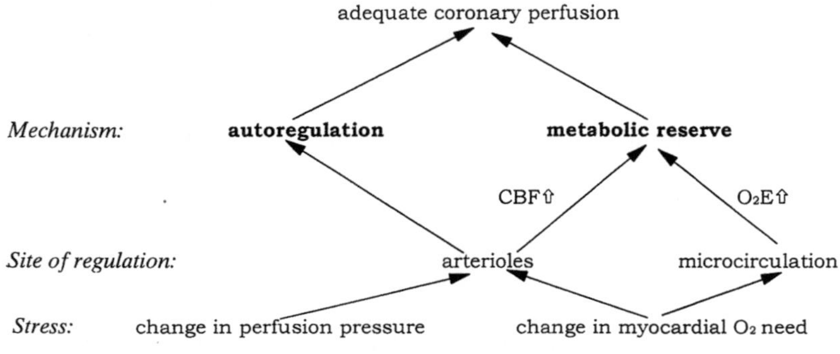

Fig. 1. The regulation of myocardial O_2 availability supports changes in perfusion pressure (autoregulation) and changes in myocardial O_2 need (metabolic regulation). *O_2E*, O_2 extraction; *CBF*, coronary blood flow

lation is not clear. It has been suggested that changes in perfusion pressure influence the arteriolar wall, which then induces vasoconstriction and vasodilation, respectively (*myogenic theory*) [24]. On the other hand, changes in coronary pressure may be followed by alterations in tissue pO_2, which could then mediate an increase in coronary blood flow (*metabolic theory*) [8, 15].

If myocardial O_2 need rises, coronary blood flow increases by vasodilation (see below). Therefore, autoregulation loses part of its ability to intervene which results in a smaller autoregulatory range. Thus, at a high coronary blood flow the autoregulatory range is smaller than 70–130 mm Hg. When coronary arterioles are maximally dilated autoregulation is lost [30].

Metabolic Regulation

Myocardial O_2 delivery is closely regulated by the heart's tissue O_2 need and can be quickly adjusted when the tissue O_2 need of the heart changes. This system can be quantified by determining the metabolic reserve of the heart [56] and consists of two components: a blood flow reserve and an O_2 extraction reserve.

The myocardial O_2 need is coupled with the coronary vasculature through mediators. Whenever there is an increase in the myocardium's O_2 need, its cells release substances (adenosine, prostacyclins) which, within 20 s, vasodilate coronary arteries and therefore support an increase in coronary blood flow [17, 18]. In order to augment coronary blood flow, cardiac output must be redistributed from "nonvital" organs, which have a higher O_2 extraction reserve than the myocardium (i.e., the gut) [1].

Since myocardial O_2 extraction is already high at rest — about 70% — the importance of myocardial O_2 extraction in contributing to this organ's metabolic reserve has been much discussed in the literature. Intravital microscopy of the beating heart shows that more capillaries can be recruited in the heart during hypoxia [41], suggesting that myocardial O_2 extraction can be increased beyond the value at rest. Feigl and coworkers argued that myocardial O_2 extraction only increases when the coronary flow "reserve" is exhausted [21]. However, it is not always possible to cover an increase in myocardial O_2 need with an increase in coronary blood flow alone, i.e., changes in α-receptor activity can partly diminish the ability to increase coronary blood flow. Under those conditions, myocardial O_2 need is partly covered by a rise in myocardial O_2 extraction (even when the coronary flow reserve is not yet exhausted) [3]. Thus, myocardial O_2 extraction reserve is an important mechanism supporting coronary circulatory reserve.

In summary, autoregulation and metabolic regulation maintain O_2 availability in the myocardium in balance with its O_2 needs. Both mechanisms depend on the intact responsiveness of arterioles, and the latter mechanism depends also on an intact coronary microcirculation.

Myocardial O_2 Availability in Sepsis

Since Cho first described, in 1972, that endotoxin directly affects coronary vessels [9], many investigators have assessed the importance of this observation on the determinants of myocardial O_2 delivery. Since it is difficult to study the regional circulation of the heart in humans, most studies addressing myocardial O_2 availability in sepsis have been conducted on animals. As our understanding of sepsis changed over the years, different animal models of sepsis have been used to study this syndrome. This may be a reason for the variety of results and sometimes diverging conclusions especially in this area. It is important to distinguish between sepsis and septic shock and we will review those studies separately.

Coronary Perfusion in Septic Shock

Most of these studies have used animal models in whom sepsis was induced by a bolus injection of endotoxin, which produced profound hypotension, or have been conducted on patients with septic shock. A summary of these studies is shown in Table 1. Both an increase [12, 25] and a decrease [6, 13, 34] in coronary blood flow have been reported during septic shock.

Since a decrease in coronary blood flow was associated with a depression

Table 1. Summary of studies investigating the effect of septic shock on myocardial O_2 availability

Author	Study design	Results
Cho [9]	Isolated hearts from endotoxemic dogs	Endotoxin constricts coronary arteries.
Bohs et al. [6]	Endotoxemic dogs	Myocardial dysfunction may be associated with cardiac ischemia.
Kleinman et al. [34]	Endotoxemic dogs	Endotoxemia is associated with non-uniform perfusion and histological damage of the heart.
Cunnion et al. [12]	Septic shock patients	Global myocardial ischemia is not the cause of myocardial depression.
Goldfarb et al. [25]	Endotoxemic pigs	Myocardial dysfunction may be due to relative hypoperfusion of the subendocardium.
D'Orio et al. [13]	Endotoxemic dogs	Coronary blood flow is sufficient to maintain myocardial O_2 need.
Dhainaut et al. [14]	Septic shock patients	Myocardial hypoxia may have participated in cardiac depression.
Groeneveld et al. [27]	Endotoxemic dogs	Increased heterogeneity of coronary blood flow may involve focal ischemia.

in cardiac contractility, it was concluded that endotoxemic shock induces cardiac hypoperfusion [6]. However, others have argued that endotoxemia reduces heart work because of a decrease in afterload. Therefore, myocardial O_2 need would fall and be followed by a decrease in coronary blood flow [13]. This would mean that the lower coronary blood flow in endotoxic shock would be adequate to maintain the myocardium's O_2 need and would not induce myocardial ischemia. However, when coronary perfusion was improved by infusion of glucose-insulin-potassium, myocardial performance in endotoxic shock was restored [7]. This study suggests that the depressed coronary blood flow during endotoxic shock may have caused the drop in myocardial performance rather than the other way around.

Clinical studies have reported an increase in coronary blood flow in patients with septic shock [12, 24]. Although it was concluded that the coronary circulation mimics the central circulation in sepsis — high blood flow, low vascular resistance, low O_2 extraction — it was also argued that myocardial dysfunction in these patients was not due to ischemia since no myocardial lactate production was observed [12]. Yet, Dhainaut and coworkers concluded that the low myocardial O_2 extraction in patients with septic shock may result in cardiac ischemia [14]. This does not contradict Cunnion's findings since it is difficult to employ the myocardial lactate metabolism as a marker of cardiac ischemia [44].

These differing observations about the behaviour of coronary blood flow in septic shock could be explained by studying the distribution of coronary blood flow inside the heart. Blood flow distribution in the heart is nonuniform in septic shock [34]. While some areas in the heart were supplied with a very high blood flow, other areas were hardly perfused at all [27]. This could lead to focal ischemia. In fact, histological damage in the heart of endotoxemic dogs was observed [34].

Coronary Perfusion in Normotensive Sepsis

These studies try to mimic the development of sepsis in the human situation by inducing sepsis with an intraperitoneal inflammatory focus and trying to avoid hypotension by adequate fluid resuscitation. Table 2 shows a summary of the cited literature. All studies found that coronary blood flow was increased in normotensive sepsis and was secondary to coronary vasodilation. However, this increase in coronary blood flow was not necessarily accompanied by a similar increase in heart work [22, 23]. A possible explanation could be that the release of vasodilating substances in sepsis leads to an inappropriate coronary vasodilation followed by overperfusion of the heart. However, Fish and coworkers found that the septic myocardium uses more O_2 per unit work than the healthy heart, thereby suggesting that the efficiency of the heart is depressed in this syndrome [22]. Thus, the high coronary blood flow in sepsis may be necessary to maintain an elevated O_2 need

Table 2. Summary of studies investigating the effect of normotensive sepsis on myocardial O_2 availability

Author	Study design	Results
Lang et al. [37]	Rats with intraperitoneal fecal inoculum	Sepsis alters myocardial efficiency.
Fish et al. [22]	Chronic endotoxemia in rats	Myocardium less efficient but metabolic control intact.
Fish et al. [23]	Chronic endotoxemia in rats	Increased coronary blood flow without increase in heart work.
Lee et al. [39]	Chronic endotoxemia in pigs	The septic myocardium is overperfused.
Bloos et al. [4]	Cecal ligation and perforation in sheep	Metabolic reserve of the heart is depressed.

of the heart. The increased coronary blood flow in sepsis is supported by a redistribution of blood flow from splanchnic organs to the heart [37].

Metabolic Coupling and Autoregulation in Sepsis

As pointed out above, an increase in coronary blood flow may reduce the autoregulatory range of the coronary circulation. In fact, it has been demonstrated that the septic heart becomes extremly sensitive to low perfusion pressures [19, 29]. Nevertheless, any increase in heart work was accompanied by an increase in coronary blood flow [4, 22] which suggests that the metabolic control is intact in sepsis. This is in agreement with our findings that septic sheep can increase their coronary blood flow during hypoxia [4]. During a severe hypoxic stress, we found that coronary flow reserve was three times larger in control sheep than in septic sheep (Table 3). Further, splanchnic organs, i.e., the small bowel, did not participate in the redistribution of cardiac output to the heart as it did in healthy animals. We observed that the hearts of septic sheep could not maintain their O_2 need when the arterial O_2 content dropped below about 80 ml O_2/ml compared to about 55 ml O_2/ml in healthy sheep [4]. This confirms the observation that in septic but not in

Table 3. Both mechanisms of the heart's metabolic reserve were depressed in normotensive hyperdynamic sheep when the coronary circulation was challenged by severe hypoxia. (From [4])

	Control sheep	Septic sheep
Coronary blood flow reserve [%]	419 ± 126*	143 ± 48*,**
Myocardial O_2 extraction reserve [%]	11 ± 5*	1 ± 4

*, Change is different from 0 with $p < 0.05$; **, $p < 0.05$ between groups, mean ± s.e.m.

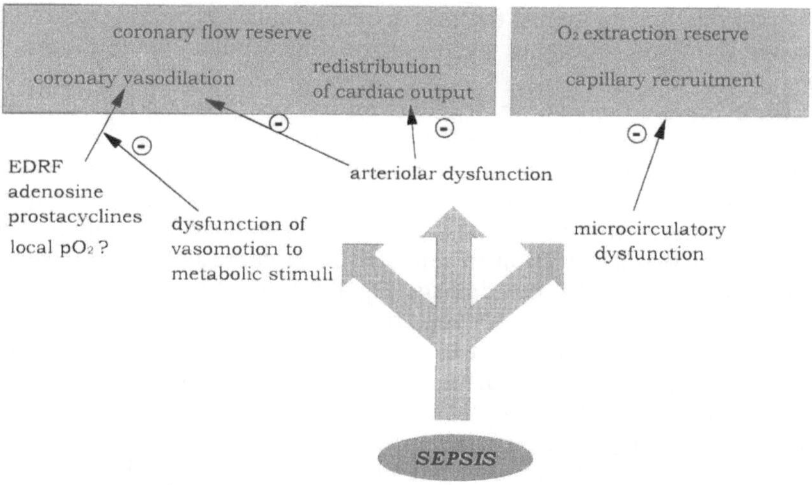

Fig. 2. Sepsis interferes with both mechanisms which maintain myocardial O_2 delivery (autoregulation and metabolic regulation) as the regional circulation is depressed both on the arteriolar and the microcirculatory level in this syndrome. EDRF, endothelium derived relaxans factor

healthy hearts, even brief hypoxia leads to a reduction of myocardial cytochrome, which is a marker of intracellular O_2 availability [53].

These studies suggest that metabolic regulation remains intact in sepsis but it's reserve is significantly depressed. As metabolic regulation depends on arteriolar function, failure of these vessels to respond to physiologic stimuli has been reported in several organs during sepsis [10, 11]. Furthermore, coronary vessels of septic animals showed an altered response to mediators, i.e., adenosine [52] and endothelium derived relaxans factor (EDRF) [35], that are important in the regulation of coronary artery tonus. These possible effects of sepsis on the coronary circulation are summarized in Fig. 2.

Coronary Microcirculation in Sepsis

Besides coronary perfusion, myocardial O_2 extraction plays an important role in the metabolic reserve of the heart. It has been reported that myocardial O_2 extraction was depressed in sepsis [12, 14]. Additionally, the septic cardiocirculation was not able to increase myocardial O_2 extraction if the heart was challenged by a severe hypoxic stress [4]. We found that, during severe hypoxia, healthy sheep but not septic sheep could increase myocardial O_2 extraction from 78% to 88% (Table 3) [4]. Thus, the septic heart shares in the O_2 extraction defect that has been demonstrated in the systemic circulation. Changes in O_2 extraction are usually associated with changes on the microcirculatory level of the circulation. Since it is difficult to employ direct observational techniques of the microcirculation to the beating heart, little is known about the coronary perfusion on the capillary level of the septic heart.

However, microcirculatory dysfunction has been demonstrated in several organs during sepsis [16, 20, 36]. The numbers of capillaries without perfusion is higher in sepsis than under normal conditions, thus reducing the density of capillaries participating in O_2 transport. This may lead to ischemia in tissue which is far from the next O_2 supplying capillary. The pathogenesis of microcirculatory dysfunction in sepsis is likely caused by several factors. It may include endothelial cell damage [2], adhesion of leukocytes to endothelial cells [55], and plugging of capillaries by stiff erythrocytes [50]. Additionally, we have shown a left-shift in the O_2 dissociation curve during hyperdynamic sepsis [5]. This may further impair the O_2 extraction defect in sepsis since an increased O_2 hemoglobin affinity could further inhibit O_2 uptake especially in underperfused capillaries.

As the sepsis syndrome is a systemic event it seems likely that the heart shares in these injuries. Biopsies from the heart of hyperdynamic septic sheep demonstrated patchy cell necrosis [28]. This kind of injury can only be reproduced when myocardial vessels are damaged on the microcirculatory level [31]. These studies suggest that a microcirculatory dysfunction exists in the septic heart which may lead to myocardial injury.

Summary and Clinical Implications

In summary, sepsis affects the myocardial O_2 metabolism in the following ways:

1. The metabolic reserve of the heart is significantly depressed in sepsis due to the inability to sufficiently increase coronary blood flow and myocardial O_2 extraction.
2. The septic myocardium works less energy efficient.
3. The septic myocardium becomes sensitive to hypoxia and hypotension.

Although the coronary perfusion in sepsis may be sufficient to maintain myocardial O_2 need at rest, any hypoxic stress or hypotension is likely to exhaust the heart's metabolic reserve followed by ischemia and a depression in cardiac performance. Although the treatment of sepsis should not be aimed at one organ alone, the following points should be taken into consideration:

- Some catecholamines (dopamine, norepinephrine) induce "O_2 wasting" [51]. Thus, they increase the basic O_2 need of the heart that is independent of heart work. In an organ which already uses O_2 less efficiently in sepsis, O_2 wasting may further depress the metabolic reserve of the heart.
- Fluid resuscitation is a key procedure in the treatment of septic patients. Although this topic goes far beyond this chapter (see Fluid Therapy in

Sepsis, W. Sibbald, this volume), the fluid type used for volume replacement may have consequences on myocardial O_2 availability. We have shown that the capillary surface area available to extract O_2 in the heart is significantly greater if a colloid rather than a crystalloid is chosen for fluid resuscitation [42].

- The O_2 availability of the healthy heart is unaffected by anemia over a large range of hematocrit due to the large metabolic reserve of this organ. However, with the metabolic reserve depressed in sepsis a normal hemoglobin might be necessary to maintain myocardial O_2 need especially in a hyperdynamic state.

In conclusion, we believe that the inability of the septic coronary circulation to sufficiently adjust myocardial perfusion to the often changing conditions of O_2 demand may result in depressed cardiac performance. More knowledge should become available as to how treatment of the sepsis syndrome could be optimized to alter this defect in a positive manner.

References

1. Adachi H, Strauss HW, Ochi H, Wagner HN Jr (1976) The effect of hypoxia on the regional distribution of cardiac output in the dog. Circ Res 39:314–319
2. Baker CH, Sutton ET, Zhou Z, Dietz JR (1990) Microvascular vasopressin effects during endotoxin shock in the rat. Circ Shock 30:81–95
3. Baran KW, Bache RJ, Dai X-Z, Schwartz JS (1992) Effect of α-adrenergic blockade with prazosin on large coronary diameter during exercise. Circ 85:1139–1145
4. Bloos F, Morisaki H, Neal A, Pitt M, Martin C, Ellis C, Sibbald WJ (1992) Is the circulatory 'reserve' supporting tissue O_2 availability depressed in normotensive hyperdynamic sepsis? Crit Care Med 20(4):S55
5. Bloos F, Neal A, Pitt M, Martin CM, Rutledge I, Ellis CG, Sibbald WJ (1993) A left-shifted O_2 dissociation curve contributes to the depressed O_2 extraction in hyperdynamic septic sheep. Chest 104(2):152S
6. Bohs CT, Turbow ME, Kolmen SN, Traber DL (1976) Coronary blood flow alterations in endotoxin shock and response to dipyridamole. Circ Shock 3(4):281–286
7. Bronsveld W, van Lambalgen AA, van Velzen D, van den Bos GC, Koopman PAR, Thijs LG (1985) Myocardial metabolic and morphometric changes during canine endotoxin shock before and after glucose-insuline-potassium. Circ Res 19:455–464
8. Broten TP, Feigl EO (1992) Role of myocardial oxygen and carbon dioxide in coronary autoregulation. Am J Physiol 262:H1231–H1237
9. Cho YW (1972) Direct cardiac action of E. coli endotoxin (36856). Proc Soc Exp Biol Med 141:705–707
10. Cryer HG, Garrison RN, Harris PD, Greenwald BH, Alsip NL (1990) Prostaglandins mediate skeletal muscle arteriole dilation in hyperdynamic bacteremia. Am J Physiol 259:H728–H734
11. Cryer HM, Unger LS, Garrison RN, Harris PD (1988) Prostaglandins maintain renal microvasular blood flow during hyperdynamic bacteremia. Circ Shock 26:71–88
12. Cunnion RE, Schaer GL, Parker MM, Natanson C, Parrillo JE (1986) The coronary circulation in human septic shock. Circulation 73(4):637–644
13. D'Orio V, El Allaf D, Vaira S, Fossion A, Juchmes J, Marcelle R (1979) Lack of defective cardiac oxidative metabolism in intact dogs subjected to a prolonged low-dose infusion of Escherichia coli endotoxin. Circ Shock 18:43–52

14. Dhainaut JF, Huyghebaert M-F, Monsallier JF et al (1987) Coronary hemodynamics and myocardial metabolism of lactate, free fatty acids, glucose, and ketones in patients with septic shock. Circulation 75(3):533–541
15. Drake-Holland AJ, Laird JD, Noble MIM, Spaan JAE, Vergroesen I (1984) Oxygen and coronary vascular resistance during autoregulation and metabolic vasodilation in the dog. J Physiol (Lond) 348:285–299
16. Drazenovic R, Samsel RW, Wylam ME, Doerschuk CM, Schumacker PT (1992) Regulation of perfused capillary density in canine intestinal mucosa during endotoxemia. J Appl Physiol 72(1):259–265
17. Edlund A, Berglund B, Kaijser L, Patrono C, Sollevi A, van Dorne D, Wennmalm Å (1983) Release of adenosine and prostacyclin from ischemic human hearts. Adv Prostaglandin Thromboxane Leukotriene Res 11:365–370
18. Edlund A, Fredholm BB, Patrignani P, Patrono C, Wennmalm Å, Wennmalm M (1983) Release of two vasodilators, adenosine and prostacyclin, from isolated rabbit hearts during controlled hypoxemia. J Physiol (Lond) 340:487–501
19. Elkins RC, McCurdy JR, Brown PP, Greenfield LJ (1973) Effects of coronary perfusion pressure on myocardial performance during endotoxin shock. Surg Gynecol Obstet 137:991–996
20. Farquhar I, Lam C, Ellis C, Tyml K, Martin C, Sibbald W (1992) Intravital microscopy of the mucosal microcirculation in sepsis. Clin Invest Med 15(4)[Suppl]:A25
21. Feigl EO, Neat GW, Huang AH (1990) Interrelations between coronary artery pressure, myocardial metabolism and coronary blood flow. J Mol Cell Cardiol 22:375–390
22. Fish RE, Burns AH, Lang CH, Spitzer JA (1985) Myocardial dysfunction in a nonlethal, nonshock model of chronic endotoxemia. Circ Shock 16:241–252
23. Fish RE, Lang CH, Spitzer JA (1986) Regional blood flow during continous low-dose endotoxin infusion. Circ Shock 18:267–275
24. Folkow B (1964) Description of the myogenic hypothesis. Circ Res 15[Suppl I]:1279–1287
25. Goldfarb RD, Nightingale LM, Kish P, Weber PB, Loegering DJ (1986) Left ventricular function during lethal and sublethal endotoxemia in swine. Am J Physiol 251:H364–H373
26. Gomez A, Wang R, Unruh H et al (1990) Hemofiltration reverses left ventricular dysfunction during sepsis in dogs. Anesthesiology 73:671–685
27. Groeneveld ABJ, van Lambalgen AA, van den Bos GC, Bronsveld W, Nauta JJP, Thijs LG (1991) Maldistribution of heterogeneous coronary blood flow during canine endotoxin shock. Cardiovasc Res 25:80–88
28. Hersch M, Gnidec AA, Bersten AD, Troster M, Rutledge FS, Sibbald WJ (1990) Histologic and ultrastructural changes in nonpulmonary organs during early hyperdynamic sepsis. Surgery 107:397–410
29. Hinshaw LB, Archer LT, Spitzer JJ, Black MR, Peyton MD, Greenfield LJ (1974) Effects of coronary hypotension and endotoxin on myocardial performance. Am J Physiol 227(5):1051–1057
30. Hoffman JIE (1984) Maximal coronary flow and the concept of coronary vascular reserve. Circulation 70(2):153–159
31. Ince C, Ashruf JF, Avontuur JAM, Wieringa PA, Spaan JAE, Bruining HA (1993) Heterogeneity of the hypoxic state in rat heart is determined at capillary level. Am J Physiol 264:H294–H301
32. Jardin F, Brun-Ney D, Auvert B, Beauchet A, Bourdarias JP (1990) Sepsis-related cardiogenic shock. Crit Care Med 18:1055–1060
33. Kanatsuka H, Lamping KG, Eastham CL, Marcus ML (1990) Heterogeneous changes in epimyocardial microvascular size during graded coronary stenosis: evidence of the microvascular site for autoregulation. Circ Res 66:389–396
34. Kleinman WM, Krause SM, Hess ML (1980) Differential subendocardial perfusion and injury during the course of gram-negative endotoxemia. Adv Shock Res 4:139–152

35. Kuo L, Chilian WM, David MJ, Laughlin MH (1992) Endotoxin impairs flow-induced vasodilation of porcine arterioles. Am J Physiol 262:H1838–H1845
36. Lam C, Tyml K, Martin C, Sibbald WJ (1991) The skeletal muscle microcirculation in sepsis. Microcirc Res 15(4):A113
37. Lang CH, Bagby GJ, Ferguson JL, Spitzer JJ (1984) Cardiac output and redistribution of organ blood flow in hypermetabolic sepsis. Am J Physiol 246:R331–R337
38. Laxson DD, Homans DC, Dai X-Z, Sublett E, Bache RJ (1989) Oxygen consumption and coronary reactivity in postischemic myocardium. Circ Res 64:9–20
39. Lee KJ, Dziuban SW Jr, van der Zee H, Goldfarb RD (1988) Cardiac function and coronary flow in chronic endotoxemic pigs (42805). Proc Soc Exp Biol Med 189:245–252
40. Liu M-W (1990) Mechanisms of myocardial membrane alterations in endotoxin shock: roles of phospholipase and phosphorylation. Circ Shock 30:43–49
41. Martini J, Honig CR (1969) Direct measurement of intercapillary distance in beating rat heart in situ under various conditions of O_2 supply. Microvasc Res 1:244–256
42. Morisaki H, Bloos F, Neal A et al (1992) Colloid infusion preserves microvascular integrety better than crystalloid in hyperdynamic sepsis. Crit Care Med 20(4)[Suppl]:S101
43. Mosher P, Ross J Jr, McFate PA, Shaw RF (1964) Control of coronary blood flow by an autoregulatory mechanism. Circ Res 14:250–259
44. Neill WA, Kremkau EL, Oxendine JM, Phelps NC (1974) Criteria for detecting ischemic myocardial hypoxia from lactate and pyruvate data during atrial pacing in humans. J Lab Clin Med 83(3):428–435
45. Nesarajah MS, Matalon S, Krasney JA, Farhi FE (1983) Cardiac output and regional oxygen transport in the acutely hypoxic conscious sheep. Respir Physiol 53:161–172
46. Ognibene FP, Parker MM, Natanson CN, Shelhamer JH, Parrillo JE (1988) Depressed left ventricular performance. Response to volume infusion in patients with sepsis and septic shock. Chest 93(5):903–910
47. Parker MM, Shelhamer JH, Bacharach SL et al (1984) Profound but reversible myocardial depression in patients with septic shock. Ann Intern Med 100:483–490
48. Parrillo JE, Burch C, Shelhamer JH, Parker MM, Natanson C, Schuette W (1985) A circulating myocardial depressant substance in humans with septic shock. J Clin Invest 76:1539–1553
49. Pawlush DG, Musch TI, Bannar SM, Martin LF (1990) Cardiac dysfunction in a rat model of chronic bacteremia. Circ Shock 31:269–279
50. Powell RJ, Machiedo GW, Rush BF Jr (1993) Decreased red blood cell deformability and impaired oxygen utilization during human sepsis. Am Surg 59:65–68
51. Rooke GA, Feigl EO (1982) Work as a correlate of canine left ventricular oxygen consumption, and the problem of catecholamine oxygen wasting effect. Circ Res 50:273–286
52. Rumsey WL, Kilpatrick L, Wilson DF, Erecinska M (1988) Myocardial metabolism during coronary flow: effects of endotoxemia. Am J Physiol 255:H1295–H1304
53. Snow TR, Dickey DT, Hinshaw LB, Taylor FB (1990) Early myocardial dysfunction induced with endotoxin in rhesus monkeys. Can J Cardiol 6(3):130–136
54. Stahl TJ, Alden PB, Ring WS, Madoff RC, Cerra FB (1990) Sepsis induced diastolic dysfunction in chronic canine peritonitis. Am J Physiol 258:H625–H633
55. Thomas JR, Harlan JM, Rice CL, Winn RK (1992) Role of leukocyte CD11/CD18 complex in endotoxic and septic shock in rabbits. J Appl Physiol 73:1510–1516
56. Weber KT, Janicki JS (1979) The metabolic demand and oxygen supply of the heart: physiologic and clinical considerations. Am J Cardiol 44(4):722–729
57. Yu P, Boughner D, Martin C, Keys J, Sibbald W (1993) Myocardial collagen damage in rats with hyperdynamic sepsis at 24 and 48 hrs. Crit Care Med 21(4)[Suppl]:S277

A Current View of Oxygen Supply Dependency

S. M. Cain

The View from the 1980s

Intensive and critical care specialists became particularly interested in oxygen uptake ($\dot{V}O_2$) and oxygen delivery (DO_2) in critically ill patients during the decade of the 1980s. This was in response to the identification of an apparent oxygen supply dependency in some patients, particularly those ill with adult respiratory distress syndrome (ARDS) or with sepsis. Although not the first to report that $\dot{V}O_2$ was unusually dependent upon DO_2, the seminal paper by Danek et al. [1] marked the beginning of increased activity in this area of investigation. Their observation was that $\dot{V}O_2$ varied directly and linearly with any change in DO_2 in ARDS patients. This was not the case in a comparable group of ventilator patients who did not have ARDS but were also in the intensive care unit. Furthermore, the apparent dependence of $\dot{V}O_2$ upon DO_2 in the ARDS patients was seen at very high levels of DO_2, well above those that were thought to be critical. Although they recognized that this observation may have had implications for the adequacy of tissue oxygenation in ARDS patients, they were unable to suggest any mechanism. Other publications followed with similar observations and I tried to summarize and to analyze what extraordinary oxygen supply dependency might mean in a review article that appeared in 1984 [2].

From experiments on anesthetized animals, $\dot{V}O_2$ was known to remain unchanged over a wide range of DO_2 by altering O_2 extraction appropriately. When the limit of compensatory changes was reached as DO_2 was progressively lowered, usually at an O_2 extraction ratio (O_2ER) of 70%–80%, $\dot{V}O_2$ would then change linearly with DO_2. This "physiologic O_2 supply dependency" was first described in a figure similar to Fig. 1 [2]. In anesthetized animals, the same critical levels of DO_2 and O_2ER were found whether DO_2 was decreased by decreasing blood flow, O_2 carrying capacity, or PO_2 in arterial blood [3]. The feature that was strikingly different in ARDS or sepsis patients and which was called "pathologic O_2 supply dependency" was the apparent inability to alter O_2 extraction appropriately with changes in DO_2 to keep $\dot{V}O_2$ constant. As a result, mixed venous PO_2 remained high even as $\dot{V}O_2$ apparently became limited by O_2 availability. The other feature in the pathological form was an increased $\dot{V}O_2$ that seemed to have no attainable upper limit in that it continued to increase with increases in DO_2.

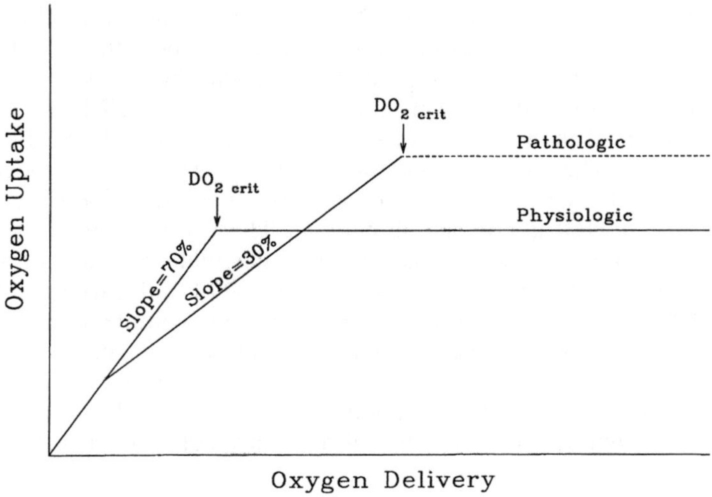

Fig. 1. Physiologic and pathologic O_2 supply dependency. The slopes show the O_2 extraction ratio (O_2ER) and DO_{2crit} designates the O_2 delivery below which O_2 uptake becomes linearly dependent upon delivery. The plateau of O_2 uptake for the pathologic case is represented by a *dashed line* because there is no evidence to prove that it exists

The plateau feature that was easily demonstrated in the physiological case was not seen in patients with ARDS or sepsis.

A decreased ability to increase O_2ER had some parallels in animal studies. For example, microembolization with microspheres caused venous PO_2 to increase in contracting dog gastrocnemius muscle because of the maldistribution of blood flow that was created [4]. An even more direct parallel was seen in studies by Landau et al. [5] and Cain et al. [6], who found that the critical DO_2 was higher and critical O_2ER lower in dog hindlimb that had been embolized by injection of microspheres. Finally, a spontaneous loss of autoregulation in dog muscle was associated with a higher $\dot{V}O_2$ and a lesser ability to extract O_2 as flow was lowered [7]. All of the animal studies pointed to the state of the microcirculation as the reason for the O_2ER defect observed in patients. In the case of ARDS, the microcirculation of the lung had already been seen to be dysfunctional. It was not a far leap of logic to think that the state of peripheral capillaries had been similarly affected by the same processes that affected the lung for the reasons cited in other overviews [8, 9].

In other representative clinical studies from the 1980s, DO_2 was altered by various means, usually by fluid loading. Typical of such studies are those of Kaufman et al. [10], Haupt et al. [11], Gilbert et al. [12] and Astiz et al. [13]. The consensus of results was that $\dot{V}O_2$ increased when DO_2 increased; additionally, lactate levels that were elevated before treatment were lowered with increased DO_2. In all cases, O_2 extraction changed little if at all. The significance of these observations was indicated by such studies as that of Gutierrez and Pohil [14], who found that patients who showed a strong supply dependency of $\dot{V}O_2$ and who were unable to increase O_2ER had a significantly lower survival than a group of similar patients who did not show these characteristics. The strongest evidence in this direction was provided by a prospective study by Bihari et al. [15], who used a potent vasodilator, prostacyclin, to increase DO_2 in critically ill patients. Those who showed a positive response $\dot{V}O_2$, 13 of 27, failed to survive their hospital stay whereas all the rest, who showed independence of $\dot{V}O_2$ from DO_2, did survive. The same study showed that prostacyclin given to normal volunteers produced the same magnitude of DO_2 increase but $\dot{V}O_2$ did not change, a response identical to that of survivors. The interpretation of these results by the authors was that pathologic O_2 supply dependency signified an occult but severe tissue hypoxia, a common view with that of many investigators at that time.

Oxygen Supply Dependency and Tissue Hypoxia

At the end of the decade of the 1980s, pathologic O_2 supply dependency and the tissue hypoxia that it was thought to represent was assumed by many to be the cause of multiple organ failure, a common consequence and putative cause of death in many ARDS and septic patients. Concurrently, O_2 supply dependency was being reported in many non-ARDS and nonseptic patients [16–19] so that its unique significance in ARDS and sepsis was laid open to question. These and similar observations led Dantzker et al. [20] to suggest that the apparent dependence of $\dot{V}O_2$ upon DO_2 was actually a normal response that was initiated by a primary increase in O_2 demand and did not necessarily mean that there was a problem in O_2ER by peripheral tissues. However, the prevailing opinion in the clinical literature as the decade of the 1980s drew to a close was that there were both sufficient disturbances in peripheral circulation and an increased O_2 demand to assume that tissue hypoxia had to be present. Elevated lactate levels in patients who showed pathologic O_2 supply dependency and increased mortality in that group reaffirmed this opinion.

The question of whether the septic state could produce an O_2ER defect was answered in animal models. The critical DO_2 (DO_{2crit}) identified in Fig. 1 as the DO_2 at which $\dot{V}O_2$ begins to fall, was used to show this. The critical O_2ER, the ratio of $\dot{V}O_2$ to DO_2 at the DO_{2crit}, provided another index of disturbed microcirculation and impaired extraction ability by the peripheral tissues. In anesthetized dogs that were hemorrhaged in steps to lower DO_2 progressively, DO_{2crit} was higher and critical O_2ER was lower in animals that had been injected with bacterial endotoxin than in controls [21]. In other similar studies, the gut was seen to be particularly susceptible to the effects of endotoxin [22], whereas resting skeletal muscle was quite resistant [23]. These animal studies showed quite convincingly that acute septic responses to endotoxin could produce an O_2 extraction defect that became evident as blood flow was decreased. The most common explanation was that disturbances in the control of blood flow through the microcirculation caused maldistribution so that hypoperfusion and hyperperfusion with respect to local O_2 needs coexisted in the same locale. Increased zones of hypoxia, therefore, caused the early failure of $\dot{V}O_2$ as DO_2 was decreased.

Although the presence of an extraction defect was highly suggestive of local tissue hypoxia, it was not direct evidence and it may not have been the case at higher blood flows. In other animal studies, Hotchkiss et al. [24] used an intracellular marker of hypoxia, [^{18}F]fluoromisonidazole, to examine the question of whether sepsis actually produced tissue hypoxia. The binding of this marker increases inside cells as PO_2 approaches lower levels. They found no evidence of cellular hypoxia in skeletal muscle, brain, liver, heart, or diaphragm of rats made septic by cecal ligation and perforation. This was true in spite of cardiac output decreases on the order of 20% in the septic animals.

Gutierrez and his group took a different approach to examine the question of tissue hypoxia in animal models. They used multipoint surface measurements in rabbit skeletal muscle to construct frequency histograms of tissue PO_2. In one study [25], they found that although the mean value was shifted downward after injection of endotoxin into the animal, the distribution of values remained Gaussian. They attributed the decrease in mean value to the hypodynamic state caused by endotoxin and interpreted the normal distribution of tissue PO_2 values to mean that there were no major maldistributive effects in skeletal muscle. In a subsequent study [26], they matched the low blood flow found in the septic group by inflating an atrial balloon in a nonseptic group. They saw exactly the same pattern of tissue PO_2 but arterial lactate values were significantly higher in the septic group.

Vallet et al. [27] used a similar approach to study tissue oxygenation in an endotoxic dog model in which the hypodynamic state was converted to a hyperdynamic one. They used the same multipoint PO_2 tissue measurement at three different sites in anesthetized dogs. They measured PO_2 frequency distributions on skeletal muscle, gut serosa, and gut mucosa before and after endotoxin infusion. To raise cardiac output and regional blood flows from the low values at the end of the endotoxin infusion period, they infused dextran continuously for 2 h. Their data are summarized in Fig. 2. The results from skeletal muscle measurements confirmed those of Gutierrez et al. [25] during the hypodynamic phase that developed with endotoxin infusion. As flow decreased, the mean tissue PO_2 decreased but the distribution retained a normal shape (results not shown). As flow was restored and then increased above preendotoxin control levels, the normal distribution was retained and the mean tissue PO_2 increased. The serosal surface of gut behaved similarly to skeletal muscle. In contrast, the gut mucosa PO_2 showed a decline toward zero that failed to recover with volume resuscitation in spite of the fact that total blood flow to the gut was at or above preendotoxin levels. This was a clear demonstration of a severe regional hypoxia. Drazenovic et al. [28] were

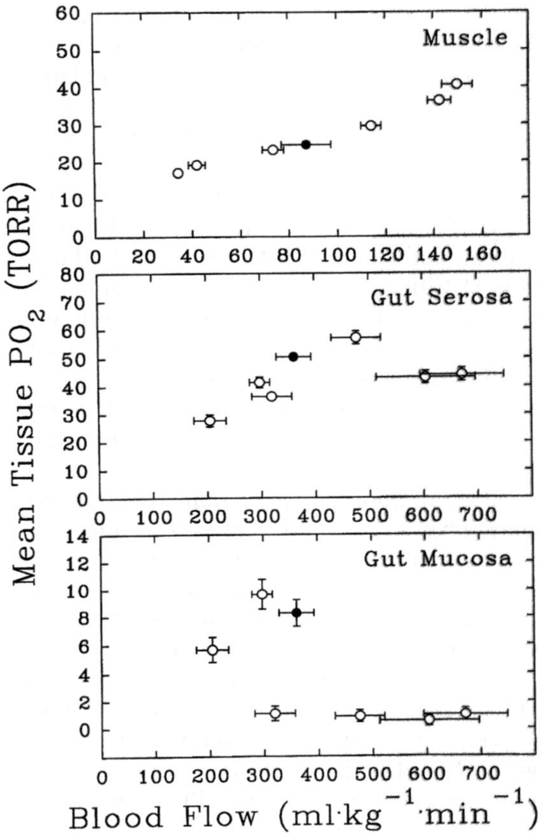

Fig. 2. Values for mean tissue PO_2 (±SE) taken from the study of Vallet et al. [44] shown as a function of mean regional blood flow (±SE) to muscle or to gut. The *filled circles* represent the preendotoxin control data; the *open circles* represent postendoxin measurements. In general, data obtained after resuscitation was begun lie close or to the right of the control points

able to show by morphological methods that circulation to canine gut mucosal villi and crypts was significantly attenuated by endotoxin injection, a finding that reinforced the validity of the mucosal PO_2 measurements.

Although it may be restricted to only one division of one organ system, the gut mucosa, tissue hypoxia is clearly an issue even when a hyperdynamic state has been established by appropriate fluid resuscitation from endotoxic shock. The old saw, that "the gut is the engine of sepsis", may enjoy a renaissance. The use of gut tonometry to calculate gut intramucosal pH (pH_i) in critically ill patients may be related to the particular vulnerability of splanchnic organs to hypoxia. Gutierrez et al. [29] claimed that persistent low pH_i was predictive of greater morbidity and mortality in such patients and even advocated the use of pH_i to guide resuscitative therapy. The route was admittedly convoluted but the original questions raised by apparent pathologic O_2 supply dependency may have led directly back to the bedside with a useful therapeutic guide. At the least it directed thought along productive pathways for basic scientists and clinicians concerned with the care of the critically ill.

The View from the 1990s

The decade of the 1990s was marked by an increasing number of challenges to the concept of pathologic O_2 supply dependency. These challenges took two general forms: (1) those that suggested that all appearances of O_2 supply dependency were really physiologic in nature and (2) those that assigned any correlation of $\dot{V}O_2$ and DO_2 to the artifactual mathematical coupling inherent when a shared variable was included, usually cardiac output estimated by thermodilution.

The first type of challenge is typified by reports such as that of Villar et al. [30], who showed that large changes in $\dot{V}O_2$ and DO_2 can occur spontaneously in critically ill patients, even those with normal arterial lactate values. Since no intervention was performed, the authors concluded that the changes they observed were instigated by changes in O_2 demand and went on to point out the difficulty that such spontaneous changes create in interpreting the presence and significance of O_2 supply dependency. A similar possibility was shown by Weissman and Kemper [31] who looked at $\dot{V}O_2/DO_2$ relationships in postoperative patients. Spontaneous activity and ICU interactions such as chest physical therapy caused both $\dot{V}O_2$ and DO_2 to increase so that there was an apparent O_2 supply dependency. Yet another study showed that an apparent O_2 supply dependency could be related to variations in sedation of critically ill patients [32]. These and other studies tended to affirm the view advanced by Dantzker et al. [20], that humans operate on a much smaller plateau of constant $\dot{V}O_2$ than do experimental animals, such as the dog, and may have a lesser ability to increase O_2ER as an initial response to primary increases in O_2 demand. As a consequence, any increase in O_2 demand is met by an increase in DO_2.

The other major challenge to the concept of pathologic O_2 supply dependency is that it can be attributed to an artifactual $\dot{V}O_2/DO_2$ relationship caused by mathematical coupling as described and illustrated by Archie [33]. This can arise when a variable and its associated error in measurement is shared between the two members of a regression analysis. The effect of any error is multiplied so that it forces an association where none may really exist. In the case of O_2 supply dependency, this was a common possibility in that many of the clinical studies used a thermodilution cardiac output to calculate both $\dot{V}O_2$ and DO_2. The practical effect of coupling error in such studies was assessed by Stratton et al. [34], who concluded that the effect was small when the range of DO_2 was sufficiently broad and if the measurement errors were of reasonable size. Nevertheless, several groups have reexamined pathologic O_2 supply dependency in the absence of a coupling error by using $\dot{V}O_2$ obtained from collection and analysis of expired gases and DO_2 as the product of thermodilution cardiac output and arterial O_2 content. Errors in $\dot{V}O_2$ and DO_2 would thus be independent of one another.

One prominent study by Ronco et al. [35] can serve as an illustration of this concern for coupling error. They selected 17 patients with ARDS but who did not have compromised cardiac function. They used expired gas analysis to calculate $\dot{V}O_2$ and thermodilution cardiac output to calculate DO_2. All methods were carefully evaluated for error sources and coefficient of variation. After a control set of measurements, 600 ml of packed red blood cells were infused over a 1 h period to raise arterial O_2 content significantly at which time another set of measurements was made. Interventions such as positive end-expiratory pressure (PEEP), inotropic agents, and the like were not changed between measurements. They found that $\dot{V}O_2$ and DO_2 increased together if both were estimated from thermodilution cardiac output but that $\dot{V}O_2$ measured by expired gas analysis did not change. Their results indicated that the apparent O_2 supply dependency seen in the first case was due to methodological error. Their conclusion was that $\dot{V}O_2$ was really independent of DO_2 in patients with ARDS and that the presence of sepsis and elevated lactate levels were not predictive of pathologic O_2 supply dependency.

As clear as the results of Ronco et al. [35] might have seemed, another interpretation was possible. All data necessary to recalculate cardiac output, by application of the Fick equation to the expired gas $\dot{V}O_2$ and the arteriovenous O_2 content difference for each of their subjects, was provided. The new values of cardiac output showed that it actually decreased with red blood cell infusion so that DO_2 did not change significantly. This response to an acute increase in hematocrit is commonly found [36]. It seemed quite credible, therefore, that $\dot{V}O_2$ did not change because there had been no real change in DO_2 with the infusion of red cells. Although they acknowledged this possibility in their discussion, Ronco et al. [35] chose to accept the thermodilution cardiac output to calculate DO_2 as the correct one because it had a better coefficient of variation than did the values obtained by direct Fick calculation. They may have elected precision over accuracy.

In Fig. 3, the differences between thermodilution cardiac output and Fick cardiac output have been graphed against the Fick cardiac outputs on the tacit assumption that the latter were the more accurate estimate of the true values. The differences were often as large as the estimate. If these two estimates purport to measure the same event, then one is probably more wrong than the other. The consistent overestimation by thermodilution suggests that it is the culprit in this case and that the conclusion of Ronco et al. [35] may have been incorrect, in that they did not succeed in their attempt to raise DO_2 in their ARDS patients. Furthermore, the large errors, or differences from the Fick derived values, when thermodilution cardiac output is used to obtain DO_2 may tend to mask any positive slope of $\dot{V}O_2/DO_2$ that might have really existed. This possibility warrants serious consideration in all future studies of this type. At the least, sufficient data should be obtained to allow both estimates of cardiac output to be made whenever feasible.

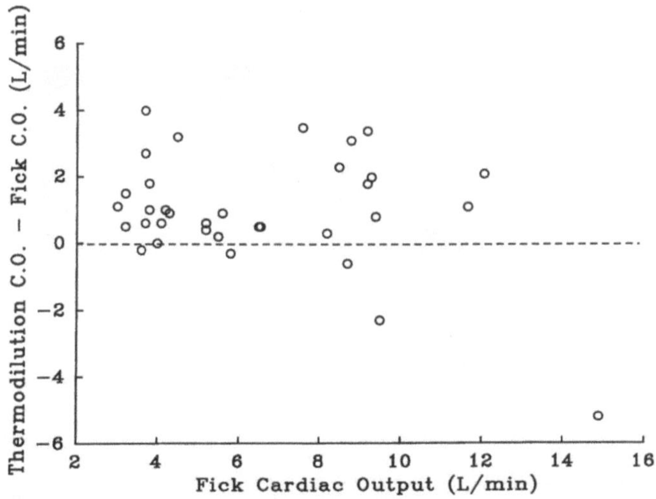

Fig. 3. Cardiac outputs (*C.O.*) were recalculated by Fick equation from data of Ronco et al. [35] and the difference from the value obtained by thermodilution was plotted against the Fick value

The question of whether $\dot{V}O_2$ is driven by DO_2 or itself drives DO_2 is still a valid issue. The question involves, to some extent, those organ systems that have flow-dependent $\dot{V}O_2$. Although the whole body of normal animals shows supply independence of $\dot{V}O_2$ above DO_{2crit}, organ systems that may be required to do more work as flow increases show a positive slope of the $\dot{V}O_2/DO_2$ relationship. The liver, for example, shows a slightly positive slope of $\dot{V}O_2/DO_2$ as flow is decreased but before the truly critical limit of DO_2 is reached [37]. Even more pronounced is the positive slope shown by the kidney which has strongly flow-dependent $\dot{V}O_2$. Nevertheless, a biphasic relationship is still seen as DO_2 is lowered to where it limits the kidney's basal energy requirements [38]. Although similar information is not presently available for the heart, it presumably would also show flow-dependent $\dot{V}O_2$ as its energy requirement for pumping is increased.

An organ system that does not normally show supply dependent behaviour of $\dot{V}O_2$ is resting skeletal muscle. In dogs that were slowly infused with endotoxin to a total dose of 2 mg/kg, however, hindlimb $\dot{V}O_2$ began to decrease as soon as DO_2 was lowered [39], as seen in Fig. 4. In these experiments, DO_2 was progressively lowered first by decreasing flow from 120 ml/kg per minute to 60 mlg/kg per minute (still within the range of normal flows observed in canine skeletal muscle) and then by decreasing inflow PO_2 with an in-line membrane oxygenator. There was no indication of O_2 supply dependency above the DO_{2crit} in a control group that was not given endotoxin (Fig. 4). The question of mathematical coupling error also did not enter into these results. Flow was measured directly with very small error and the range

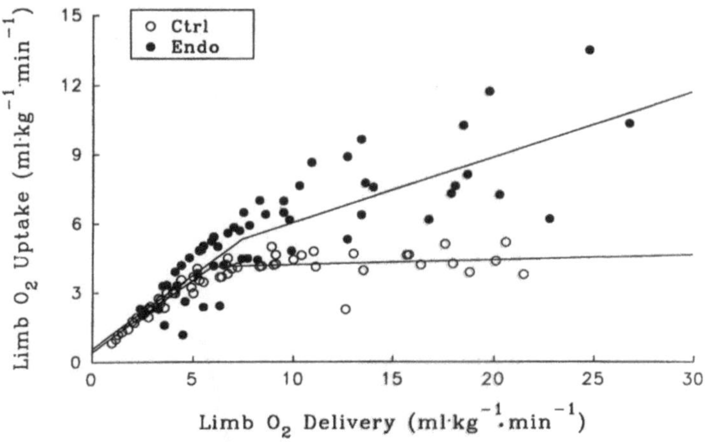

Fig. 4. Individual measurements of limb muscle O_2 uptake as a function of the corresponding O_2 delivery in normal control animals (*open circles*) and in endotoxemic animals (*filled circles*). (From [39])

of DO_2 values was up to four-fold above critical, which more than satisfied the criteria of Straton et al. [34]. The significance of these observations is that they may explain why pathologic O_2 supply dependency can be observed in certain groups of patients.

In addition to the O_2 supply dependency above the critical value so evident in Fig. 4, there was also an increased O_2 demand in the limb muscle of endotoxic dogs. Taken as the average $\dot{V}O_2$ above DO_{2crit}, the increase was over 80%. If that result is extrapolated to the rest of the muscles, it is more than sufficient to account for the approximately 25% increase in whole body $\dot{V}O_2$ measured in those experiments. In other words, O_2 supply dependency above the DO_{2crit} may occur mostly if not entirely in skeletal muscle of endotoxic dogs. The implication is that skeletal muscle may be the source of O_2 supply dependency in ARDS and septic patients. Whatever else it implies, it represents an abnormal flow dependency of $\dot{V}O_2$ for which the reasons remain obscure.

A Current View of Old and New Questions

The original review article in 1984 [2] offered an interpretation of pathologic O_2 supply dependency that centered attention on the state of the peripheral circulation. This led to widespread speculation that multiorgan failure, the often fatal consequence to ARDS and sepsis, was directly related to pervasive and profound tissue hypoxia. Based on results from experimental models of endotoxemia, the extent to which that is true except in selected organ systems such as the gut is still questionable. Nevertheless, there is a prevalent view among clinicians that tissue hypoxia is a key factor in the morbidity and mortality rates associated with ARDS and sepsis. One feature that helps to convince them is the elevated lactate levels in such patients, particularly those with a poor outcome. Some rely more on lactate to predict outcome than they do on any other measured variable [40–42]. The assumption is that the lactate is caused by tissue hypoxia [43]. Contrary to this idea is the experimental evidence that the rise in lactate is primarily due to inactivation of pyruvate dehydrogenase because treatment with dichloroacetate, an activator of the enzyme, completely reversed hyperlactatemia in endotoxic dogs [44]. To confuse further the issue of whether or not tissue hypoxia is a life threatening problem in ARDS and sepsis patients, several investigators have shown that increased DO_2 levels are associated with improved survival [45–47]. Clearly, the reality of tissue hypoxia in these patients still requires definitive solution.

There is, however, sufficient evidence to believe that the microcirculation and ability of peripheral tissue to extract O_2 is adversely affected by the cytokines and immune cascades activated in these disease states. Accordingly, a new picture of pathologic O_2 supply dependency is offered for the 1990s in Fig. 5. Regional differences and decreased adaptability of the microcirculation to changes in DO_2 are proposed to smear the point of intersection at DO_{2crit} and to exaggerate the curvilinear nature of the relationship with $\dot{V}O_2$ which is probably closer to the truth. No plateau is shown because none has yet been demonstrated. Instead, every increase in DO_2 is accompanied by an increase in $\dot{V}O_2$ and we do not know which takes precedence in that relationship.

If we assume that the increase in O_2 demand mandates the increase, either spontaneous or sponsored, in DO_2, then further questions arise. Where is the increased $\dot{V}O_2$ being used and for what purpose? Several possibilities can be suggested. Extramitochondrial pathways for O_2 use are probably greatly in-

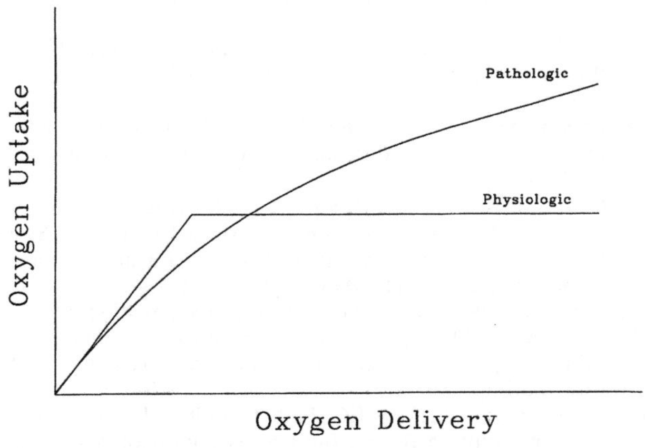

Fig. 5. A new representation of pathologic O_2 supply dependency (see text)

creased. For example, the amount of O_2 used in respiratory bursts to form reactive O_2 species has never been well quantified. We now know that molecular O_2 is used to form nitric oxide, the production of which greatly increases with the induction of nitric oxide synthase as part of the septic syndrome [48]. These extramitochondrial oxidases may require higher tissue PO_2 because of their lesser affinity for O_2 relative to mitochondrial oxidases. That would explain the continued increase in $\dot{V}O_2$ with increased DO_2. The results of Curtis et al. [39] would suggest skeletal muscle, which comprises 40%–50% of total body weight, figures prominently as the site of the increase. Finally, the effect of many of the cytokines and associated processes is to disturb the integrity of the membranes. Increased activity of membrane ATPases in response to the resultant imbalances of ions across the membrane would require increased energy production. These explanations for increased $\dot{V}O_2$ in ARDS and sepsis need to be evaluated and related to the possible effects on outcome.

It is now 20 years since Powers et al. [49] first reported what came to be called pathologic O_2 supply dependency. Although much has been learned about its occurrence and possible significance, the unanswered questions still leave much room for doubt and provide much reason to continue research in this area.

References

1. Danek S, Lynch JP, Weg JG, Dantzker DR (1980) The dependence of oxygen uptake on oxygen delivery in the adult respiratory distress syndrome. Am Rev Respir Dis 122:387–395
2. Cain SM (1984) Supply dependency of oxygen uptake in ARDS: myth or reality? Am J Med Sci 288:119–124
3. Cilley RE, Scharenberg AM, Bongiorno PF, Guire KE, Bartlett RH (1991) Low oxygen delivery produced by anemia, hypoxia, and low cardiac output. J Surg Res 51:425–433
4. Gaehtgens P, Benner KU, Schickendantz S (1976) Nutritive and non-nutritive blood flow in canine skeletal muscle after partial microembolization. Pflugers Arch 361:183–189
5. Landau SE, Alexander RS, Powers SR Jr, Stratton HS, Goldfarb RD (1982) Tissue oxygen exchange and reactive hyperemia following microembolization. J Surg Res 32:38–43
6. Cain SM, King CE, Chapler CK (1988) Effects of time and microembolization on O_2 extraction by dog hindlimb in hypoxia. J Crit Care 3:89–95
7. Duran WN, Renkin EM (1974) Oxygen consumption and blood flow in resting mammalian skeletal muscle. Am J Pysiol 226:173–177
8. Cain SM (1986) Assessment of tissue oxygenation. Crit Care Clin 2:537–550
9. Cain SM (1989) Supply dependency of oxygen uptake. In: Reinhart K, Eyrich K (eds) Clinical aspects of O_2 transport and tissue oxygenation. Springer, Berlin, Heidelberg, New York, pp 80–91
10. Kaufman BS, Rackow EC, Falk JL (1984) The relationship between oxygen delivery and consumption during fluid resuscitation of hypovolemic and septic shock. Chest 85:336–340

11. Haupt MT, Gilbert EM, Carlson RW (1985) Fluid loading increases oxygen consumption in septic patients with lactic acidosis. Am Rev Respir Dis 131:912–916
12. Gilbert EM, Haupt MT, Mandanas RY, Huaringa AJ, Carlson RW (1986) The effect of fluid loading, blood transfusion, and catecholamine infusion on oxygen delivery and consumption in patients with sepsis. Am Rev Respir Dis 134:873–878
13. Astiz ME, Rackow EC, Falk JL, Kaufman BS, Weil MH (1987) Oxygen delivery and consumption in patients with hyperdynamic septic shock. Crit Care Med 15:26–28
14. Gutierrez G, Pohil RJ (1986) Oxygen consumption is linearly related to O_2 supply in critically ill patients. J Crit Care 1:45–53
15. Bihari D, Smithies M. Gimson A, Tinker J (1987) The effects of vasodilation with prostacyclin on oxygen delivery and uptake in critically ill patients. N Engl J Med 317:397–403
16. Albert RK, Schrijen F, Poincelot F (1986) Oxygen consumption and transport in stable patients with chronic obstructive pulmonary disease. Am Rev Respir Dis 134:678–682
17. Mohsenifar Z, Amin D, Jasper AC, Shah PK, Koerner SK (1987) Dependence of oxygen consumption on oxygen delivery in patients with chronic congestive heart failure. Chest 92:447–450
18. Dorinsky PM, Costello JL, Gadek JE (1988) Relationships of oxygen uptake and oxygen delivery in respiratory failure not due to the adult respiratory distress syndrome. Chest 93:1013–1019
19. Williams AJ, Mohsenifar Z (1989) Oxygen supply dependency in patients with obstructive sleep apnea and its reversal after therapy with nasal continuous positive airway pressure. Am Rev Respir Dis 140:1308–1311
20. Dantzker DR; Foresman B, Gutierrez G (1991) Oxygen supply and utilization relationships. A reevaluation. Am Rev Respir Dis 143:675–679
21. Nelson DP, Beyer C, Samsel RW, Wood LDH, Schumacker PT (1987) Pathological supply dependence of O_2 uptake during bacteremia in dogs. J Appl Physiol 63:1487–1492
22. Nelson DP, Samsel RW, Wood LDH, Schumacker PT (1988) Pathological supply dependence of systemic and intestinal O_2 uptake during endotoxemia. J Appl Physiol 64:2410–2419
23. Samsel RW, Nelson DP, Sanders WM, Wood LDH, Schumacker PT (1988) Effect of endotoxin on systemic and skeletal muscle O_2 extraction. J Appl Physiol 65:1377–1382
24. Hotchkiss RS; Rust RS, Dence CS et al (1991) Evaluation of the role of cellular hypoxia in sepsis by the hypoxic marker [^{18}F]fluoromisonidazole. Am J Physiol 261:R965–R972
25. Gutierrez G, Lund N, Palizas F (1991) Rabbit skeletal muscle PO_2 during hypodynamic sepsis. Chest 99:224–229
26. Hurtado FJ, Gutierrez AM, Silva N, Fernandez E, Khan AE, Gutierrez G (1992) Role of tissue hypoxia as the mechanism of lactic acidosis during E. coli endotoxemia. J Appl Physiol 72:1895–1901
27. Vallet B, Lund N, Curtis SE, Kelly DR, Cain SM (1993) Gut and muscle tissue PO_2 in endotoxemic dogs during shock and resuscitation. Am Rev Respir Dis 147:A618
28. Drazenovic R, Samsel R, Wylam ME, Doerschuk CM, Schumacker PT (1992) Regulation of perfused capillary density in canine intestinal mucosa during endotoxemia. J Appl Physiol 72:259–265
29. Gutierrez G, Palizas F, Doglio G et al (1992) Gastric intramucosal pH as a therapeutic index of tissue oxygenation in critically ill patients. Lancet 339:195–199
30. Villar J, Slutsky AS, Hew E, Aberman A (1990) Oxygen transport and oxygen consumption in ciritically ill patients. Chest 98:687–692
31. Weissman C, Kemper M (1991) The oxygen uptake-oxygen delivery relationship during ICU interventions. Chest 99:430–435
32. Boyd O, Grounds M, Bennett D (1992) The dependency of oxygen consumption on oxygen delivery in critically ill postoperative patients is mimicked by variations in sedation. Chest 101:1619–1624

33. Archie JP (1981) Mathematic coupling of data – a common source of error. Ann Surg 193:296–303
34. Stratton HH, Feustel PJ, Newell JC (1987) Regression of calculated variables in the presence of shared measurement error. J Appl Physiol 62:2083–2093
35. Ronco JJ, Phang PT, Walley KR, Wiggs B, Fenwick JC, Russell JA (1991) Oxygen consumption is independent of changes in oxygen delivery in severe adult respiratory distress syndrome. Am Rev Respir Dis 143:1267–1273
36. Stork RL, Bredle DL, Chapler CK, Cain SM (1988) Regional hemodynamic responses to hypoxia in polycythemic dogs. J Appl Physiol 65:2069–2074
37. Schlichtig R, Kramer DJ, Pinsky MR (1991) Flow redistribution during progressive hemorrhage is a determinant of critical O_2 delivery. J Appl Physiol 70:169–178
38. Schlichtig R, Kramer DJ, Boston JR, Pinsky MR (1991) Renal O_2 consumption during progressive hemorrhage. J Appl Physiol 70:1957–1962
39. Curtis SE, Bradley WE, Cain SM (1992) Effects of endotoxin on canine skeletal muscle oxygen delivery-uptake relations during progressive hypoxic hypoxia. Adv Exp Med Biol 317:751–757
40. Bakker J, Coffernils M, Leon M. Gris P, Vincent J-L (1991) Blood lactate levels are superior to oxygen-derived variables in predicting outcome in human septic shock. Chest 99:956–962
41. Fenwick JC, Dodek PM, Ronco JJ, Phang PT, Wiggs B, Russell JA (1990) Increased concentrations of plasma lactate predict pathologic dependence of oxygen consumption on oxygen delivery in patients with adult respiratory distress syndrome. J Crit Care 5:81–86
42. Kruse JA, Haupt MT, Puri VK, Carlson RW (1990) Lactate levels as predictors of the relationship between oxygen delivery and consumption in ARDS. Chest 98:959–962
43. Vincent J-L (1993) Oxygen transport in severe sepsis. Acta Anaesthesiol Scand 37 [Suppl 98]:29–31
44. Curtis SE, Cain SM (1992) Regional and systemic oxygen delivery/uptake relations and lactate flux in hyperdynamic, endotoxin-treated dogs. Am Rev Respir Dis 145:348–354
45. Hayes MA, Yau EHS, Timmins AC, Hinds CJ, Watson D (1993) Response of critically ill patients to treatment aimed at achieving supranormal oxygen delivery and consumption. Chest 103:886–895
46. Russell JA, Ronco JJ, Lockhat D, Belzberg A, Kiess M, Dodek PM (1990) Oxygen delivery and consumption and ventricular preload are greater in survivors than in non-survivors of the adult respiratory distress syndrome. Am Rev Respir Dis 141:659–665
47. Tuchschmidt J, Fried J, Astiz M, Rackow E (1992) Elevation of cardiac output and oxygen delivery improves outcome in septic shock. Chest 102:216–220
48. Shibano T, Vanhoutte PM (1993) Induction of NO production by TNF-α and lipopolysaccharide in porcine coronary arteries without endothelium. Am J Physiol 264:H403–H407
49. Powers SR Jr, Mannal R, Neclerio M et al (1973) Physiologic consequences of positive end-expiratory pressure (PEEP) ventilation. Ann Surg 178:265–272

Sepsis and Nutritional Blood Flow

M. D. Menger, B. Vollmar and K. Messmer

Introduction

Despite the great progress that has been made in intensive care medicine, the incidence of sepsis and its sequelae has not diminished and still carries high mortality [1, 2]. Although the pathogenesis is not completely understood, sepsis is generally known to be caused by the activation of inflammatory cells and the release of endogenous humoral mediators in response to bacterial products, in particular endotoxins [3]. Evidence is slowly accumulating that excessively activated endogenous inflammatory cells and their compounds may be responsible for structural damage and functional deterioration of remote vital organ systems [4]. However, besides the activation of neutrophils and macrophages and the actions of cytokines, arachidonic acid metabolites, complement products, proteolytic enzymes and toxic oxygen radicals, impaired nutritional blood flow has been advocated as a key determinant for the development of organ dysfunction and subsequent multiple organ failure in septic shock [5, 6].

The initial phase of endotoxemia and sepsis is characterized by a high-flow (hyperdynamic circulatory) state with low systemic vascular resistance and baroreceptor reflex-mediated increase of cardiac output, which at later time turns into hypodynamic septic shock [7] with failure to sustain appropriate cardiac output values and to guarantee adequate oxygen supply to tissues. Inadequacy and maldistribution of nutrional flow in the early hyperdynamic circulatory state have been proposed to determine the transition into the hypodynamic state with the progression of the septic shock syndrome and development of irreversible tissue damage [8]. Therefore, efficient therapeutic strategies in septic shock must be associated with early diagnosis, e.g., during the hyperdynamic circulatory state.

To investigate the pathologic mechanisms which cause deterioration of nutritional perfusion, experimental models must approximate the characteristic time course of clinical septicemia including establishment of a hyper- and hypodynamic circulatory state. Various studies have confirmed that several of the pathophysiological states characteristic of sepsis and septic shock in patients can be simulated experimentally by:

a) ligation and puncture of the cecum [9],

b) peritoneal administration of pooled fecal inoculum [10] or discrete numbers of live *E. coli* organisms [11], and in particular
c) slow rate intravenous infusion of endotoxins/lipopolysaccharides (LPSs) [12, 13].

Regional Blood Flow

The hyperdynamic state after endotoxin challenge is characterized by high cardiac output and low peripheral vascular resistance [5] associated with enhanced systemic oxygen delivery but reduced whole body oxygen extraction [14]. Initially, global organ blood flow is maintained to brain, heart, skin, muscle, spleen, kidney and gastrointestinal tract as well as to liver and adipose tissue [12, 15]. The maintenance of blood flow to metabolically active tissues, coexistent with demonstrated alterations of *in vitro* cellular metabolism and *in vivo* function, has been found consistent with the concept that the earliest pathophysiological consequences of endotoxemia are intracellular and metabolic in nature rather than hemodynamic [15, 16]. However, Kreimeier et al. [12] have demonstrated that, although global organ blood flow to heart and kidney is maintained during the hyperdynamic phase of porcine endotoxemia, maldistribution of intraorgan blood flow may be a key factor in the development of endotoxin-induced organ failure.

Analysis of regional myocardial blood flow revealed a significant redirection of nutritive perfusion away from the subendocardium concomitant with the reduced subendocardial/subepicardial blood flow ratio [12]. Hence, the depression of ventricular performance at high myocardial blood perfusion during endotoxemia [17, 18] appears further aggravated by hypoxia-induced changes of cell structure due to redistribution of transmural blood flow, as observed in the course of clinical sepsis [19, 20].

Endotoxin-induced maldistribution of regional blood flow within the kidney is characterized by enhanced perfusion of the medulla at the expense of the cortical layer [19]. Since deterioration of renal function during hyperdynamic endotoxemia correlates with the redistribution of intrarenal blood flow [21], restricted perfusion of the renal cortex may represent a major factor in the development of oliguria and anuria in endotoxemic patients.

Today, circulatory disturbances rather than alterations in cellular metabolism are considered as major determinants of tissue oxygen uptake and cellular ischemia in septic shock [5]. Heterogeneity and maldistribution of regional blood flow due to disturbed autoregulation and opening of anatomic arteriovenous shunts [22, 23] with subsequent peripheral shunting of oxygen are presumably responsible for diminished oxygen extraction, as reflected by the narrowed arteriovenous oxygen difference. This phenomenon is supposedly responsible for the pathologic dependency of oxygen consumption on oxygen delivery and for lactacidemia in septic shock and underlines the predominant role of microcirculatory disturbances in the pathogenesis of organ failure in endotoxemia and sepsis.

Microcirculation

Although it is widely accepted that the endotoxin-induced sequence of events is primarily vascular in origin, the underlying mechanisms and the exact role of endotoxins have not been clearly established. Hypotheses range from vasomotor instability, vasoconstriction and vasodilation, hypo- and hyperreactivity to catecholamines, to disturbances in blood barriers and increased microvascular permeability [see 24]. There are two conflicting schools of thought, one providing evidence for arterial constriction and the other for arterial dilation. Moreover, Cryer et al [25, 26] reported differential arteriolar response during live *E. coli* bacteremia-induced high cardiac output (hyperdynamic) phase of sepsis, i.e., constriction of large (A_1) arterioles but dilation of small (A_3, A_4) arterioles. The most detailed description of the microcirculatory responses to endotoxin was given by Brånemark and Urbaschek [27]. Using *in vivo* microscopic techniques these authors reported arterial constriction and venular dilation 10 min after endotoxin administration with additional lumenal narrowing of the arterioles due to swelling of pericytes and endothelial cells [27]. However, initial arterial vasoconstriction was followed in 10–15 min by degranulation of mast cells and subsequent loss of arterial tone [27, 28]. These observations are in agreement with previous studies of Zweifach et al. [29] demonstrating dose-dependent induction of both an endotoxin-induced increase and a decrease in vascular reactivity to catecholamines, culminating in a complete absence of reactivity. It has been advocated that secondary arterial vasodilation comes as a result of tissue release of several vasoactive mediators including histamine, serotonin and bradykinin (see [30]), but also of prostanoids [25, 30] and endothelium-derived relaxing factor (nitric oxide) [31, 32]. Recent studies have confirmed marked suppression of sensitivity and maximum contraction of vascular tissue (rat aorta) to norepinephrine after exposure of endotoxin and septic sera from humans and dogs *in vitro* [33, 34] and during endotoxin shock *in vivo* [35].

Besides alteration of local vasomotor control, endotoxins have been demonstrated to induce microcirculatory disorders by capillary engorgement, endothelial swelling and intravascular hemoconcentration [36]. *In vivo* microscopic studies of the liver [37, 38] revealed significant perfusion failure of individual sinusoids upon endotoxin exposure, probably due to swelling of endothelial and Kupffer cells. Impairment of nutritional flow results in tissue hypoxia [39], depletion of energy stores [40] and, consequently, damage of parenchymal cells. In addition, tissue damage may also be induced directly by cellular uptake of endotoxins or toxic lipid component A with impairment of oxidative phosphorylation by degradation of cytochromes [41, 42].

In parallel with the deterioration of nutritional flow, *in vivo* microscopy revealed endotoxin-induced accumulation of leukocytes within the microvasculature and their adherence to the endothelial lining, in particular of post-capillary venules [37, 38, 43].

The extent of microcirculatory disturbances seems to be dependent upon:

a) the numbers of leukocytes interacting with the endothelial surface and tissue sessile macrophages,
b) the state of activation of these cells, and
c) the release of their potentially toxic mediators. Aggregation and adhesion of platelets with formation of microthrombi and adhesion of lymphocytes to macrophages (Kupffer cells) may further contribute to the breakdown of the microcirculation in endotoxic shock [37].

Polymorphonuclear Leukocytes

Endotoxin challenge is associated with a dramatic drop of circulating neutrophils [44], probably due to activation and emigration out of the vascular bed [45]. Neutrophils may be activated directly by:

a) endotoxins alone [46],
b) macrophage-derived products [47], or
c) the alternative complement pathway [48], all initiating the formation of aggregates and enhanced adhesiveness to microvascular endothelium [49].

Polymorphonuclear leukocyte (PMN)-endothelium interaction is the prerequisite for transendothelial emigration and infiltration into tissue. Using *in vivo* fluorescence microscopy Vollmar et al. [38] have demonstrated in the hepatic microvasculature that adherence of PMNs is observed as early as 20 min after endotoxin exposure, predominantly at the venular segments of the microcirculation. The process of PMN adherence after endotoxin exposure seems to involve specific adhesion molecules including the CD11b/CD18 glycoprotein complex on the surface of PMNs [50–52] and E-selectin (ELAM-1) on the surface of endothelial cells [53].

The microvasculature is the primary target for the initial damage in endotoxemia, which is characterized by loss of endothelial integrity and increased microvascular permeability [44, 54, 55]. Endotoxin-mediated increase of microvascular permeability is primarily dependent upon leukocyte accumulation and adherence. This view is supported by the results from *in vivo* microscopy experiments in the hamster cheek pouch, which revealed a significant correlation between the number of leukocytes and microvascular permeability [56], and by experiments demonstrating that neutrophil depletion prevents the endotoxin-induced increase of vascular permeability [54].

PMNs may not only affect the microvasculature, but have also been proposed to induce parenchymal cell injury by several mechanisms. Activated PMNs release reactive oxygen metabolites including superoxide anion and hydrogen peroxide [57]. These cytotoxic substances can initiate peroxidation of lipids and oxidation of protein thiols that might contribute to tissue injury [40]. This hypothesis has been confirmed by experiments, in which products of lipid peroxidation were detected upon LPS exposure [40], and supports the view that reactive oxygen metabolites released from activated PMNs contribute to endotoxin-induced tissue injury [58, 59]. Apart from toxic oxygen metabolites, lysosomal enzymes have been implicated in certain instances of PMN-mediated tissue injury [60].

Several studies revealed that: (1) after endotoxin exposure there is an early sequestration and accumulation of leukocytes in proximity to damaged tissue [47, 54] and (2) neutrophil depletion or blockade of leukocyte adherence affords protection against endotoxin-induced hepatic tissue damage [50, 52, 61] and prevention of multiple organ failure [62]. These results further confirmed the pivotal role of leukocytes in causing endotoxin-induced organ tissue damage.

Macrophages

Sessile tissue macrophages, in particular Kupffer cells, are the principal site of endotoxin detoxification via unspecific pinocytosis rather than receptor-mediated endocytosis [41]. Endotoxin challenge leads to increased phagocytic activity [63], proliferation of macrophages [41], and recruitment of mononuclear phagocytes from bone marrow [64]. However, apart from endotoxin clearance activated macrophages may contribute to systemic endotoxin toxicity by release of chemotactic factors/mediators, i.e., cytokines, eicosanoids, complement, procoagulant factors and reactive oxygen metabolites [64–66] which additionally elicit both adverse effects on the microcirculation and tissue destructive properties, predisposing to failure of remote organ systems [55].

Endotoxin-induced stimulation of macrophages leads to the release of cytokines including tumor necrosis factor-α (TNF-α) [52, 66, 67], interleukin-1 (IL-1) [68], interleukin-6 (IL-6) [69] and transforming growth factor-β (TGF-β) [70], which may potentially affect nutritional microcirculation. TNF-α increases vascular permeability [71] and procoagulant activity [72], depresses mitochondrial respiration [73] and triggers the release of platelet activating factor (PAF) from endothelial cells [74]. Both TNF-α and IL-1 synergistically induce up-regulation of adhesion molecules on the endothelial cell surface (ELAM-1 [75], ICAM-1 [76]), thus promoting leukocyte adherence to microvascular endothelium. Accumulation and adherence of leukocytes may be augmented by the action of TGF-β, which, although reducing cytokine production, exerts strong chemoattractant properties on monocytes, macrophages and neutrophils [77–79]. By contrast, interleukin-10 (IL-10), which is produced as a result of immune activation by subpopulations of T helper cells [80], B cells [81] and macrophages/monocytes [82, 83], decreases endotoxin-induced TNF-α release and provides protection from lethal endotoxemia [84].

Apart from the actions of cytokines, an imbalance of arachidonic acid metabolites, i.e., prostanoids such as prostaglandins E_1 and -E_2 (PGE_1, PGE_2), prostaglandin I_2 (PGI_2), and thromboxane A_2 (TXA_2) and leukotrienes (LTB_4, -C_4, -D_4, -E_4), with preferential synthesis of the latter may account for the manifestation of endotoxin-induced microvascular injury [85]. *In vitro* and *in vivo* studies have shown that LTB_4 exerts powerful chemotactic activities and promotes leukocyte adhesion to and emigration across the endothelial wall of postcapillary venules [86, 87], whereas the cysteinyl leukotrienes LTC_4, LTD_4, and LTE_4 are implicated in the regulation of vessel permeability and the induction of macromolecular leakage [86, 88]. In addition, both leukotrienes and TXA_2 induce arteriolar vasoconstriction [89], which further aggravates nutritional perfusion failure and focal ischemia [7].

The pathogenesis of microvascular injury following endotoxemia may also involve humoral mediators, in particular complement 5a (C5a). Activation of the complement system occurs via endotoxin stimulation or TNF-α release, alters the endothelial barrier function of the microvessel wall with an increase of vascular permeability, and stimulates neutrophils to release cytotoxic oxidants and proteases (see [90]). The reactive oxygen metabolites released from both leukocytes and macrophages after endotoxin exposure initiate further leukocyte accumulation and release of potent mediators, and thus constitute a self-sustaining vicious circle. Finally, all PAF, TXA_2 and procoagulant factors may be operative in the initiation of endotoxin-induced endothelial damage, platelet and fibrin deposition and diffuse coagulative changes, in severe cases resulting in disseminated intravascular coagulation [DIC] with breakdown of the microcirculation and organ failure [91].

Conclusion

Early sepsis and endotoxemia are characterized by a transient hyperdynamic circulatory state associated with an enhanced cardiac output, reduced systemic vascular resistance and narrowed arteriovenous oxygen difference, indicating impaired peripheral oxygen extraction. The defect in oxygen extraction may, in part, be due to inadequate nutritional tissue perfusion, resulting in tissue ischemia. Microvascular injury is a primary step in the development of endotoxin-induced organ failure and is characterized by accumulation and adherence of leukocytes to the endothelial lining with increased microvascular permeability and release of a variety of toxic mediators (cytokines, eicosanoids, lipid mediators, procoagulant factors and reactive oxygen metabolites). Therefore, therapeutic strategies to prevent endotoxin-associated microvascular injury should inhibit leukocyte accumulation or adherence [50, 52, 61], and block the synthesis, release and/or action of individual mediators [40, 92–94]. One should, however, keep in mind that successful therapeutic strategies in septic shock have to include early and efficient elimination of endotoxins from the circulation.

References

1. Bone RC, Fisher CJ, Clemmer TP, Slotman GJ, Metz CA, Balk RA (1989) The methylprednisolone severe study group: Sepsis syndrome: a valid clinical entity. Crit Care Med 17:389–393
2. Harris RL, Musher DM, Bloom K et al (1987) Manifestations of sepsis. Arch Intern Med 147:1895–1906
3. Morrison DC, Ulevitch RJ (1978) The effects of bacterial endotoxins in host mediation systems. Am J Pathol 93:527–617
4. Goris RJA (1990) Mediators of multiple organ failure. Intensive Care Med 16:S192–S196
5. Thijs LG, Schneider AJ, Groeneveld ABJ (1990) The haemodynamics of septic shock. Intensive Care Med 16:S182–S186
6. Kreimeier U, Ruiz-Morales M, Messmer K (1993) Comparison of the effects of volume resuscitation with dextran 60 vs Ringers's lactate on central hemodynamics, regional blood flow, pulmonary function, and blood composition during hyperdynamic endotoxemia. Circ Shock 39:89–99
7. Messmer K, Kreimeier U, Hammersen F (1988) Multiple organ failure: clinical implications to macro- and microcirculation. In: Manabe H, Zweifach BW, Messmer K (eds) Microcirculation in circulatory disorders. Springer, Berlin Heidelberg New York, pp 147–157
8. Thijs LG, Groeneveld ABJ (1987) The circulatory defect of septic shock. In: Vincent JL, Thijs LG (eds) Septic shock. Springer, Berlin Heidelberg New York, pp 161–178
9. Baker CC, Chaudry IH, Gaines HO, Baue AE (1983) Evaluation of factors affecting mortality rate after sepsis in murine cecal ligation and puncture model. Surgery 94:331–335
10. Lang CH, Bagby GJ, Bornside GH, Vial LJ, Spitzer JJ (1983) Sustained hypermetabolic sepsis in rats: characterization of the model. J Surg Res 35:201–210
11. Short BL, Gardiner WM, Walker RI, Fletcher JR, Rogers JE (1983) Rat intraperitoneal sepsis – a clinically relevant model. Circ Shock 10:351–359
12. Kreimeier U, Hammersen F, Ruiz-Morales M, Yang Zh, Messmer K (1991) Redistribution of intraorgan blood flow in acute, hyperdynamic porcine endotoxemia. Eur Surg Res 23:85–99
13. Wichtermann KA, Baue AE, Chaudry IA (1980) Sepsis and septic shock – a review of laboratory models and a proposal. J Surg Res 29:189–201
14. Bersten AD, Gnidec AA, Rutledge FS, Sibbald WJ (1990) Hyperdynamic sepsis modifies a PEEP-mediated redistribution in organ blood flows. Am Rev Respir Dis 141:1198–1208
15. Fish RE, Lang CH, Spitzer JA (1986) Regional blood flow during continuous low-dose endotoxin infusion. Circ Shock 18:267–275
16. Wang P, Zhou M, Rana MW, Ba ZF, Chaudry IH (1992) Differential alterations in microvascular perfusion in various organs during early and late sepsis. Am J Physiol 263:G38–G43
17. Abel FL (1989) Myocardial function in sepsis and endotoxin shock. Am J Physiol 26:R1265–R1281
18. Lang CH, Bagby GJ, Ferguson JL, Spitzer JJ (1984) Cardiac output and redistribution of organ blood flow in hypermetabolic sepsis. Am J Physiol 246:R331–R337
19. Parker MM, Shelhammer JH, Bacharach SL et al (1984) Profound but reversible myocardial depression in patients with septic shock. Ann Intern Med 100:483–490
20. Weisel RD, Vito L, Dennis RC (1977) Myocardial depression during sepsis. Am J Surg 133:512–521
21. Frey L, Kreimeier U, Schwarz G, von Hirschhausen E, Messmer K (1990) Deterioration of renal function during hyperdynamic endotoxemia correlates with redistribution of intrarenal blood flow. Eur Surg Res 22:66 (abstract)

22. Cunnion RE, Schaer GL, Parker MM, Natanson C, Parillo JE (1986) The coronary circulation in human septic shock. Circulation 73:637–644
23. Oettinger W, Roscher R, Jonescu J, Beger HG (1986) Renal prostaglandin-release, blood flow, and function in porcine endotoxic shock. Langenbecks Arch Chir 187–190
24. Nagler AL (1980) The circulatory manifestations of bacterial endotoxemia. In: Kaley G, Altura BM (eds) Microcirculation. University Park Press, Baltimore, pp 107–117
25. Cryer HG, Garrison RN, Harris PD, Greenwald BH, Alsip NL (1990) Prostaglandins mediate skeletal muscle arteriole dilation in hyperdynamic bacteremia. Am J Physiol 259:H728–H734
26. Cryer HM, Garrison RN, Harris PD (1988) Role of muscle microvasculature during hyperdynamic and hypodynamic phases of endotoxin shock in decerebrate rats. J Trauma 28:312–318
27. Brånemark PI, Urbaschek B (1967) Endotoxins in tissue injury. Vital microscopic studies on the effect of endotoxin from E. coli on the microcirculation. Angiology 18:667–671
28. Urbaschek B, Huth K, Krech HJ (1969) Endotoxin-induced microcirculatory disturbances and interaction to various metabolic parameters including the coagulation system. Bibl Anat 10:442–448
29. Zweifach BW, Nagler AL, Thomas L (1956) The role of epinephrine in the reactions produced by endotoxins of gram negative bacteria. The changes produced by endotoxin in the vascular reactivity of epinephrine in the rat mesoappendix and the isolated, perfused rabbit ear. J Exp Med 104:881–896
30. Bond RF (1985) Peripheral circulatory responses to endotoxin. In: Hinshaw LB (ed) Pathophysiology of endotoxin. Elsevier Science, Amsterdam, pp 36–75 (Handbook of endotoxin, vol 2)
31. Lübbe AS, Garrison RN, Cryer HM, Alsip NL, Harris PD (1992) EDRF as a possible mediator of sepsis-induced arteriolar dilation in skeletal muscle. Am J Physiol 262:H880–H887
32. Wright CE, Rees DD, Moncada S (1992) Protective and pathological role of nitric oxide in endotoxin shock. Cardiovasc Res 26:48–57
33. Hollenberg SM, Cunnion RE, Parrillo JE (1992) Effect of septic serum on vascular smooth muscle: In vitro studies using rat aortic rings. Crit Care Med 20:993–998
34. McKenna TM (1992) Recovery of vascular tissue contractile function during sustained endotoxin exposure. Am J Physiol 263:H1628–H1631
35. Baker CH, Sutton ET, Zhou Z, Dietz JR (1990) Microvascular vasopressin effects during endotoxin shock in the rat. Circ Shock 30:81–95
36. Balis JU, Rappaport ES, Gerber L, Fareed J, Buddingh F, Messmore HL (1978) A primate model for prolonged endotoxin shock. Blood-vascular reactions and effects of glucocorticoid treatment. Lab Invest 38:511–523
37. McCuskey RS (1993) Hepatic microvascular responses to endotoxinemia and sepsis. Prog Appl Microcirc 19:76–84
38. Vollmar B, Glasz J, Senkel A, Menger MD, Messmer K (1993) Role of leukocytes in the initial hepatic microvascular response to endotoxemia. Zentralbl Chir 118:691–696
39. Gutierrez G, Lund N, Palizas F (1991) Rabbit skeletal muscle PO_2 during hypodynamic sepsis. Chest 99:224–229
40. Sugino K, Dohi K, Yamada K, Kawasaki T (1987) The role of lipid peroxidation in endotoxin-induced hepatic damage and the protective effect of antioxidants. Surgery 101:746–752
41. Nolan JP (1981) Endotoxin, reticuloendothelial function, and liver injury. Hepatology 1:458–465
42. Schaefer CF, Biber B, Lerner MR, Vliet J-V, Fagraeus L (1991) Rapid reduction of intestinal cytochrome a_1a_3 during lethal endotoxemia. J Surg Res 51:382–391
43. Kawasaki K, Galla TJ, Lehr HA, Meßmer K (1990) Endotoxin verstärkt das Leukozytensticking in der Mikrozirkulation des postischämischen Skelettmuskels. Langenbecks Arch Chir Forum 90:29–32

44. Snapper JR, Bernard GR, Hinson JM, Hutchinson AA, Loyd JE, Ogletree ML, Brigham KL (1983) Endotoxemia-induced leukopenia in sheep. Am Rev Respir Dis 127:306–309
45. Grisham MB, Everse J, Janssen HF (1988) Endotoxemia and neutrophil infiltration in vivo. Am J Physiol 254:H1017–H1022
46. Dahinden C, Galanos C, Fehr J (1983) Granulocyte activation by endotoxin I. J Immunol 130:857–862
47. Issekutz AC, Megyeri P, Issekutz TB (1987) Role for macrophage products in endotoxin-induced polymorphonuclear leukocyte accumulation during inflammation. Lab Invest 56:49–59
48. Wilson ME (1985) Effects of bacterial endotoxins on neutrophil function. Rev Infect Dis 7:404–418
49. Meyrick BO (1986) Endotoxin-mediated pulmonary endothelial cell injury. Federation Proc 45:19–24
50. Jaeschke H, Farhood A, Smith CW (1991) Neutrophil-induced liver cell injury in endotoxin shock is a CD11b/CD18-dependent mechanism. Am J Physiol 261:G1051–G1056
51. Simms HH, D'Amico R (1991) Increased PMN CD11b/CD18 expression following posttraumatic ARDS. J Surg Res 50:362–367
52. Windsor ACJ, Walsh CJ, Mullen PG et al (1993) Tumor necrosis factor-α blockade prevents neutrophil CD18 receptor upregulation and attenuates acute lung injury in porcine sepsis without inhibition of neutrophil oxygen radical generation. J Clin Invest 91:1459–1468
53. Engelberts I, Samyo SK, Leuwenberg JFM, van der Linden C, Buurman WA (1992) A role of ELAM-1 in the pathogenesis of MOF during septic shock. J Surg Res 53:136–144
54. Heflin AC, Brigham KL (1981) Prevention of granulocyte depletion of increased vascular permeability of sheep lung following endotoxemia. J Clin Invest 68:1253–1260
55. Koike K, Moore FA, Moore EE, Poggetti RS, Tudre RM, Banerjee A (1992) Endotoxin after gut ischemia/reperfusion causes irreversible lung injury. J Surg Res 52:656–662
56. Matsuda T, Rubinstein I, Robbins RA, Koyama S, Joyner WL, Rennard SI (1991) Role of neutrophils in endotoxin-mediated microvascular injury in hamsters. J Appl Physiol 71:307–313
57. Fantone JC, Ward PA (1982) Role of oxygen-derived free radicals and metabolites in leukocyte-dependent inflammatory reactions. Am J Pathol 107:397–418
58. Bautista AP, Spitzer JJ (1990) Superoxide anion generation by in situ perfused rat liver: effect of in vivo endotoxin. Am J Physiol 259:G907–G912
59. Mayer AMS, Spitzer JA (1991) Continuous infusion of escherichia coli endotoxin in vivo primes in vitro superoxide anion release in rat polymorphonuclear leukocytes and Kupffer cells in a time-dependent manner. Infect Immun 59:4590–4598
60. Mavier P, Preaux A-M, Guigui B, Lescs M-C, Zafrani E-S, Dhumeaux D (1988) In vitro toxicity of polymorphonuclear neutrophils to rat hepatocytes: evidence for a proteinase-mediated mechanism. Hepatology 8:254–258
61. Hewett JA, Schultze E, VanCise S, Roth RA (1992) Neutrophil depletion protects against liver injury from bacterial endotoxin. Lab Invest 68:347–361
62. Mallick AA, Ishizaka A, Stephens KE, Hatherill JR, Tazelaar HD, Raffin TA (1989) Multiple organ damage caused by tumor necrosis factor and prevented by prior neutrophil depletion. Chest 95:1114–1120
63. Arredondo MI, Kampschmidt RF (1962) Effect of endotoxins on phagocytic activity of the reticuloendothelial system of the rat. PSEBM 112:78–81
64. Pilaro AM, Laskin DL (1986) Accumulation of activated mononuclear phagocytes in the liver following lipopolysaccharides treatment of rats. J Leukoc Biol 40:29–41
65. Decker K (1990) Biologically active products of stimulated liver macrophages (Kupffer cells). Eur J Biochem 192:245–261
66. Monden K, Arii S, Itai S et al (1991) Enhancement and hepatocyte-modulating effect

of chemical mediators and monokines produced by hepatic macrophages in rats with induced sepsis. Res Exp Med 191:177–187
67. Karck U, Peters T, Decker K (1988) The release of tumor necrosis factor from endotoxin-stimulated rat Kupffer cells is regulated by prostaglandin E_2 and dexamethasone. J Hepatol 7:352–361
68. Dinarello CA (1984) Interleukin-1. Rev Infect Dis 6:51–95
69. Callery MP, Mangino MJ, Kamei T, Flye MW (1990) Interleukin-6 production by endotoxin-stimulated Kupffer cells is regulated by prostaglandin E2. J Surg Res 48:523–527
70. Assoian RK, Fleurdelys BE, Stevenson HC et al. (1987) Expression and secretion of type β transforming growth factor by activated human macrophages. Proc Natl Acad Sci USA 84:6020–6024
71. Remick DG, Kunkel RG, Larrick JW, Kunkel SL (1987) Acute in vivo effects of human recombinant tumor necrosis factor. Lab Invest 56:583–590
72. Bevilacqua MP, Pober JS, Majeau GR, Fiers W, Cotran RS, Gimbrone MA (1986) Recombinant tumor necrosis factor induces procoagulant activity in cultured human vascular endothelium: characterization and comparison with the actions of interleukin 1. Proc Natl Acad Sci USA 83:4533–4537
73. Stadler J, Billiar TR, Curran RD, Stuehr DJ, Ochoa JB, Simmons RL (1991) Effect of exogenous and endogenous nitric oxide on mitochondrial respiration of rat hepatocytes. Am J Physiol 260:C910–C916
74. Braquet P, Hosford D (1989) The potential role of platelet-activating factor (PAF) in shock, sepsis and adult respiratory distress syndrome (ARDS). Prog Clin Biol Res 308:425–439
75. Bevilacqua MP, Pober JS, Mendrick DL, Cotran RS, Gimbrone MA (1987) Identification of an inducible endothelial-leukocyte adhesion molecule. Proc Natl Acad Sci USA 84:9238–9242
76. Pober JS, Gimbrone MA, Lapierre LA, Mendrick DL, Fiers W, Rothlein R, Springer TA (1986) Overlapping patterns of activation of human endothelial cells by interleukin 1, tumor necrosis factor, and immune interferon. J Immunol 137:1893–1896
77. Drake WT, Issekutz AC (1993) Transforming growth factor-β1 enhances polymorphonuclear leukocyte accumulation in dermal inflammation and transendothelial migration by a priming action. Immunology 78:197–204
78. Reibman J, Meixler S, Lee TL et al (1991) Transforming growth factor β1, a potent chemoattractant for human neutrophils, bypasses classic signal-transduction pathway. Proc Natl Acad Sci USA 88:6805–6809
79. Wiseman DM, Polverini PJ, Kamp DW, Leibovich SJ (1988) Transforming growth factor-beta (TGFβ) is chemotactic for human monocytes and induces their expression of angiogenic activity. Biochem Biophys Res Commun 157:793–800
80. Fiorentino DF, Bond MW, Mosmann TR (1989) Two types of mouse T helper cell: IV. Th2 clones secrete a factor that inhibits cytokine production by Th1 clones. J Exp Med 170:2081–2095
81. O'Garra A, Chang R, Hastings R, Go N, Haughton G, Howard M (1992) Ly1 B (B-1) cells are the main source of B-cell derived IL-10. Eur J Immunol 22:711–717
82. de Waal Malefyt R, Abrams J, Bennett B, Figdor C, de Vries JE (1991) IL-10 inhibits cytokine synthesis by human monocytes: an autoregulatory role of IL-10 produced by monocytes. J Exp Med 174:1209–1220
83. Fiorentino DF, Zlotnik A, Mosmann TR, Howard M, O'Garra A (1991) IL-10 inhibits cytokine production by activated macrophages. J Immunol 147:3815–3822
84. Howard M, Muchamuel T, Andrade S, Menon S (1993) Interleukin 10 protects mice from lethal endotoxemia. J Exp Med 177:1205–1208
85. Ogletree ML, Oates JA, Brigham KL, Hubbard WC (1982) Evidence for pulmonary release of 5-hydroxyeicosatetraenoic acid (5-HETE) during endotoxemia in unanesthetized sheep. Prostaglandins 23:459–468
86. Dahlen SE, Björk J, Hedqvist P, Arfors KE, Hammarström S, Lindgren JA, Samuelsson B (1981) Leukotriene promotes plasma leakage and leukocyte adhesion in postca-

pillary venules: in vivo effects with relevance to the acute inflammatory response. Proc Natl Acad Sci USA 78:3887–3891
87. Ford-Hutchinson AW, Bray MA, Doig MV, Shipley ME, Smith MJH (1980) Leukotriene B4, a potent chemokinetic and aggregating substance released from polymorphonuclear leukocytes. Nature 286:264–265
88. Hua XY, Dahlen SE, Lundberg JM, Hammarström S, Hedqvist P (1985) Leukotrienes C_4, D_4, and E_4 cause widespread and extensive plasma extravasation in the guinea pig. Naunyn-Schmiedebergs Arch Pharmacol 330:136–141
89. Piper PJ (1984) Formation and action of leukotrienes. Physiol Rev 64:744–761
90. Bone RC (1992) Inhibitors of complement and neutrophils: a critical evaluation of their role in the treatment of sepsis. Crit Care Med 20:891–898
91. Harkema JM, Chaudry IH (1992) Magnesium-adenosine triphosphate in the treatment of shock, ischemia and sepsis. Crit Care Med 20:263–275
92. Alexander HR, Doherty GH, Buresh CM, Venzon DJ, Norton JA (1991) A recombinant human receptor antagonist to interleukin 1 improves survival after lethal endotoxemia in mice. J Exp Med 173:1029–1032
93. Beutler B, Milsark IW, Cerami A (1985) Passive immunization against cachectin/tumor necrosis factor protects mice from lethal effect of endotoxin. Science 229:869–871
94. Kopaniak MM, Movat HZ (1983) Kinetics of acute inflammation induced by Escherichia coli in rabbits II. The effect of hyperimmunization, complement depletion, and depletion of leukocytes. Am J Pathol 110:13–29

Endothelial Cell Function in the Critically Ill

J.-L. Vincent, J. C. Preiser, G. Friedman and H. Zhang

Introduction

Our concepts have changed markedly since W. Harvey's original description of the vasculature as a passive conduit for blood to the vital organs. The endothelium of the vasculature represents a complex organ synthesizing a number of mediators and interacting actively with other cellular elements including circulating white blood cells and platelets and infiltrating macrophages. The endothelium can directly influence the vascular smooth muscle, thereby regulating the distribution of blood flow to the cells. The total endothelium surface area is estimated to cover six tennis courts and to weigh 1–1.5 kg in an adult.

The endothelium contributes to the metabolism of vasoactive substances such as bradykinin, inflammatory mediators such as platelet activating factor (PAF) and hemostatic factors such as thrombin. Many of the influences of the endothelial cells act in opposing ways, representing the "ying" and "yang" of several important processes. The endothelium releases vasoconstrictive substances (such as endothelin, thromboxin and superoxide anions) and vasodilating substances (such as nitric oxide or prostacyclin). It releases procoagulant and anticoagulant substances. It releases both growth factors and inhibitors; it releases proinflammatory and antiinflammatory substances. Hence, alteration in endothelial cell function will result in an imbalance between these opposing elements.

This chapter will focus on the importance of the endothelium in regulating the microcirculation and on the interactions between endothelial cells and polymorphonuclear leukocytes in the inflammatory response.

Regulation of the Microcirculation

The endothelium is strategically located to control the microvascular blood supply. An increase in blood flow and in particular in shear stress can result in an increased release of nitric oxide (NO) and prostaglandins and a reduced release of endothelin [1, 2]. The increased shear stress will also induce a realignment of cells in the direction of flow [3], increase the release of tissue plasminogen activator [4] and reduce fibronectin synthesis. The endothelial cells will also respond to an increase in microvascular pressure via a stretch activated channel [5].

A number of substances can also induce vasodilation via the release of NO. These include bradykinin, thrombin, serotonin, vasopressin and adenosine diphosphate (ADP). These substances can act by several pathways. For instance, thrombin acts by a pertussin toxin sensitive pathway but bradykinin acts by another pathway. Nevertheless, the final mechanism usually involves a change in phosphoinositol metabolism resulting in alterations in intracellular calcium availability.

The Role of Nitric Oxide in the Septic Patient

The discovery of endothelium derived relaxing factor (EDRF) resulted from the important experience by Furchgott and Zawadzki [6] showing that acetylcholine-induced relaxation by isolated preparations of arteries previously contracted by norepinephrine was observed only when endothelial cells were present. These fundamental experiments implicated the presence of muscarinic receptors on the endothelial cells. Subsequent studies showed that EDRF and an aqueous solution of NO had identical effects and induced an identical spectral shift in the absorbance of hemoglobin [7, 8]. Palmer et al. [9] demonstrated that NO is produced from the oxidation of L-arginine in the presence of NADP. Other investigators showed that NO may be released as a more stable compound such as nitrosocysteine [10]. There may also be EDRF substances other than NO that are released from endothelial cells [11]. The presence of hemoglobin or superoxide free radicals markedly reduces the release of EDRF. Hence, the presence of superoxide dismutase is necessary to control the cellular superoxide levels [12].

As a small gas molecule NO can easily penetrate into the smooth muscle cells where it binds to soluble guanylate cylase to increase the intracellular levels of cyclic guanidine monophosphate (cGMP). This in turn reduces calcium availability in the cells by several possible mechanisms including reduced entry of calcium via calcium channels, increased calcium uptake by the sarcoplasmic reticulum and reduced sensitivity of myosin for calcium.

An increase in blood flow may also activate potassium channels resulting in the hyperpolarization of smooth muscle cells [13] and the release of nitrovasodilators [14].

Interestingly, hypoxia has been shown to trigger the release of EDRF in several models but anoxia may abolish its release. This may explain how NO may be released in excessive amounts in some forms of acute circulatory failure but perhaps become deficient in some areas of the body when oxygen is no longer available to the cells.

Several studies have clearly established increased expression of the inducible NO synthase by endotoxin or cytokines such as tumor necrosis factor (TNF), interleukin-1 (IL-1) or interferon-γ. This increased release of NO has been incriminated in the sepsis-induced vasodilation. Administration of lipopolysaccharide (LPS) to animals increases their urinary nitrate excretion [15] and monomethyl-L-arginine (L-NMMA), an inhibitor of the NO synthase, has been shown to increase vascular tone following the administration of LPS [16] or TNF [17]. However, these effects may not be very specific since L-NMMA can increase arterial pressure in normal individuals or immediately after endotoxin administration before NO synthase can be induced [18].

This topic remains quite controversial since a number of studies have questioned the beneficial effects of L-NMMA or other NO synthase inhibitors in endotoxic shock. In some studies, these substances increased blood pressure and systemic vascular resistance but reduced cardiac output [19] or increased mortality rates [20]. These different observations may be explained by differences in models and timing of intervention. It is also important to realize that NO is a very important cell messenger with multiple physiologic actions. It also has an important role in host defense mechanisms so that complete blockade of its activity could be very harmful. This concept is illustrated by the different effects obtained according to the dose of inhibitor used. Nava et al. [21, 22] observed that, in endotoxic rats, an intermediate dose of L-NMMA (10 mg/kg) could prevent a fall in blood pressure and reduce the mortality rate but a higher dose (300 mg/kg), which also increased blood pressure, increased the mortality rate.

There have been preliminary reports on the administration of L-NMMA in humans [23]. These observations suggested that blockade of the NO synthase may increase blood pressure but not cardiac output. The administration of methylene blue may represent another way to interfere with the hemodynamic effects of NO. Methylene blue is an inhibitor of the guanylate cyclase which can therefore block the vasodilating effects of NO on the vascular smooth muscle while preserving the activity of NO as a cell-to-cell messenger and an antimicrobial substance. In a recent study including 14 patients with severe septic shock requiring adrenergic therapy, we observed that methylene blue at a dose of 2 mg/kg could substantially increase mean arterial pressure. However, this intervention had no significant effect on cardiac output, oxygen delivery or oxygen consumption. There was, however, a significant reduction in blood lactate levels but this could be due to the reducing effects of methylene blue [24].

These mechanisms can also account for some of the effects of corticosteroids in septic shock. Corticosteroids have been shown to inhibit the induction of NO synthase by endotoxin [25]. Such a mechanism may explain why corticosteroids have been found effective when administered before or very early during the septic challenge but not when administered later as a therapeutic intervention.

Role of Adhesion Molecules

Endothelial cells play a very important role in the activation of leukocytes. They present a number of adhesion molecules that can interact with circulating cells. Endotoxin itself and cytokines such as TNF of IL-1 exert a profound influence on the adhesion molecules. This fundamental interaction between endothelial cells and inflammatory cells is illustrated by the fact that TNF can induce degranulation of polynuclear neutrophils only if adhesion molecules are expressed [26].

Adhesion molecules present in three different forms:

1) The immunoglobulin superfamily, which includes the antigen-specific receptors of T and B lymphocytes and the intercellular adhesion molecule 1 (ICAM-1) whose induction is sustained in sepsis.
2) The selectins, which interact with neutrophils and lymphocytes. An important selectin in the context of sepsis is the endothelial cells leukocyte adhesion molecule 1 (ELAM-1), which is induced by TNF and IL-1 3–8 h after endotoxin administration.
3) The integrin family, which interferes with leukocyte activation, platelet adhesion and cell migration. It includes several leukocyte membrane proteins such as the CD11b/CD18 glycoprotein complex which regulates important leukocyte function. These adhesion molecules are expressed under the influence of various constituents including not only cytokines but also complement C5a, leukotrienes and PAF.

Recent biotechnological developments have made antibodies to adhesion molecules available. Monoclonal antibodies to the CD11b/CD18 complex have been administered to animals in an attempt to reduce leukocyte mediated injury during hemorrhagic shock in primates [27] or rabbits [28]. The administration of these antibodies has been shown to reduce organ damage. They have also been shown to attenuate myocardial reperfusion injury in dogs [29].

These antibodies have also been shown to be protective in some models of sepsis. In dogs given TNF, antibody to CD11b increased PaO2 and improved the survival rate [30]. In a pig model of sepsis induced by live Pseudomonas, these antibodies attenuated neutropenia and reduced alveolar capillary membrane damage [31]. Nevertheless, there may be a risk of increased infection. In a study by Sharrar et al. [32], an antibody to CD18 did not increase the septic response but increased the size of abscess due to Staphylococcus in rabbits. Recently, Eichacker et al. [30] studied the effects of a murine monoclonal antibody to CD18 in a model of intraperitoneal sepsis in conscious dogs otherwise treated with antibiotics and intravenous fluids. Although the differences were not statistically significant, the survival time was shorter in the animals treated with this antibody. These animals showed worse cardiovascular function (lower mean arterial pressure, lower cardiac index, lower cardiac filling pressures), a more severe lactic acidosis, a greater increase in endotoxin levels, a lower glucose concentration and higher levels of blood urea nitrogen (BUN) and alkaline phosphatase (AP). All these elements suggested that the antibody aggravated rather than attenuated the signs of sepsis. This could be explained by a reduced recruitement of polynuclear neutrophils at the site of infection. It is important to note that due to a genetic defect, some humans do not express these integrins. These individuals are more prone to develop severe infections [33]. *In vitro* studies indicated that neutrophils deficient in the CD11b/CD18 complex or treated with an antibody to this complex have an impaired ability to phagocytose bacteria and endotoxin [34, 35].

These controversial elements again underline the "ying" and "yang" nature of the relation between endothelial cells and leukocytes. An excessive activation of neutrophils can result in permeability alterations and organ damage. By their release of oxygen free radicals, various proteases and arachidonic acid metabolites, polynuclear neutrophils have been largely implicated in the development of nonhemodynamic pulmonary edema (adult respiratory distress syndrome). However, these cells also play an essential role in the phagocytosis of particles and in the clearance of microbiological products.

Instead of acting on the leukocyte itself, one could interfere with the expression of ELAM-1 on endothelial cells. This may preserve the leukocyte's ability to phagocytose bacteria and their products. We have started a phase II trial on the use of an antibody to ELAM-1 in patients with septic shock. Our ultimate goal is to maintain host defense mechanisms against the invasive organisms while trying to prevent the damaging effects of leukocytes on the host.

References

1. Cooke JP, Stamler J, Andon N, Davies PF, McKinley G, Loscalzo J (1990) Flow stimulates endothelial cells to release a nitrovasodilator that is potentiated by reduced thiol. Am J Physiol 259:H804–H812
2. Frangos JA, Eskin SG, McIntire LV, Ives CL (1985) Flow effects on prostacyclin production by cultured human endothelial cells. Science 227:1477–1479
3. Davies PF, Dewey CJ, Bussolari SR, Gordon EJ (1984) Influence of hemodynamic forces on vascular endothelial function: in vitro studies of shear stress and pinocytosis in bovine aortic cells. J Clin Invest 73:1121–1129
4. Diamond SE, Eskin SG, McIntire LV (1989) Fluid flow stimulates tissue plasminogen activator secretion by cultured human endothelial cells. Science 243:1483–1485
5. Dzau VJ, Gibbons GH, Cooke JP, Omoigui N (1993) Vascular biology and medicine in the 1990s: scope, concepts, potentials, and perspectives. Circulation 83:705–719
6. Furchgott RF, Zawadzki JV (1980) The obligatory role of endothelial cells in the relaxation of arterial smooth muscle by acetylcholine. Nature 288:373–376
7. Ignarro LJ, Byrns RE, Buga GM, Wood KS (1987) Endothelium-derived relaxing factor from pulmonary artery and vein possesses pharmacologic and chemical properties identical to those of nitric oxide radical. Circ Res 61:866–879
8. Palmer RM, Ferrige AG, Moncada S (1987) Nitric oxide release accounts for the biological activity of endothelium-derived relaxing factor. Nature 327:524–526
9. Palmer RM, Ashton DS, Moncada S (1988) Vascular endothelial cells synthesize nitric oxide from L-arginine. Nature 333:664–666
10. Mayers I, Johnson D, Hurst T, To T (1991) Interactions of tumor necrosis factor and granulocytes with pulmonary vascular resistance. J Appl Physiol 71:2338–2345

11. Sembowicz A, Hecker M, MacArthur H, Sessa WC, Vane JR (1991) Nitric oxide and another potent vasodilator are formed from NG-hydroxy-L-arginine by cultured endothelial cells. Proc Natl Acad Sci USA 88:11172–11176
12. Omar HA, Cherry PD, Mortelliti MP, Burke-Wolin T, Wolin MS (1991) Inhibition of coronary artery superoxide dismutase attenuates endothelium-dependent and -independent nitrovasodilatator relaxation. Circ Res 69:601–608
13. Olesen SP, Chapham DE, Davies PF (1988) Haemodynamic shear stress activates a K+ current in vascular endothelial cells. Nature 331:168–170
14. Cooke JP, Rossitch E, Andon NA, Loscalzo J, Dzau VJ (1991) Flow activates an endothelial potassium channel to release an endogenous nitrovasodilator. J Clin Invest 88:1663–1671
15. Granger DL, Hibbs JB, Broadnax LM (1991) Urinary nitrate excretion in relation to murine macrophage activation: influence of dietary L-arginine and oral NG-monomethym-L-arginine. J Immunol 146:1294–1302
16. Julou-Schaeffer G, Gray GA, Fleming I, Schott C, Parratt JR, Stoclet JC (1990) Loss of vascular responsiveness induced by endotoxin involves L-arginine pathway. Am J Physiol 259:H1038–H1043
17. Kilbourn RG, Jubran A, Gross SS et al (1990) Reversal of endotoxin-mediated shock by NG-methyl-L-arginine, an inhibitor of nitric oxide synthesis. Biochem Biophys Res Commun 172:1132–1138
18. Preiser C, Zhang H, Wachel D, Boeynaems JM, Buurman W, Vincent JL (1993) Is the endotoxin-induced hypotension related to nitric oxide formation? Eur Surg Res (in press)
19. Klabunde RE, Ritger RC (1991) NG-monomethyl-L-arginine (NMA) restores arterial blood pressure but reduces cardiac output in a canine model of endotoxic shock. Biochem Biophys Res Commun 178:1135–1140
20. Wright CH, Rees DD, Moncada S (1992) Protective and pathological roles of nitric oxide in endotoxin shock. Cardiovasc Res 26:48–57
21. Nava E, Palmer RM, Moncada S (1991) Inhibition of nitric oxide synthesis in septic shock: how much is beneficial? Lancet 338:1555–1557
22. Nava E, Palmer RM, Moncada S (1992) The role of nitric oxide in endotoxic shock: effects of NG-monomethyl-L-arginine. J Cardiovasc Pharmacol 20:S132–S134
23. Petros A, Bennett D, Vallance P (1991) Effect of nitric oxide synthase inhibitors on hypotension in patients with septic shock. Lancet 338:1557–1558
24. Preiser JC, Lejeune P, Roman A, Carlier E, Leeman M, Vincent JL (1993) Use of methylene blue in patients with refractory septic shock. Circ Shock S2:68 (abstract)
25. Rees DD, Cellek S, Palmer RM, Moncada S (1990) Dexamethasone prevents the induction by endotoxin of a nitric oxide synthase and the associated effects on vascular tone: an insight into endotoxin shock. Biochem Biophys Res Commun 173:541–547
26. Richter J, Ng-Sikorski J, Olsson I, Andersson T (1990) Tumor necrosis factor-induced degranulation in adherent neutrophils is dependent on CD11b/CD18-integrin-triggered oscillations of cytosolic free Ca2+. Proc Natl Acad Sci USA 87:9472–9476
27. Mileski WJ, Winn RK, Vedder NB, Pohlman TH, Harlan JM (1990) Inhibition of CD-18 dependent neutrophil adherence reduces organ injury after hemorrhagic shock in primates. Surgery 108:206–212
28. Vedder NB, Winn RK, Rice CL, Chi EY, Arfors KE, Harlan JM (1988) A monoclonal antibody to the adherence-promoting leukocyte glycoprotein, CD18, reduces organ injury and improves survival from hemorrhagic shock and resuscitation in rabbits. J Clin Invest 81:939–944
29. Simpson PJ, Todd RF, Fantone JC, Mickelson JK, Griffin JD, Lucchesi BR (1988) Reduction of experimental canine myocardial reperfusion injury by a monoclonal antibody (anti-MO1, anti-CD11b) that inhibits leukocyte adhesion. J Clin Invest 81:624–629
30. Eichacker PQ, Farese A, Hoffman WD et al (1992) Leukocyte CD11b/18 antigen-directed monoclonal antibody improves early survival and decreases hypoxemia in dogs challenged with tumor necrosis factor. Am Rev Respir Dis 145:1023–1029

31. Walsh CJ, Carey PD, Cook DJ, Bechard DE, Fowler AA, Sugerman HJ (1991) Anti-CD18 antibody attenuates neutropenia and alveolar capillary-membrane injury during gram-negative sepsis. Surgery 110:205–212
32. Sharrar SR, Winn RK, Nurry CE, Harlan JM, Rice CL (1991) A CD18 monoclonal antibody increases the incidence and severity of subcutaneous abscess formation after high-dose staphylococcus aureus injection in rabbits. Surgery 110:213–220
33. Todd RF, Freyer DR (1988) The CD11/18 leukocyte glycoprotein deficiency. Hematol Oncol Clin North Am 2:13–31
34. Anderson DC, Schmalsteig FC, Arnaout MA (1989) Abnormalities of polymorphonuclear leukocyte function associated with a heritable deficiency of high molecular weight surface glucoproteins (GP138): common relationship to diminished cell adherence. J Clin Invest 74:536–551
35. Wright SD, Levin SM, Jung MT, Chad Z, Kabbash LG (1989) CR-3 (CD11b/CD18) expresses one binding site for Arg-Gly-Asp containing peptides and a second site for bacterial lipopolysaccharide. J Exp Med 169:175–183

Sepsis and Cellular Metabolism

G. Gutierrez

Introduction

The cellular and molecular mechanisms of sepsis are unknown. Intense research in the areas of physiology, biochemistry, and cell biology has provided clearer understanding of the causal relationship between bacteria, neutrophils, cytokines, and target cells in sepsis. Knowledge of cellular cytokine interaction [1] has changed our concept of sepsis as an infective process to the more encompassing notion of systemic inflammatory response syndrome (SIRS) [2].

As a result of this increased knowledge, numerous clinical trials currently are under way testing the efficacy of monoclonal blocking agents to endotoxin, tumor necrosis factor α (TNFα), and interleukin-1 (IL-1) receptor antagonists. I will not dwell on the merits of this type of therapy in sepsis [3, 4]; the answer will be provided by the results of clinical trials. The purpose of this chapter is to discuss our current understanding of the basic cellular defect in sepsis and to speculate on the possible cellular mechanisms set in motion by the message bearing cytokines. In order to understand the cellular mechanisms of sepsis, ultimately we must find the answers to the following questions: Which biochemical pathways are affected? How are they disrupted? What are the molecular alterations associated with sepsis? Can they be reversed by genetic or by chemical means? In my opinion, finding the answer to these and other related questions should be the ultimate goal of sepsis research.

Does Sepsis Represent a Failure of Microvascular Control?

There is overwhelming evidence of blood flow redistribution among the different organs in sepsis. Rabbits injected with endotoxin show decreases in flow to the kidney and hepatic artery [5], whereas in pigs [6] and monkeys [7] endotoxin reduces blood flow to the cerebrum, kidney, spleen, and skeletal muscle.

The infusion of *Escherichia coli* endotoxin in rats results in marked reductions in blood flow to skeletal muscle [8]. Endotoxin exerts a profound effect on the rat diaphragmatic microvasculature, manifested by constriction of arterioles and impaired capillary perfusion [9]. In a rat Langendorff preparation exposed to endotoxin, Rumsey et al. [10] found diminished capacity of the heart's vasculature to adjust blood flow to energy needs. They also noted a *hyperdynamic, hypermetabolic* state characterized by increases in myocardial O_2 consumption.

Several experimental studies have singled out the intestines as a target organ of sepsis. It appears that the ability of the gut to extract O_2 is impaired [11] and Drazenovic et al. [12] found evidence that the intestinal microvasculature may be disrupted. They administered *E. coli* endotoxin to an exteriorized segment of dog small intestine labeled with colloidal carbon and found a decreased perfused capillary density in the mucosal vili and crypts of the septic gut segments. There may be a differential microvascular response to sepsis among tissues, with skeletal muscle being more resilient than the gut. Gutierrez et al. [13] examined the effect of *E. coli* endotoxin administration on rabbit hindlimb skeletal muscle oxygenation measured with surface PO_2 microelectrodes. They noted decreased O_2 transport with endotoxin and the development of tissue hypoxia. The distribution of the tissue PO_2 histograms remained constant for 2 h following the infusion of endotoxin, implying that increases in skeletal muscle microcirculatory heterogeneity does not increase in early sepsis. These findings agree with those of Kopp et al. [14], who measured muscle PO_2 in pigs and concluded that microcirculatory changes do not take place in skeletal muscle during the first 2 h of septic shock.

It is not clear how endotoxin or other septic mediators alter the microvascular response to sepsis. The role played by endothelial derived vascular mediators has received considerable attention recently. Beasley et al. [15] measured smooth muscle contractility in intact and endothelium denuded thoracic aortic rings from rats. They found an endothelium dependent inhibition to contraction after a 1 h exposure to endotoxin. In contrast, after a 3 h exposure to endotoxin, aortic ring contraction was inhibited to a similar degree in rings with or without endothelium.

It appears that endothelium derived nitric oxide (NO) may play an important role in vascular reactivity during sepsis, perhaps by the activation of soluble guanylate cyclase into guanosine 3′,5′-cyclic monophosphate [16, 17], a potent intracellular mediator of vasodilation [18]. Evidence is accumulating pointing towards NO induced guanylate cyclase activation as the mediator of the vascular manifestations of sepsis [19]. Should this prove to be the case, substances that inhibit endothelial NO synthesis may become the "magic bullets" in the treatment of sepsis. On the basis of this hypothesis, that is, that vascular changes in sepsis are related to the overproduction of NO, Kilbourn et al. [20, 21] infused N^{G}-methyl-L-arginine, an inhibitor of NO synthesis, to dogs following the administration of either *E. coli* endotoxin or TNFα. In both cases they noted the reversal of the hypotensive response to these agents. Meyer et al. [22] found that the intravenous administration of N^{ω}-nitro-L-arginine methyl ester to septic ewes increased mean arterial pressure and decreased the pulmonary shunt fraction. It appears that NO also may exert a direct effect on myocardial contractility in sepsis [23].

Isolated guinea pig cardiac ventricular myocytes from endotoxin treated animals show decreased contractility. This effect of endotoxin is reversed by N^{G}-methyl-L-arginine.

Although preliminary data are promising, there are no studies demonstrating either improved animal mortality or a reduction in organ system failure, by the infusion of NO synthesis inhibitors in sepsis. Moreover, inhibitors of NO synthesis produce decreases in cardiac output [22], perhaps by an acute rise in afterload. This implies that the restoration of blood pressure by inhibitors of NO synthesis may be the result of nonselective systemic vasoconstriction, perhaps to the detriment of nutritive flow to individual tissues. In my opinion, NO probably plays a very important role in mediating the systemic vasodilation of sepsis; however, these vascular abnormalities may be the manifestation, not the cause, of cellular metabolic damage set in motion by sepsis related cytokines. In other words, the initial insult is directed to the tissue cells which, in turn, signal the endothelium to produce NO and perhaps other vasodilator substances.

Are the Cellular Manifestations of Sepsis the Result of Hypoxia?

The answer to this question appears to be no. At least during the early stages of sepsis, cellular alterations in sepsis do not appear to be the result of hypoxia. Hurtado et al. [24] compared the hemodynamic and metabolic changes in rabbits subjected to comparable decreases in cardiac output produced by the intravenous administration of endotoxin or by inflating a balloon placed in the right ventricle. The idea was to differentiate the hypodynamic condition, with its resulting hyperfusion and tissue hypoxia, from the effects that could be attributed directly to endotoxin. Both groups experienced similar decreases in O_2 transport, O_2 consumption, and skeletal muscle PO_2, but the septic group had greater increases in arterial lactate concentration. This finding suggests that lactate production in sepsis may be unrelated to changes in systemic O_2 transport. Moreover, force-frequency curves showed decreased force generation by the hindlimb of the septic animals 90 min after the infusion of endotoxin. Hotchkiss et al. [25] used [^{18}F]fluoromisonidazole as a marker of tissue hypoxia in rats made septic by cecal ligation and perforation. They found no evidence of tissue hypoxia in skeletal muscle, brain, liver, heart, or diaphragm of septic rats. Tresadern et al. [26] found no changes in creatine phosphate concentration in muscle biopsies obtained from 31 patients with sepsis and concluded that tissue hypoxia was not present in these patients.

Are Cellular Bioenergetics Disrupted in Sepsis?

Again, the answer appears to be no. The majority of studies in septic animals do not show decreases in the levels of ATP. However, almost uniformly, there are increases in arterial lactate concentration.

Cellular energy metabolism refers to the series of biochemical reactions responsible for providing the cell with adequate energy for protein synthesis and the maintenance of adequate membrane permeability. Under aerobic conditions, the formation of ATP is coupled to the consumption of oxygen in the mitochondria. The reducing equivalents (NADH and FADH) required by the cytochrome chain derive from the fermentation of glucose or glycogen and fatty acid oxidation. The ATP molecules move from the mitochondria into the cytosol where they undergo hydrolysis liberating the energy required for cellular function. The hydrolysis of ATP produces ADP, inorganic phosphate (Pi), and hydrogen ions. These metabolites do not accumulate in the cytosol, but are reutilized in the formation of additional ATP.

When the delivery of O_2 to the cells falters, several mechanisms are set in motion to maintain a balance between cellular ATP production and cellular energy needs. The first mechanism employed by the tissues in the defense of aerobic metabolism is an increase in the fraction of O_2 extracted from capillary blood, defined as the O_2 extraction ratio (ERO_2 = O_2 consumption/O_2 transport). Increases in ERO_2 are effected by increasing the number of perfused capillaries for a given volume of tissue, thus reducing the diffusion distance from capillaries to cells. This mechanism is suited to organs capable of large increases in capillarity, such as skeletal muscle, and to a lesser extent the myocardium. Organs with poor capillary reserve, or those with counter current arteriovenous microvascular arrangements, such as the intestinal vili and the ascending loop of Henle in the kidney, fare less well. With severe decreases in O_2 transport, increases in ERO_2 may not be sufficient to provide the mitochondria with the O_2 required to sustain aerobic metabolism. At this juncture the cell must turn to anaerobic sources of energy to produce ATP. The disadvantage of anaerobiasis as an alternate source of ATP is that the products of ATP hydrolysis, ADP, Pi, and H^+, accumulate in the cytosol. The three sources of anaerobic ATP production are the lactic dehydrogenase reaction, the adenylate kinase reaction, and the creatine kinase reaction. The lactic dehydrogenase reaction produces lactate, the adenylate kinase reaction results in increases of AMP and its derivatives xanthine and uric acid, and the creatine kinase reaction decreases the concentration of creatine phosphate in skeletal muscle, heart, and brain. These byproducts of anaerobic metabolism provide markers with which to judge the severity of tissue hypoxia.

Metabolic Manifestations of Sepsis

Increased Glucose Utilization

The enhanced glycolytic effect of sepsis is not well understood. The infusion of endotoxin to dogs results in increased glucose uptake and lactate release by the dog hindlimb [27, 28]. As shown by Amaral et al. [29] increase in skeletal muscle glucose uptake produced by endotoxin requires incubation in plasma. This implies that the presence of a cytokine, such as TNF or IL-1, is needed, perhaps, to act on the regulatory enzymes of glycolysis. The initial response to endotoxin administration is the immediate rise in blood glucose, followed by a steady decrease as glucose is consumed [30, 31]. Increased glucose utilization may lead to hypoglycemia [32] and decreases in muscle glycogen [33] in rabbits. Romanosky et al. [28] found decreases in arterial glucose concentration following endotoxemia that were accompanied by increases in skeletal muscle glucose, despite normal levels of plasma insulin. These findings suggest that endotoxin may have an "insulin-like" effect, or potentiate the sensitivity of tissues to insulin, perhaps mediated by changes in membrane glucose transporter. This is the mechanism proposed by Zeller et al. [34], who noted increases in messenger RNA coding for the Glut 1 glucose transporter in endotoxemic rats.

Control of Glycolysis and Lactate Production

Phosphofructokinase (PFK) is an important glycolytic regulatory enzyme that is activated by ADP, AMP, and Pi and inhibited by ATP. Perhaps sepsis results in increased glycolytic flux by activating PFK, with resulting pyruvate accumulation, and lactate and alanine production [35]. Although attractive, this theory has not been supported by experimental evidence. On the contrary, Lundsgaard-Hansen et al. [36] found PFK inhibition in rabbits injected with endotoxin.

Another possible metabolic target to endotoxin is pyruvate dehydrogenase (PDH), the enzyme that regulates the rate of pyruvate oxidation by the mitochondria. The conversion of pyruvate to acetyl-CoA by this reaction regulates the utilization of glucose or glycogen by the mitochondria. There are two isozymes of PDH, active and inactive. Active PDH is phosphorylated into the inactive form by PDH kinase. This reaction is enhanced by high ratios of ATP/ADP and $NADH^+$/NAD. The converse reaction is promoted by PDH phosphatase, a step facilitated by Ca^{2+} and Mg^{2+} and low levels of intramitochondrial ATP. It has been proposed that endotoxin stimulates the conversion of the active to the inactive form of PDH [37], resulting in the accumulation of pyruvate and the formation of lactate by a mass action phenomenon. Vary et al. [37] found a threefold increase in inactive PDH in sepsis and Kilpatrick-Smith and Erecinska [38] noted a 54% decrease in PDH activity in endotoxin treated neuroblastoma cells. Dichloroacetate (DCA) promotes the formation of active PDH and decreases the lactic acidosis in sepsis [39]. The cellular benefits accruing from this action are controversial [40]. Curtis and Cain [41] administered endotoxin to dogs and noted the development of significant lactic acidosis although whole body, limb, and gut O_2 transport levels remained above reported critical values. Therapy with DCA reversed this lactic acidosis but did not affect O_2 consumption, implying that elevated arterial lactate levels may be more a function of PDH activity than of tissue hypoxia. Furthermore, this study adds to the body of literature supporting the notion that blood lactate levels may be a poor marker of hypoxia in sepsis. In a recently completed, placebo-controlled, randomized trial [42], intravenous DCA was administered to 252 patients with lactic acidosis. The arterial blood lactate concentration decreased significantly in 66% of the patients who received DCA and in 36% of the patients who received placebo. The arterial blood pH also increased more in the DCA-treated patients. These changes were not associated with improvement in hemodynamics or survival. Only 12% of the DCA-treated patients and 17% of the placebo patients survived to be discharged from the hospital.

Results from a study by Fink et al. [43] support the hypothesis that the lactic acidosis of sepsis may not be related to a state of cellular anaerobiasis. Using an intestinal PCO_2 silastic tonometer they measured intraluminal pH in pigs following the injection of *E. coli* endotoxin. Calculations of the intestinal mucosal pH were made using the method of Fiddian-Green et al. [44]. They found that intestinal mucosal pH increases following the administration of endotoxin, although intestinal O_2 consumption remained constant.

Control of Mitochondrial Respiration

It has been hypothesized that endotoxin inhibits mitochondrial respiration [45], and defective skeletal muscle mitochondrial O_2 consumption has been noted in patients with septic shock [46]. However, Dawson et al. [47] found enhanced respiration in rat liver mitochondria following lethal doses of *E. coli* endotoxin. To date, there is little evidence that sepsis results in mitochondrial dysfunction.

A slower turnover rate of the tricarboxylic acid (TCA) cycle has been implicated as the cause of decreased O_2 consumption ($\dot{V}O_2$) during sepsis [48]. However, Hotchkiss et al. [49], using ^{31}P nuclear magnetic resonance spectroscopy and fluorometric enzymatic methods, found no differences in TCA cycle intermediates or high energy phosphates when comparing septic rat myocardium to a nonseptic control.

Changes in Adenine Nucleotides and Cellular Energetics

Sepsis affects the levels of O_2 consumption and organ function, but the cellular concentrations of high energy phosphates, ATP, ADP, AMP, phosphocreatine (PCr), and Pi, remain unaltered. Pappova et al. [33] found no changes in adenine nucleotides concentration in rabbits given endotoxin intravenously. Chaudry et al. [50] also measured tissue adenine nucleotides in liver, kidney, diaphragm and skeletal muscle from rats in which sepsis was produced by cecal ligation. They found no changes in blood flow or in adenine nucleotides in early sepsis, 10 h after cecal ligation. During late sepsis, 16–24 h, ATP and ADP were decreased in liver and kidney, but not in diaphragm or gastrocnemius muscle. Pasque et al. [51] noted an *increase* in myocardial ATP in rats 18 h after cecal ligation, which was attributed to an increase in energy production by a sepsis-stimulated myocardium. Myrvold et al. [52] also found increases in skeletal muscle ATP in endotoxin-treated dogs and concluded that tissue hypoxia does not occur during the initial period of endotoxemia.

The above studies have been complemented by experiments in septic animals using ^{31}P magnetic resonance spectroscopy. This technique allows the measurement of high energy phosphates ATP, PCr, and Pi in a noninvasive manner. Therefore, sequential measurements can be taken in the same experimental preparation. Jepson et al. [8] found decreases in blood flow and $\dot{V}O_2$ in skeletal muscle of rats given *E. coli* endotoxin, but no changes in the levels of high energy phosphates. The lack of effect of endotoxin on skeletal muscle ATP and PCr levels was corroborated by Gutierrez and Dubin [53] in rabbit skeletal muscle.

Alterations in Cellular Membrane Function

A possible cellular target in sepsis is the cell membrane. The propagation of the action potential at the sarcolemmal membrane is an energy-requiring step that requires a resting membrane potential of -80 mV. This membrane potential is maintained by Na^+-K^+ ATPases whose function is the bidirectional transport of Na^+ out and K^+ into the cell. Failure of these pumps is manifested by increased K^+ efflux from the cells, lower transmembrane potential, and decreased magnitude of the action potential [54]. Consequently, less Ca^{2+} is released from the sarcoplasmic reticulum and muscle tension is reduced. Illner and Shires [55] measured skeletal muscle resting membrane potential in rabbits given i.v. *E. coli* endotoxin and found that depolarization of the cell membrane occurred before the rabbits became hypotensive. They also found that the concentration of high energy phosphates was unaffected by endotoxin.

Leon et al. [56] found decreases in transdiaphragmatic pressures and in resting membrane potential in rats given i.v. *E. coli* endotoxin. Kilpatrick-Smith and Erecinska [38] noted decreases in intracellular K^+ in culture mouse neuroblastoma cells exposed to *E. coli* endotoxin, although the transmembrane potential was greater in the endotoxin treated cells. It is possible that endotoxin may have increased the rate of K^+ loss from the myocytes, resulting in a smaller action potential and greater muscular fatigue in the endotoxin-treated rabbits.

Conclusions

Sepsis results in a fairly predictable pattern of metabolic alterations consisting of increased glucose utilization and increased lactate production. These changes occur under apparently adequate conditions of O_2 transport and tissue oxygenation for most organs [57]. It is possible that selected organs with a low injury threshold to hypoxia, such as the gut and the kidney, may be responsible for initiating a cascade of events leading to these abnormalities. However, another possibility is that the cytokines associated with endotoxemia. TNFα, Il-1 etc., set in motion a series of intracellular events leading to a preprogrammed cellular reaction to stress.

Perhaps cellular reaction to stress represents a uniform pattern of physiological and biochemical actions aimed at increasing the activity of organs involved in locomotion as part of the "flight or flight" reaction. Therefore, it is not surprising that some of the changes that characterize exercise also are found in sepsis. These include a hyperdynamic condition, increases in arterial glucose, and greater capillary recruitment. Thus, the systemic manifestations to the stress imposed by sepsis may be a misdirected effort of the organism to flee from danger. This concept may be useful as a point of departure in our efforts to unravel the more puzzling aspects of the septic response.

References

1. Mizel SB (1989) The interleukins. FASEB J 3:2379–2388
2. American College of Chest Physicians/Society of Critical Care Medicine Consensus Conference (1992) Definitions for sepsis and organ failure and guidelines for the use of innovative therapies in sepsis. Crit Care Med 20:864–874
3. Ziegler E, Fisher C, Sprung C et al (1991) Treatment of gram negative bacteremia and septic shock with HA-1A human monoclonal antibody against endotoxin. N Engl J Med 324:429–436
4. Warren SH, Danner RL, Munford RS (1992) Anti-endotoxin monoclonal antibodies. N Engl J Med 326:1153–1157
5. Fink MP, Fiallo V, Stein KL et al (1987) Systemic and regional hemodynamic changes after intraperitoneal endotoxin in rabbits. Circ Shock 22:73–81
6. Nishijima MK, Breslow MJ, Miller CF et al (1988) Effect of naloxone and ibuprofen on organ blood flow during endotoxin shock in pig. Am J Physiol 255:H177–H184
7. Weiner DE (1970) Effects of endotoxin on cerebral blood flow in the monkey. Am J Physiol 218:160–164
8. Jepson MM, Cox M, Bates PC et al (1987) Regional blood flow and skeletal muscle energy status in endotoxemic rats. Am J Physiol 253:E581–E587
9. Boczkowski J, Vicaut E, Aubier M (1992) In vivo effects of Escherichia coli endotoxemia on diaphragmatic microcirculation in rats. J Appl Physiol 72:2219–2224
10. Rumsey WL, Kilpatrick L, Wilson DF, Erecinska M (1988) Myocardial metabolism and coronary flow: effects of endotoxemia. Am J Physiol 255:H1295–H1304
11. Nelson DP, Samsel RW, Wood L et al (1988) Pathological supply dependence of systemic and intestinal O_2 utake during endotoxemia. J Appl Physiol 64:2410–2419
12. Drazenovic R, Samsel RW, Wylam ME et al (1992) Regulation of perfused capillary density in canine intestinal mucosa during endotoxemia. J Appl Physiol 72:259–265
13. Gutierrez G, Lund N, Palizas F (1991) Rabbit skeletal muscle PO_2 during hypodynamic sepsis. Chest 99:224–229
14. Kopp KH, Sinagowitz E, Muller H (1984) Oxygen supply of skeletal muscle in experimental septic shock. In: Lubbers DW, Acker H, Leniger-Follert E, Goldstick TK (eds) Oxygen transport to tissue, vol V. Plenum, New York, pp 467–476
15. Beasley D, Cohen R, Levinsky N (1990) Endotoxin inhibits contraction of vascular smooth muscle in vitro. Am J Physiol 258:H1187–H1192

16. Beasley D (1990) Interleukin 1 and endotoxin activate soluble guanylate cyclase in vascular smooth muscle. Am J Physiol 259:R38–R44
17. Lamas S, Michel T, Brenner BM et al (1991) Nitric oxide synthesis in endothelial cells: evidence for a pathway inducible by TNF-α. Am J Physiol 261:C634–C641
18. Murad F (1986) Cyclic guanosine monophosphate as a mediator of vasodilation. J Clin Invest 78:1–5
19. Julou-Schaeffer G, Gray G, Fleming I et al (1990) Loss of vascular responsiveness induced by endotoxin involves L-arginine pathway. Am J Physiol 259:H1038–H1042
20. Kilbourn RG, Jubran A, Gross SS et al (1990) Reversal of endotoxin-mediated shock by N^G-Methyl-L-arginine, an inhibitor of nitric oxide synthesis. Biochem Biophys Res Commun 172:1132–1138
21. Kilbourn RG, Gross SS, Jubran A et al (1990) N^G-Methyl-L-arginine inhibits tumor necrosis factor-induced hypotension: implications for the involvement of nitric oxide. Proc Natl Acad Sci USA 87:3629–3632
22. Meyer J, Traber LD, Nelson S et al (1992) Reversal of hyperdynamic response to continuous endotoxin administration by inhibition of NO synthesis. J Appl Physiol 73:324–328
23. Brady AJB, Poole-Wilson PA, Harding SE et al (1992) Nitric oxide production within cardiac myocytes reduces their contractility in endotoxemia. Am J Physiol 263:H1963–H1966
24. Hurtado FJ, Gutierrez AM, Silva N et al (1992) Role of tissue hypoxia as the mechanism of lactic acidosis during E. coli endotoxemia. J Appl Physiol 72:1895–1901
25. Hotchkiss RS, Rust RS, Dence CS et al (1991) Evaluation of the role of cellular hypoxia in sepsis by the hypoxic marker [^{18}F]fluoromisonidazole. Am J Physiol 261:R965–R972
26. Tresadern JC, Threlfall CJ, Wilford K et al (1988) Muscle adenosine 5′triphosphate and creatine phosphate concentrations in relation to nutritional status and sepsis in man. Clin Sci 75:233–242
27. Raymond RM, Harkema JM, Emerson TE et al (1981) Mechanisms of increased glucose uptake by skeletal muscle during Escherichia coli endotoxin shock in the dog. Circ Shock 8:77–83
28. Romanosky AJ, Bagby GJ, Bockman EL et al (1980) Increased muscle glucose uptake and lactate release after endotoxin administration. Am J Physiol 239:E311–E316
29. Amaral J, Shearer J, Mastrofrancesco B (1989) The effect of endotoxin on glucose metabolism in skeletal muscle requires the presence of plasma. Arch Surg 124:727–732
30. Wolfe RR, Dariush E, Spitzer JJ (1977) Glucose and lactate kinetics after endotoxin administration in dogs. Am J Physiol 232:E180–E185
31. Merril GF, Spitzer JJ (1978) Glucose and lactate kinetics in guinea pigs following Escherichia coli endotoxin administration. Circ Shock 5:11–21
32. Hinshaw LB, Beller BK, Archer LT et al (1976) Hypoglycemic response of blood to live Escherichia coli organisms and endotoxin. J Surg Res 21:141–150
33. Pappova E, Urbaschek B, Heitmann L et al (1971) Energy-rich phosphates ad glucose metabolism in early endotoxin shock. J Surg Res 11:506–512
34. Zeller WP, The SM, Sweet M et al (1991) Altered glucose transporter mRNA abundance in a rat model of endotoxic shock. Biochem Biophys Res Commun 176:535–540
35. Marrou A, Turner D, Oglethorpe N (1981) Fructose 1,6-Diphosphate: an agent for treatment of experimental endotoxin shock. Surgery 90:482–488
36. Lundsgaard-Hansen P, Pappova E, Urbaschek B et al (1972) Circulatory deterioration as the determinant of oxygen energy metabolism in endotoxin shock. J Surg Res 13:282–288
37. Vary TC, Siegel JH, Nakatani T et al (1986) Effect of sepsis on activity of PDH complex in skeletal muscle and liver. Am J Physiol 250:E634–E640
38. Kilpatrick-Smith L, Erecinska M (1983) Cellular effects of endotoxin in vitro. I. Effect

of endotoxin on mitochondrial substrate metabolism and intracellular calcium. Circ Shock 11:85–99
39. Park R, Arieff AI (1982) Treatment of lactic acidosis with dichloroacetate in dogs. J Clin Invest 70:853–862
40. Vary TC, Siegel JH, Tall BD et al (1988) Metabolic effect of partial reversal of pyruvate dehydrogenase activity by dichloroacetate in sepsis. Circ Shock 24:3–38
41. Curtis SE, Cain SM (1992) Regional and systemic delivery/uptake relations and lactate flux in hyperdynamic, endotoxin-treated dogs. Am Rev Respir Dis 145:348–354
42. Stacpoole PW, Wright EC, Baumgartner TG et al (1992) A controlled clinical trial of dichloroacetate for treatment of lactic acidosis in adults. The Dichloroacetate-Lactic Acidosis Study Group. N Engl J Med 327:1564–1569
43. Fink MP, Cohn SM, Lee PC et al (1989) Effect of lipopolysaccharide on intestinal mucosal hydrogen concentration in pigs: evidence of gut ischemia in a normodynamic model of septic shock. Crit Care Med 17:641–646
44. Fiddian-Green R, Pittenger G, Whitehouse WM (1982) Back-diffusion of CO_2 and its influence on the intramural pH in gastric mucosa. J Surg Res 33:39–46
45. Mela L, Bacalzo LV, Miller LD (1971) Defective oxidative metabolism of rat liver mitochondria in hemorrhagic and endotoxin shock. Am J Physiol 220:571–576
46. Poderoso JJ, Boveris A, Jorge MA et al (1978) Function mitochondrial en el shock septico. Medicinal (Firenze) 38:371–377
47. Dawson KL, Geller ER, Kirkpatrick JR (1988) Enhancement of mitochondrial function in sepsis. Arch Surg 123:241–246
48. Clowes GHA, O'Donnell TF, Ryan NT et al (1974) Energy metabolism in sepsis. Treatment based on different patterns in shock and high output stage. Ann Surg 179:684–696
49. Hotchkiss R, Long R, Hall J (1989) An in vivo examination of rat brain during sepsis with ^{31}P-NMR spectroscopy. Am J Physiol 257:C1055–C1059
50. Chaudry IH, Wichterman KA, Baue AE (1979) Effect of sepsis on tissue adenine nucleotide levels. Surgery 85:205–211
51. Pasque MK, Murphy CE, van Tright P et al (1983) Myocardial adenosine triphosphate levels during early sepsis. Arch Surg 118:1437–1440
52. Myrvold HE, Enger E, Haljamae H (1975) Early effect of endotoxin on tissue phosphagen levels in skeletal muscle and liver of the dog. Eur Surg Res 7:181–192
53. Gutierrez G, Dubin A (1990) Cellular metabolism in sepsis. In: Vincent JL (ed) Update in intensive care and emergency medicine, vol 12. Springer, Berlin Heidelberg New York, pp 227–241
54. Sjogaard G (1990) Exercise-induced muscle fatigue: the significance of potassium. Acta Physiol Scand [Suppl] 593:1–63
55. Illner HP, Shires T (1981) Membrane defect and energy status in rabbit skeletal muscle cells in sepsis and septic shock. Arch Surg 116:1302–1305
56. Leon A, Boczkowski J, Dureuil B et al (1992) Effects of endotoxic shock on diaphragmatic function in mechanically ventilated rats. J Appl Physiol 72:1466–1472
57. Hotchkiss RS, Karl IE (1992) Reevaluation of the role of cellular hypoxia and bioenergetic failure in sepsis. JAMA 267:1503–1510

IV. Monitoring

Monitoring of O_2 Transport and Tissue Oxygenation in Septic Shock

K. Reinhart, L. Hannemann, A. Meier-Hellmann and M. Specht

Introduction

Tissue hypoxia plays an important role in the pathogenesis of sepsis and multiple organ dysfunction syndrome [1]. Hypoxia may not only result from the various insults that initiate sepsis but may itself perpetuate the septic process by enhancement of cytokine production and release of other mediators (Fig. 1). Prevention of tissue hypoxia is therefore a crucial part of the supportive treatment in patients with sepsis and septic shock. Figure 2 depicts various factors that may contribute to the impairment of cellular O_2 supply in septic shock. It is obvious that tissue hypoxia may result not only from inadequate global oxygen transport but also from regional mismatch between supply and demand and especially from the impairment of gas and substrate exchange due to pathologic alterations on the microcirculatory level.

There are some studies suggesting that improving tissue oxygenation by increasing cardiac output in critically ill patients, including those in septic shock, improves outcome [2–4]. Ideally we should consider alterations of the determinants of cellular O_2 supply on all levels. However, in the clinical set-

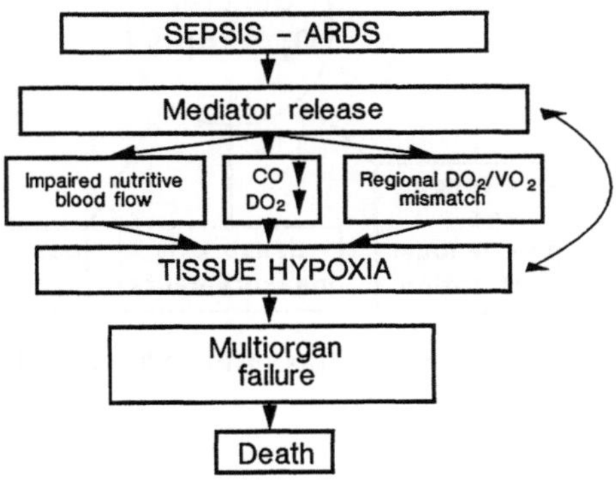

Fig. 1. Sequelae of mediator release in sepsis and adult respiratory distress syndrome (*ARDS*). *CO*, cardiac output; DO_2, oxygen transport; $\dot{V}O_2$, oxygen consumption

ting that is not easy to achieve. At present we are just beginning to appreciate the need and possibilities for monitoring on the regional and tissue levels [5–7], but we still largely depend on global indicators of the adequacy of cellular O_2 supply. As long as direct information on cellular status, as determined by nuclear magnetic resonance (NMR) spectroscopy or near infrared spectroscopy, remains difficult to obtain at the bedside [8, 9], we will be limited to indirect indicators of tissue oxygenation [10] (Fig. 3).

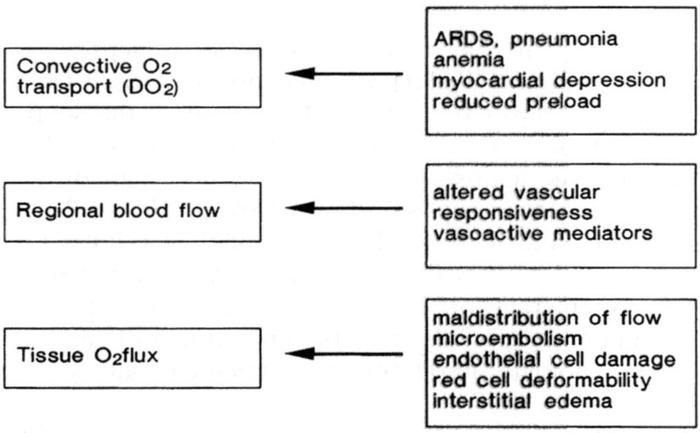

Fig. 2. Factors that may contribute to the deterioration of cellular O_2 supply in the critically ill patient. *ARDS,* adult respiratory distress syndrome

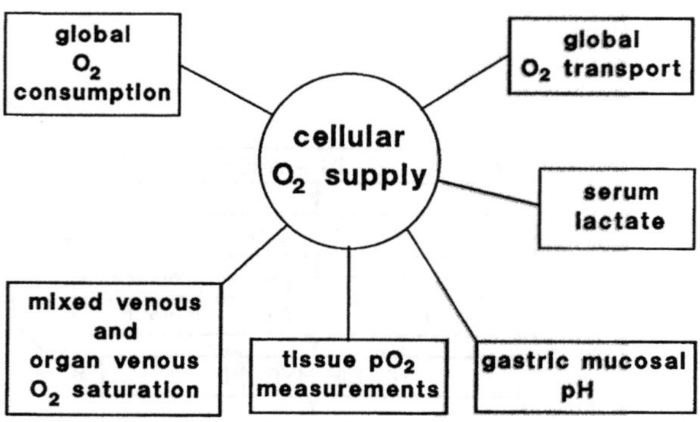

Fig. 3. Indirect indicators of the adequacy of tissue oxygenation, obtainable at the bedside

Global Parameters for the Assessment of Tissue Oxygenation

Oxygen Transport

Oxygen transport (DO_2) is calculated from the product of cardiac index and arterial oxygen content and is one of the main determinants of cellular O_2 supply. Values can be calculated at the bedside and this is the parameter that is manipulated most in attempts to optimize tissue oxygenation [11–13]. Therefore, invasive hemodynamic monitoring with pulmonary artery (PA) catheters is practiced in most patients with severe sepsis and septic shock. PA catheters not only allow cardiac output measurements and better assessment of left heart filling pressures, but also provide mixed venous blood samples. In patients with septic shock correlation between central venous pressure (CVP) and pulmonary capillary wedge pressure (PCWP) is poor (Fig. 4). Conventional basic hemodynamic parameters like systemic blood pressure and heart rate are only poor indicators of DO_2 (Fig. 5), and thus are of little help in optimizing DO_2 in septic shock patients.

Oxygen Consumption and the "Oxygen Flux Test"

Oxygen consumption ($\dot{V}O_2$) is typically higher in septic patients than in non-septic individuals, and a higher than normal DO_2 is required to guarantee cellular supply in sepsis. The term "pathologic O_2 supply dependency of O_2 consumption" was coined from this phenomenon [14]. This concept was pri-

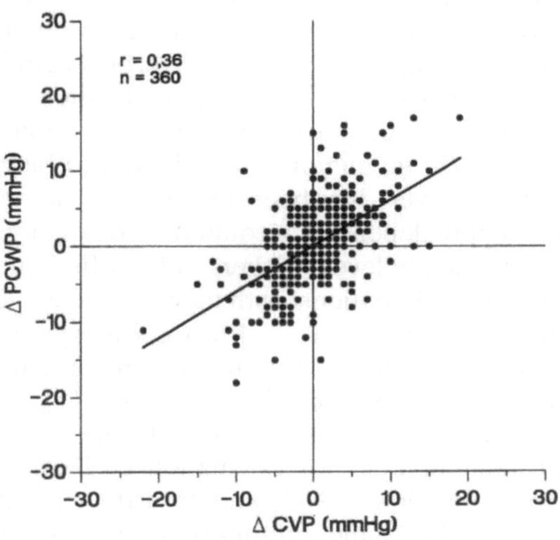

Fig. 4. Correlation of changes between pulmonary capillary wedge pressure (*PCWP*) and central venous pressure (*CVP*)

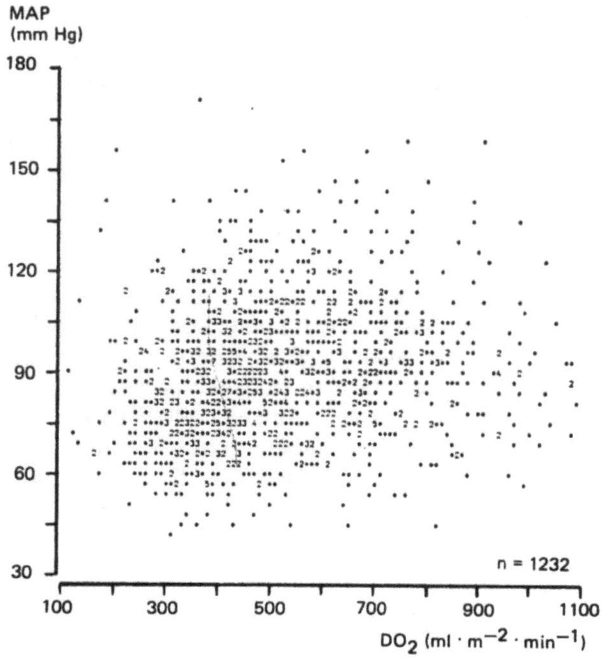

Fig. 5. Correlation between mean arterial pressure (*MAP*) and oxygen transport (*DO_2*)

marily based on the observation that in animal models of sepsis a decrease in DO_2 resulted in a greater decrease in $\dot{V}O_2$ than in nonseptic controls [14]. Additionally, in some clinical studies, it was found that patients with septic shock and low DO_2 increased $\dot{V}O_2$ after increasing DO_2, which was interpreted as improvement of a covert O_2 debt [11]. Measurements of $\dot{V}O_2$ after increasing DO_2, the so-called "O_2 flux test", are therefore used for the assessment of the adequacy of tissue oxygenation, and an increase in $\dot{V}O_2$ by more than 10–20 ml/min/m^2 is considered to be clinically relevant [13]. This concept however, has been questioned. Some authors found that pathologic O_2 supply dependency could only be demonstrated in patients with elevated serum lactate levels. Others did not find an increase in $\dot{V}O_2$ after improving DO_2, even in patients with elevated lactate levels, particularly when $\dot{V}O_2$ was measured directly from the respiratory gases and not calculated indirectly from arterial mixed venous oxygen content difference multiplied by the cardiac output (indirect Fick principle) [15].

Mathematical combination of data by using cardiac output and arterial O_2 content both for calculation of DO_2 and $\dot{V}O_2$ might contribute to an overestimation of $\dot{V}O_2$ and an artificially high correlation between delivery and uptake. Some authors therefore consider it necessary to measure $\dot{V}O_2$ independently when performing an "O_2 flux test" [15].

There are several other methodological problems with $\dot{V}O_2$ measurements in critically ill patients. One is that considerable $\dot{V}O_2$ fluctuations may occur, caused by unrest, fever, shivering, etc. It is crucial therefore that all these situations be taken into consideration when an "O_2 flux test" is performed. An increase in $\dot{V}O_2$ for spurious reasons should not be interpreted as an improvement of tissue oxygenation, because under these circumstances it results only from an increase in O_2 demand. Another limitation in the interpretability of an "O_2 flux test" exists if catecholamines are used to increase DO_2, because it is difficult to separate their potential calorigenic effects from their potential effects on $\dot{V}O_2$ by improving tissue oxygenation.

There are some conceptual limitations to the "O_2 flux test". We can only measure the actual O_2 consumption which does not necessarily reflect the actual O_2 needs! If $\dot{V}O_2$ does not increase after increasing DO_2 this may not rule out tissue hypoxia because whole body measurements may be too insensitive to reflect conditions on regional levels. We recently monitored gastric mucosal pH as an indicator of gastrointestinal tissue oxygenation in septic shock patients challenged with 1200 ml hydroxyethylstarch. DO_2 increased 15% but whole body $\dot{V}O_2$ was unchanged. Gastric mucosal pH improved but remained low (<7.32). Thus, a negative "O_2 flux test" failed to identify an improved, yet still inadequate, oxygenation of a specific region [16].

Arteriovenous Oxygen Content Difference, Oxygen Extraction Ratio, Oxygen Demand/Supply Ratio, Mixed Venous Oxygen Saturation

All these parameters convey information on the degree to which the arterial blood is desaturated during its course through the various organs and tissues. Under normal nonseptic conditions these parameters select the extent to

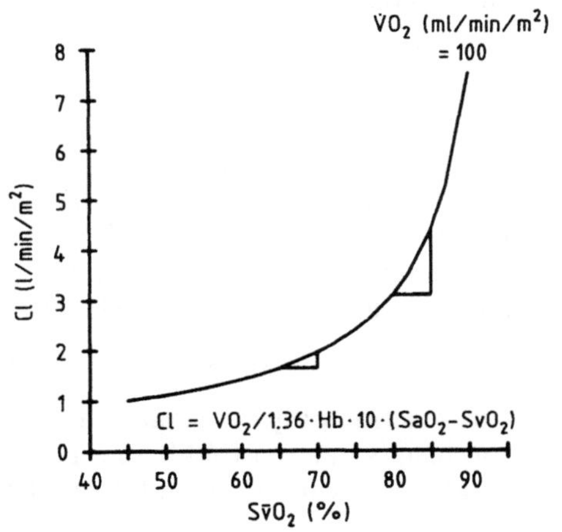

Fig. 6. Relationship between cardiac index (*CI*) and mixed venous O_2 saturation ($S\bar{v}O_2$) when O_2 consumption ($\dot{V}O_2$) remains stable

which the physiological compensatory mechanisms maintain cellular O_2 supply, when changes in DO_2 and or $\dot{V}O_2$ occur. For clinical purposes arteriovenous (av) DO_2, O_2 extraction ratio and $DO_2/\dot{V}O_2$ can be replaced by mixed venous O_2 saturation ($S\bar{v}O_2$) monitoring which is easily performed at the bedside, can be monitored continuously, and does not require serial blood gas measurements and calculations [10, 17]. Due to the curvilinear relationship between cardiac index (CI) and $S\bar{v}O_2$ provided $\dot{V}O_2$ remains stable [10], a drop in $S\bar{v}O_2$ in the high range, for example from 85% to 80%, indicates a much greater decline in CI than a drop of $S\bar{v}O_2$ from 70% to 65% (Fig. 6). As $S\bar{v}O_2$ in hyperdynamic septic shock patients is in the upper range of normal, or even supernormal, its continuous monitoring can be helpful for early detection of changes in DO_2.

Limitations of mixed venous oxygen saturation monitoring in septic shock. The principal limitation of $S\bar{v}O_2$ monitoring is that it only reflects global O_2 extraction and gives no information about the regional level, where tissue hypoxia may exist despite normal $S\bar{v}O_2$ values. This becomes all the more problematic for the patient in septic shock. Due to changes between various regional O_2 supply/demand relationships which occur especially in the hepatic-splanchnic region during sepsis, $S\bar{v}O_2$ may be up to 40% higher than hepatic venous O_2 saturation.

Blood lactate. Hyperlactatemia is defined as a moderate, persistent increase in blood lactate concentration (2–5 mmol/l) without metabolic acidosis, whereas lactic acidosis is characterized by persistently increased blood lactate levels (>5 mmol/l) in association with metabolic acidosis [18].

The organs which produce the largest amount of lactate are the muscle and the skin. Another important source of lactate is the erythrocytes, because they lack an oxidizing system to metabolize pyruvate.

Lactate is produced entirely from glucose metabolism. Glucose metabolism ends up in aerobic and anaerobic conditions forming pyruvate. Pyruvate can be metabolized in three possible ways [19].

1. Pyruvate dehydrogenase (PDH) mediates the transformation into acetyl-coA, which enters the citric acid cycle for complete oxidation. This is an irreversible reaction.
2. The alanine aminotransferase (AAT) can transaminate pyruvate with glutamate to form alanine and L-ketoglutarate. This is a reversible reaction in the liver and the kidney, thus contributing to gluconeogenesis.
3. The lactate dehydrogenase (LDH) can decrease pyruvate by nicotinamide adenine dinucleotide (NADH) into lactate, according to the reaction:

$$\text{Pyruvate} + \text{NADH} + \text{H}^+ \leftrightarrow \text{Lactate} + \text{NAD}^+.$$

This reaction only takes place in the cytosol. The equilibrium of this reaction results in a ten-fold higher lactate to pyruvate ratio and therefore the lactate level within the cell is regulated by the pyruvate and H^+ concentrations and by the redox state of the cytosol. During oxidative metabolism, the NADH formed is used by the mitochondrial electron transport chain to produce adenosine triphosphate (ATP) and can regenerate NAD^+, whereas hypoxia prevents the NAD^+ formation and thus increases the $NADH/NAD^+$ ratio and increases lactate levels.

Blood lactate levels can be easily determined using automated analyzers that can be placed at the bedside. The major organs removing lactate are the liver (50%) and the kidney (30%). The heart also contributes to lactate utilization.

Lactate as an end product can only be metabolized by conversion into pyruvate when oxygen is available. Then lactate is either oxidized or utilized for gluconeogenesis in the liver and the kidney.

During hypoxia, glucose is used preferentially, this is because the amount of ATP produced per mole of oxygen is higher with glucose than with other nutrients. The accumulation of adenosine monophosphate (AMP) in the cytosol also stimulates glycolysis ("Pasteur effect"). Thus, the accumulation of lactate can be due not only to anaerobic metabolism, but also in part to glycolytic flux.

The widely accepted classification system of Cohen and Woods [20] separated lactic acidosis (LA) into two categories: Type A is LA occurring in association with chemical evidence of poor tissue perfusion or oxygenation of blood (e.g., different types of shock, severe hypoxemia, severe anemia). Type B is LA occurring when clinical evidence of poor tissue perfusion or oxygenation is absent (B_1: LA occurring in association with an underlying disease; B_2: LA due to drugs/toxins; B_3: LA due to congenital errors of metabolism). Thus, the distinction between types A and B of LA is based on the presence or absence of clinical evidence of tissue hypoperfusion.

In experimental studies in which oxygen supply was acutely reduced by hypoxic hypoxia, stagnant hypoxia (low flow), and anemic hypoxia, blood lactate levels have been shown to closely correlate with the oxygen deficit [21–23]. The critical systemic oxygen supply is similar in the presence of anemia and hypoxemia; in both cases, the blood lactate levels start to rise as soon as the critical DO_2 value is reached.

In several septic shock studies it has been clearly demonstrated that the uptake/supply dependency phenomenon is associated with LA. It has been documented that elevated blood lactate levels predicted an increase in $\dot{V}O_2$ in response to an increase in DO_2 associated with fluid administration [24]. In another study [25], in which two subgroups of patients were investigated according to the presence or absence of LA, $\dot{V}O_2$ increased significantly only in those patients with LA. In this clinical trial the effects of dopamine and dobutamine at various doses were also studied. The constant finding was that in patients with LA $\dot{V}O_2$ increased to a significantly higher level after catecholamine administration than in those with normal lactate levels. These observations were attributed to direct stimulating effects of the catecholamines on cellular metabolism in patients with normal lactate levels. It should be noted that in these studies initial DO_2 before administration of volume and/or catecholamines was within normal or upper normal ranges, so that hyperdynamic circulation with above normal convective O_2 transport had not been achieved [24, 25].

There are several other studies whose data indicate that the uptake/supply dependency phenomenon is usually associated with the development of anaerobic metabolism with increased blood lactate levels. In one study with four patient groups according to the cardiac or septic nature of their disease, and also according to lactate levels, it has been demonstrated that in both groups of patients the $\dot{V}O_2$ only increased in patients with elevated lactate levels [26]. In a recent study in adult respiratory distress syndrome (ARDS) patients it has been demonstrated that $\dot{V}O_2$ only increased significantly after blood transfusion when blood lactate levels were increased [27]. In addition, Annat et al. observed no correlation between $\dot{V}O_2$ and DO_2 in ARDS patients with normal lactate levels [28].

Evidently the results of these studies are relevant arguments against the hypothesis that the uptake/supply dependency phenomenon reflects the use of oxygen by extramitochondrial or non-ATP producing systems. The oxygen used by these mechanisms activated by the inflammatory process may be deleterious, because it can contribute to the disturbances within the microcirculatory blood flow. However, the affinity of oxygen for the extramitochondrial systems is much lower than for the cytochrome aa_3 oxidase of the mitochondrial electron transport chain. Therefore, any increase in oxygen supply within the hypoxic cell will be preferentially used by the mitochondria. Thus it seems to be plausible that an increase in O_2 supply to the cells is probably desired in the presence of LA in septic patients without "supranormal" DO_2 levels, and O_2 is not likely to "fuel the fire" by increasing the release of toxic products.

Nonetheless, the use of lactate as an index of tissue perfusion has several limitations. There are various causes of type B LA which may produce hyperlactatemia and LA in the absence of tissue hypoperfusion. It has been demonstrated in a recent study of septic patients with normal or increased plasma lactate levels that increased concentration of plasma lactate did not predict dependence of $\dot{V}O_2$ on DO_2 after increasing DO_2 by dobutamine infusion [15]. Recent research has focused on the splanchnic circulation [6, 11, 29]. In a study of patients undergoing cardiac surgery, it has been demonstrated that transient episodes of intraoperative splanchnic ischemia, manifested by a decrease in gastric mucosal pH, was linearly related to lactate concentration in the hepatic vein and also predicted postoperative complications [5].

These data confirm some limitations of blood lactate as a reliable index of tissue hypoxia:

1. In hemodynamically stabilized patients with sepsis, the increased lactate concentration may be a marker of previous and resolved tissue hypoxia

after fluid and vasopressor administration rather than a marker of tissue hypoxia.
2. For significant increases in blood lactate to occur, lactate must not only accumulate in tissues and spill into the systemic circulation, but its rate of production must exceed hepatic, renal and skeletal muscle uptake [30]. Thus, delayed clearance of plasma lactate due to liver dysfunction with decreased hepatic clearance rather than anaerobic production may be responsible for increased blood lactate levels.
3. Increased lactate levels may be due to inhibition of pyruvate dehydrogenase enzyme by endotoxin [31, 32].
4. Accelerated aerobic glycolysis rather than anaerobic glycolysis may cause hyperlactatemia [33, 34].
5. Increases in blood lactate may be due to effects of increased endogeneous and infused catecholamines [35].

Therefore, both adequate tissue perfusion and regional hypoperfusion may be present despite elevated or normal blood lactate concentration. The blood lactate values are in this respect, like DO_2 and $\dot{V}O_2$, only global metabolic parameters, which insufficiently reflect regional tissue oxygenation.

It has been suggested that a "lactate washout" phenomenon may be a potential limitation of the interpretation of blood lactate levels. Undoubtedly, such a phenomenon can occur in reperfused organs [16, 36], and may indicate, as explained, an improved perfusion of hypoxic areas rather than a worsening of cellular hypoxia. Even after cardiac arrest, the "lactate washout" phenomenon did not exceed 4–8 min [37]. Thus, despite the existence of such a phenomenon, it does not interfere with the interpretation of blood lactate analysis.

The frequency of blood lactate level determinations appears to be of relevance. A patient with uncontrolled sepsis may demonstrate only moderate LA which may persist or even increase with time. If the interpretation of blood lactate levels remains difficult, the "O_2 flux test" or "$\dot{V}O_2$ challenge test", keeping in mind their limitations, can clarify whether a relevant global uptake/supply dependency phenomenon exists [12].

Elevated blood lactate levels reflect the severity of circulatory failure. Therapy must therefore be directed towards the eradication of the cause of circulatory failure. Administration of sodium bicarbonate in LA has been seriously challenged [38]. The effect is limited by rapid transformation, and in experimental LA, sodium bicarbonate resulted in deleterious hemodynamic effects, probably related to a more rapid passage of the transformed carbon dioxide into the myocardial cells [39] with a further decrease in intramyocardial pH and worsening of myocardial contractility.

In septic experimental models it has been shown that the pyruvate dehydrogenase activity was reduced [31]. Sodium dichloroacetate, an activator of pyruvate dehydrogenase, has been demonstrated to effectively reduce blood lactate levels under these experimental conditions. However, in a recent animal study of endotoxic shock, although able to decrease blood lactate levels dichloroacetate could not alter the hemodynamic parameters including the DO_2 related variables [40]. Thus, the beneficial effects of the substance remain doubtful.

In summary, lactate levels are useful indexes reflecting the severity of tissue hypoxia in severe septic shock with evidence of hypoperfusion and in septic patients without hyperdynamic circulation. Frequent evaluation of blood lactate levels may be helpful in controlling the efficiency of the therapeutic approach. A possible "washout" phenomenon may be of short duration and reflects the adequacy of therapy rather than playing down the clinical value of blood lactate measurements.

In hyperdynamic, stable shock the interpretation of blood lactate values may be more difficult and evidently has some limitations. Normal lactate levels do not exclude discrete regional tissue hypoxia and increased lactate levels are not necessarily due to tissue hypoxia. Increased lactate values may at least in part be due to the inhibition of enzyme systems (PDH), to red blood cell lactate production, to decreased lactate clearance, to a "washout" phenomenon after resuscitation, to accelerated aerobic glycolysis, and to increased catecholamines. Thus, several clinical conditions beyond tissue hypoxia may cause elevated lactate levels in septic patients.

Future Perspectives in the Monitoring of Global Oxygen Transport Related Variables

Even in well staffed and equipped intensive care units (ICU), the measurement of DO_2 and $\dot{V}O_2$ is usually limited to a few times daily because it is time consuming. Only $S\bar{v}O_2$ measurements are available on a continuous basis with fiber optic PA catheters [10, 17]. However, various methods for continuous cardiac output measurements are currently being clinically tested [41, 42] and will probably soon be available. Their accuracy seems to be sufficient for clinical purposes [41]. The combination of continuous cardiac output (CO), fiber optic mixed venous O_2 saturation ($S\bar{v}O_2$) measurements and pulse oximetry O_2 saturation (SaO_2) allows continuous calculation and dis-

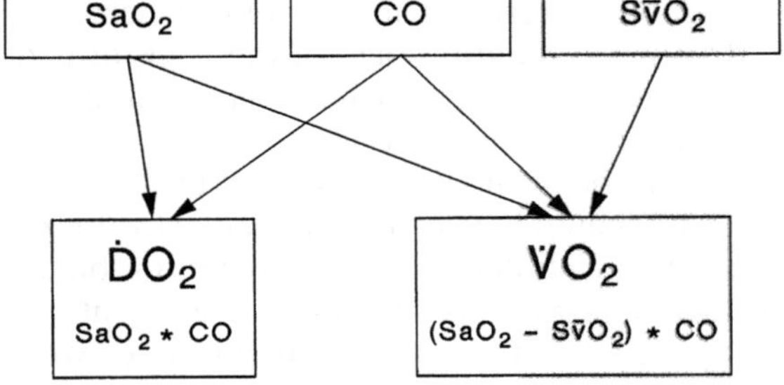

Fig. 7. Parameters for continuous calculation of O_2 transport (*DO_2*) and O_2 consumption (*$\dot{V}O_2$*), obtainable at the bedside. [*SaO_2*, pulse oximetry O_2 saturation; *CO*, cardiac output; *$S\bar{v}O_2$*, mixed venous O_2 saturation; *PAC*, pulmonary artery catheter]

play of DO_2 and $\dot{V}O_2$ [41] (Fig. 7). The continuous display of DO_2, $\dot{V}O_2$, $S\bar{v}O_2$, and SaO_2 is superior to continuous $S\bar{v}O_2$ alone, as it quickly depicts whether a change in $S\bar{v}O_2$ has resulted from changes in $\dot{V}O_2$, DO_2 or SaO_2 or a combination of these parameters (Fig. 8). For example, Fig. 8 shows that a change in the catecholamine regimen from dobutamine plus norepinephrine to norepinephrine alone resulted in no change in global $\dot{V}O_2$ despite a sharp decrease in DO_2. If it can be shown in future studies that errors made by calculating DO_2 and $\dot{V}O_2$ are tolerable for clinical purposes, these methods would make the optimization of DO_2 and $\dot{V}O_2$ easier in the clinical setting.

Parameters for the Assessment of Regional Tissue Oxygenation

As already outlined, the global parameters for the assessment of tissue oxygenation have some limitations in their ability to reflect the specific situation on the regional level. Clinically applicable methods for the assessment of regional O_2 supply and tissue oxygenation are therefore warranted.

Tissue Oxygen Tension Measurements

Direct measurements of oxygen tension (PO_2) by polarographictype needle probes are possible in the clinical setting [43, 44]. However, it is limited to measurements in areas such as muscle and subcutaneous tissue. In preliminary

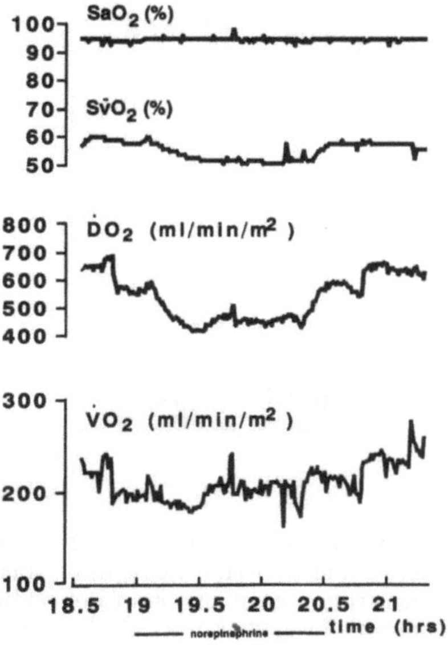

Fig. 8. Continuous display of pulse oximetry measured O_2 saturation (*SaO_2*), mixed venous O_2 saturation (*$S\bar{v}O_2$*), O_2 transport (*DO_2*) and O_2 consumption (*$\dot{V}O_2$*) by changes in the catecholamine regimen (dobutamine plus norepinephrine; norepinephrine alone; dobutamine plus norepinephrine)

studies we found lower muscle tissue PO_2 despite higher DO_2 and $S\bar{v}O_2$ in patients with septic shock than in patients without sepsis who had higher muscle tissue PO_2 despite lower DO_2 and $S\bar{v}O_2$ [45]. However, when we extended these measurements to patients with even higher baseline levels of DO_2, we found normally distributed tissue PO_2 histograms and even slightly elevated mean values for tissue PO_2 that could not be further elevated by further increasing DO_2 (Fig. 9). Data from other investigators exist which confirm that muscle tissue oxygenation does not suffer in adequately treated patients with hyperdynamic septic shock [43]. These direct tissue PO_2 measurements are not very helpful in optimizing tissue oxygenation in these types of patients, because the tissues that remain most vulnerable despite high DO_2 levels (such as the gut) are not currently measurable with these devices.

Hepatic Venous Oxygen Saturation Measurements

Hepatic venous O_2 saturation ($Sh\bar{v}O_2$) is similar to $S\bar{v}O_2$ as a marker of the relationship between O_2 supply and consumption. However the information supplied about this relationship comes from a region which is especially important for the pathogenesis of sepsis. $Sh\bar{v}O_2$ has been monitored during liver surgery [46, 47] and in critically ill patients with and without septic shock [48, 49], but to date it is not yet routinely used in these types of patients. In some studies, in which whole body DO_2 changed due to hypoxia or treatment with dobutamine, parallel changes were observed between $S\bar{v}O_2$ and $Sh\bar{v}O_2$ [48, 50].

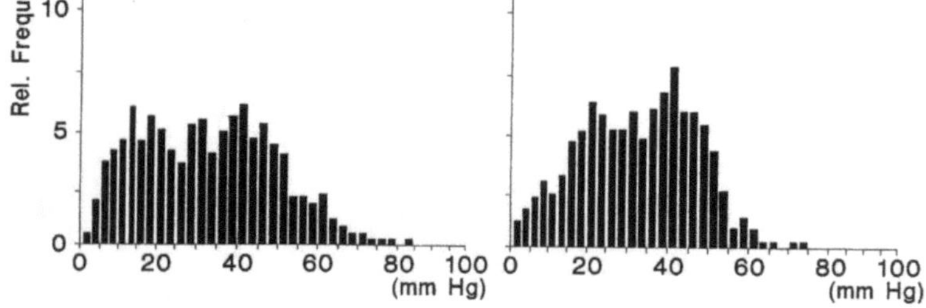

Fig. 9. Pooled oxygen tension (*PO_2*) histograms of patients in hyperdynamic septic shock before and after an increase of O_2 transport (*DO_2*) by a change in the catecholamine regimen from a combination of dobutamine and norepinephrine to dopamine. The dose of dopamine was chosen to achieve the same mean arterial pressure as before

Measurements in patients with septic shock yielded 15% lower mean values for $Sh\bar{v}O_2$ than for $S\bar{v}O_2$, while no differences were found in patients without septic shock [48]. That study [48] and our own results in 29 septic patients, demonstrates that a great variation exists in the difference between $S\bar{v}O_2$ and $Sh\bar{v}O_2$. The smallest individual difference in our patients was 0.5%, the largest 36.7% (Fig. 10). $S\bar{v}O_2$ within a normal range can therefore not exclude a greatly decreased $Sh\bar{v}O_2$. The relevance of a decreased $Sh\bar{v}O_2$ in the clinical setting is demonstrated by Kainuma et al., who found that in post hepatectomy patients an intraoperative $Sh\bar{v}O_2$ below 40% correlated to a postoperative increase in liver transaminases and subsequent liver failure [47]. The critical value for $Sh\bar{v}O_2$ in patients in septic shock, however, is not yet established. In animal models with endotoxic shock a higher critical level for regional DO_2, i.e., O_2 supply dependency of O_2 uptake, was shown in the gut [51]. One might therefore conclude that the hepatic-splanchnic region might suffer from inadequate regional O_2 supply when $Sh\bar{v}O_2$ is still above the critical level of 40% for $Sh\bar{v}O_2$, which has been found in patients with liver surgery [47].

The lower $Sh\bar{v}O_2$ in septic patients results from an increase in $\dot{V}O_2$ in the splanchnic region that may comprise more than 50% of whole body $\dot{V}O_2$, compared to only 20%–30% in nonseptic conditions [49]. Obviously, the increased $\dot{V}O_2$ is not fully matched by an increase in O_2 supply to this region.

Hepatic Venous vs Mixed Venous Oxygen Saturation

As depicted in Fig. 10, the difference between $S\bar{v}O_2$ and $Sh\bar{v}O_2$ can be considerable. Additionally, the question arises as to what extent changes in patients' condition or therapy are reflected in $S\bar{v}O_2$ and $Sh\bar{v}O_2$. Therapeutic interventions such as the use of positive end-expiratory pressure (PEEP) [52, 53] or the infusion of catecholamines or vasoactive drugs [54] may alter both regional blood flow and regional $\dot{V}O_2$. It has been reported that a drop in arterial PO_2 during bronchoscopy was reflected by a parallel decrease in

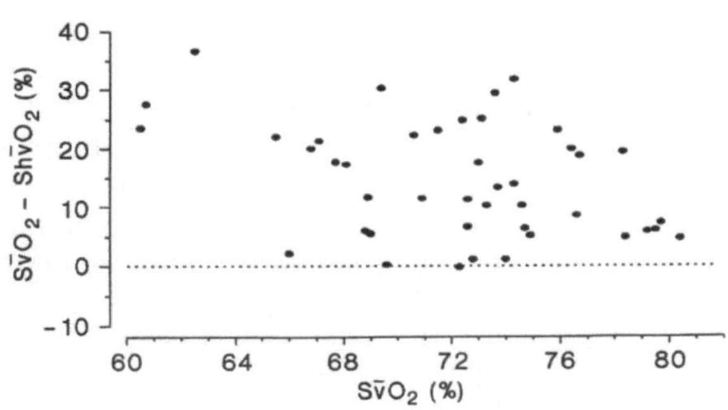

Fig. 10. Difference between mixed venous O_2 saturation ($S\bar{v}O_2$) and hepatic venous O_2 saturation ($Sh\bar{v}O_2$) in fully resuscitated hyperdynamic septic shock patients

$S\bar{v}O_2$ and $Sh\bar{v}O_2$ and that increasing DO_2 in critically ill patients with dobutamine resulted in a parallel increase in both $S\bar{v}O_2$ and $Sh\bar{v}O_2$ [50]. However, this may not be true for all clinical situations.

We compared a combination of dobutamine and norepinephrine to norepinephrine or epinephrine alone at doses to achieve equal mean arterial pressures. With norepinephrine we found a decrease in $S\bar{v}O_2$ from 75% ±5% to 69% ±5% and in $Sh\bar{v}O_2$ from 62% ±13% to 49% ±13%. With epinephrine the $S\bar{v}O_2$ remained unchanged but the $Sh\bar{v}O_2$ decreased to the same extent as it had with norepinephrine, from 64% ±8% to 54% ±10%. With vasopressor as monotherapy, the difference between $S\bar{v}O_2$ and $Sh\bar{v}O_2$ increased (see Fig. 1, Meier-Hellmann and Reinhart, this volume), indicating a deterioration of O_2 supply/consumption relationship in the splanchnic region. In the case of epinephrine this was associated with a decrease in O_2 uptake in splanchnic region, whereas whole body $\dot{V}O_2$ remained unchanged. In contrast, both whole body and splanchnic O_2 uptake remained unchanged with norepinephrine (unpublished data).

The addition of low dose dopamine (3 μg/kg/min) or dopexamine (2 μg/kg/min) to the combination of dobutamine with norepinephrine resulted in no significant changes in the difference between $S\bar{v}O_2$ and $Sh\bar{v}O_2$ (see Fig. 1, Meier-Hellmann and Reinhart, this volume). This indicates that the increase in CO achieved by these drugs results in a parallel increase in global and splanchnic DO_2. With dopamine $S\bar{v}O_2$ increased from 69% ±4% to 74% ±4% and $Sh\bar{v}O_2$ from 53% ±13% to 64% ±10%. Dopexamine had no effect on venous O_2 saturation with values from 75% ±5% to 77% ±3% for $S\bar{v}O_2$ and from 58% ±12% to 59% ±13% for $Sh\bar{v}O_2$, respectively. These results demonstrate that changes in $S\bar{v}O_2$ reflect changes in a global O_2 supply/consumption relationship and do not necessarily reflect parallel changes in $DO_2/\dot{V}O_2$ in the individual organs. Vasoactive drugs may have varying effects in different organs interfering with regional blood flow and/or regional $\dot{V}O_2$ [54].

The interpretation of a change in $Sh\bar{v}O_2$ includes the same limitations as for $S\bar{v}O_2$. A relatively greater increase in $Sh\bar{v}O_2$ as compared to the $S\bar{v}O_2$ could be due to a relatively increased splanchnic perfusion or decreased splanchnic oxygen consumption. Low-dose dopamine has been demonstrated to improve perfusion of the splanchnic area. However, Giraud et al. [55] demonstrated that dopamine increases the perfusion in the superior mesenteric artery but decreases the perfusion of the intestinal mucosa with a net result of decreased $\dot{V}O_2$ by the gut. Therefore from the increase of $Sh\bar{v}O_2$ after infusion of dopamine, it cannot be concluded with certainty that tissue oxygenation in the splanchnic region was improved. It cannot be ruled out that there was decreased perfusion or an increased arteriovenous shunting to some tissues at the expense of decreased blood flow to others. Thus, to differentiate whether changes in $Sh\bar{v}O_2$ indicate improvement or impairment of tissue oxygenation, splanchnic perfusion needs to be measured together with $Sh\bar{v}O_2$ to determine the $\dot{V}O_2$. This, however, is not easily done in the clinical setting.

These limitations do not imply that $Sh\bar{v}O_2$ monitoring is of no value in septic patients. Figures 11 and 12 indicate the importance of $Sh\bar{v}O_2$ monitoring in a patient with septic shock. The conversion from dobutamine to epinephrine leads to a slight increase in DO_2 and $\dot{V}O_2$ (Fig. 11). The $S\bar{v}O_2$ remained unchanged, but the $Sh\bar{v}O_2$ markedly decreased (Fig. 12). In this case the simultaneous measurement of splanchnic blood flow and the calculation of splanchnic oxygen consumption revealed a decrease in both these para-

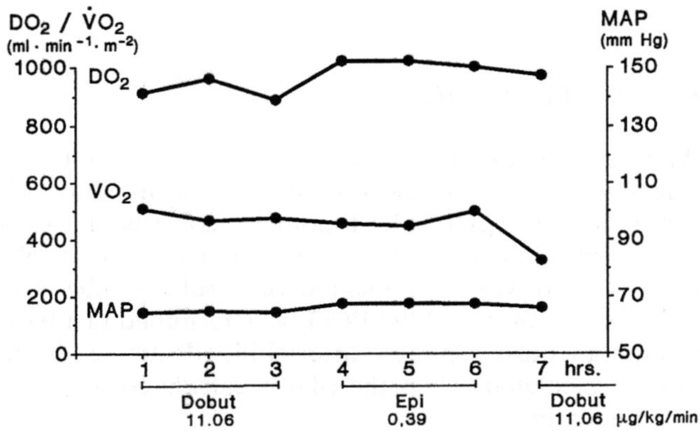

Fig. 11. Changes in O_2 transport (*DO_2*) and O_2 consumption (*$\dot{V}O_2$*) after changes in the catecholamine regimen (*dobut,* dobutamine; *epi,* epinephrine) in a patient with hyperdynamic septic shock. The dose of epinephrine was chosen to achieve the same mean arterial pressure (*MAP*) as before

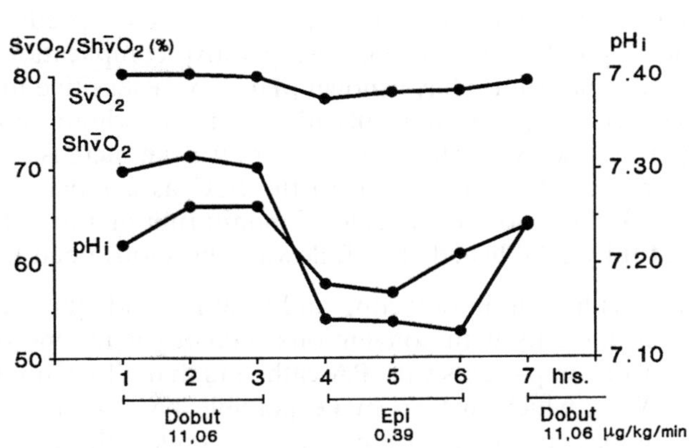

Fig. 12. Changes in mixed venous O_2 saturation (*$S\bar{v}O_2$*), hepatic venous O_2 saturation (*$Sh\bar{v}O_2$*) and gastric mucosal pH (*pHi*) after changes in catecholamine regimen (*dobut,* dobutamine; *epi,* epinephrine) in a patient with hyperdynamic septic shock. The dose of epinephrine was chosen to achieve the same mean arterial pressure (MAP) as before

meters. In this patient the change in catecholamine treatment induced a deterioration in splanchnic oxygenation indicated by $Sh\bar{v}O_2$ monitoring but not by the $S\bar{v}O_2$ or the "O_2 flux test". Therefore, monitoring $Sh\bar{v}O_2$ may prove helpful in the management of patients with severe septic shock by detection of a disturbed relationship between oxygen supply and consumption in the splanchnic area. A positive "O_2 flux test" is not always a reliable indicator of an improvement in tissue oxygenation. Further investigations are necessary to more clearly define the circumstances in which changes of $Sh\bar{v}O_2$ are not similarly reflected by changes in $S\bar{v}O_2$. These are the situations where monitoring of $Sh\bar{v}O_2$ may be most helpful for the management of critically ill patients.

Gastric Mucosal pH

Another method of assessing the adequacy of tissue oxygenation in the splanchnic area is by the tonometric determination of the pH value in the gastric mucosa (pHi). The tonometer consists of a polyester elastomer tube with a silastic balloon close to its tip. The balloon, placed in the gastric lumen, is filled with 2.5 ml saline via a rubber tube. After equilibriation, the saline is aspirated and the PCO_2 is determined in a blood gas analyzer. From a simultaneously aspirated arterial blood sample the bicarbonate concentration is calculated. Then the pHi is calculated using the Henderson-Hasselbalch equation:

$$pHi = 6.1 + \log (HCO_3\text{-}/PCO_2 \times 0.003)$$

Equilibriation across the tonometer balloon takes 90 min so a correction factor for the equilibrium time must be used in the equation. Gastric tonometry has demonstrated a high specificity for predicting patient survival [7, 56, 57] and for predicting postoperative complications in the ICU [6].

Several studies have shown pHi to be a sensitive marker for gastric mucosal hypoxia [5]. In critically ill patients, in whom DO_2 was raised whenever pHi fell below normal levels, there was an increased mortality if pHi values were <7.35 on admission to the ICU as compared with initial pHi values >7.35 [56]. So far, the role of monitoring pHi in critically ill patients is not yet fully established. The following questions need to be answered:

1) It is helpful in detecting and treating inadequate tissue oxygenation only in patients with conventional hemodynamic monitoring, or is it also of value in patients with PA catheters that allow monitoring $S\bar{v}O_2$, DO_2, and VO_2, which in turn make possible an "O_2 flux test"? Does it have an impact on patient outcome in patients with septic shock in whom extensive hemodynamic monitoring is used?

2) Is it helpful only in the early detection of deterioration of gut mucosal oxygenation, or also when gut mucosal hypoxia has already been established?

To answer some of these questions we measured pHi together with the DO_2 related variables. In ten patients with hyperdynamic septic shock and with pHi values <7.35 indicating regional tissue hypoxia we further increased DO_2 with colloidal volume substitution. This caused a significant rise in the pHi from 7.20±0.05 to 7.25±0.05 but did not change $\dot{V}O_2$ [58] (Fig. 13). In these patients the criteria for a negative "O_2 flux test" were fulfilled, but the increased pHi indicated an improvement in the oxygenation of gastric mucosa. Meanwhile there is a brief report that prostacyclin (PGI2), though not increasing $\dot{V}O_2$ despite an increase in DO_2, significantly improved pHi [59]. Once again, a negative "O_2 flux test" does not exclude regional tissue hypoxia and an increase in DO_2 may improve tissue oxygenation without measurable changes in $\dot{V}O_2$.

Figures 11 and 12 demonstrate a change in pHi without a change in $S\dot{v}O_2$, DO_2 and $\dot{V}O_2$. The conversion from dobutamine to epinephrine induced a decrease in pHi and after reconversion to dobutamine the pHi increased to the previous level. The pHi, similar to the $Sh\dot{v}O_2$, indicated a deterioration in splanchnic oxygenation.

Conclusion

Global indices of the adequacy of tissue oxygenation have several limitations in the assessment of actual regional tissue oxygenation.

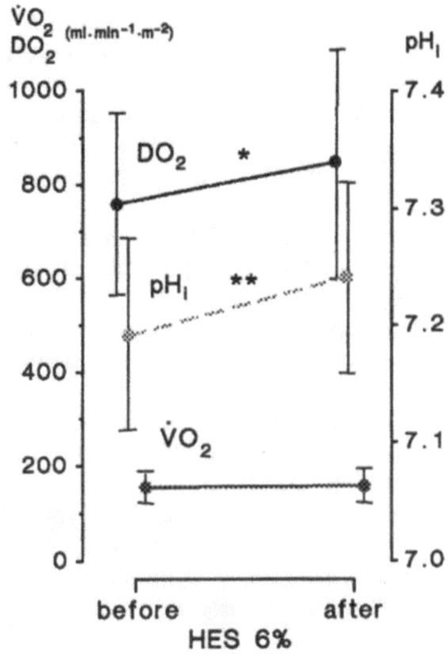

Fig. 13. Changes in O_2 transport (*DO_2*), O_2 consumption (*$\dot{V}O_2$*) and gastric mucosal pH (*pHi*) after colloidal volume substitution with hydroxyethylstarch 6% (*HES 6%*) in a patient with hyperdynamic septic shock. (From [58])

Monitoring of hepatic venous O_2 saturation, even if not combined with regional flow and consumption measurements, may prove helpful in the detection of mismatches between regional O_2 supply and consumption and guiding therapeutic interventions. The best indications for hepatic venous O_2 saturation monitoring, however, have not yet been completely defined. The disadvantages of this method are that it is invasive, expensive, and requires fluroscopic control of the catheter tip.

In contrast to hepatic venous O_2 saturation monitoring, the gastric tonometer is easy to use. An abnormally low pHi is associated with increased morbidity and mortality in patients undergoing major surgery and in patients admitted to the ICU. Early intervention using pHi as a therapeutic index is associated with better survival of patients admitted to the ICU with normal pHi. However, no benefit in outcome was demonstrable when the admission pHi was abnormally low. Some evidence suggests that pHi offers important additional information on the adequacy of tissue oxygenation even in patients with PA catheters. Further studies are necessary to define the subgroups of patients that may benefit most from the monitoring of pHi in terms of reduction of morbidity and mortality.

References

1. Sibbald WJ, Bersten A, Rutledge FS (1989) The role of tissue hypoxia in multiple organ failure. In: Reinhart K, Eyrich K (eds) Clinical aspects of oxygen transport and tissue oxygenation. Springer, Berlin Heidelberg New York, pp 102–114
2. Edwards D et al (1989) Use of survivors' cardiorespiratory values as therapeutic goals in septic shock. Crit Care Med 17:1098–1103
3. Shoemaker WC, Appel PL, Kram HB, Waxman K, Lee TS (1988) Prospective trial of supranormal values of survivors as therapeutic goals in high risk surgical patients. Chest 94:1176–1186
4. Tuchschmidt J, Fried J, Astiz M, Rackow E (1992) Elevation of cardiac output and oxygen delivery improves outcome in septic shock. Chest 102:216–220
5. Fiddian-Green RG (1991) Should measurements of tissue pH and PO_2 be included in the routine monitoring of intensive care unit patients? Crit Care Med 19:141–143
6. Fiddian-Green RG, Baker S (1987) Predictive value of the stomach wall pH for complications after cardiac operations: comparison with other monitoring. Crit Care Med 15:153–156
7. Gutierrez G, Palizas F, Doglio G et al (1992) Gastric intramucosal pH as a therapeutic index of tissue oxygenation in critically ill patients. Lancet 339:195–199
8. Gutierrez G, Pohil RJ (1987) Assessment of hypoxia by magnetic resonance spectroscopy and positron emmission tomography. In: Bryan Brown CW, Ayre SM (eds) Oxygen transport and utilization. New Horizons, Society of Critical Care Medicine, Fullerton, pp 171–214
9. Jöbsis FF (1977) Noninvasive infrared monitoring of cerebral and myocardial oxygen sufficiency and circulatory parameters. Science 198:1264–1267
10. Reinhart K (1989) Monitoring of O_2 transport and tissue oxygenation in critically ill patients. In: Reinhart K, Eyrich K (eds) Clinical aspects of O_2 transport and tissue oxygenation. Springer, Berlin Heidelberg New York, pp 195–211
11. Bihari DJ (1989) Multiple organ failure: role of tissue hypoxia. In: Bihari DJ, Cerra FB (eds) Multiple organ failure. Society of Critical Care Medicine, Fullerton, pp 25–36

12. Bihari D, Smithies M, Gimson A, Tinker J (1987) The effects of vasodilation with prostacyclin on oxygen delivery and uptake in critically ill patients. N Engl J Med 317:397–403
13. Dhainaut JF, Edwards JD, Grootendorst AF, Nightingale P, Pinky MR, Reinhart K, Shoemaker WC, Vincent JL (1990) Practical aspects of oxygen transport: conclusions and recommendations of the Round Table Conference. Intensive Care Med 16:179–180
14. Cain SM (1989) Supply dependency of oxygen uptake. In: Reinhart K, Eyrich K (eds) Clinical aspects of O_2 transport and tissue oxygenation. Springer, Berlin Heidelberg New York, pp 80–91
15. Ronco JJ, Fenwick JC, Wiggs BR, Phang TP, Russell JA, Tweeddale MG (1993) Oxygen consumption is independent of increases in oxygen delivery by dobutamine in septic patients who have normal or increased plasma lactate. Am Rev Respir Dis 147:25–31
16. Haljamae H, Enger E (1975) Human skeletal muscle energy metabolism during and after complete tourniquet ischemia. Ann Surg 18–27
17. Reinhart K, Schäfer M, Rudolph T, Specht M (1989) Mixed venous oxygen saturation. Appl Cardiopulmon Pathophysiol 2:315–325
18. Krebs HG, Woods HG, Alberti KGMM (1975) Hyperlactatemia and lactic acidosis. Essays Med Biochem 1:81–103
19. Kreisberg RA (1980) Lactate homeostasis and lactic acidosis. Ann Intern Med 92:227–237
20. Cohen RD, Woods HF (1976) Clinical and biochemical aspects of lactic acidosis. Blackwell Scientific, Boston
21. Alpert NR, Kayne H, Haslett W (1958) Relationship among recovery O_2, O_2 missed, lactate production and lactate removal during and following severe hypoxia in the unanesthetized dog. Am J Physiol 192:585–591
22. Cain SM (1965) Appearance of excess lactate in anesthetized dogs during anemic and hypoxic hypoxia. Am J Physiol 209:604–608
23. Moss M, Moreau G, Lister G (1987) Oxygen transport and metabolism in the conscious lamb: the effects of hypoxemia. Pediatr Res 22:177–183
24. Haupt MT, Gilbert EM, Carlson RW (1985) Fluid loading increases oxygen consumption in septic patients with lactic acidosis. Am Rev Respir Dis 131:912–916
25. Gilbert EM, Haupt MT, Mandanas RY, Huaringa AJ, Carlson RW (1986) The effect of fluid loading, blood transfusion, and catecholamine infusion on oxygen delivery and consumption in patients with sepsis. Am Rev Respir Dis 134:873–878
26. Vincent JL, Roman A, De Backer D, Kahn RJ (1990) Oxygen uptake/supply dependency: Effects of short-term dobutamine infusion. Am Rev Respir Dis 142:2–7
27. Fenwick JC, Dodek PM, Ronco JJ, Phang PT, Wiggs B, Russell JA (1993) Increased concentrations of plasma lactate predict pathologic dependence of oxygen consumption on oxygen delivery in patients with adult respiratory distress syndrome. J Crit Care
28. Annat G, Viale JP, Percival C, Froment M, Motin J (1986) Oxygen delivery and uptake in the adult respiratory distress syndrome: lack of relationship when measured independently in patients with normal blood lactate concentrations. Am Rev Respir Dis 133:999–1001
29. Haglund U, Fiddian-Green RG (1989) Assessment of adequate tissue oxygenation in shock and critical illness: oxygen transport in sepsis. Intensive Care Med 15:475–477
30. Kruse JA, Carlson RW (1987) Lactate metabolism. Crit Care Clin 3:725–746
31. Curtis SE, Cain SM (1992) Regional and systemic lactate flux in hyperdynamic endotoxin-treated dogs. Am Rev Respir Dis 145:348–354
32. Vary TC, Siegel JH, Nakatani T, Sato T, Aoyama H (1986) Effect of sepsis on activity of pyruvate dehydrogenase complex in skeletal muscle and liver. Am Physiol 250:E634–E640
33. Cerra FB (1987) Hypermetabolism, organ failure, and metabolic support. Surgery 101:1–14

34. Hargrove DM, Bagby GJ, Lang CH, Spitzer JJ (1988) Adrenergic blockade does not abolish elevated glucose turnover during bacterial infection. Am J Physiol 254:E16–E22
35. Bessey PQ, Watters JM, Aoki TT, Wilmore DW (1984) Combined hormonal infusion simulates the metabolic response to injury. Ann Surg 200:264–280
36. Apstein CS, Gravino FN, Haudenschild CC (1983) Determinants of a protective effect of glucose and insulin on the ischemic myocardium: effects on contractile function, diastolic compliance, metabolism, and ultrastructure during ischemia and reperfusion. Circ Res 52:512–526
37. Leavy JA, Weil MH, Rackow EC (1988) "Lactate washout" following circulatory arrest. JAMA 260:662–664
38. Steenbergen C, Deleeuw KG, Rich T et al (1977) Effects of acidosis and ischemia on contractility and intracellular pH of rat heart. Circ Res 41:849–858
39. Bersin RM, Arieff AI (1988) Improved hemodynamic function during hypoxia with carbicarb, a new agent for the management of acidosis. Circulation 77:227–233
40. Preiser JC, Moulart D, Vincent JL (1990) Dichloroacetate administration in the treatment of endotoxin shock. Circ Shock 30:221–228
41. Specht M, Wichmann K, Apenburg C, Johnson RW, Reinhart K (1991) Continuous measurement of oxygen supply and oxygen consumption-first data on a new monitoring concept. Anesthesiology V75 3A:A456
42. Yelderman M (1990) Continuous measurement of cardiac output with the use of stochastic system identification techniques. J Clin Monit 6:322–332
43. Boekstegers P, Weidenhöfer St, Pilz G, Werdan K (1991) Peripheral oxygen availability within skeletal muscle in sepsis and septic shock: comparison to limited infection and cardiogenic shock. Infection 5:317–323
44. Kersting Th, Reinhart K, Dennhardt R, Fleckenstein W, Eyrich K (1985) Effect of low dose dopamine on muscle PO_2 in healthy volunteers and intensive care patients. Eur J Anaesthesiol 2:143–148
45. Reinhart K, Bloos F, König F, Hannemann L, Kuss B (1989) Oxygen transport and muscle tissue oxygenation in hyperdynamic septic shock. Anesthesiology 71:A379
46. Kainuma M, Nakashima K, Sakuma I et al (1991) Monitoring hepatic venous hemoglobin oxygen saturation in patients undergoing liver surgery. Anesthesiology 75:49–52
47. Kainuma M, Nakashima K, Sakuma I et al (1992) Hepatic venous hemoglobin oxygen saturation predicts liver dysfunction after hepatectomy. Anesthesiology 76:379–386
48. Dahn MS, Lange MP, Jacobs LA (1988) Central mixed and splanchnic venous oxygen saturation monitoring. Intensive Care Med 14:373–376
49. Dahn MS, Lange P, Lobdell K, Hans B, Jacobs LA, Mitchell RA (1987) Splanchnic and total body oxygen consumption differences in septic and injured patients. Surgery 101:69–80
50. Ruokonen E, Takala J, Uusaro A (1991) Effect of vasoactive treatment on the relationship between mixed venous and regional oxygen saturation. Crit Care Med 19:1365–1369
51. Nelson DP, Samsel RW, Wood LD, Schumacker PT (1988) Pathologic supply dependence of systemic and intestinal O_2 uptake during endotoxemia. J Appl Physiol 64:2410–2419
52. Matuschak GM, Pinsky MR, Rogers RM (1987) Effects of positive end-expiratory pressure on hepatic blood flow and performance. J Appl Physiol 62:1377–1383
53. Winsö O, Biber B, Gustavsson B, Holm C, Milsom I, Niemand D (1986) Portal blood flow in man during graded positive end-expiratory pressure ventilation. Intensive Care Med 12:80–85
54. Roytblat L, Gelman S, Bradley EL, Henderson T, Parks D (1990) Dopamine and hepatic oxygen supply-demand relationship. Can J Physiol Pharmacol 68:1165–1169
55. Giraud GD, MacCannell KL (1984) Decreased nutrient flow during dopamine and epinephrine induced intestinal vasodilation. J Pharmacol Exp Ther 230:214–230

56. Doglio GR, Pusajo JF et al (1991) Gastric mucosal pH as a prognostic index of mortality in critically ill patients. Crit Care Med 19:1037–1040
57. Gys T, Hubens A, Neels H, Lauwers LF, Peeters R (1988) Prognostic value of gastric intramural pH in surgical intensive care patients. Crit Care Med 16:1222–1224
58. Hannemann L, Meier-Hellmann A, Specht M, Spies C, Reinhart K (1993) O_2-Angebot, O_2-Verbrauch und Mukosa pH-Wert des Magens. Indikatoren der Gewebeoxygenierung. Anaesthesist 42:11–14
59. Radermacher P, Buhl R, Santak B (1993) Prostacyclin improves gastric intramucosal pH in patients with septic shock. Clin Intensive Care 4 [Suppl 2]:7

V. Therapy

Sepsis-Related Problems in Pediatric Patients

J.A. Hazelzet and R. de Groot

Introduction

The physiologic changes that constitute the process of sepsis are induced by microbial agents during bloodstream infection or by the toxic products of pathogens that are released from sites of focal infection. This process involves changes generated by the immune system and controlled by hormones, cytokines and enzymes. There are many host and microbial factors that may unfavorably influence this complex immune response. Underlying diseases with immunosuppressive effects, surgery, state of nutrition, immunomodulatory therapy and site of infection increase the risk for development of invasive disease and determine the extent of the immune response [1–3]. However, sepsis in the pediatric population occurs very frequently in previously healthy children. Also, in comparison with adults, the sepsis is more overwhelming. Mortality is mainly confined to the first 48 h of the disease. In children vs adults, different pathogens are involved and the quality and quantity of the immune response depend on the age of the child. These differences are probably caused by developmental aspects of several organ systems and may have special consequences for management and therapy.

Epidemiology

The incidence of sepsis in children shows a bimodal distribution. The first peak is in the neonatal period (defined as infants <1 month of age): 4.3/1000 newborns, from which 60% in the first 5 days and an overall mortality of about 20% [4], and a second peak around the age of 2 years. These periods are two milestones in the development of immunocompetence of the child. In children 1–4 years of age sepsis represents the ninth leading cause of death with an estimated annual mortality rate of 0.5/100000 population. The pathogens involved in this age group are in the first 2 months mainly *group B Streptococci* and *Escherichia coli* [4, 5], and later on *Neisseria meningitidis, Haemophilus influenzae, Streptococcus pneumoniae* (all of them encapsulated microorganisms which are protected against complement mediated phagocytosis and killing), *Streptococcus pyogenes* and *Staphylococcus aureus.* In addition an extensive list of other pathogens is involved in nosocomial infections [6]. Host factors predisposing to nosocomial infections are similar to those in adults [3, 7].

Sepsis in young children caused by severe meningococcal disease is rapidly progressive, overwhelming and its mortality is high (20%–60%) in the first 24–48 h. Late mortality seems to be rare [8].

Recognition

Clarification of current terminology is important to understand the pathophysiology of the septic process. A definition for sepsis in infants and children has been suggested [1] which was adapted from guidelines proposed for older patients (Table 1). We believe that the diastolic blood pressure should be included, because in the early phase of sepsis patients are sometimes able to maintain their systolic, but not their diastolic, blood pressure. This results in a low mean blood pressure and an altered organ perfusion leading to organ dysfunction.

Clinical signs and symptoms of sepsis in the pediatric population depend very much on the age of the child. Especially in the first 6 months the symptoms are nonspecific. In contrast to most adults or older children, a variety of thermal responses are seen in this age group. Apnea, leading to respiratory insufficiency, is an important sign. Extension of the bacteremia to the meninges is seen in 30% of patients with sepsis. Seizures and focal findings are often associated with the presence of meningitis. The hemodynamic signs in patients with sepsis include tachycardia, hypotension (systolic and diastolic) and cold extremities indicating an increased systemic vascular resistance (SVR).

The early stages of warm septic shock in infants and older children are

Table 1. Definition for sepsis in pediatric patients[a]

Bacteremia	Presence of viable bacteria in the circulating blood confirmed by culture
Sepsis	Clinical suspicion of infection and evidence of systemic response to infection (tachycardia, tachypnea, hyperthermia or hypothermia)[b]
Sepsis syndrome	Sepsis plus evidence of altered organ perfusion with at least one of the following: acute change in mental status[c], oliguria[d], elevated blood lactate and hypoxemia
Septic shock	Sepsis syndrome with hypotension[e] requiring fluid resuscitation and/or vasopressor support

[a] Adapted from Jafari [1].
[b] Tachycardia and tachypnea >2 standard deviations (SD) for age; hyperthermia >38.5 °C; hypothermia <36 °C.
[c] A reduction by at least 3 points from baseline value in Glasgow coma score (GCS).
[d] Diuresis <0.8 ml/kg/h.
[e] Systolic *or* diastolic blood pressure <SD for age.

heralded by signs of hypoperfusion. The earliest signs are a change in mental status and a decreased urine output. Other signs include tachycardia, a widened pulse pressure with an increase in cardiac output and a decrease in SVR. The rapid progression of the disease and the early exhaustion are characteristic. The remainder of the clinical picture in this age group is comparable with that in adults.

There are several clinical syndromes in pediatric patients which show much resemblance to the clinical picture of septic shock. Their relation with toxins is either established or hypothesized. Examples of these are toxic shock syndrome [9], necrotizing enterocolitis [9], hemorrhagic shock and encephalopathy syndrome [10].

Pathophysiology

The interaction between microbial and host factors may partly explain the differences in immune response between children and adults.

Microbial Factors

Group B streptococci (GBS) are among the leading causes of overwhelming neonatal sepsis. Although other microorganisms may cause similar clinical syndromes, most investigators have used experimental animal models of GBS infection to study the pulmonary and cardiac hemodynamics of neonatal septic shock. Gram-positive bacteria such as GBS do not have endotoxin. Two different polysaccharide toxins of GBS have been described [11]. The polysaccharide capsule may also contribute to the organism's virulence through its protection from host phagocytosis. Although the presence of neutralizing maternal IgG antibodies to the capsular polysaccharide correlates with protection against disease in neonates, the age-related risk of GBS in newborns has not been fully explained.

Severe meningococcal disease is the most frequent cause of sepsis in children above 3 months of age and in teenagers without underlying disease. In several countries in Europe the incidence has increased during the last decade. The clinical picture includes an overwhelming septic shock with purpura. The mortality remains high, in spite of extensive research especially regarding the pathogenetic role of endotoxin [12]. The reason for this specific clinical picture has still not been completely elucidated. The endotoxin or lipopolysaccharides (LPSs) of many nonenteric gram-negative organisms, such as *Neisseria meningitidis* and *Haemophilus influenzae,* lack the outer polysaccharide O-chain and contain only the oligosaccharide and the lipid A region often referred to as lipo-oligosaccharides (LOSs). The lipid A region is considered to be the most bioactive and toxic part and extensive investigative efforts have been directed towards developing anti-lipid A antibodies. However, in animal experiments there are differences in lethality and in neutralization by polymyxin B between LOS and LPS from *E. coli* [13] and the lipid A cores of gram-negative organisms are known to be heterogenous. Furthermore, meningococcus contains surface components and secretes molecules and complex vesicle structures (blebs) that may modulate or deflect the immune system. The bacterium can undergo phase and antigenic variation and is able to use host factors for its own protection and growth [14]. The blebs are shed through the body and contain LOS, and other membrane parts which may also have antigenic properties. Ultracentrifugation studies on plasma specimens from patients with severe meningococcal disease suggest that most of the circulating LOSs are present as large fragments or aggregates [8] which make recognition by the immune system probably more difficult.

Host Factors

Immune response. Developmental aspects of the pediatric immune response are still unknown to a large extent. The majority of the work has been performed in the neonate. Much less is known about the growing child. At birth, a child is protected against a variety of bacterial and viral agents by maternal antibodies and remains less susceptible for many infections until the age of 6 months. Immunoglobulin synthesis of infants increases until at the age of 2 years about 75% of adult values are reached. The IgG and IgA synthesis produced after a certain antigenic stimulus is limited until the age of 2–4 years. Polysaccharide capsule does not give an appropriate immune response and does not induce immunological memory. This is due to an immature T cell function. These problems can be circumvented by covalently linking the polysaccharide antigens to proteins, the principle used in the production of conjugate vaccines [12, 15]. There are many differences between the neonatal polymorphonuclear leukocyte (PMN) and the adult PMN. The response of the neonatal PMN to chemotactic signals initiated by infectious agents is poor. Further disaggregation of PMN and migration to the infected tissues are markedly depressed. Depletion of circulating neutrophils with the exhaustion of the neutrophil storage pool in the bone marrow is more likely to occur because the storage pool is low (14% of the adult pool) and the turnover rate is high [16]. In comparison with adults, there are differences in the cytokine production of mononuclear cells when they are stimulated in vitro [17]. Several studies over the past 5 years have indicated the possible benefit of hematopoietic colony-stimulating factors (CSFs). These cytokines may in fact enhance neonatal myeloid progenitor proliferation, modulate neonatal bone marrow neutrophil storage, proliferate bone marrow neutrophil pools, and enhance neonatal host defense against overwhelming bacterial infection [18]. The characteristics of the PMN of the growing child have not been studied in detail.

Results of studies regarding age-related differences in susceptibility to and mortality of sepsis between infant and adult animals are controversial and probably depend on the experimental model [7, 19], the exact age [20] and the pathogen involved [7].

Metabolic response. Sepsis may lead to pronounced metabolic alterations. Elevations of plasma glucose, lactate, insulin, and free fatty acids concentrations and increased muscle protein breakdown are well known changes during the early phase of sepsis in the adult patient. The differences in metabolic response to sepsis between infants and adults are not completely understood. Muscle protein metabolism data from experimental studies suggest that despite prominent differences in basal protein turnover rates between infant and adult rats the effect of sepsis on muscle protein metabolism is not age-dependent [20, 21]. The glucoregulatory changes in the developing human and animal are different from the adult. In young infants during sepsis, there is an increased glucose disappearance rate without hyperinsulinemia [7, 22, 23]. In an experimental sepsis model in rats studying age-related differences, the adult rats became hyperglycemic, while young animals were hypoglycemic 8 h after cecal ligation but normalized after 16 h [21]. Human infants with severe septic shock often have a hypoglycemia which necessitates correction.

Cardiovascular system. Clinical studies in adults have demonstrated that myocardial dysfunction begins within hours of sepsis and peaks in 1–2 days, with survivors returning to normal function in a 7–10 day period. Hyperdynamic circulatory state in survivors is probably maintained by ventricular dilatation. Again, studies in adults present conflicting results regarding coronary perfusion during sepsis. Similar studies in children are not available. However, there are several experimental studies which have demonstrated the presence of age-related differences between neonatal and adult animals in myocardial reserve (which increases because of an improving diastolic compliance), relation between contractile and noncontractile myocardial elements, metabolic substrates (from carbohydrates to free fatty acids), sensitivity for hypoxemia, maturation of the pulmonary vasculature and sensitivity of sympathic receptors to catecholamines [24–27]. Our group is preparing an experimental septic shock model in young piglets using meningococcal endotoxin to study the differences between young and adult pigs. Only a small number of studies have been published about the myocardial dysfunction during septic shock in children [28–30]. These studies were performed in pediatric patients with meningoccal sepsis. They revealed hypovolemia and severe disturbances in cardiac function as indicated by left ventricular shortening fraction (echocardiography) and cardiac output (thermodilution). Myocardial dysfunction in septic shock in children reaches a maximum within hours and is the main cause of early mortality. Recovery takes 1–3 days. Cardiac output (CO) in infants is classically thought to be more rate- than stroke volume-dependent which is probably the reason for cardiac frequencies of sometimes over 180 beats/min. It is unknown to what extent ventricular dilatation is useful in the maintainance of a possible hyperdynamic state. It is also not known whether there is a hyperdynamic state in infants [30]. CO in infants is very much preload-dependent. Therefore fluid resuscitation is an important step in the initial management of children with septic shock to overcome the hypovolemia on the basis of a diffuse capillary leak [31, 32]. Altered vascular tone and flow-oxygen utilization relationships are considered a hallmark of sepsis in children. An altered vascular tone leads to decreased peripheral vascular resistance. This results in a lowered diastolic aorta pressure. It is this pressure, in combination with the duration of the diastole, which are the two main determinants of coronary perfusion and indeed, coronary ischemia may be seen in children even in the first 24 h after admission.

Coagulation system. Especially in meningococcal sepsis, but also in other forms of pediatric and neonatal sepsis, thrombopenia and dissiminated intravascular coagulation [DIC] can be found leading to petecchiae and ecchymoses. At birth several clottingfactors are present at serum levels much lower than in adults. This possibly explains why the balance is easily switched towards coagulation. During the first 2 years of life these serum levels increase until adult values are reached [33, 34]. In meningococcal sepsis in children, there is an extreme depletion of anticoagulatory factors like proteins C and S [35] as opposed to adults in which a depletion of anti-thrombin III predominates. Protein C has gained interest because of its possible role in sepsis and its protective effect in experimental sepsis [36]. The combination of extreme capillary vasoconstriction, caused by mediators like endothelin, and the increased deposition of fibrin, caused by the hypercoagulatory state and decreased fibrinolysis, will lead to increased formation of microthrombi and in this way to autoinfarction and gangrene.

Therefore an important part of the volume supplementation which is administered in our hospital during the acute phase of sepsis comprises fresh frozen plasma (FFP), which still is the only balanced substitute of clotting factors in this situation. However, there have been no controlled studies to prove the superiority of FFP over other colloids in this situation. On the contrary, recently a study was published in experimental sepsis which indicated the presence of deleterious effects of plasma therapy [37].

Management Aspects

Cardiovascular Function

The abnormal microcirculation and a decreased aortic diastolic pressure cause a compromised coronary perfusion in children with septic shock. Together with possible depressing mediators this will lead to a severely depressed myocardial function with a decreased stroke volume. Here, α- and β-adrenergic support may possibly restore a normal mean arterial pressure and systemic vascular resistance. To inhibit or improve capillary vasoconstriction, a local vasodilatator could be added. Recently Heyderman et al. [38] presented findings suggesting that a deficiency of prostacyclin (PGI_2) may have a role in the pathogenesis of meningococcal shock and that exogenous PGI_2 may be of therapeutic benefit. There is no consensus on which particular inotropic drugs are most useful. Especially in children, the pharmacodynamics of these drugs are still not well known. The combination we use is norepinephrine, dopamine and PGI_2, with the lowest possible α-agonist dose to achieve a mean arterial blood pressure which enables an adequate urine ouput and no further increase in oxygen consumption.

Fluid Resuscitation and Monitoring

The importance of fluid resuscitation to overcome the hypovolemia caused by capillary leak has already been mentioned. Sometimes 100–200 ml/kg of colloids (like FFP) are needed during the first day of treatment. Due to several reasons it is not daily practice to insert pulmonary artery catheters in every patient but central venous pressure monitoring and echocardiography are indicated and frequently used [29, 30, 32, 39]. Lactate and several coagulation parameters are used as a tool to monitor the condition of the patient.

Respiratory Function

More than 60% of critically ill children with septic shock are intubated and ventilated within 24 h after admission. Indications for intubation are hypoxia, apnea, acidosis, increased work of breathing (WOB) and neuromuscular blockade for invasive procedures. About 40% of these patients develop acute respiratory distress syndrome (ARDS). In children with heart failure, WOB can require as much as 25% of oxygen consumption. Extrapolating a similar effect of cardiac dysfunction and increased WOB to ARDS in sepsis leads to the general recommendation to intubate and ventilate in an early stage and not to wait until a disease stage in which intubation becomes a dangerous procedure. Delicate handling of the fluid balance because of increased extravascular lung water is necessary.

Prognostic Factors

Several prognostic factors have been related to nonsurvival:

1. Increased levels of: serum endotoxin [8], tumor necrosis factor, interleukin-1 [40], interleukin-6 [41–44], interleukin-8 [45], lactate [44], plasmino-

gen activator inhibitor-1 [46], intercellular adhesion molecule (ICAM-1) [47], procalcitonin [48], elastase-α_1-proteinase inhibitor [49, 50]
2. Decreased levels of: C-reactive protein [44, 51], fibrinogen, glucose, protein C [35], leukocytes, platelets [52]
3. Several scoring systems also exist [51, 53, 54]

The morbidity of sepsis in pediatric patients depends on the age and the causative pathogen. In the neonate and infant the neurologic sequelae can be more severe especially if meningitis is present. Chronic renal failure after a septic period is rare in children. In particular, in severe meningococcal disease the morbidity is relatively low and is limited to skin lesions and amputations of extremities.

Future Therapy

Prevention is still superior to treatment. Progress has been made in the field of active immunization. In several countries in Europe immunization has been started against *H. influenzae.* It will take at least another 5 years to develop a vaccine against *N. meningitidis* group B. Passive immunization using either pooled plasma or pathogen-specific immunoglobulins has been used in neonates. A limited number of studies have been performed and they suggest a beneficial effect in GBS infections [55]. Administration of neutrophils to infants with significant neutropenia has been suggested as an approach [4]. The European multicenter trial using human monoclonal antibody to the lipid A domain of endotoxin (HA-1A) in pediatric patients with septic shock and purpura is still ongoing. More than 170 patients are included. Until this trial has been concluded, a recommendation for the use of HA-1A in these patients can not be given. Concerning the extensive list of other possible immunomodulative therapies, it is important to realize that on admission of a septic child, the process is in a well advanced stage, so that influencing the momentary endotoxin level only will have a limited influence on outcome. Trials should be directed to influence the microcirculation. Currently, a trial with recombinant protein C is in preparation.

Conclusions

- There is only limited epidemiological and clinical data available on children with septic shock. There is a need for a universal definition for children with sepsis. This definition may be adapted from guidelines proposed for adults.
- Septic shock in neonates and infants is more overwhelming than in adults. The highest mortality is in the first 48 h and does often occur in previously healthy children.

- Specific sepsis-related differences between adults and pediatric patients are probably caused by developmental aspects especially in the cardiovascular and coagulation system, and the immune and metabolic response.
- Pathophysiologic aspects of sepsis, especially in the infant age range, should be the subjects of further research.

References

1. Jafari HS, McCracken GHJ (1992) Sepsis and septic shock: a review for clinicians. Pediatr Infect Dis J 11(9):739–748
2. Bell LM, Baker MD, Beatty D, Taylor L (1992) Infections in severely traumatized children. J Pediatr Surg 27(11):1394–1398
3. Ashkenazi S, Leibovici L, Samra Z, Konisberger H, Drucker M (1992) Risk factors for mortality due to bacteremia and fungemia in childhood. Clin Infect Dis 14(4):949–951
4. Ferrieri P (1990) Neonatal susceptibility and immunity to major bacterial pathogens. Rev Infect Dis 12 [Suppl 4]:S394–S400
5. Zangwill KM, Schuchat A, Wenger JD (1992) Group B streptococcal disease in the United States, 1990: report from a multistate active surveillance system. MMWR CDC Surveill Summ 41(6):25–32
6. Jacobs RF, Sowell MK, Moss MM, Fiser DH (1990) Septic shock in children: bacterial etiologies and temporal relationships. Pediatr Infect Dis J 9(3):196–200
7. Pryor RW, Hinshaw LB (1989) Sepsis/septic shock in adults and children. Pathol Immunopathol Res 8(5–6):222–230
8. Brandtzaeg P, Kierulf P, Gaustad P, Skulberg A, Bruun JN, Halvorsen S, Sorensen E (1989) Plasma endotoxin as a predictor of multiple organ failure and death in systemic meningococcal disease. J Infect Dis 159(2):195–204
9. Bayston K, Cohen J (1990) Bacterial endotoxin and current concepts in the diagnosis and treatment of endotoxaemia. J Med Microbiol 31:73–83
10. Chesney P, Chesney R (1989) Hemorrhagic shock and encephalopathy: reflections about a new devastating disorder that affects normal children. J Pediatr 114(2):254–256
11. Hellerqvist C, Sundell H, Gettins P (1987) Molecular basis for group B beta-hemolytic streptococcal disease. Proc Natl Acad Sci USA 84:51
12. Verheul AF, van Gaans JA, Wiertz EJ, Snippe H, Verhoef J, Poolman JT (1993) Meningococcal lipopolysaccharide (LPS)-derived oligosaccharide-protein conjugates evoke outer membrane protein but not LPS-specific bactericidal antibodies in mice: influence of adjuvants. Infect Immun 61(1):187–196
13. Baldwin G, Alpert G, Caputo GL et al (1991) Effect of polymyxin B on experimental shock from meningococcal and Escherichia coli endotoxins. J Infect Dis 164(3):542–549
14. Verheul A, Snippe H, Poolman J (1993) Meningococcal lipopolysaccharides: virulence factor and potential vaccine component. Microbiol Rev 57(1):34–49
15. Poolman JT (1988) Meningococcal vaccines. J Med Microbiol 26(3):170–172
16. Cairo MS (1989) Neonatal neutrophil host defense. Prospects for immunologic enhancement during neonatal sepsis. Am J Dis Child 143(1):40–46
17. English BK, Burchett SK, English JD, Ammann AJ, Wara DW, Wilson CB (1988) Production of lymphotoxin and tumor necrosis factor by human neonatal mononuclear cells. Pediatr Res 24(6):717–722
18. Cairo M (1991) Cytokines: a new Immunotherapy. Clin Perinatol 18(2):343–359
19. Wei C, Gilliam M, Cohen M, Cornell J, Moazam F (1987) A preliminary study of age-related difference in resistance to sepsis in the rat model. J Surg Res 43:460–467

20. Zamir O, Hasselgren PO, Frederick JA, Fischer JE (1992) Is the metabolic response to sepsis in skeletal muscle different in infants and adults? An experimental study in rats. J Pediatr Surg 27(11):1399–1403
21. Pedersen PV, Warner BW, Bjornson HS et al (1989) Hemodynamic and metabolic alterations during experimental sepsis in young and adult rats. Surg Gynecol Obstet 168(2):148–156
22. Fitzgerald MJ, Goto M, Myers TF, Zeller WP (1992) Early metabolic effects of sepsis in the preterm infant: lactic acidosis and increased glucose requirement. J Pediatr 121(6):951–955
23. Zeller WP, Goto M, Hurley RM (1988) Endotoxin in newborn septic shock: significance, metabolic, and cardiovascular changes. Ann Clin Lab Sci 18(3):253–259
24. Horton JW, Coln D (1985) Cardiovascular function and fluid compartments in newborn canine hemorrhagic shock. Am J Physiol 248 (6, 2):R724–R731
25. Agata Y, Hiraishi S, Oguchi K et al (1991) Changes in left ventricular output from fetal to early neonatal life (see comments). J Pediatr 119(3):441–445
26. Fiser DH, Fewell JE, Hill DE, Brown AL (1988) Cardiovascular and renal effects of dopamine and dobutamine in healthy, conscious piglets. Crit Care Med 16(4):340–345
27. Shavit G, Sagy M, Nadler E, Vidne BA, Gitter S (1989) Myocardial response to alpha-agonist (phenylephrine) in relation to age. Crit Care Med 17(12):1324–1327
28. Monsalve F, Rucabado L, Salvador A, Bonastre J, Cuñat J, Ruano M (1984) Myocardial depression in septic shock caused by meningococcal infection. Crit Care Med 12(12):1021–1023
29. Boucek MM, Boerth RC, Artman M, Graham TP, Boucek RJ (1984) Myocardial dysfunction in children with acute meningococcemia. J Pediatr 105:538–542
30. Mercier J-C, Beaufils F, Hartmann J-F, Azéma D (1988) Hemodynamic patterns of meningococcal shock in children. Crit Care Med 16(1):27–33
31. Carcillo JA, Davis AL, Zaritsky A (1991) Role of early fluid resuscitation in pediatric septic shock. JAMA 266(9):1242–1245
32. Carcillo JA, Pollack MM, Ruttimann UE, Fields AI (1989) Sequential physiologic interactions in pediatric cardiogenic and septic shock. Crit Care Med 17(1):12–16
33. van Teunenbroek A, Peters M, Sturk A, Borm JJ, Breederveld C (1990) Protein C activity and antigen levels in childhood. Eur J Pediatr 149(11):774–778
34. Andrew M, Paes B, Milner R, Johnston M, Mitchell L, Tollefsen DM, Powers P (1987) Development of the human coagulation system in the full-term infant. Blood 70(1):165–172
35. Leclerc F, Hazelzet J, Jude B, Hofhuis W, Hue V, Martinot A, van der Voort E (1992) Protein C and S deficiency in severe infectious purpura of children: a collaborative study of 40 cases. Intensive Care Med 18(4):202–205
36. Taylor FBJ, Chang A, Esmon CT, D'Angelo A, Vigano-D'Angelo S, Blick KE (1987) Protein C prevents the coagulopathic and lethal effects of Escherichia coli infusion in the baboon. J Clin Invest 79(3):918–925
37. Busund R, Lindsetmo R, Balteskard L, Rekvig O, Revhaug A (1993) Repeated plasma therapy induces fatal shock in experimental septicemia. Circ Shock 40:268–275
38. Heyderman RS, Klein NJ, Shennan GI, Levin M (1991) Deficiency of prostacyclin production in meningococcal shock. Arch Dis Child 66(11):1296–1299
39. Gill AB, Weindling AM (1993) Echocardiographic assessment of cardiac function in shocked very low birthweight infants. Arch Dis Child 68 [Suppl 1]:17–21
40. Waage A, Halstensen A, Shalaby R, Brandtzaeg P, Kierulf P, Espevik T (1989) Local production of tumor necrosis factor alpha, interleukin 1, and interleukin 6 in meningococcal meningitis. Relation to the inflammatory response. J Exp Med 170(6):1859–1867
41. Waage A, Brandtzaeg P, Halstensen A, Kierulf P, Espevik T (1989) The complex pattern of cytokines in serum from patients with meningococcal septic shock. Association between interleukin 6, interleukin 1, and fatal outcome. J Exp Med 169(1):333–338

42. Saladino R, Erikson M, Levy N, Bachman D, Silber GR, Fleisher GR (1992) Utility of serum interleukin-6 for diagnosis of invasive bacterial disease in children. Ann Emerg Med 21(12):1413–1417
43. Sullivan JS, Kilpatrick L, Costarino ATJ, Lee SC, Harris MC (1992) Correlation of plasma cytokine elevations with mortality rate in children with sepsis. J Pediatr 120 (4, 1):510–515
44. Hazelzet JA, van den Voort E, Lindemans J, ter Heerdt PGJ, Neyens HJ (1993) Relation between cytokines and routine laboratory parameters in children with septic shock and purpurae. Intensive Care Med (in press)
45. Halstensen A, Ceska M, Brandtzaeg P, Redl H, Naess A, Waage A (1993) Interleukin-8 in serum and cerebrospinal fluid from patients with meningococcal disease. J Infect Dis 167(2):471–475
46. Brandtzaeg P, Joo GB, Brusletto B, Kierulf P (1990) Plasminogen activator inhibitor 1 and 2, alpha-2-antiplasmin, plasminogen, and endotoxin levels in systemic meningococcal disease. Thromb Res 57(2):271–278
47. Kuster H, Degitz K (1993) Circulating ICAM-1 in neonatal sepsis (letter). Lancet 341(8843):506
48. Assicot M, Gendrel D, Carsin H, Raymond J, Guilbaud J, Bohuon C (1993) High serum procalcitonin concentrations in patients with sepsis and infection. Lancet 341(8844):515–518
49. Speer CP, Rethwilm N, Gahr M (1987) Elastase-α1-proteinase inhibitor: an early indicator of septicaemia and bacterial meningitis in children. J Pediatr 111:667–671
50. Tegtmeyer FK, Horn C, Richter A, van Wees J (1992) Elastase alpha 1 proteinase inhibitor complex, granulocyte count, ratio of immature to total granulocyte count, and C-reactive protein in neonatal septicaemia. Eur J Pediatr 151(5):353–356
51. Leclerc F, Chenaud M, Delepoulle F, Francois DJ, Alain M, Valerie H (1991) Prognostic value of C-reactive protein level in severe infectious purpura: a comparison with eight other scores. Crit Care Med 19(3):430–432
52. Housinger TA, Brinkerhoff C, Warden GD (1993) The relationship between platelet count, sepsis, and survival in pediatric burn patients. Arch Surg 128(1):65–66
53. Pollack M, Ruttimann U, Getson P (1988) Pediatric risk of mortality (PRISM) score. Crit Care Med 16:1110–1116
54. Leclerc F, Beuscart R, Guillois B et al (1985) Prognostic factors of severe infectious purpura in children. Intensive Care Med 11(3):140–143
55. Fischer GW (1988) Immunoglobulin therapy of neonatal group B streptococcal infections: an overview. Pediatr Infect Dis J 7 [Suppl 5]:S13–S16

Definitions and Therapy of Sepsis

R. C. Bone

The syndrome of multiple systems organ failure (MSOF) is defined as the presence of two or more organ systems with impaired function. MSOF is characterized by a hyperdynamic, hypermetabolic state identical to that seen in the septic syndrome. The mortality rate associated with MSOF exceeds 60% and the emergence of MSOF and the septic syndrome as important clinical entities is related to improvements in the technology of life support systems.

Sepsis

While many advances have occurred recently in our understanding of the pathogenetic mechanisms and treatment of septic shock, our ability to rescue a patient from it has unfortunately lagged behind. Its definition is simply the deranged metabolic state that arises from systemic sepsis in a hypotensive patient unresponsive to fluid management. Septic shock may be precipitated by a variety of organisms. Invasion into the bloodstream by bacteria or their toxic metabolites triggers various pathophysiologic sequelae that eventually lead to hypotension and MSOF.

Gram-negative sepsis is now a major concern in immunosuppressed patients. Each year in the United States there are an estimated 300000–500000 cases of gram-negative sepsis, with mortality rates ranging from 20% to 75%. Given that sepsis is more often considered a complication of disease rather than the lethal end point of a serious underlying disease, these mortality figures may be underestimated. The literature on gram-negative sepsis is limited to case reports from the preantibiotic era. Today, gram-negative sepsis accounts for 1% of all university hospital admissions.

Septic shock should not be viewed as a single entity, since a vast array of organisms presenting in a variety of fashions may culminate in moribund patients (Table 1). Vasomotor collapse can result from decreased intravascular volume (as in patients with cholera). Organisms (e.g., meningococcemia, Rocky Mountain spotted fever, viral myocarditis) may invade the myocardium and lead to hypotension. The myriad of organisms that cause endocarditis may cause shock from progressive destruction of endovalvular structures.

Table 1. Mechanisms of shock in sepsis

– Decreased intravascular volume (e.g., cholera, toxic shock syndrome, dengue)
– Myocardial depression
– Myocardial cell invasion or pump failure (e.g., meningococcemia, viral myocarditis, diphtheria)
– Endovalvular destruction (e.g., endocarditis)
– Decreased venous return to heart (e.g., gram-negative sepsis)

Probably the most intensely studied form of shock – and one of increasing importance – is that of gram-negative sepsis. Shock with this form of sepsis is linked to activation of several inherent metabolic pathways, which will be discussed later.

Perhaps the single most important determinant of outcome in patients with septic shock is severity of underlying disease. Patients with malignancies or cirrhosis, asplenics, and those of advanced age or with multiple diseases (diabetes, renal failure, heart disease, etc.), or patients treated with immunosuppressive agents are at greatest risk of dying from septic shock. The source of infection and virulence of the organism have significant effects on patient outcome. Nosocomial infections and sepsis due to gram-negative bacilli are associated with higher mortality rates than community-acquired infections and gram-positive infections.

In the summer of 1991, a consensus conference jointly sponsored by the American College of Chest Physicians and the Society of Critical Care Medicine was held to develop a set of definitions of sepsis and related terms that could be used by both clinicians and investigators. The results of that conference were published in the June, 1992 issue of both *Chest* and *Critical Care Medicine* [1]. It is hoped that a more universally accepted set of definitions will aid research into the pathophysiologic mechanisms of sepsis and the methods and agents for intervening in that process, thereby improving patient outcomes (Table 2).

Clinical Aspects

The clinical presentation of a patient in septic shock may evolve over days or may take an explosive course (as in meningococcemia), killing the patient in a matter of hours. One of the keys to successful therapy, therefore, is to recognize septic shock as quickly as possible. The earliest changes may occur in the patient's vital signs or mental status. The presence of fever or hypothermia, tachycardia, hyperventilation or a change in mental status (none of which are specific for septic shock) should prompt acquisition of several blood cultures and possible initiation of therapy. Early in its course, blood pressure may be normal or slightly reduced, and perfusion to the extremities

Table 2. Definitions

Infection
Microbial phenomenon characterized by an inflammatory response to the presence of microorganisms or the invasion of normally sterile host tissue by those organisms.

Bacteremia
The presence of viable bacteria in the blood.

Systemic inflammatory response syndrome (SIRS)
The systemic inflammatory response to a variety of insults is manifested by two or more of the following conditions:
Temperature >38°C or <36°C
Heart rate >90 beats per minute
Respiratory rate >20 breaths per minute or $PaCO_2$<32 mm Hg
White blood cell count >12000 cells/ml^3, <4000 cells/ml^3, or >10% immature (band) forms

Sepsis
The systemic response to infection is manifested by two or more of the following conditions:
Temperature >38°C or <36°C
Heart rate >90 beats per minute
Respiratory rate >20 breaths per minute or $PaCO_2$<32 mm Hg
White blood cell count >12000 cells/ml^3, <4000 cells/ml^3, or >10% immature (band) forms

Severe sepsis
Sepsis associated with organ dysfunction, hypoperfusion, or hypotension. Hypoperfusion and perfusion abnormalities may include, but are not limited to lactic acidosis, oliguria, or an acute alteration in mental status.

Septic shock
Sepsis with hypotension, despite adequate fluid resuscitation, in conjunction with the presence of perfusion abnormalities, which may include, but are not limited to lactic acidosis, oliguria, or an acute alteration in mental status. Patients who are on inotropic or vasopressor agents may not be hypotensive at the time that perfusion abnormalities are measured.

Hypotension
A systolic blood pressure <90 mm Hg or a reduction of >40 mm Hg from baseline in the absence of other causes for hypotension.

Multiple organ dysfunction syndrome (MODS)
Presence of altered organ function in an acutely ill patient such that homeostasis can not be maintained without intervention.

is usually adequate; as septic shock progresses, hypotension results, and as perfusion to the extremities drops, the skin becomes mottled, cyanotic, and cold. The skin in occasional patients may show classic changes as the ecthyma gangrenosum lesion of bacteremia with *Pseudomonas aeruginosa,* and sometimes, *Aeromonas hydrophila.* Bullae and desquamation of the palms and soles may suggest toxic shock syndrome in menstruating women or post-surgical patients. Petechiae occur with several types of bacteremia; however, with gram-negative bacilli they are less common. They may accompany pneumococcal sepsis in asplenic patients. Meningococcemia may present rather dramatically, with diffuse petechial, purpuric, and ecchymotic lesions. Petechiae should also alert clinicians to the possibility of disseminated intravascular coagulation (DIC). If the coagulation cascade is activated (as with gram-negative bacteremia), DIC may result. DIC is characterized by thrombocytopenia, coagulation factor consumption, fibrin split products, decreased fibrinogen levels, and often, significant hemorrhaging (most frequently in the gastrointestinal tract, lungs, and skin). DIC is viewed by many to be an incidental preterminal event. Janeway lesions, Osler nodes, splinter hemorrhages, palatal and conjunctival petechiae would, of course, suggest endocarditis, but these are seen in only a minority of cases (Table 3).

With the wide availability of Swan-Ganz monitoring, the cardiovascular changes of septic shock have been well-documented. Traditionally, these changes have been characterized by a spectrum, beginning with decreased systemic vascular resistance and increased cardiac output (warm shock), then progressing to decreased cardiac output and increased systemic vascular resistance (cold shock). Even though patients are best managed with hemodynamic monitoring, a reasonable assessment of tissue perfusion can be made quickly by feeling the temperature of the extremities and looking for mottling, cyanosis, etc. Lactic acid levels have been followed in septic patients. High levels are associated with hypoperfusion and ineffective aerobic glycolysis; decreasing levels correlate with improvement of the septic state.

Pulmonary manifestations of septic shock may include dyspnea, tachypnea, and diffuse rales. Early on, arterial blood gases usually show respiratory alkalosis, with or without hypoxemia. This proceeds to respiratory and metabolic acidosis as the patient further decompensates. Shunt physiology is present when 100% FIO_2 fails to correct the hypoxemia. Chest X-rays may show diffuse pulmonary infiltrates. A diagnosis of adult respiratory distress syndrome (ARDS) – or noncardiogenic pulmonary edema – can be made if these factors are present in conjunction with a normal wedge pressure. Some series document ARDS in 20% of patients in septic shock.

Acute tubular necrosis and oliguric renal failure may develop in patients with septic shock. Optimal fluid management to simultaneously maintain renal perfusion and avoid congestive heart failure further argues for invasive hemodynamic monitoring. The liver may acutely show striking elevations in transaminase levels if significant hypotension is present. SGOT and SGPT

Table 3. Clinical manifestations of septic shock

- Vital signs: hypotension, tachycardia, tachypnea, hypo or hyperthermia, chills
- Skin: petechiae, ecthyma gangrenosum, bullae, ecchymoses, purpurae, mottling, cyanosis
- Coagulation abnormalities: bleeding, DIC
- Hematologic: granulocytosis with left shift, thrombocytopenia, leukopenia
- Multiorgan failure: lung, liver, kidney, heart

usually fall as quickly as they rise if blood pressure is restored and the patient survives. Elevated bilirubin levels should alert physicians to bacteremia with *Bacteroides* species or hemolysis as occurs with *Clostridial* infections or DIC.

Therapy

One way of organizing a treatment strategy is to divide various modalities into the following groups:

1) *Essential,* including antibiotics, fluids, oxygen, and cardiotropic agents;
2) *Controversial,* including heparin, opiate antagonists, steroids, and cyclooxygenase inhibitors; and
3) *Future,* including monoclonal antibodies and passive immunizations for bacterial antigens and toxins, which may, some day, come into clinical usage.

Essential Therapy

Treatment of patients with septic shock should be started immediately. Several studies have shown the mortality rate of bacteremia can be reduced with appropriate use of antibiotics. They should be begun empirically and in maximum doses *before* culture results are available. Antibiotic coverage should include gram-positive and gram-negative organisms, as well as those suggested by the clinical situation. These might include anaerobes if a pelvic or gastrointestinal source of infection is suspected. Metronidazole and clindamycin are drugs that would be added to cover for anaerobic bacteria. *Pseudomonas aeruginosa* in cancer patients or those with ecthyma gangrenosum skin lesions, *Streptococcus pneumoniae* in asplenics, or *Staphylococcus aureus* pneumonia complicating influenza epidemics, for example, would necessitate utilization of antibiotics to cover these organisms. Combination therapy with a third-generation cephalosporin or anti-pseudomonal β-lactam and an aminoglycoside has theoretical advantages of increased spectrum, more rapid killing, prevention of resistance, and synergy. These concepts, however, have not been proven in clinical studies, and except for *Pseudomonas* infections in immunocompromised hosts, have not been universally accepted. Newer antibiotics with broad spectra of activity (including against *Pseudomonas aeruginosa*) are ceftazadime and imipenim-cilastatin. If blood cultures become positive, therapy can be adjusted to include antibiotics with lower toxicity and narrower spectra. Narrowing the spectrum of coverage is important, since prolonged use of broad-spectrum agents is more often associated with superinfections, bleeding, pseudomembranous colitis, etc. In immunosuppressed patients, vancomycin is sometimes used empirically to cover coagulase-negative staphylococci and *Corynebacterium JK* bacilli; both of these skin organisms may become invasive in the presence of intravenous lines and Hickman catheters.

The hypotension of sepsis should first be corrected with volume. We prefer crystalloid (0.9 normal saline or Ringer lactate) to colloid because crystalloids are less expensive, do not activate the kallikrein-kinin system, and do not cause bleeding. The proper amount of IV crystalloid to administer is best judged with the clinical response or with Swan-Ganz monitoring. In patients with underlying heart disease, right heart filling pressures should be kept at levels that maximize cardiac output. Pulmonary capillary wedge pressures should be kept below 18 mm Hg (in the absence of obvious heart disease). Studies are under way to evaluate the efficacy of hypertonic albuminated fluids.

As septic shock progresses, volume administration becomes inadequate to maintain normal blood pressure, and cardiotropic agents are needed. Dopamine is probably the drug of choice, since at low infusion rates (2–3 μg/kg per minute) it increases renal, mesenteric, cerebral, and coronary flow. At higher levels (20–50 μg/kg per minute), greater α-adrenergic vasoconstrictive action is seen. Dobutamine enhances cardiac output, decreases systemic vascular resistance (with little change in heart rate), and may be used synergistically with dopamine in some cases. α-Adrenergic agents (such as phenylephrine and methoxamine) are not usually dependable in septic shock, since tissue perfusion is not elevated (especially in acidosis) and tissues are unresponsive to these sympathomimetic amines.

Vasodilators like nitroprusside may be indicated in the setting of congestive heart failure and high systemic vascular resistance. Digitalis has not proven useful in septic shock, with the possible exception of meningococcemia sepsis. In some refractory cases, intraaortic balloon pump counterpulsations may be necessary until other measures control the septic state.

The last two therapies in the essential group include oxygen in hypoxemic patients and bicarbonate in acidotic patients. Arterial blood gas levels should be obtained serially and hypoxemia corrected, with increasing concentrations of inspired oxygen (FIO_2) and positive end-expiratory pressure (PEEP), if necessary. Caution with both of these modalities must be taken; prolonged use of O_2 at high concentrations ($>50\%$ over several days) can lead to irreversible pulmonary fibrosis, and PEEP can decrease cardiac output. With increasing PEEP (>20 cm H_2O), the risk of pneumothorax increases. The PaO_2/FIO_2 ratio and its response to therapy can be used as an index of survival (Fig. 1).

Controversial Therapy

Controversial therapies of septic shock include the use of heparin, opiate antagonists, steroids, and cyclooxygenase inhibitors. In order to discuss each of these properly, a knowledge of drug actions on the underlying pathophysiologic mechanisms and metabolic pathways activated in septic shock is

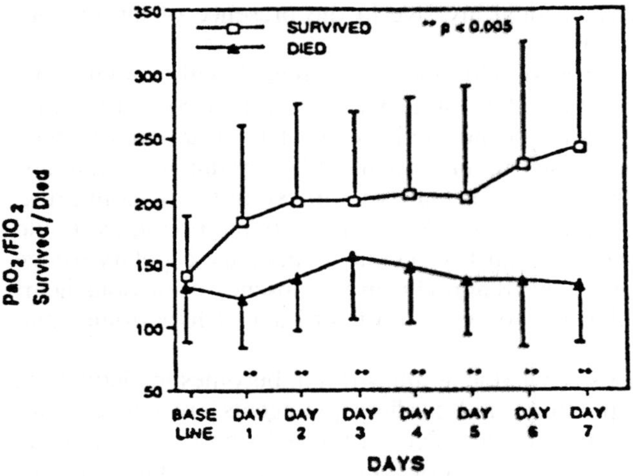

Fig. 1. PaO_2/FIO_2 ratio and survival in acute respiratory failure

necessary. Most of the studies to date have dealt with shock associated with experimental gram-negative rod bacteremia for several reasons. The incidence of shock in patients with gram-negative bacteremia is much greater than with gram-positive organisms. Shock seems to be a more integral part of gram-negative sepsis, not only because of its frequency, but its timing as well – occurring much earlier (within 4–10 h). Experimental infusion of minute amounts of endotoxin released from gram-negative bacteria have reproduced the clinical manifestations and metabolic changes of septic shock. There are many problems correlating these studies with clinical septic shock, but the mechanism of their deleterious effect in animals provides hope for future therapies in controlled human trials.

Endotoxin (lipopolysaccharide) is thought to be an initiating factor in gram-negative septic shock. After entry into the bloodstream, endotoxin ac-

Table 4. Proposed mediators in septic shock

- Complement components C_3A, C_5A
- Coagulation factors
- Kinins
- Endorphins
- Histamine
- Prostaglandins
- Lysosomal enzymes
- Macrophage products (interleukins, monokines)
- Catecholamines, acetylcholine
- Glucocorticoids

tivates several proposed mediators, which are, in turn, responsible for the pathophysiologic changes observed (Table 4).

Both endotoxin and intact gram-negative bacilli are capable of activating the complement system, through both the classical and alternate (properdin) pathways. The latter pathway is thought to be a first-line of defense and does not require antibody to initiate the complement cascade. This may account for some of the early clinical differences between gram-positive and gram-negative sepsis. Two vasodilatory anaphylotoxins, C_3A and C_5A, are released after activation of the complement cascade. C_3A induces histamine release (mast cell degranulation); resulting vasodilation constitutes the first wave of inflammation. C_5A and the terminal (C_3–C_9) complex activate polymorphonuclear cells (PMNs). Arachidonic acid products, lysosomal enzymes, and oxygen radicals released from these PMNs create a capillary leak syndrome and thus comprise the second wave of inflammation.

Endotoxin also initiates the coagulation system through its affects on Hageman factor. If the compensatory fibrinolytic mechanisms fail, a state of DIC – with coagulation factor consumption, bleeding, and ischemia – may ensue. The kallikrein-kinin system is also activated by Hageman factor, causing production of the very potent vasodilator bradykinin. One of the major inhibitors of Hageman factor is antithrombin III, whose activity is enhanced by heparin.

Lastly, the vasodilatory properties of endotoxin may be due to activation of phagocytic cells that produce various compounds (e.g., leukocyte endogenous mediator, endogenous pyrogen, lymphocyte activating factor). These substances, in turn, induce endorphin release from the pituitary gland, reset the hypothalamic thermostat, suppress granulopoiesis and neutrophil release, and set in motion a variety of metabolic activities in the liver, pancreas, and muscle.

The controversial therapeutic modalities used in septic shock are known to act on the above-mentioned pathways. It was hoped that heparin could be used to inhibit coagulation factor consumption and activation of the kallikrein-kinin system, but the efficacy of heparin in accomplishing these effects has never been proven. There is a definite risk of bleeding with heparin use, so we very rarely advocate its use for septic shock other than to use it in low doses to prevent pulmonary emboli.

Naloxone, an opiate antagonist, has been used in septic shock because animal models suggest that the hypotension of endotoxin shock is at least partly mediated by endogenous opiates (endorphins). Naloxone increases mean systolic blood pressure in laboratory animals in shock, but has no effect on normal controls. Several prospective, randomized, double-blinded studies in humans, however, have failed to demonstrate any significant effect on blood pressure or clinical outcome. However, in these studies, no dose-response curve was generated to define an efficacious dose. Thyroid-releasing hormone has similar actions on hypotensive laboratory animals as naloxone, but it does not reverse analgesia – which has some theoretical advantages in the treatment of patients. Steroids may also block endorphin release because of their inhibition of ACTH (a relative of β-lipotropin).

A spin-off of complement activation is C_5A, which is chemotactic for PMNs. These cells, in the presence of C_5A, become more adhesive. Aggregation and degranulation then occur. Release of toxic metabolites (oxygen radicals, neutral proteases, and arachidonic acid metabolites) leads to tissue injury and greater influx of PMNs. Prostaglandins produced in endothelial cells may also account for some of the tissue damage. It seems that the host must pay the price of a small amount of tissue damage from normal inflammatory processes in order to control microbial invasion. Steroids have been used in septic shock in attempts to control the host response to the inciting stimulus. In high concentrations steroids are believed to: (1) block binding of chemotactic substances to PMNs; (2) blunt the effects of activated complement on PMNs; (3) inhibit lysosomal degranulation; and (4) block phospholipase A_2.

High dose steroids have been shown to reduce mortality from lethal doses of endotoxin in some experimental animal models. In other animals, however, the LD_{50} of infused organisms is lowered by steroid administration. The results of several human studies are equally contradictory. The results of two recent multicenter, prospective, randomized trials did not show decreased mortality rate in "steroid" groups.

Leukotriene infusion produces a shock-like scenario when given to experimental animals. Antiprostaglandin therapy has had success in reducing the mortality of experimental septic shock in various animal models. Aspirin and nonsteroidal agents improve survival in dogs given otherwise lethal doses of endotoxin or gram-negative bacteria. Many studies suggest that thromboxane A_2 (TxA_2) is responsible for the pulmonary hypertension, capillary leakage, and leukocyte activation seen in the lungs of humans with ARDS. Prostacyclin (PGI_2), a membrane stabilizer and inhibitor of platelet aggregation, appears to counteract the activities of thromboxane products. The balance between PGI_2 and TxA_2 may therefore be important in determining the degree of lung injury in septic shock. Infusion of PGI_2 30 min after endotoxin administration increases survival in experimental animals. Thromboxane synthetase and cyclooxygenase inhibitors (nonsteroidal anti-inflammatory drugs) have the same effect. Studies are now under way to evaluate various prostaglandin inhibitors and their ability to halt the metabolic pathways triggered by sepsis in experimental animals.

Future Therapy

In the future, therapies for septic shock will most likely include forms of passive immunization (e.g., human antisera, monoclonal antibodies to common bacterial antigens). Several researchers are studying antisera to endotoxin. In general, bacterial lipopolysaccharides are composed of oligosaccharide side chains, core polysaccharide, and lipid A. Development of antiserum to the

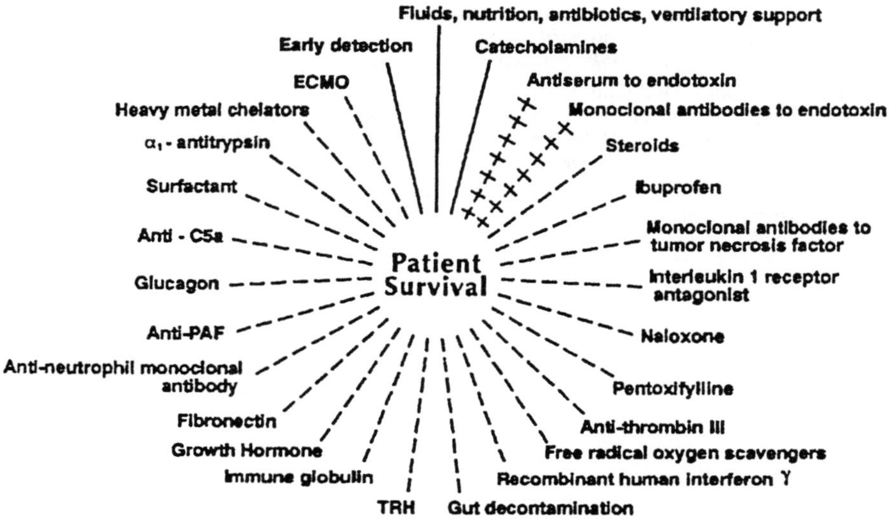

Fig. 2. Conventional and proposed treatment of septic shock and multiorgan failure. Conventional therapies are represented by *solid lines. Dashed lines* indicate agents currently subjected to animal studies or clinical trials

side chains would be difficult because of variation from strain to strain. The core polysaccharide-lipid A complex, however, is much more uniform amongst species of *Enterobacteriaceae.*

Antiserum to a mutant strain of *E. Coli* (the core moiety is exposed for greater immunogeneity) has been shown to reduce mortality in a randomized, controlled study of more than 200 gram-negative bacteremic patients. This approach is appealing, in that the effects of endotoxin are neutralized quickly and the harmful inflammatory reactions are avoided. Monoclonal antibody therapy may, one day, prove to be a cost-effective and efficacious manner of treating septic shock.

Therapies currently under investigation are illustrated in Fig. 2.

References

1. Bone RC, Balk RA, Cerra FB et al (1992) American College of Chest Physicians/Society of Critical Care Medicine Consensus Conference: definitions for sepsis and organ failure and guidelines for the use of innovative therapies in sepsis. Crit Care Med 20:864–874
2. Bone RC, Fisher CJ Jr, Clemmer TP, Slotman GJ, Metz CA, Balk RA (1987) A controlled clinical trial of high-dose methylprednisolone in the treatment of severe sepsis and septic shock. N Engl J Med 317(11):653–658
3. Goris RJ, Nuytinck HK, Redl H (1987) Scoring systems and predictors of ARDS and MOF. Prog Clin Biol Res 236B:3–15

4. Jacobs ER, Bone RC (1983) Sepsis. In: Bone RC (ed) Pulmonary disease reviews, vol IV. Wiley, New York, pp 99–117
5. Jacobs ER, Bone RC (1986) Clinical indicators in sepsis and septic adult respiratory distress syndrome. Med Clin North Am 70(4):921–932
6. Schuster HP (1987) Multisystem organ failure. Prog Clin Biol Res 236A:459–462
7. Schwartz DB, Bone RC, Balk RA, Szidon JP (1989) Hepatic dysfunction in the adult respiratory distress syndrome. Chest 95(4):871–875
8. Tracey KJ, Lowry SM, Cerami A (1988) Cachetin/TNF-alpha in septic shock and septic adult respiratory distress syndrome. Am Rev Respir Dis 138(6):1377–1379

Role of Surgical Intervention in the Prevention and Therapy of Sepsis

W. Teichmann, B. Herbig and M. Weidner

Sepsis Caused by Intraabdominal Infections

Due to almost two square meters of surface, peritoneal inflammation caused by intraabdominal septic foci quickly leads to involvement of the entire organism within the disease process. If the significant peritoneal host defense mechanisms fail, its enormous surface turns into a threatening opponent. Assimilation of several liters of fluid leads to decreased intravascular volume and hypovolemic shock. Increased intraabdominal pressure, through peritoneal edema, produces compression of the lower lung. Both mechanisms lead to hypoxia and thereby insufficient tissue perfusion. In connection with cellular and humoral reactions permeability of the bowel wall increases resulting in penetration of bacteria and endotoxins into the bloodstream with consecutive failure of multiple organ systems. Thus, the disease process is not limited to its origin, rather, it spreads to become a disorder of the entire organism, i.e., a sepsis syndrome.

Prevention of Intraabdominal Infections from the Operative Standpoint

The majority of intraabdominal infections are caused by spontaneous perforations of the gastrointestinal tract and by postoperative complications such as disruption of a surgical anastomosis.

Furthermore, with increasing numbers of major and risky abdominal operations, especially in the older age group, there is a need to counter septic complications by effective prevention.

The clinical assessment of coexisting risk factors when deciding on an elective abdominal operation plays an important role in the success of the surgery. In addition to patient age, magnitude of the intended surgery and cardiac and respiratory insufficiencies, metabolic disorders like diabetes, liver cirrhosis or tumor cachexia are to be considered. If necessary efforts to improve the patients initial situation can still be made.

For elective surgery of the gastrointestinal tract preoperative orthograde bowel lavage has been established to reduce bacteria. The question whether selective bowel decontamination is useful has not been answered so far.

In acute abdominal illness an immediate decision for surgical treatment is crucial for limitation of the intraabdominal infection. If preoperative orthograde bowel lavage is not indicated (stenosis, ileus situation, perforation), intraoperative bowel lavage should be performed even in an emergency setting.

A crucial part in preventing complications is a skillful and atraumatic operative technique, including intraoperative control of intestinal anastomosis sites for insufficiencies. Prophylactic antibiotics, given as a single dose, are almost regarded as a standard today. Antibiotics added to lavage fluid at the end of an operation should be avoided as the rate of resorption cannot be calculated. Under these conditions, the questionable effectiveness and risk of developing resistance should be considered.

In the postoperative period, suspicion of a septic complication justifies early reintervention. As commonly known, obtaining pertinent laboratory data trails behind spreading of the infectious process and undue delay may lead to fatal outcome. Therefore, clinical experience and the decision of the surgeon for reoperation remain vital.

Surgical Concepts in Treatment of Intraabdominal Infections

An improved pathophysiological understanding of the disease process of intraabdominal infections and advances in intensive care medicine (mechanical ventilation, alimentation, hemofiltration) have led to the development of new surgical treatment concepts within the past one and a half decades. More aggressive surgical treatment of septic foci has been made possible. Besides important prognostic criteria, such as localization and characterization of the infectious source and duration of the infection, it has been acknowledged that the quality of surgical performance is vital for the outcome of intraabdominal infections.

Most cases of peritonitis may be treated successfully following the concept, laid down by Martin Kirschner in 1926, referred to as the standard form of treatment. Standard therapy includes sufficient removal of septic foci and intraoperative lavage with debridement of necrotic tissue prior to definite closure of the abdomen (with or without local drainage). In postoperative peritonitis though mortality rates of up to 60% have been reported [1].

In the general surgical setting approximately 10%–15% of intraabdominal infections may only be controlled by more aggressive surgical treatment forms. This is based on the perception that in cases of diffuse peritonitis the abdominal cavity cannot be drained locally and the infectious process cannot be controlled by a single operation.

The following concepts of treatment currently compete for dealing with the severe forms of peritonitis:

- Closed, continuous, postoperative peritoneal lavage
- Open package

- Open, continuous, dorsoventral peritoneal lavage
- Programmed peritoneal lavage (staged four quadrant lavage)

Closed, Continuous, Postoperative Peritoneal Lavage

After conclusion of the primary surgical procedure four to six *Tenkhof* style catheters are placed within the abdominal cavity (subphrenically, subhepatically, paracolic and in the pouch of Douglas). Different types of rinsing solutions have been tested as a continuous lavage, usually runing for 2–7 days. Return of clear lavage fluid and negative endotoxin determinations (if available) are used as indicators for discontinuing therapy. In spite of good experiences, mainly described by Beger et al. [2] and Berger et al. [3], in cases of diffuse peritonitis this method has not proven itself to be profitable in clinical practice.

A reduced rate of relaparotomy, less aggressive therapeutic concept and possibly more cost effectiveness have been proclaimed as advantages of this procedure. However, the severe disadvantages include: absorption of fluid by peritoneal defects, loss of electrolytes and protein and dilution of host defense factors. If not administered correctly closed, continuous, postoperative peritoneal lavage may easily lead to catheter blockade and formation of lavage streaks along the catheters. The drainages themselves can cause specific problems such as erosions. High intraabdominal pressure diminishes respiratory function. By the time relaparotomy is considered inevitable it is generally too late, since the appearance of clinical symptoms trails far behind the spreading of the infectious process.

Open Package

The high mortality rates in diffuse peritonitis have led to the development of diverse concepts. In contrast to continuous lavage of the closed abdominal cavity the open package concept follows the rule of thumb in septic surgery: keeping the infected wound open after removal of the septic focus. This idea had already been suggested by Miculicz at the turn of the century, only failing because of the technical deficiencies of that time. Hay et al. [4] and Hollender et al. [5] were the first to apply the laparostoma in the treatment of diffuse peritonitis. In the 1970s this concept was favored by surgeons in France and the United States. Mortality rates were between 30% and 60%, largely influenced by a negative selection.

The purpose of the open package is broad drainage of the entire abdominal cavity and removal of remaining abscesses or secretions. The abdomen remains wide open with only temporary coverage.

Advantages are good evacuation of peritoneal pus, early recognition of arising complications and reduced intraabdominal pressure, improving ventilation. Disadvantages are a significant loss of electrolytes and protein (comparable to that of burn patients), frequent formation of small bowel fistula (15%–30%) and the inevitable need for major reconstructive surgery of the abdominal wall.

Open, Continuous, Dorsoventral Peritoneal Lavage

The open dorsoventral lavage was developed as a combination of open package and continuous lavage in order to take advantage of both concepts. In 1978 Neidhard and Rousson [6] published their results on continuous dorsoventral lavage, using a Marlex mesh for coverage. A similar approach was made by Pichlmayr et al. [7], placing large-bore drainage tubes dorsally and smaller drainages ventrally for recovery of lavage fluid. The abdomen is then covered by silastic drains. In the meantime this procedure has been expanded by combining it with the concept of programmed peritoneal lavage. Coverage of the abdomen is now achieved by adhesive operating drapes.

Taking only the most severe forms of peritonitis into account, Pichlmayr et al. reported a mortality rate of about 40% in 1985. The addition of programmed daily reexploration lowered mortality rates in his patients to 30% [7].

Programmed Peritoneal Lavage (Staged Four Quadrant Lavage)

The term already implies the basic idea that in diffuse peritonitis the infectious problem cannot be solved by a single operation rather than stepwise, that is, in stages [8–10].

Elimination of septic foci continues to be the most important part of surgical intervention. Given the often critical general condition of the patient, there is no need to pressurize such procedures in the very beginning of programmed peritoneal lavage. Initially the abdominal cavity of patients suffering from multiple system organ failure can be treated as an open wound and laid out with saline gauzes. After stabilization of the patients condition with mechanical ventilation and hemofiltration, a definite surgical therapy of septic foci is performed, offering much better general conditions.

For the semiopen technique of programmed peritoneal lavage a temporary wound closure is necessary. To achieve this a special sliding tab (Ethizip), consisting of polyester covered with polyethylene, was developed. Advantages are convenient attachment to the peritoneum and fascial layers by uninterrupted sutures and individual adjustment to wound size. At first it can be applied generously allowing for lower intraabdominal pressure. As peritoneal edema decreases it is reattached in a tighter fashion every 2–3 days. Thereby a step by step readaptation of the commonly deviating wound edges is achieved. It is the base for final closure of the fascial layers even after prolonged therapy. This is a particular advantage of the Ethizip closure over other forms of temporary wound closure.

Initially reoperations are performed on a day to day basis. Thus direct control of the intraabdominal situation is guaranteed. All intraabdominal spaces are irrigated and recently formed adhesions between bowel loops are removed, reducing the risk of abscess formation (especially interenteric). Surgical anastomosis sites and transfixations can be inspected for insufficiencies (i.e., by decreasing edema) and promptly be taken care of if nesessary. Thus the share of primary anastomosis can be increased without risk. Following each lavage the small bowel is arranged in parallel coops, offering a safe prophylaxis against mechanical ileus. To prevent rigid adhesions between the abdominal wall and loops of small bowel, the latter is covered with a polyethylene layer. The development of small bowel fistula can be reduced to a minimum.

After about a week the operation interval is increased to 48 h, depending on the local situation. Once the abdominal cavity is clean the abdomen may be closed. In some cases step by step readaptation of the wound edges must precede closure. This also allows the respiratory system to accommodate the increasing intraabdominal pressure. Fascia and peritoneum are closed using either a continuous absorbable suture or by deep interrupted absorbable sutures. With exception of pancreatic or bile fistulae no intraabdominal drainages are used. Only in exceptional cases may the closure of the abdominal wall not be successful. The remaining fascial dehiscence must be tolerated. As soon as the small bowel is covered by granulation tissue the subcutis is mobilized for final wound closure. In these cases reconstructive surgery of the abdominal wall must be performed later on.

Advantages of the programmed peritoneal lavage concept are a fixed point of time for relaparotomy leading to early recognition of new complications frequently seen in severe intraabdominal sepsis, low intraabdominal pressure and minimal dilution of host defense components. A disadvantage is the requirement of a high degree of surgical skill, limiting its use to surgeons who are familiar with septic abdominal surgery. High treatment costs and the required operating room capacities are additional problems.

Discussion

Numerous preventive surgical actions are taken today to reduce the incidence of intraabdominal infection. Still some postoperative cases as well as spontaneous perforations cause severe diffuse peritonitis.

Indisputably, surgical elimination of septic foci remains the groundwork of successful treatment. The majority of all patients with peritonitis can be sufficiently treated by standard therapy. In 15% of severe diffuse peritonitis though different surgical approaches are required to lower the unreasonably high mortality rate. Advances in intensive care treatment (mechanical ventilation, antimicrobial chemotherapy, hemofiltration) of secondary injuries due to the infection have given way to a more aggressive surgical therapy.

Currently, different open and closed treatment concepts compete. The dynamic process of sepsis is the reason for numerous complications during its course. When using the closed treatment forms one has to rely on indirect clinical symptoms and laboratory data. The time point for necessary relaparotomy is generally chosen too late and is mainly responsible for the high mortality. In spite of a few good results [2] many arguments oppose closed treatment concepts. New immunological investigations of peritoneal exudate have shown the dilution of host defense components by continuous lavage [11].

Although competent comparative studies of surgical treatment forms are missing, there is an obvious preferation for semiopen therapy [8, 9, 12–15]. In weighing pros and contras towards continuous lavage important arguments favor programmed lavage.

Optimized postoperative control of intraabdominal sepsis seems to be a substantial advantage of programmed lavage. New complications in the course of the disease can be diagnosed in time and treated accordingly. The combination of constant lavage with planned relaparotomy tries to join the questionable advantage of continuous dilution of bacteria with aggressive control of sepsis [7, 14, 15]. This concept though is in opposition to recent investigations by Billing [11], who even suggests local addition of opsonins and proteinase inhibitors at the end of each programmed lavage.

The assessment of the significance of different therapy forms is only possible if the severity of the disease can be described exactly in order to form treatment groups of patients with a similar risk. So far several efforts of classifying the severity of peritonitis by scoring systems (APACHE II [16], Mannheimer Peritonitis Index [17]) have been insufficient. Besides ethical reasons the lack of comparability between the heterogenous groups of patients is responsible for the absence of controlled randomized studies.

Disadvantageous to all treatment forms are missing indication criteria, the requirement for highly skilled personnel, and the potential danger of nosocomial infections. However, the treatment concepts described above have evidently proven, successful in the treatment of those cases of diffuse peritonitis with a high mortality rate. Future studies should be aimed at showing the value or superiority of new surgical methods in a more objective way.

References

1. Altunbay S, Bleiler HJ, Heil T (1982) Die postoperative Peritonitis. Fortschr Med 100:560–565
2. Beger HG, Krantzberger W, Bittner R (1983) Die Therapie der diffusen bakteriellen Peritonitis mit kontinuierlicher postoperativer Peritoneal-Lavage. Chirurg 54:311–315
3. Berger D, Beger HG (1992) Pathophysiologische Grundlagen der Peritonitistherapie. Chirurg 63:147–152
4. Hay JM, Duchatelle P, Elman A, Flamant Y, Maillard N (1979) Les ventres laisses ouverts. Chirurgie 105:508–510
5. Hollender LF, Bur F, Schwenk D, Pigache P (1983) Das offen gelassene Abdomen. Technik, Indikation und Resultate. Chirurg 54:316–319

6. Neidhard JH, Rousson B (1978) Peritonitis aihues generali sec post operatoives. In. Patel J (ed) Chirurgie abdominale et digestive. Masson, Paris
7. Pichlmayr R, Weimann A, Klempnauer J (1992) Kontinuierliche Spülung oder Etappenlavage bei Peritonitis. Chirurg 63:162–168
8. Herbig B, Teichmann W (1992) Etappenlavage-Therapie bei diffuser Peritonitis – ein Erfahrungsbericht. In: Köckerling F (ed) Therapie schwerer intraabdomineller Infektionen. Zuckschwerdt, Munich, pp 18–25
9. Teichmann W, Wittmann DH, Andreone PA (1986) Scheduled reoperations (Etappenlavage) for diffuse peritonitis. Arch Surg 121:147–152
10. Teichmann W, Herbig B (1992) Etappenlavage. 109th Congress of Deutsche Gesellschaft für Chirurgie, Munich
11. Billing A (1991) Immunologische Probleme der Peritonitis. Aktuel Chir 26:41
12. Bartels H, Barthlen W, Sifert JR (1992) Therapie-Ergebnisse der programmierten Relaparotomie bei der diffusen Peritonitis. Chirurg 63:174
13. Dollinger P, Harnoss BU, Berger G, Häring R (1992) Die postoperative Peritonitis. Aktuel Chir 3:52
14. Köckerling F, Neumann U, Gall FP (1992) Diffuse Peritonitis – kontinuierliche offene Peritoneallavage. 109th Congress of Deutsche Gesellschaft für Chirurgie, Munich
15. Waclawiczek HW, Boeckl O (1992) Die geschlossene kontinuierliche Peritoneallavage mit geplanter Relaparotomie. 109th Congress of Deutsche Gesellschaft für Chirurgie, Munich
16. Knaus WA, Draper EA, Wagner DP, Zimmerman JE (1985) APACHE II: a severity of disease classification system. Crit Care Med 13:818–830
17. Linder MM, Wacha H, Feldmann U (1987) Der Mannheimer Peritonitis Index. Chirurg 58:84–92

Antibacterial Treatment of Sepsis

D. Adam and B. Gerlach

Introduction

Sepsis is an inflammatory process of increasing importance due to the changing patient population: patients are more often elderly, immunocompromised, and suffering from severe underlying diseases. The incidence of sepsis largely depends on the type of hospital and patient population and varies in a range from 4 to 21 episodes per 1000 admissions in European and North American university hospitals, according to an analysis of several studies in the 1970s and 1980s [1]. In spite of improved supportive care and a wide range of potent antimicrobials, sepsis may still be fatal in 20%–30% of cases. In the presence of septic shock which develops in 20%–40% of episodes, mortality rises to about 50% [2].

This chapter outlines the bacterial producers of the exogenous mediators involved in the different types of sepsis, their prevalence and pathogenicity, and the considerations for a rational antibiotic regimen in the treatment of sepsis.

Origin of Septic Processes

Although sepsis may arise without a preceding local infection or a detectable portal of entry (9%–19% [1]); rare in community-acquired sepsis but up to 25% in hospital-acquired cases [3], in the vast majority of cases it arises as a complication of disease. Bacteria or their toxins are distributed in the bloodstream from the original location of infection to secondary sites. These metastatic foci often are difficult to localize and thus complicate the progress of sepsis.

There have been several shifts in the prevalence of gram-positive and gram-negative pathogens. In the pre-antibiotic era, nearly nine-tenths of all episodes of sepsis were caused by gram-positive pathogens. With the introduction of penicillin and streptomycin in clinical practice, *Staphylococcus aureus* and especially gram-negative pathogens increasingly replaced the streptococci prevalent previously. Until the mid 1970s, this trend continued and the percentage of gram-positive pathogens dropped to 32%–35% [4, 5]. With the development and use of antibiotics high effective against gram-negative organisms and the increasing use of selective decontamination of the digestive tract, the situation reversed again and is now nearly balanced depending on the antibiotic prophylaxis and therapy.

Several factors predispose patients to sepsis:

- Age (>50% are over 60 years old)
- Major operation
- Polytrauma
- Immunosuppression
- Cancer chemotherapy
- Diabetes mellitus
- Congestive heart failure
- Uremia
- Prolonged indwelling devices (urinary, respiratory, and intravascular devices)
- Premature birth

Most of these factors predispose to sepsis caused by gram-negative pathogens, with the exception of vascular devices and skin or soft tissue infections.

In most cases, sepsis results from **urinary tract infections** (20%–50% of community-acquired cases, 20% of nosocomial cases [3]). In community-acquired urosepsis, the vast majority of pathogens consists of *Escherichia coli* and *Proteus* spp., whereas in nosocomial urosepsis multiresistant *Klebsiella* spp., *Enterobacter* spp., *Serratia marcescens, Proteus* spp., *Providencia* spp., and *Pseudomonas* spp. dominate. According to Geerdes et al. [1], these latter pathogens as well as enterococci are involved in urosepsis at a frequency of 5%–7% each.

As the second-most frequent portal of entry, Geerdes et al. [1] identified **intravascular devices.** This type of sepsis occurs only in hospitals and represents 16% of all cases. It is caused mainly by *S. aureus* (42%) and coagulase-negative staphylococci (30%). Less frequently, enterococci (9%) and gram-negative pathogens (10%) are causative agents.

As in the case of urinary tract infections, the etiology of sepsis as a complication of **respiratory tract infections** depends completely on the environment. For the most part, community-acquired sepsis of this kind is caused by gram-positive pathogens, predominantly by pneumococci (up to 40%). In contrast, the sepsis which frequently accompanies nosocomial pneumonias originates from gram-negative pathogens in about 67% of cases [3]: *Klebsiella* spp., *Enterobacter* spp., *P. aeruginosa, E. coli, S. marcescens,* and *Acinetobacter* spp., which often are acquired from the multiresistant hospital flora. In combination with the often severe underlying disease, pneumonial gram-negative sepsis has a high mortality rate.

Another 10%–20% of cases of sepsis originate from **intra-abdominal foci** primarily infected by *E. coli* (24%), enterococci (14%), *Salmonella* spp. (13%), and anaerobes (10%) [1]. In nosocomial peritonitis-related sepis, *Klebsiella* spp., *Enterobacter* spp., and *P. aeruginosa* also occur [3]. In cases of cholangiogenic location, *E. coli* is causative in as much as 59% of cases, other enterobacteria in 17%, while the prevalence of enterococci remains unchanged.

Whereas sepsis is commonly caused by a single pathogen, it is often polymicrobial if it derives from peritonitis involving lesions of the gastrointestinal tract.

Mortality is high in infections caused by pathogens that produce exotoxins, i.e., *P. aeruginosa* and staphylococci (40%–60% and 24%–48%, respectively). For *Klebsiella* spp., *Enterobacter* spp., and *Proteus* spp., mortality rates of 20%–30% have been reported; for *E. coli,* pneumococci, and viridans streptococci, mortality is lower, in a range of 15%–25%. But mortality rates also depend on the underlying disease, as was observed by Watanakunakorn and Weber [6] and Feldman et al. [7]. In patients with nosocomial pneumonia or other diseases predisposing for sepsis, mortality increased drastically with *Klebsiella* spp., *Enterobacter* spp., and *Proteus* spp. to 55%–69%. An explanation of this observation could be that in times of reduced immune competence, liberated endotoxin can no longer be neutralized by circulating antibodies, thus inducing the harmful effects of the sepsis cascade. Mortality is also increased in case of polymicrobial sepsis.

Aspects of the Antibacterial Treatment of Sepsis

In the course of sepsis, it is of primary importance to cope with the physiological status of the patient to prevent escalation to septic shock and multiorgan dysfunction syndrome. If complications arise in intra-abdominal sepsis, early surgical intervention is indicated. However, since the patient is often in a state of more or less pronounced immune incompetence, early and effective antibiotic therapy is mandatory as well. Considerations should not only include which possible pathogens are to be expected, according to the probable portal of entry, but also whether the infection was hospital- or community-acquired, which pathogens are prevalent in the hospital setting, their resistance profiles, and, last but not least, the underlying condition of the patient. Especially with neutropenic and cancer patients, antibiotic therapy should cover *P. aeruginosa,* and *Enterobacter* spp. and should take into account the increasing incidence of gram-positive pathogens such as staphylococci [1]. Therefore, empiric therapy should cover a broad spectrum. As soon as the causative pathogen is identified and its antibiotic resistance determined, therapy may be switched to a more specific agent or combination.

But in the light of recent research, there is a further aspect of antibiotic therapy that deserves consideration: antibiotic-induced release of endotoxin. Endotoxin is a component of the cell wall of gram-negative bacteria which is released during rapid cell growth and in larger amounts during cell lysis. During infection, endotoxin can be detected in the circulation. Free endotoxin can stimulate monocytes and macrophages to release tumor necrosis factor (TNF) and a variety of cytokines which act as inflammatory mediators, thus activating the sepsis cascade. In excessive volumes, this often leads to septic shock with or without multiorgan dysfunction syndrome. In other words, antibiotic-induced endotoxin release during treatment of septicemia can potentiate TNF toxicity and tissue damage and may therefore be clinically significant. We therefore should avoid any therapy that would provoke large amounts of endotoxin. Minimization of additional endotoxin release could improve the patient's outcome.

Antibiotic-Induced Release of Endotoxin from Gram-Negative Bacteria in Vitro

Several investigators have analyzed the potential of different classes of antibiotics to liberate endotoxin from several bacterial species. In general, they found that more endotoxin was released in the presence of antibiotics damaging the cell wall than in the presence of other bactericidal antibiotics not attacking the cell wall.

In 1991, Dofferhoff et al. [8] observed differences in endotoxin release associated with the bactericidal test agents aztreonam, ceftazidime, cefuroxime, imipenem, and tobramycin. Free endotoxin concentrations measured after 4 h were lowest for imipenem, and 2–30 times higher for the other agents investigated. The highest endotoxin release was found with cefuroxime and aztreonam (Table 1). These phenomena result from the different site of action of the β-lactams. Whereas imipenem preferentially binds to penicillin-binding protein (PBP) 2 and also PBP 1, resulting in spheroplast formation with little endotoxin content and release, and rapid killing, cephalosporins and penicillins preferentially bind to PBP 3, leading to the formation of long

Table 1. Antibiotic-induced release of endotoxin from an *in vitro* culture of *E. coli*

Antibiotic/ Controls	Endotoxin (ng/ml) release after		
	1 h	2 h	4 h
Imipenem	109±23	141± 12	149± 34
Tobramycin	39±13	109± 25	278± 51
Ceftazidime	122±18	259± 17	379± 53
Cefuroxime	24± 1.7	298±138	2215±163
Aztreonam	21± 1.7	81± 24	4188±172
Heated cultures[a]	83±13	88± 18	79± 13
Untreated controls	23± 0.8	47± 8	363± 59

Adapted from [8]. Results are expressed as the mean ±SEM.
[a] Heated cultures indicate the potentially releasable endotoxin that is not degraded during the 4 h of experiment.

endotoxin-rich filaments and slower cell death. In their study, the authors clearly demonstrated that the antibiotic used determines the total amount of endotoxin release as well as the rate of its release over time.

In 1993, Eng et al. [9] found similar effects for *K. pneumoniae, E. cloacae,* and *P. aeruginosa* as well. But there were species-specific differences in liberation potential of the agents investigated, as seen in Fig. 1 for *K. pneumoniae* and *E. cloacae.* In all species, imipenem revealed the most rapid killing accompanied by the lowest release of endotoxin compared to the other agents and antibiotic free cultures.

According to their findings, both groups of investigators therefore advocated the use of antimicrobials that provide rapid bacterial killing and minimize endotoxin release, so as to keep host damage as low as possible.

Jackson and Kropp [10] observed in 1992, in a comparison of the action of imipenem and ceftazidime on *P. aeruginosa,* that ceftazidime induced strong filamentation, and release of endotoxin was up to 14 times higher than for imipenem-treated cells (Fig. 2). In a mouse model, Jackson and Kropp [10] determined the toxic effects of liberated endotoxin by injecting various tenfold serial dilutions of culture filtrates from untreated cultures and cultures treated with either imipenem at 100 × minimal inhibitory concentration (MIC) or ceftazidime at 50 × MIC into the tail vein of mice sensitized for endotoxin. Ceftazidime-derived culture filtrates proved to be 70- to 80-fold more lethal than both imipenem-treated and untreated culture filtrates which demonstrated equivalent toxicity (Fig. 3).

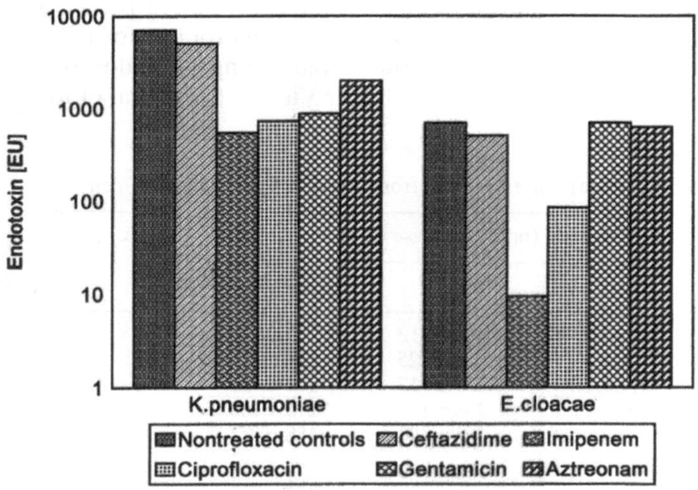

Fig. 1. Endotoxin release from *K. pneumoniae* and *E. cloacae* incubated in the presence of different antibiotics at serum-achievable concentrations for 6 h (Adapted from [9]).
EU, Endotoxin unit as defined by the Food and Drug Administration endotoxin reference lot EC-5 by cross-reference titration of limulus gelatinization bioreactivity. (Adapted from [9])

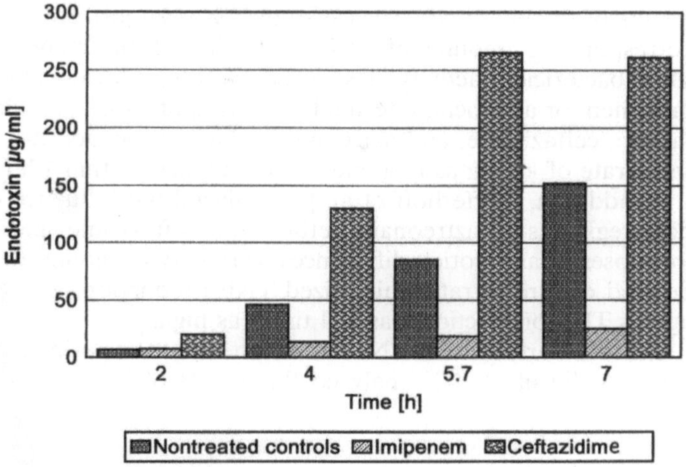

Fig. 2. Endotoxin release from *P. aeruginosa* incubated without antibiotics or with 2 µg/ml imipenem or 4 µg/ml ceftazidime, respectively, for the time indicated. (Derived from [10])

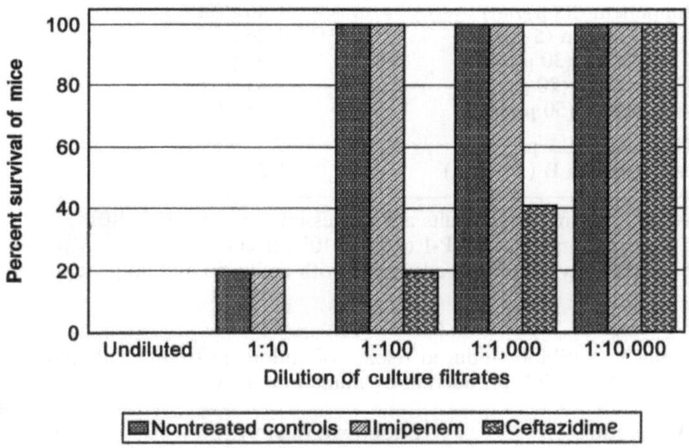

Fig. 3. Survival of mice after injection of serially diluted *P. aeruginosa* culture filtrates derived from untreated, imipenem-treated (at 100×MIC), and ceftazidime-treated (at 50×MIC) cultures, respectively. (Adapted from [10])

Endotoxin-Induced TNF Production in Vitro and ex Vivo

Simon et al. [11] and Dofferhoff et al. [8] persued closer to the sepsis process in their investigations by analyzing the TNF production of human monocytes induced by antibiotic treatment-derived culture filtrates of *E. coli*. Like the results of the endotoxin release studies *in vitro* just presented, they showed corresponding amounts of TNF production (Table 2 and 3). In spite of the same bactericidal activity, TNF production was lowest after treatment with imipenem or amikacin, intermediate with quinolones, and highest with cefotaxime, ceftazidime, and aztreonam, which all needed 2–4 h to achieve the same rate of killing as imipenem and amikacin within 1 h (Table 2) [11].

In addition, Dofferhoff et al. [8] analyzed the influence of low and high-dose regimens for aztreonam, ceftazidime, cefuroxime, and imipenem. Using low doses of antibiotics, differences were very pronounced. Only imipenem-derived culture filtrates minimized TNF production, whereas for the other agents TNF production was 3–4 times as high.

To avoid artefacts of TNF induction due to experimental *in vitro* conditions, Arditi et al. [12] analyzed the effects of imipenem- and ceftriaxone-

Table 2. TNF production by cells of the human monocyte/macrophage cell line THP-1 stimulated by culture filtrates of antibiotic-treated *E. coli*

Antibiotic/controls	*n*	TNF (ng/ml)[a]
Amikacin (25 μg/ml)	9	0.46±0.15
Imipenem (33 μg/ml)	8	0.46±0.19
Ciprofloxacin (5 μg/ml)	5	1.26±0.53
Cefotaxime (30 μg/ml)	3	1.62±0.13[b]
Ceftazidime (20 μg/ml)	9	2.33±0.63[b]
Aztreonam (50 μg/ml)	3	2.75±0.95[b]
Endotoxin (0.1 μg/ml)	9	2.38±0.31
+Polymyxin B (5 μg/ml)	5	0.23±0.03

Adapted from [11]. Results are expressed as the mean ±SEM.
[a] Concentrations of THP-1 cells = 5.10^5 cells/ml.
[b] Statistically significant compared with amikacin and imipenem.

Table 3. Antibiotic-induced release of endotoxin from *E.coli* and its stimulating effect on extracellular TNF production by human monocytes

Antibiotic/ controls	Endotoxin (ng/ml) release after		TNF (ng/ml) production after	
	4 h	24 h	4 h	24 h
Imipenem (100 μg/ml)	100±4.2	67±6.3	0.507±0.054	0.381±0.053
Ceftazidime (100 μg/ml)	303±19	219±2.8	0.576±0.098	0.846±0.107
Aztreonam (100 μg/ml)	238±49	394±60	0.524±0.062	5.969±1.145
Cefuroxime (75 μg/ml)	353±42	483±84	0.478±0.175	6.440±0.942
Controls[a]	0.07±0.004	0.09±0.003	0.119±0.007	0.08±0.007

Adapted from [8]. Results are expressed as the mean ± SEM of triplicate cultures from one monocyte donor.
[a] Controls consisted of monocyte cultures without the addition of *E. coli* and antibiotics.

treated *Haemophilus influenzae* type B on human peripheral blood cells in heparinized blood only separated by a filter. Regardless of the *H. influenzae* inoculum, mean TNF concentrations were significantly higher after 6 h with ceftriaxone.

Effects of Antibiotic-Induced Endotoxin Release in the Treatment of Experimental and Clinical Sepsis

Different groups of investigators have demonstrated in experimental infections or observed retrospectively in clinical therapy of sepsis and septic shock that an increase in endotoxin concentration can be associated with a higher mortality rate at least in some cases [13 (benzylpenicillin), 14 (kanamycin), 15 (moxalactam), 16 (gentamicin), 17 (gentamicin)]. Their results, achieved with different antibiotics, reflect individual differences in other factors influencing the inflammatory response. In addition, Rokke et al. [16] observed a negative correlation of endotoxin increase and cardiac performance in a porcine sepsis model.

Proposals for a Rational Antibacterial Treatment of Sepsis

There is no doubt that high levels of endotoxin and TNF play a detrimental role in the process of sepsis.

In mild to moderate infections, the impact of endotoxin is not so decisive. Therapy using an aminopenicillin with β-lactamase inhibitor (for example, piperacillin/tazobactam, ticarcillin/clavulanic acid) or a second or third generation cephalosporin all in combination with an aminoglycoside should cover the expected pathogens such as *E. coli*, *Klebsiella* spp., staphylococci, and streptococci. If necessary, also anaerobic coverage in intra-abdominal infections should be achieved.

In severe and life-threatening infections, all the considerations described above gain importance. Furthermore, antibiotics should be preferred that not only cover the broad spectrum of often multi-resistant potential pathogens, but that are also rapidly bactericidal and minimize endotoxin release. At least *in vitro*, aminoglycosides were able to reduce the endotoxin release of cephalosporins drastically, but there is no clinical evidence so far that this is also true *in vivo*. Quinolones may also be used in combination with anti-anaerobic agents and additional gram-positive coverage, since the quinolones clinically available do not kill anaerobes and show increasing resistance against gram-positive pathogens such as staphylococci. At present, the antibiotics that best meet all requirements, even in the case of renal insufficiency, are imipenem or other carbapenems that do not bind PBP 3. If *P. aeruginosa* is the causative pathogen, they can be combined with an aminoglycoside. After pathogen identification and antibiogram determination, therapy may be shifted to another drug. In severe cases of sepsis due to gram-positive organisms as *MRSA/MRSE* or penicillin-resistant enterococci, vancomycin or teicoplanin alone or in combination with other antibiotics should be administered.

In the future, treatment of septic shock will include methods that enable down-regulation of TNF and cytokine production to a favorable level. What can be done at present via antibiotic therapy is to try to reduce as much as possible factors leading to the inflammatory overresponse cascade.

References

1. Geerdes HF, Ziegler D, Lode H, Hund M, Loehr A, Fangmann W, Wagner J (1992) Septicemia in 980 patients at a university hospital in Berlin: prospective studies during 4 selected years between 1979 and 1989. Clin Infect Dis 15:991–1002
2. Kreger BE, Craven DE, McCabe WR (1980) Gram-negative bacteremia IV. Re-evaluation of clinical features and treatment in 612 patients. Am J Med 68:344–355
3. Dofferhoff ASM (1991) Release of endotoxin and other mediators during the treatment of gram-negative sepsis. Gram-negative sepsis — an introduction. Rijksuniversity Groningen, pp 1–32
4. McGowan JE Jr, Parrott PL, Duty VP (1977) Nosocomial bacteremia. Potential for prevention of procedure-related cases. JAMA 237:2727–2729
5. Scheckler WE (1977) Septicemia in a community hospital, 1970 through 1973. JAMA 237:1938–1941
6. Watanakunakorn C, Weber J (1989) Enterobacter bacteremia: a review of 58 episodes. Scand J Infect Dis 21:1–8
7. Feldman C, Smith C, Levy H, Ginsburg P, Miller SD, Koornhof JH (1990) Klebsiella pneumoniae bacteremia at an urban general hospital. J Infect 20:21–31
8. Dofferhoff ASM, Esselink MT, de Vries-Hospers HG, van Zanten A, Bom VJJ, Weits J, Vellenga E (1993) The release of endotoxin from antibiotic-treated Escherichia coli and the production of tumour necrosis factor by human monocytes. J Antimicrob Chemother 31:373–384
9. Eng RHK, Smith SM, Fan-Havard P, Ogbara T (1993) Effect of antibiotics on endotoxin release from gram-negative bacteria. Diagn Microbiol Infect Dis 16:185–189
10. Jackson JJ, Kropp H (1992) β-Lactam antibiotic induced release of free endotoxin: in vitro comparison of penicillin-binding protein (PBP) 2-specific imipenem and PBP 3-specific ceftazidime. J Infect Dis 165:1033–1041
11. Simon DM, Koenig G, Trenholme GM (1991) Differences in release of tumor necrosis factor from THP-1 cells stimulated by filtrates of antibiotic-killed Escherichia coli. J Infect Dis 164:800–802
12. Arditi M, Kabat W, Yogev R (1989) Antibiotic-induced bacterial killing stimulates tumor necrosis factor-α release in whole blood. J Infect Dis 160:818–825
13. Andersen BM, Solberg O (1984) Effect of benzylpenicillin in mice infected with endotoxin-liberating or non-liberating variant strains of Neisseria meningitidis. Scand J Infect Dis 16:257–266
14. Johnston CA, Greisman SE (1984) Endotoxemia induced by antibiotic therapy: a mechanism for adrenal corticosteroid protection in gram-negative sepsis. Trans Assoc Am Physicians 97:172–181
15. Shenep JK, Barton RP, Mogan KA (1985) Role of antibiotic class in the rate of liberation of endotoxin during therapy for experimental gram-negative bacterial sepsis. J Infect Dis 151:1012–1018

16. Rokke O, Revhaug A, Osterud B, Giercksky KE (1988) Increased plasma levels of endotoxin and corresponding changes in circulatory performance in a porcine sepsis model: the effect of antibiotic administration. Prog Clin Biol Res 272:247–262
17. Mustafa MM, Mertsola J, Ramilo O, Saez-Llorens X, Risser RC, McCracken GH (1989) Increased endotoxin and interleukin-1β concentrations in cerebrospinal fluid of infants with coliform meningitis and ventriculitis associated with intraventricular gentamicin therapy. J Infect Dis 160:891–895

Diagnostic and Therapeutic Approach in Invasive Fungal Infections of Intensive Care Unit Patients

M. Petri, H. Lode and T. Schaberg

Introduction

Fungal infections are not the most common infections in intensive care unit (ICU) patients but they often represent a most serious complication. Data collected by the NNIS (National Nosocomial Surveillance System) in the United States pointed out that 8% of all nosocomial infections between 1980 and 1990 were caused by fungi; *Candida* spp. accounted for almost 80% of these fungal isolates [1]. The reported mortality among patients with candidemia ranged from 60% to 80% overall. In long-time ICU patients isolation of *Candida* spp. in tracheal secretions, urine and serum is a frequent microbiological finding but the clinical significance is not yet clear.

Whereas most fungal infections were previously thought to be due to *Candida* or *Aspergillus* spp., recent reports also emphasize the contribution of uncommon fungi like *Fusarium* spp. (all patients reported with disseminated *Fusarium* infections have either been neutropenic or had extensive burns) and *Trichosporon* spp. However, this summary will concentrate on invasive mycosis caused by *Aspergillus* and *Candida* spp.

Disposing Factors

The factors predisposing and the patients predisposed to fungal infections are:

a) endogenous: (post)transplantation patients, neonates, hematological malignancies, solid tumors, hyperglycemia, chronic diseases;
b) exogenous: (poly)trauma, burns, drug addiction;
c) iatrogenic: intensive care, mechanical ventilation, intravascular catheters, extensive surgery, hyperalimentation, (poly)chemotherapy (immunosuppressive, antibiotic, cytostatic).

The most two common cases that emerge are:

1) the debilitated surgical patient hospitalized for a week or two who has received broad-spectrum antibiotics, prolonged parenteral hyperalimentation and has undergone surgical procedures (often more than one) that have violated the integrity of the gastrointestinal tract and

2) the granulocytopenic patient with underlying hematological malignancy receiving (mucosal-disrupting) chemotherapy and broad-spectrum antibiotics during a prolonged period of severe neutropenia.

Epidemiological studies are hampered by the fact that most septic patients dying in the ICU do not undergo autopsy. On the other hand autopsy studies indicate that invasive candidiasis is frequently not diagnosed antemortem and therefore not treated prior the patients demise.

Diagnosis

Signs and symptoms of most fungal infections are nonspecific; cultures may be negative or it can take several days to grow. Furthermore the significance of some isolates may be difficult to interpret. Unfortunately, serological assays have only shown clinical utility in a few cases (latex agglutination test for cryptococcal antigen). Fungi are frequently cultured from urine specimens of hospitalized patients but the significance of these findings is not yet clear [2]. At present, the distinction between fungal colonization and fungal infection of the bladder still must be based on symptoms and signs.

Demonstration of circulating antibodies is considered an important criterion in the diagnosis of fungi-induced diseases. However, currently available antigen and antibody detection methods are not satisfactory and need to be improved for dependable results. The major reasons for the nonavailability of standardized antigens are as follows:

a) Antigen preparations are highly variable; culture filtrates and mycelial extracts show considerable differences in their antigenic components.
b) Antigens show cross-reactivity.
c) Dependable serological methods are lacking.
d) Toxins and enzymes may be present.

In light of these problems, purified or semipurified and standardized antigens are essential for the development of reliable and sensitive immunoassays. In an immunocompromised patient, antibody detection methods are usually not helpful since the humoral response may be variable or absent. In these instances antigen detection systems may provide more information helpful in diagnosing the disease.

Candida spp.

Several studies have confirmed the substantial increase in frequency of candidemia and the parallel increase of disseminated candidiasis. Fungal infections were diagnosed in only 3% of patients with acute leukemia in the 1940s. Some 20 years later the frequency of candidiasis alone had increased to 20%. At present, in most cancer centers 20%–30% of all patients with acute leukemia die of *candida infections* [3]. Candidiasis is also increasing in frequency in patients with other hematological malignancies but it remains an infrequent cause of infection in patients with solid tumors. Estimates for the prevalence of *candida infection* amount to 0.5–0.8 cases of disseminated infection per 100 hospitalizations [4]. The increase is multifactorial in origin and reflects increased recognition, a growing population of patients at risk, and the improved survival of patients with underlying neoplasms and immunosuppressed patients. The majority of *candida infections* are due to *Candida albicans,* but in recent years there have been growing numbers of infections due to other *Candida* spp. *Candida parapsilosis* is emerging as an important nosocomial pathogen with strong association with total parenteral nutrition and prosthetic devices.

Candida may be part of the normal oral, upper respiratory, vaginal and gastrointestinal flora of the adult. Oral and fecal *Candida albicans* prevalence is approximately 10% for normal adults, the isolation frequency of *C. albicans* is 15% for vaginal specimens from healthy women and 10% for urine specimens [5, 6]. The presence of other microorganisms appears to inhibit adhesion, colonization, and dissemination of *Candida* spp. from the gastrointestinal tract. Induction of granulocytopenia (by cytotoxic chemotherapy) commonly causes disruption of mucosal barriers of the gastrointestinal tract, thereby permitting *Candida* and other yeast-like fungi to invade more readily across the altered mucosal surface. Also approximately 50% of patients with disseminated candidiasis have had abdominal surgery [7]. *Candida* colonizes mucosal tissues of the gastrointestinal tract in a mycelial form, although yeast forms can also be seen in tissues. The presence in a tissue biopsy of mycelial and budding yeast is pathognomic of *Candida infection.* In a recent study of 30% of mechanically ventilated patients with highly *Candida*-contaminated trachial secretions developed pulmonary infections after 3–6 days [8].

The main problem is how to discriminate between colonization and invasive candidiasis. Some patients who are heavily colonized are without the need for systemic antifungal therapy. Candiduria may signify contamination of the urine specimen, reflect colonization (catheter and lower urinary tract) or may indicate an invasive infection of the lower and/or upper urinary tract. Even the presence of *Candida* spp. in the urine $>10^5$/ml may only represent colonization. Although a single positive blood culture for *Candida* spp. may reflect contamination it is never appropriate to assume this in neutropenic or other high-risk patients, especially following major surgery. Initial management should include removal of possible foci of infection, including removal of intravascular lines. The only patients requiring additional observation pending the results of additional blood cultures are those afebrile patients with no history of recent surgery and those who are not immunocompromised in any way. When *Candida invasion* occurs through the gastrointestinal tract, candidemia of the portal circulation can result in seeding in the liver. Dissemination through the blood stream can result in other metastatic infections. These include *candida* enophthalmitis (white cotton puff-balls of the retinal surface). Recent autopsy data demonstrated that disseminated *Candida* infections may involve the lung more than is appreciated [9].

Disseminated candidiasis can be acute or chronic. Acute disseminated *candidiasis* refers to infection with *Candida* at two or more noncontiguous sites seeded from the gastrointestinal tract or through an intravenous line. Clinical deterioration will be rapid, with fever, skin lesions and sometimes shock. The organs and tissues that are the most frequent foci for *Candida* localization during hematogenous dissemination are the kidneys, lungs, liver, spleen, brain, heart, skin, skeletal muscle, and bone. Chronic disseminated candidiasis almost always occurs in neutropenic patients and probably follows weeks to months after acute infection with *Candida* organisms. Neutropenic patients may develop macroabscesses in the liver, spleen and pancreas which are large enough to be diagnosed by contrast radiography [10]. Extensive investigative efforts have been made to develop a serodiagnosis test for disseminated candidiasis. Serodiagnostic methods for detecting antibodies to *Candida* spp. have included immunoelectrophoresis, counterimmunoelectrophoresis, double diffusion, radioimmunoassay and enzyme-linked immunosorbent assay (ELISA). The sensitivity of these assays in diagnosing systemic candidiasis has ranged from 50% to 92% for immunocompetent patients. As mentioned above *Candida* antibodies are often falsely negative in immunocompromised patients with serious *Candida* infections. False-positive results occur in patients with minor *Candida* infection, colonization and controls with other fungal diseases. Likewise there is no accurate assay for *Candida* antigens. At present no available test has to be considered a reliable indicator of disseminated candidiasis. In a multicenter prospective study in 409 nonneutropenic long-time ICU patients serological analyses (antibody, i. e., indirect hemagglutination, immunofluorescence, and antigen measurements, i.e., latexagglutination) were of no importance to clinical diagnosis of invasive mycosis [11].

Trichosporon spp. can cause disseminated infection that resembles disseminated candidiasis. Both acute and chronic forms of disseminated *Trichosporon* infections can be seen and imitate acute and chronic disseminated candidiasis.

Aspergillus spp.

Aspergillus fumigatus is the species of *Aspergillus* most frequently isolated from human beings with saprophytic, allergic, or invasive disease manifestations. The predominant species involved with invasive *aspergillosis* is *A. fumigatus*, but other species have also been implicated. In the environment *Aspergillus* spores are ubiquitous and they may become concentrated in hospital ventilation systems. In the normal host *Aspergillus* spp. can be isolated from the oropharynx and gastrointestinal tract. The hospital may serve as source for microepidemics of aspergillosis. Construction within the hospital or at adjacent sites may be associated with microepidemics. High efficiency air filters and laminar air flow rooms can reduce the risk of nosocomial aspergillosis. Hematogenous spread from sites such as the gastrointestinal tract or intravenous catheters results in multiple miliary microabscesses throughout all organs.

In the past, invasive aspergillosis occurred almost exclusively in patients with hematological malignancies, especially acute leucemia. In recent years the spectrum has been expanding, infection is now common in patients with leukemia and other hematological malignancies, in patients undergoing organ transplantation and in chronic granulomatous diseases of childhood. An increase in prevalence of invasive aspergillosis has been noted in bone marrow transplant recipients. Predisposing factors for the development of invasive aspergillosis in immunocompromised patients are manifold. They include granulocytopenia, underlying chronic diseases and treatments such as those with corticosteroids, broad-spectrum antibiotics and cytotoxic drugs. Although invasive aspergillosis has been considered an infection exclusively of immunocompromised patients, sporadic cases have been reported even in normal hosts – maybe due to unrecognized subtle immunological defects, tissue damage, viral infections or antibiotic therapy for a bacterial infection. Infections in the normal host may follow surgical procedures, trauma or prosthetic devices. Most prosthetic device infections are due to the introduction of *Aspergillus* spores at the time of surgery. In a few instances, infections have been traced to defective ventilation in operating rooms. Recovery of *Aspergillus* spp. from a normal host is not indicative of infection, even if recovered repeatedly. Nevertheless, if a patient with pulmonary infection fails to respond to antibacterial therapy and has multiple positive *Aspergillus* cultures, invasive procedures should be performed. Several cases of osteomyelitis have been reported either due to hematogenous dissemination or contiguous spread from a pulmonary infection. A few cases of disseminated infection have even occurred in patients without any apparent deficiencies in host defense mechanisms. The mortality rate is substantial despite antifungal therapy.

The symptoms of invasive aspergillosis are mostly nonspecific. They include coughing, wheezing, dyspnea and fever. Until more effective diagnostic measures become available, therapy will have to be initiated in a substantial number of patients based upon a high probability of infection being present. Patients with acute leukemia and bone marrow transplant recipients are at highest risk. The most important predisposing factors are prolonged severe neutropenia ($<100/mm^3$ for >1 week), chronic corticosteroid administration, and tissue damage from preexistent infection. Among these susceptible patients antifungal therapy should be administered if any of the following conditions exist:

a) eschar on the nose or palate or progressive sinusitis unresponsive to antibacterial agents;
b) symptoms suggestive of acute pulmonary embolism, especially if associated with pleural friction rub;

c) characteristic lesions on chest X-ray examination which include wedge-shaped infarcts, nodular densities, new cavitary lesions or fungus balls;
d) persistent fever with or without pulmonary infiltrates that fails to respond to antibacterial therapy;
e) any clinical manifestation suggestive of an acute vascular event associated with fever.

The isolation of *Aspergillus* spp. from respiratory tract secretions in any of these settings should be considered confirmatory evidence [12].

The widespread radiological infiltrates give an indication how extensively the disease has spread. The differential diagnosis of invasive aspergillosis includes infections such as those due to *Pneumocystis carinii* or *Nocardia, Candida, Mycobacterium* or *Mycoplasma* spp. as well as some of the common bacterial infections. In host tissue, the *Fusarium* spp. resemble *Aspergillus* spp. in that they induce similar clinical features and histopathologic lesions. Serological tests serve as important aids in the effective diagnosis of various types of aspergillosis. Circulating antibodies against. *A. fumigatus* or other species of *Aspergillus* can be readily detected in immunocompetent patients. The immunodiffusion test is useful for diagnosing invasive aspergillosis when the patient is not receiving extensive immunosuppressive therapy.

Due to the high mortality of invasive aspergillosis and the need for early diagnosis which is often difficult because major clinical symptoms are nonspecific and blood cultures are usually negative, the interest in developing rapid serological methods for the diagnosis of invasive aspergillosis has increased. Due to the of lack of a functionally normal immune system resulting from malignancy or intentional immunosuppression as in organ transplantation there is very little or no antibody response in these patients. The usual serological studies therefore have not been useful in the diagnosis of invasive aspergillosis.

A variety of tests with diverse sensitivities have been developed to detect circulating antibodies to aspergilli:
a) Immunodiffusion: because of its simplicity and ease of performance it is still the most widely used technique. However, the immunodiffusion test lacks sensitivity and gives no quantitive information on antibody concentrations.
b) Immunogold assay: this method is similar to indirect immunofluorescence but more sensitive and does not need any special equipment.
c) Radioimmunoassay (RIA): several investigators have developed and utilized RIA as a reliable tool for detecting antibodies in patients with aspergillosis. RIA has several disadvantages including limited storage life of the radioisotopes, length of time required to complete the assay, and the need for expensive radioactivity detectors.
d) ELISA: because of its high sensitivity, reliability and versatility the ELISA is being widely used in the serodiagnosis of various forms of aspergillosis. Although the sensitivity of the ELISA system depends on many variables, the nature and type of antigens used and their abilities to bind to surfaces are of prime importance.

e) Immunoblotting has been used with great success in detecting specific antibodies to *Aspergillus* spp.

Several other diagnostic procedures that have also been developed for detecting aspergillosis include immunoelectrophoresis (counterimmunoelectrophoresis has been widely used, mainly because of the short time required to obtain results), passive hemagglutination, indirect immunofluorescence, latex agglutination and complement fixation [13]. Apart from the use of immunoelectrophoresis in the characterization of antigens, the use of other tests is fairly limited because of factors such as false-positives, instability of antigen-treated erythrocytes and the recent availability of more versatile and more sensitive detection methods. All tests for *Aspergillus* antibodies and antigens have been extensively evaluated for rapid diagnose of invasive pulmonary aspergillosis but their diagnostic role remains unproven. Antigen detection assays have not yet been proved to be accurate and useful [14].

Treatment and Prophylaxis

There are several problems in the treatment of fungal infections. The diagnosis of fungal infection is often not exact and it is not evident when to start therapy. Duration of therapy predominantly depends on the host's immune status and not on the treated fungus. Antifungal agents may be ineffective *in vivo* despite *in vitro* inhibition or killing.

Candida spp.

Amphotericin B. Amphotericin B remains the drug of choice for treatment of life-threatening fungal infections, but the toxicity rates are high, particularly for nephrotoxicity. In numerous patients, the glomerular filtration rate is reduced to 60% of normal soon after beginning of therapy. Amphotericin B is seldom effective in patients with persistent neutropenia, hence, recovery of the neutrophil count is a critical factor in response to therapy. After a test dose of 1 mg of amphotericin B the candidemic immunocompromised patient should receive therapeutic concentrations of amphotericin B administered over 3–6 h. In less ill patients amphotericin B can be initially given as a 5 mg infusion and repeated every 8 h with progressive 5 mg increments until 1 mg/kg has been reached. The total dose should be influenced by the duration of fungemia prior to therapy, the response to antifungal therapy, the underlying status of the patient and whether disseminated visceral disease is documented. Disseminated candidiasis requires a higher total dose of 1.5–2.0 g of amphotericin B.

Liposomal preparations of amphotericin B seem to be an alternative to the conventional preparation. Liposomal amphotericin B is substantially less toxic and shows more efficacy against experimentally induced candidiasis.

More than 50% patients with *Candida* or *Aspergillus* infections that have failed to respond to conventional amphotericin B achieved complete or partial response with liposomal amphotericin B (dose increase up to 3 mg/kg possible). Amphotericin B-induced nephrotoxicity has improved during therapy with the liposomal preparation.

Flucytosine. Flucytosine is a potentially important antifungal agent when used in combination with amphotericin B in cryptococcal meningitis and disseminated candidiasis. Since the clinical response rate of amphotericin B in fungemic patients with underlying malignancies is poor, combination therapy of amphotericin B and flucytosine (100–150 mg/kg/day) should be considered. The risk of hematologic toxicity can be reduced substantially by careful monitoring of serum flucytosine levels and dose adjustment (2 h postdose levels below 100 mg/l).

Fluconazole. Like itraconazole, fluconazole is a triazole that is well absorbed after oral administration, but food does not affect its absorption. There is an increasing body of information on the positive results obtained with fluconazole therapy in invasive *Candida* infections; however, the effective dosages are high and could reach 1000–1600 mg per day [15].

The high mortality associated with fungal infections and the high morbidity associated with their treatment have induced multiple studies to examine the role of antifungal agents given prophylactically to prevent or delay the occurrence of fungal infection. A low dose regimen with amphotericin B in patients undergoing bone marrow transplantation was associated with significant increased survival but this could not be attributed to the prevention of fungal infections. Fluconazole was also given as prophylaxis in bone marrow transplant patients and decreased the number of systemic fungal infections but survival rates between the treatment and placebo group were not significant.

Aspergillus spp.

The therapy of invasive aspergillosis has been not very encouraging. This is due in part to the inability to diagnose the infection antemortem in a substantial number of cases. Several reports have suggested that early diagnosis and administration of antifungal therapy results in higher response rates.

Amphotericin B. Amphotericin B is the antifungal agent with established activity against infection with *Aspergillus* spp. The response of normal hosts with aspergillosis is much more frequent than in patients with underlying diseases associated with impaired host defenses. The proper dosage schedule of amphotericin B therapy has not been clearly established. Since *Aspergillus* spp. are often only moderately susceptible to amphotericin B, full doses of 1 mg/kg/day should be administered at least until significant nephrotoxicity occurs (serum creatinine >3.0 mg/dl). Some investigators have attempted therapy with doses even higher than 1 mg/kg/day. There are also reports of patients who have acquired aspergillosis while receiving daily doses of 0.5–0.6 mg/kg/day. Furthermore failure of amphotericin B therapy due to resistance, either inherent or acquired during therapy, is observed. Even the proper duration of therapy has also not been clearly defined.

Itraconazole. Clinical responses have been reported in patients with systemic mycoses, including coccidiomycosis, sporotrichosis, chromoblastomycosis and aspergillosis. The most exciting prospect for itraconazole use is in the treatment of *Aspergillus* infections. Aspergillosis has been difficult to treat even with amphotericin B and has not been responsive to oral agents. Itraconazole is a lipophilic compound that, like ketoconazole, is better absorbed in the presence of food. Usual treatment regimens with itraconazole have included daily doses at 400 mg or less. Few adverse effects have been noted in the treatment of human mycoses with doses of up to 400 mg/day. The optimal dose for the treatment of severe systemic mycoses has yet to be determined. Selected patients might benefit from 600 mg of itraconazole per day. Like ketoconazole, itraconazole interferes with the metabolism of cyclosporine. Thus, when the two drugs are given concomitantly, cyclosporine levels may quickly rise, leading to toxicity.

Conclusion

The diagnosis of a systemic fungal infection has to be based upon a combination of clinical and laboratory findings. Clinical and radiologic studies enable a presumptive diagnosis and laboratory procedures are necessary to confirm this diagnosis. Proper interpretation of test results or observations is enhanced if the laboratory has access to information on the patients clinical history, symptoms, treatment, occupation, history of travel and residence. It requires confirmation by histopathology (characteristic organisms seen in the appropriate clinical specimens) and/or fungal cultures. The success in detecting antigenemia in a patients serum mainly depends on the frequent monitoring of samples. When two or more serum samples were tested the frequency of detection increases up to more than five-fold compared with single testing. The evaluation of invasive fungal infection should be based on unequivocal definitions:

1) exact clinical definition of invasive mycosis,
2) laboratory and microbiological findings,
3) histology/obduction findings.

Diagnosis of invasive mycosis is only to be accepted if at least two of the three conditions are definitely positive.

The prognosis of systemic mycosis remains poor despite modern antifungal therapy.

References

1. Jarvis WR et al (1992) 3rd international conference on nosocomial infections, Atlanta
2. Wong-Beringer A, Jacobs RA, Guglielmo BJ (1992) Treatment of funguria. JAMA 267:2780–2785
3. Horn R, Wong B, Kiehn TE, Armstrong D (1985) Fungemia in a cancer hospital: changing frequency, earlier onset and results of therapy. Rev Infect Dis 7:646–655
4. Maksymiuk AW, Thongprasert S, Hopfer R, Luna M, Fainstein V, Bodey GP (1984) Systemic candidiasis in cancer patients. Am J Med 77:20–27
5. Odds FD (1979) Candida and candidosis. University Park Press
6. Andersen LI, Frederiksen HJ, Appleyard M (1992) Prevalence of esophageal candida colonization in a Danish population: special reference to esophageal symptoms. Benign esophageal disorders and pulmonary disease. J Infect Dis 165:389–392
7. Edwards JE (1989) Candidemia and candida catheter-associated sepsis. In: Holmberg K, Meyer RD (eds) Diagnosis and therapy of systemic fungal infections. Raven, New York pp 39–46
8. Füssle R, Biscoping D, Zeiler D, Michaelis G, Sziegoleit A (1991) Mikrobiologische Betreuung von beatmeten Intensivpatienten. Anaesthesist 91:491–496
9. Fraser VJ, Jones M, Dunkel J, Storfer S, Medoff G, Dunagan WC (1992) Candidemia in a tertiary hospital: epidemiological risk factors and predictors of mortality. Clin Infect Dis 15:414–421
10. Thales M, Tastakia B, Shawker TH et al (1988) Hepatic candidiasis in cancer patients: the evolving picture of the syndrome. Ann Intern Med 108:88–100
11. Petri M, Moecke HP, Gramm HJ et al (1993) Epidemiologie invasiver Mykosen auf Intensivstationen. 2. Deutscher Konreß für Infektions- und Tropenmedizin
12. Bodey GP, Vartivarian S (1989) Aspergillosis. Eur J Microbiol Infect Dis 8:413–437
13. Kurup VP, Kumar A (1991) Immunodiagnosis of Aspergillosis. Clin Microbiol Rev 4:439–456
14. Wheat LJ (1993) The role of the serologic diagnostic laboratory and the diagnosis of fungal disease. In: Sarosi GE, Davies FD (eds) Fungal diseases of the lung, 2nd edn. Raven, New York pp 29–38
15. Anaissia E, Kontoyiannas C, Huls C, Prince R, Bosso JA, Bodey GP (1993) Efficacy, safety and pharmakokinetics of high dose fuconazol in patients with fungal infections. Z Chemother 1:6 (abstract)

Fluid Therapy in Sepsis

W. J. Sibbald

Introduction

Sepsis is a systemic illness characterized by an uncontrolled host inflammatory response, usually to severe infection [1]. Patients with sepsis are frequently admitted to the ICU for life-support of multiple organ dysfunction, and circulatory failure is the most frequent clinical manifestation of this complication. While it is estimated that greater than 500000 patients develop this syndrome in North America annually, its incidence continues to increase as sepsis is a complication of applying new medical and surgical technologies to our aging population.

The circulation is an early target organ for injury by the uncontrolled systemic inflammatory processes which are typical of sepsis. Myocardial contractility is depressed and arterial resistance vessels are hyporesponsive in sepsis, both of which may contribute to the maldistribution of organ blood flows observed in this syndrome (reviewed in [2]). It is also believed that progressive microcirculatory dysfunction complicates sepsis and impairs the normal metabolic coupling of tissue O_2 delivery (QO_2) with O_2 needs [3]. For example, a depression in maximal O_2 extraction (O_2E) is taken as evidence of microcirculatory dysfunction in the septic gut [4] (Fig. 1).

Treatment of sepsis is both definitive and supportive. Given the positive correlation between death and failure to maintain elevated systemic QO_2's

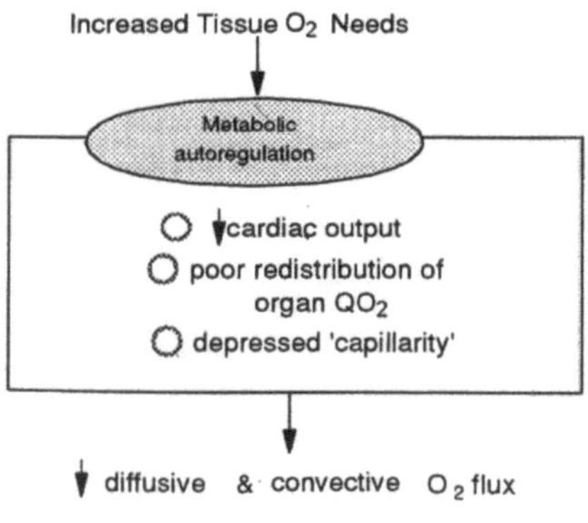

Fig. 1. In sepsis, circulatory dysfunction contributes to impaired diffusive and convective tissue O_2 flux.
QO_2, O_2 delivery

[5, 6], recommendations for supportive therapy include maintaining supranormal systemic QO_2's. Examination of the systemic QO_2 equation:

$$\text{Systemic } QO_2 = [\text{cardiac index} \times (\text{hemoglobin}) \times SaO_2 \times 1.34] + [PaO_2 \times 0.003]/100$$

demonstrates that augmenting both cardiac output and/or arterial O_2 content (CaO_2) increases QO_2. Clinically, cardiac output is augmented by volume infusion or inotropic therapy, and CaO_2 is augmented by red blood cell (RBC) transfusions, as well as by measures which improved arterial oxygenation (e.g., positive end-expiratory pressure and/or increased inspired O_2 concentrations).

This chapter will review current issues regarding fluid and transfusion therapy in sepsis.

Fluid Therapy: Crystalloid or Colloid?

Background

Maintenance of the intravascular volume is fundamental to supporting the hyperdynamic circulatory state typical of surviving septic patients. However, there is no apparent consensus on whether unique clinical benefits can be ascribed to any of the different parenteral solutions available for intravascular volume replacement therapy in this syndrome.

Three structures influence fluid and solute flux between the intravascular and interstitial compartments: (1) the microvascular membrane; (2) the interstitium; and (3) the lymphatic vessels. Fluid and protein flux across this microvascular membrane occurs by diffusion and the rate of fluid flux at any time may be described by the modified Starling equation as a product of the net driving pressure across the membrane and the conductance, or ease, of fluid transport.

Thus,

$$J_v = K_{FC}[(P_c - P_t) - J_c(\pi_c - \pi_i)]$$

where J_V is the rate of fluid movement into or out of the microcirculation; K_{FC} is the capillary filtration coefficient of the microcirculatory bed, a function of both its perfused surface area and its unique permeability to solute; P_c is the hydrostatic pressure within the vessel, while P_t is the hydrostatic pressure within the interstitium; and π_c is the osmotic pressure in the capillary, while π is the osmotic pressure in the interstitium.

Following an increase in fluid flux across a microvascular membrane, defense mechanisms become operative to minimize the accumulation of interstitial fluid. An increase in the P_t initially reduces the effective magnitude of the P_c. Concurrently, an increase in transmicrovascular water flux induces a protein washout from the interstitium; the $p_c - p_t$ gradient thence widens and serves to further minimize the effect of any increase in the P_c. Other mechanisms which protect the interstitium from excessive fluid accumulation (i.e., edema) are equally as important, particularly the lymphatic vessels and the interstitial space itself.

Although initially described in the pulmonary microcirculation [7, 8], it is now recognized that the systemic microcirculation is also injured during the evolution of sepsis [9]. Thus, widespread tissue edema complicates this syndrome, primarily due to an abnormal increase in microvascular permeability in both the lung [8] and extrapulmonary [9, 10] organs. Due to this alteration in microvascular integrity, the initial restoration and subsequent maintenance of intravascular volume with parenteral fluid therapy in septic patients will be accompanied by an obligate increase in transmicrovascular fluid flux. The increase in microvascular permeability permits an increase in fluid flux from the intravascular to interstitial compartments. At the same time, depressed lymphatic efficiency reduces the interstitial clearance of fluid which has egressed the intravascular compartment.

Clinical strategies to reduce the degree of interstitial edema in sepsis have focused on two broad issues: (1) ameliorate the microvascular permeability defect, and (2) manage the Starling hydrostatic and colloid osmotic pressures. When comparing crystalloid vs colloid therapy, the principle being tested is that widening the colloid osmotic pressure gradient across the microvascular membrane, while at the same time minimizing an increase in the microvascular hydrostatic pressure, will reduce the abnormal increase in microvascular fluid flux which occurs in sepsis. However, studies which have evaluated the potential for clinically significant differences between crystalloid and colloid therapy in sepsis have generally focused on the lung. For example, a clinical strategy to minimize lung water accumulation in patients with adult respiratory distress syndrome was accompanied by improved survival [11]. Despite the increase in microvascular permeability in sepsis, such data suggest that therapy which widens the microvascular hydrostatic pressure minus colloid osmotic pressure gradient might have a significant clinical effect in this syndrome. As outcome from sepsis is determined by the effects of this syndrome on extrapulmonary organ function, it is now germane to ask whether different types of fluid therapy of sepsis could modify extrapulmonary organ injury which complicates this syndrome. Furthermore, as factors contributing to edemagenesis vary to some extent between organs, it is inappropriate to transfer concepts regarding fluid therapy gained from study of the pulmonary circulation to the extrapulmonary circulation without explicit confirmatory experiments.

A problem with previous studies which have evaluated the interaction of various fluid therapies and microvascular fluid flux on organ function in sepsis is the adoption of study designs which measured outcome variables only in the short-term, i.e., in hours. As the circulatory response changes in therapy probably require a longer period of time to reach new steady state conditions [12], the clinical relevance of such studies requires assessment over a longer period of study.

Experimental Approach

We tested the hypothesis that the type of fluid infused for long-term maintenance of intravascular volumes would modify both microvascular integrity and cellular structure in extrapulmonary organs in hyperdynamic sepsis. Following cecal ligation and perforation, awake sheep were treated for 48 h with 10% Pentastarch ($n=9$), or Ringer's lactate ($n=8$), titrated to maintain a constant left atrial pressure. Pentastarch is a commercially available artificial colloid solution. After 48 h of fluid therapy, biopsy samples were taken from the left ventricle and gastrocnemius for electron microscopy. Some 48 h following cecal ligation and perforation, all groups demonstrated similar hyperdynamic circulatory responses, systemic O_2 utilization, and regional blood flows (measured by the radioactive microsphere technique). However, greater capillary luminal area with less endothelial swelling and less parenchymal injury were found with Pentastarch infusion than with Ringer's lactate in both muscle types.

Summary and Clinical Implications

In a large animal model of normotensive hyperdynamic sepsis, we evaluated microvascular and ultrastructural parenchymal alterations in both the myocardium and skeletal muscle following treatment with the clinically available synthetic colloid Pentastarch (10%) or a conventional crystalloid, Ringer's lactate, for 48 h. Despite similarities in calculated O_2 delivery at both the central and regional levels of the circulation, greater preservation of microvascular architecture in the Pentastarch vs Ringer's lactate treated animals is consistent with the conclusion that 10% Pentastarch ameliorated a depression in the microvascular surface area available for O_2 exchange. Pentastarch also retarded the progression of parenchymal ultrastructural injury in both muscle types studied.

A number of interesting questions arise from these data. For example, do the ultrastructural alterations in the myocardium demonstrated in this study, including mitochondrial damage, reduce glycogen storage and myofibrillar edema, account for the myocardial dysfunction reported in sepsis? An excellent correlation between the functional and ultrastructural alterations in isolated canine heart has been demonstrated; a gradual decrease in myocardial function depending on the degree of ischemia was accompanied by progressive destruction of subcellular components [13]. In addition, a recent study suggested that myocardial edema itself compromised myocardial systolic and diastolic function [14]. It is therefore possible that the systemic microcirculatory lesion of sepsis, leading to excessive interstitial edema and depressed microvascular surface area for O_2 exchange, may be directly related to the progression of multiple organ dysfunction which characterizes this syndrome. Furthermore, we believe that colloid therapy, which minimizes organ edema in sepsis, will retard the emergence of clinical multiple organ dysfunction.

Fluid Therapy – Red Blood Cell Transfusions?

Background

A growing body of evidence supports the belief that elevated tissue O_2 needs in sepsis are not consistently matched by parallel increases in O_2 delivery. Perhaps the most compelling validation of this concept are data which have linked high levels of systemic oxygen delivery with survival [5, 6]. Indeed, therapeutic guidelines increasingly emphasize the need to maintain systemic O_2 delivery at supranormal levels.

Transfusing packed RBCs to maintain a normal hemoglobin concentration has been proposed to represent the most effective means of increasing systemic O_2 delivery in sepsis [15]. If a tissue O_2 debt characterizes this syndrome, increasing systemic O_2 delivery with RBC transfusion should be accompanied by an increase in systemic O_2 uptake. However, current clinical guidelines regarding transfusion therapy deemphasize routine blood transfusions until the hemoglobin concentration is approximately <70 g/L [16–18].

Generally, low hematocrits can be safely tolerated since systemic and organ QO_2's are well-maintained between hematocrits of 40%–60% (reviewed in [19]). Compensation to maintain systemic O_2 consumption ($\dot{V}O_2$) involves all levels of the circulation. This includes both flow recruitment within the microcirculation and changes in hemoglobin O_2 affinity. Increasing the number of capillaries with RBC flow when hematocrits are depressed permits tissues to extract more of the available O_2 since: (a) increased capillary density reduces the diffusion distance for O_2; (b) increased numbers of perfused capillaries augment surface area to muscle fibre-volume available for O_2 diffusion; and (c) reduced RBC velocity within each capillary elevates O_2 diffusion time.

A number of observations, however, support the notion that circulatory dysfunction in sepsis might limit the ability to maintain tissue O_2 uptake during modest anemia. First, the microcirculatory injury we have shown to be typical of sepsis could depress the microcirculatory compensation required to maintain tissue O_2 uptake when hemoglobin is depressed. Second, during sepsis, arterioles may be depressed in their ability to respond to metabolic needs of tissue under conditions of reduced QO_2. This would limit required arteriolar vasodilation during anemia. Third, we also found that depressed vasoreactivity in sepsis limits the ability to redistribute blood flow (Q) from the splanchnic to the vital circulations [2] as is normally required to augment Q to the myocardium and thereby maintain this organ's QO_2 during anemia.

The impact of the sepsis-associated regional and microregional circulatory abnormalities during anemia may be a particularly relevant issue in the myocardium. Thus, in health, myocardial $\dot{V}O_2$ does not usually increase during modest depressions in hemoglobin concentration [20]. In contrast, we recently found that depressed hemoglobin concentrations (to levels currently recommended as clinically tolerable) augmented myocardial $\dot{V}O_2$ needs in sepsis [21]. Paradoxically, however, it is probable that sepsis simultaneously depresses the normal circulatory compensation which is required to maintain (appropriate) parallel increases in O_2 availability. Therefore, we believe that depressed hemoglobin concentrations in sepsis reduce the *margin of safety* (or reserve) of myocardial O_2 availability, a process which normally permits moment-to-moment alterations in the heart's metabolic demands to be satisfied (Fig. 2).

Experimental Approach

We designed a study to examine whether sepsis modifies the host's ability to maintain regional QO_2 and whether regional Q and QO_2 reserve under hypoxic stress would be altered in sepsis across a clinically relevant range of hematocrits. A total of 90 rats were randomly allocated to cecal ligation and perforation (CLP) or a sham (SHAM) procedure, which was followed by random isovolemic transfusion into three different hematocrit subgroups; low (21%–28%), middle (33%–40%), and high (45%–52%) with either rat plasma, whole blood or packed RBCs, respectively. At 24 h postlaparotomy, all CLP groups showed a normotensive, hyperdynamic hemodynamic state. There was no unique effect of sepsis on regional Q and QO_2 to organs across this range of hematocrits. All rats were then subjected to a hypoxic stress state. The low hematocrit group in the CLP rats demonstrated a loss of Q and QO_2 reserve to heart and brain, mainly due to poor redistribution of QO_2 from splanchnic organs. In this model of sepsis, we concluded that, under a hypoxic stress in sepsis, depressed hematocrit may reduce physiological QO_2 reserve to vital organs.

Given that transfusion therapy to normalize hematocrits may therefore be important to maintain QO_2 at supranormal levels in sepsis, we then determined the effect of transfusing "old" RBCs on whole body and organ O_2 uptake in this syndrome.

In 23 critically ill septic patients undergoing mechanical ventilation, sys-

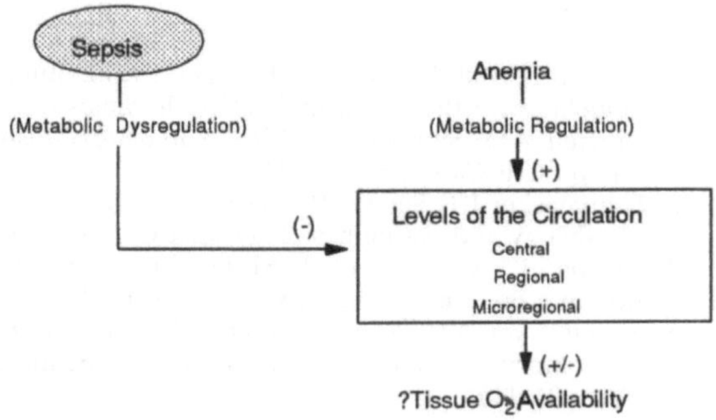

Fig. 2. In sepsis, circulatory dysfunction may limit the degree of anemia normally tolerated by the patient

temic O_2 uptake was both measured by indirect calorimetry and calculated by the Fick method. Gastrointestinal pH (pHi) measured with tonometry was used to assess changes in splanchnic oxygen availability. Measurements were made prior to transfusion of three units of packed RBCs. These were then repeated immediately posttransfusion as well as then 3 and 6 h later. There was no increase in systemic O_2 uptake measured by indirect calorimetry in any of the patients studied for up to 6 h posttransfusion (including those patients with an elevated arterial lactate). However, the calculated systemic O_2 uptake increased in parallel with O_2 delivery in all the patients. We also found a inverse correlation between the change in pHi and the age of the transfused blood ($r=0.71$; $p=0.001$). In those patients receiving blood which had been stored for greater than 15 days, the pHi consistently fell following RBC transfusion. We believe that a loss in RBC deformability (which occurs with prolonged storage) may lead to microvascular obstruction when RBCs are transfused and, therefore, may lead to depressed organ QO_2's.

Summary

1. Sepsis is a syndrome characterized by increased O_2 needs.
2. Increasing cardiac output is currently the most effective clinical method to increase tissue O_2 availability.
3. When colloid is used to augment cardiac preload (to elevate cardiac output), less tissue edema is observed and extrapulmonary organs show less overall sepsis-induced injury.
4. Circulatory dysfunction in sepsis likely necessitates maintaining a higher hemoglobin level than is currently recommended for other critically ill patients (i.e., >100 g/L).
5. When transfusing RBCs, consider that changes in RBC rigidity in sepsis may contribute to the microvascular defect in O_2 extraction typical of this syndrome.

References

1. Bone RC, Balk RA, Cerra FB et al (1992) Definitions for sepsis and organ failure and guidelines for the use of innovative therapies in sepsis. Chest 101:1644
2. Bersten AD, Sibbald WJ (1989) Circulatory disturbances in multiple systems organ failure. Crit Care Clinics 5:233
3. Schumacker PT, Samsel RW (1989) Oxygen delivery and uptake by peripheral tissues: physiology and pathophysiology. Crit Care Clin 5:255
4. Nelson DP, King CE, Dodd SL (1987) Systemic and intestinal limits of oxygen extraction in a dog during endotoxemia. J Appl Physiol 63:387
5. Shoemacker WC, Appel P, Kram HB, Waxman K, Lee TS (1988) Prospective trial of "supranormal" values of survivors as therapeutic goals and high risk surgical patients. Chest 94:1176

6. Tuchschmidt J, Fried J, Astiz M, Rackow E (1992) Elevation of cardiac output and oxygen delivery improves outcome in septic shock. Chest 102:216
7. Anderson RR, Holliday RL, Driedger AA, Lefcoe M, Reid B, Sibbald WJ (1979) Documentation of pulmonary capillary permeability in human adult respiratory distress syndrome (ARDS) secondary to sepsis. Am Rev Respir Dis 119:869
8. Judges D, Sharkey P, Cheng H, Craig I, Driedger AA, Sibbald WJ, Finley R (1986) Pulmonary microvascular fluid flux in a large model of sepsis: evidence for increased pulmonary endothelial permeability accompanying surgically induced peritonitis in sheep. Surgery 99:222
9. Hersch M, Gnidec A, Bersten AD, Troster M, Groom A, Sibbald WJ (1990) Histologic and ultrastructural changes in non-pulmonary organs during early hyperdynamic sepsis. Surgery 107:397
10. Harada H, Ishizaka A, Yonemaru M et al (1989) The effects of aminophylline and pentoxifylline on multiple organ damage after escherichia coli sepsis. Am Rev Respir Dis 140:974
11. Mitchell JP, Schuller P, Calardino FS, Schuster PP (1992) Improved outcome based on fluid management in critically ill patients requiring pulmonary artery catheterization. Am Rev Respir Dis 145:990
12. Metting PJ, Strader JR, Briton SL (1988) Evaluation of whole body autoregulation in conscious dogs. Am J Physiol 255:H44
13. Schaper J, Mulch J, Winkler B, Schaper W (1979) Ultrastructural, functional and biochemical criteria for estimation for reversibility of ischemic injury: a study on the effect of global ischemia on the isolated dog heart. J Mol Cell Cardiol 11:521
14. Laine GA, Allen SJ (1991) Left ventricular myocardial edema: lymph flow, interstitial fibrosis, and cardiac dysfunction. Circ Res 68:1713
15. Weg JG (1991) Oxygen transport in adult respiratory distress syndrome and other acute circulatory problems: the relationship of oxygen delivery and oxygen consumption. Crit Care Med 19:650
16. Office of Medical Applications Research (1988) Peri-operative red cell transfusion. JAMA 260:1700
17. Welch GH, Meehan KR, Goodnough LT (1992) Prudent strategies for red blood cell transfusion. Ann Intern Med 116:393
18. Cain RD (1990) Hemoglobin: how much is enough? Crit Care Med 18:1046
19. Chappler CK, Cain SM (1986) The physiologic reserve in oxygen carrying capacity: Studies in experimental hemodilution. Can J Physiol Pharmacol 64:7
20. Baer RW, Vlahakes GJ, Uhlig PN, Hoffman JIE (1987) Maximum myocardial oxygen transport during anemia and polycythemia in dogs. Am J Physiol (Heart Circ Physiol) 252:H908
21. Bersten AD, Gnidec A, Rutledge FS, Sibbald WJ (1990) Hyperdynamic sepsis modifies a PEEP-mediated redistribution in organ blood flows. Am Rev Respir Dis 141:1198

Influence of Catecholamines on Regional Perfusion and Tissue Oxygenation in Septic Shock Patients

A. Meier-Hellmann and K. Reinhart

Introduction

Multiple organ failure (MOF) is the major cause of death in patients with sepsis [1]. Macro- and microcirculatory maldistribution of blood flow to the tissues and hypoxia of certain organs play an important role in the pathogenesis of sepsis [2, 3]. In addition, an oxygen extraction deficit is at present being researched. Therefore a supranormal oxygen delivery (DO_2) is required to guarantee adequate tissue oxygenation [4, 5]. Sufficient volume substitution and treatment with catecholamines is usually required to achieve a supranormal DO_2 and an adequate systemic perfusion pressure. Despite this, the mortality rate of sepsis and the incidence of MOF remains persistantly high [6]. It is obvious that under the conditions of a supranormal DO_2 tissue hypoxia in different tissues may occur [2, 4]. Information regarding perfusion and oxygenation in different regions of the body is mandatory for the detection of regional tissue hypoxia. Intensive care regimens, particulary, treatment with catecholamines and their influence on perfusion and oxygenation in different organs and tissues, are not fully understood and require further investigation.

Renal and gastrointestinal failure are major complications in sepsis [7–9]. Bacterial translocation from the gut is considered by some authors to induce and maintain sepsis [10–12]. Nelson et al. [13] demonstrated that the critical DO_2 of the small intestine in septic sheep was higher than whole body DO_2. The achievement of critical whole body DO_2 does not exclude oxygen supply dependency in different tissues [13].

Previous studies do not confirm the reduction of splanchnic perfusion in sepsis. One reason for this may be that different methods were used to measure splanchnic perfusion [14]. In septic patients, Dahn et al. [15] demonstrated that splanchnic perfusion increased to the same extent as the cardiac output (CO), although the splanchnic oxygen consumption ($\dot{V}O_2hep$) increased to a far greater extent than whole body oxygen consumption ($\dot{V}O_2$). In experimental settings [16, 17] it has been reported that redistribution of blood flow and relative improvement of hepatic and small intestine perfusion occurrs. In healthy individuals, an infusion of endotoxin doubled splanchnic blood flow [18]. We found that 60% of the CO in septic patients was distributed through the splanchnic region, in comparison to 18%–30% in healthy individuals [19, 20].

Little is known about the influence of different catecholamines on regional blood flow and oxygenation [21, 22]. The catecholamines mostly used in the clinical setting, e.g., dobutamine, dopamine, norepinephrine, epinephrine, and dopexamine, were mostly investigated in patients without sepsis or not in septic shock (Tables 1, 2).

Dobutamine

Many authors suggest that due to its β 1 receptor mediated effects dobutamine is the catecholamine of choice for increasing myocardial contractility and achieving supranormal CO and DO_2 levels [23–26]. Animal investigations [27] and clinical studies [4, 28] have shown that an increase in DO_2 induced by dobutamine infusion leads to an increased $\dot{V}O_2$. Furthermore, it is hypothesized that the β 2 mediated effects counteract peripheral vasoconstriction and hence improve tissue oxygenation [26]. Under the conditions of an adequate volume replacement, dobutamine increases CO and DO_2 to a greater extent than dopamine [27]. Vincent et al [28] demonstrated that an infusion of dobutamine at 5 μg/kg/min in adequately volume replaced septic patients increases the DO_2 by 29% and $\dot{V}O_2$ by 18%. To our knowledge it is

Table 1. Effects of the different catecholamines on the different receptors

Catecholamine	α 1	α 2	β 1	β 2	DA 1	DA 2
Dobutamine	++	0	+++	++	0	0
Epinephrine	+++	+++	++	+++	0	0
Norepinephrine	+++	+++	++	+	0	0
Dopamine						
0–3 μg/kg/min	0	+	0	0	+++	++
2–10 μg/kg/min	+	+	++	+	++	++
>10 μg/kg/min	++	++	++	+	+	+
Dopexamine	0	0	+	+++	++	+

Table 2. Effects of the different catecholamines on regional blood flow

Catecholamine	Kidney	Brain	Heart	Splanchnic	Muscle	Skin
Dobutamine	+	+	+	+	++	+
Epinephrine	−/+	+	+	−/+	+/0	−
Norepinephrine	−/+	+	+	−/+	−/0	0
Dopamine						
0–3 μg/kg/min	+++	+	0	+++	0	0
2–10 μg/kg/min	++/+	+	+	++/+	0	0
>10 μg/kg/min	−/+	+	+	−/+	−	−
Dopexamine	+++	+	+	+++	+	+

not clear whether dobutamine selectively influences splanchnic or renal perfusion. Improvement in splanchnic oxygenation is supported by the results of Silverman et al. [29], who found that infusion of dobutamine at 5 μg/kg/min increased a pathologically reduced gastric mucosal pH (pHi). In contrast, blood transfusion did not influence pHi but increased DO_2 to a similar extent. In septic pigs Schneider et al. [30] found that adequate volume substitution alone restored a decreased CO and led to redistribution of blood flow in favor of the splanchnic region. An additional infusion of dobutamine did not influence the distribution of blood flow to the kidneys and the splanchnic region. In patients with congestive heart failure, Leier [31] found that those who received dobutamine at 7.5 μg/kg/min experienced an increase in CO accompanied by a decrease in splanchnic perfusion. In the same study renal perfusion was increased to a lesser extent than CO. Mousdale et al. [32] were able to measure only a minor increase in renal blood flow under dobutamine and dopexamine. However, different doses of dopamine induced remarkable increases in renal blood flow.

In conclusion, if dobutamine is used to increase DO_2 there is some evidence of an improvement in tissue oxygenation. Whether dobutamine selectively influences regional blood flow is unknown. Management of septic shock with dobutamine alone is often not sufficient to restore adequate blood pressure. Whether the combination of dobutamine and norepinephrine is superior to the treatment with dopamine alone has not yet been investigated.

Norepinephrine

Norepinephrine has only moderate β 1 and β 2 mimetic effects. In experimental models it increases splanchnic vascular resistance and decreases splanchnic blood flow [33]. Norepinephrine is used in animal studies to induce renal failure [34]. Consequently, norepinephrine is often only used as a last resort if hemodynamic stabilization is not achieved with other catecholamines [35].

Melchior et al. [36] found that an infusion of 0.5 and 1.0 μg/kg/min norepinephrine did not change whole body $\dot{V}O_2$ despite an increased cardiac index (CI) and mean arterial pressure (MAP). They drew the conclusion that the beneficial β mimetic effects of norepinephrine outweigh the possible deleterious effects mediated by α receptors. In septic dogs, Bakker and Vincent [37] demonstrated an increase of right and left ventricular stroke work index with an infusion of norepinephrine ranging from 0.1 to 0.2 μg/kg/min and an increase of DO_2 and $\dot{V}O_2$ with an infusion of norepinephrine from 0.5 to 1.0 μg/kg/min. Schneider et al. [30] recommended norepinephrine in favor of dobutamine for the treatment of right heart failure in septic shock since an increase in diastolic blood pressure improves myocardial perfusion. Schreuder et al. [38] reported that a norepinephrine infusion in patients in septic shock increased $\dot{V}O_2$ but did not change the DO_2. However it remains unknown whether the increase in $\dot{V}O_2$ in caused by an improvement in perfusion pressure which increased simultaneously from 57 mm Hg to 75 mm Hg. This finding underlines the importance of an adequate perfusion pressure and shows that treatment with norepinephrine is indicated if an adequate perfusion pressure cannot be maintained with volume substitution and dobutamine or dopamine. In six patients with septic shock in whom hemodynamic stabilization by dopamine or dobutamine infusion was not achieved, DO_2 and $\dot{V}O_2$ values were inconsistent when they were treated with norepinephrine [39]. In our own investigations [40], the change in catecholamine treatment from dobutamine to norepinephrine in patients with septic shock led to a decrease in DO_2 but $\dot{V}O_2$ remained unchanged. The unchanged $\dot{V}O_2$ can be explained by an unchanged tissue oxygenation. However, redistribution of blood flow with norepinephrine treatment alone, undetected by the measurement of the global O_2 transport related variables, cannot be excluded.

Different authors have demonstrated an increase in urine output in patients with septic shock treated with norepinephrine [41–43]. However, it should be emphasized that these patients had markedly decreased blood pressures. In the study from Desjars et al. [41] the infusion of 0.5–1.0 μg/kg/min norepinephrine increased the MAP from 48 mm Hg to 62 mm Hg. Hesselvik and Brodin [42] reported an increase in MAP from 50 mm Hg to 69 mm Hg after the infusion of 0.5 μg/kg/min norepinephrine. The principal mechanism of improved renal function in these studies is the increase of perfusion pressure to an adequate level. Redl-Wenzl et al. [44] reported an increase in the creatinine clearance after treatment with norepinephrine in 56 patients with septic shock. However, in this study the patients also had an inadequate perfusion pressure of 56 mm Hg before treatment with norepinephrine. There is a lack of kowledge about whether treatment with norepinephrine has beneficial effects on the renal function in the presence of an adequate perfusion pressure. Fukuoka et al. [45] reported in septic patients with lactate levels in a normal range that a norepinephrine infusion increased urine output and did not change creatinine clearance, whereas in patients with elevated lactate levels norepinephrine had no effect on urine output but decreased creatinine clearance.

The findings concerning the effects of norepinephrine on splanchnic perfusion are inconsistent. Bersten et al. [46] compared the effects of different catecholamines on regional blood flow in septic and nonseptic sheep. In the nonseptic animals there was a redistribution of blood flow measured by microsphere technique to the heart away from brain, kidneys, liver and pancreas with norepinephrine, dobutamine, dopamine, dopexamine or salbutamol treatment. A deleterious effect of norepinephrine on splanchnic perfusion is demonstrated in this study. In contrast, in septic animals the reported redistribution of regional blood flow was not found. The authors explained these findings by a decreased sensibility of α receptors and a direct sepsis associated vasodilation [47–51].

Schneider et al. [30] infused pigs with *Escherichia coli* and stabilized the animals initially only by volume substitution. Further treatment with dobutamine or norepinephrine did not influence the distribution of the given volume. Measured with radiolabeled erythrocytes, there was a decreased pooling of blood in the legs after norepinephrine infusion. Breslow et al. [52] infused pigs with *E. coli* and kept the pulmonary capillary wedge pressure within the normal range by infusing isotonic solutions. Under these conditions norepinephrine, dopamine and phenylepinephrine given in doses to achieve MAP of 75 mm Hg were without selective effects on regional blood flow.

In our investigation [53] in patients with septic shock, the hepatic venous O_2 saturation ($Sh\bar{v}O_2$) decreased rapidly by changing the catecholamine management from dobutamine to norepinephrine, whereas the mixed venous O_2 saturation ($S\bar{v}O_2$) decreased only slightly. The difference therefore between $S\bar{v}O_2$ and $Sh\bar{v}O_2$ increased significanctly (Fig. 1). This effect may be explained due to a decrease in splanchnic perfusion mediated by intestinal α receptors [33, 54, 55]. This finding is in contrast to the reported animal studies [46] which demonstrated unchanged splanchnic perfusion with norepinephrine. In our study the selective decrease in $Sh\bar{v}O_2$ could be a marker for a deterioration in splanchnic oxygenation. To demonstrate this interpretation of a changed $Sh\bar{v}O_2$ the splanchnic blood flow has to be measured and the DO_2 and $\dot{V}O_2$ in the splanchnic region have to be calculated.

We measured the splanchnic blood flow in ten patients with septic shock by the green dye dilution technique. After changing the catecholamine treatment from a combination of dobutamine with norepinephrine to norepinephrine alone we observed the previously reported changes in $S\bar{v}O_2$ and

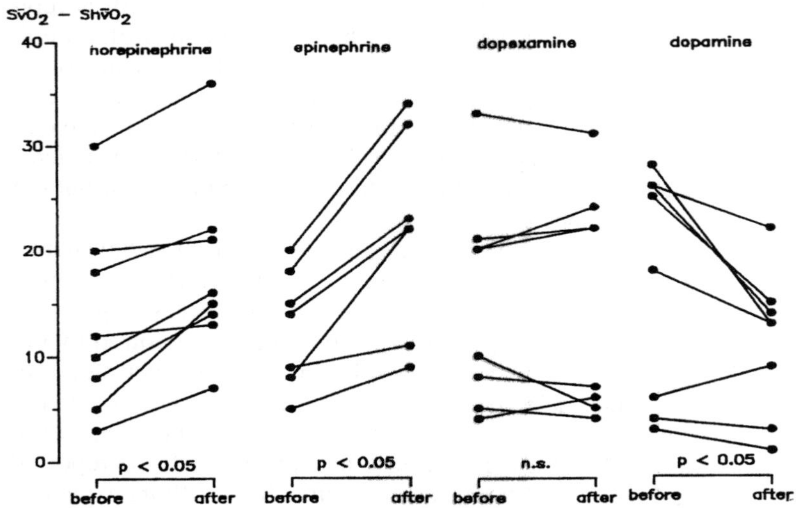

Fig. 1. Effects of norepinephrine, epinephrine, dopexamine and dopamine on the difference between mixed venous O_2 saturation (*$S\bar{v}O_2$*) and hepatic venous O_2 saturation (*$Sh\bar{v}O_2$*)

$Sh\bar{v}O_2$. Treatment with norepinephrine alone led to a parallel decrease in splanchnic perfusion and CO. The relationship between splanchnic perfusion and CO remained unchanged. Furthermore, the splanchnic $\dot{V}O_2$ remained unchanged (Table 3). Due to the decrease in splanchnic DO_2 hepatic venous O_2 extraction increased. Therefore, in situations where there is a further decrease in splanchnic DO_2, there is an increased risk that splanchnic $\dot{V}O_2$ becomes supply dependent with norepinephrine treatment alone.

In conclusion it should be pointed out that treatment with vasopressors is often indispensable in the therapeutical management of septic shock. Provided that the DO_2 is in a supranormal range, treatment with norepinephrine alone is without negative tissue oxygenation effects. Animal studies have shown that the negative effect of norepinephrine on splanchnic perfusion is only seen in nonseptic conditions.

Epinephrine

Epinephrine is advocated in the treatment of septic shock [56–58] because it leads to a β receptor mediated increase in CO and an α receptor mediated increase in perfusion pressure. Low doses of epinephrine have predominantly β mimetic effects and only in higher doses do the α mimetic effects become predominant [59]. Bollaert et al. [56] investigated the effects of epinephrine in doses between 0.5 and 1.0 μg/kg/min in 13 patients with septic shock that could not be stabilized by 15 μg/kg/min dopamine. Epinephrine increased MAP, systemic vascular resistance and CO in these patients. Furthermore the DO_2 and $\dot{V}O_2$ increased. Elevated arterial lactate levels were

Table 3. Effects of changing catecholamine treatment from a combination of dobutamine with norepinephrine to norepinephrine alone

	Dobutamine/ norephinephrine	Norepinephrine alone	Significance
DO_2 (ml/min/m^2)	796 ±151	598 ±113	*
$\dot{V}O_2$ (ml/min/m^2)	159 ± 27	152 ± 26	n.s.
CI (l/min/m^2)	6.0 ± 1.2	4.3 ± 0.8	*
DO_2hep (ml/min/m^2)	210 ±108	171 ± 88	*
$\dot{V}O_2$hep (ml/min/m^2)	77 ± 41	72 ± 21	n.s.
HBF (l/min/m^2)	1.6 ± 0.8	1.1 ± 0.6	*
DO_2/DO_2hep	4.3 ± 1.4	4.1 ± 1.7	n.s.
$\dot{V}O_2$/$\dot{V}O_2$hep	4.9 ± 2.5	4.8 ± 1.3	n.s.
CI/HBF	4.3 ± 1.4	4.1 ± 1.7	n.s.
$S\bar{v}O_2$ (%)	76 ± 4	71 ± 6	*
$Sh\bar{v}O_2$ (%)	58 ± 13	49 ± 15	*

DO_2, oxygen delivery; $\dot{V}O_2$, oxygen consumption; CI, cardiac index; DO_2hep, splanchnic oxygen delivery; $\dot{V}O_2$hep, splanchnic oxygen consumption; HBF, hepatic blood flow; $S\bar{v}O_2$, mixed venous O_2 saturation; $Sh\bar{v}O_2$, hepatic venous O_2 saturation; *, statistically significant; n.s., not significant.

interpreteted as a metabolic effect due to epinephrine. Moran et al. [60] reported an increase in DO_2 from 481 to 531 ml/min/m^2 and an increase in $\dot{V}O_2$ from 165 to 193 ml/min/m^2 with an epinephrine infusion in doses up to 18 μg/kg/min in patients with septic shock. According to the dose dependent effects of epinephrine both a reduction [61–63] and an improvement [64] of splanchnic perfusion are reported in animal studies. Little is known about the effects of epinephrine on splanchnic and renal perfusion in septic shock states.

In our investigations, changing the catecholamine treatment from a combination of dobutamine and norepinephrine to epinephrine alone decreased the $Sh\bar{v}O_2$ but did not change the $S\bar{v}O_2$, so the difference between the two was significantly increased [53]. Dahn et al. [65] reported a parallel decrease in $Sh\bar{v}O_2$ and $S\bar{v}O_2$ under hypoxia. In contrast, in 33 patients undergoing liver surgery the $Sh\bar{v}O_2$ decreased and the $S\bar{v}O_2$ did not change after skin incision [66]. The authors explained this discrepancy as being a selective decrease in splanchnic perfusion mediated by endogeneous catecholamines liberated following skin incision. The selective decrease in $Sh\bar{v}O_2$ seems to be a marker for deterioration in splanchnic oxygenation. We measured splanchnic perfusion, DO_2 and $\dot{V}O_2$ in three patients with septic shock treated with epinephrine. Figure 2 demonstrates the changes in DO_2 and $\dot{V}O_2$ during the change of catecholamine treatment from a combination of dobutamine and norepinephrine to epinephrine alone. MAP was maintained during the change. Epinephrine decreased the splanchnic perfusion in the presence of

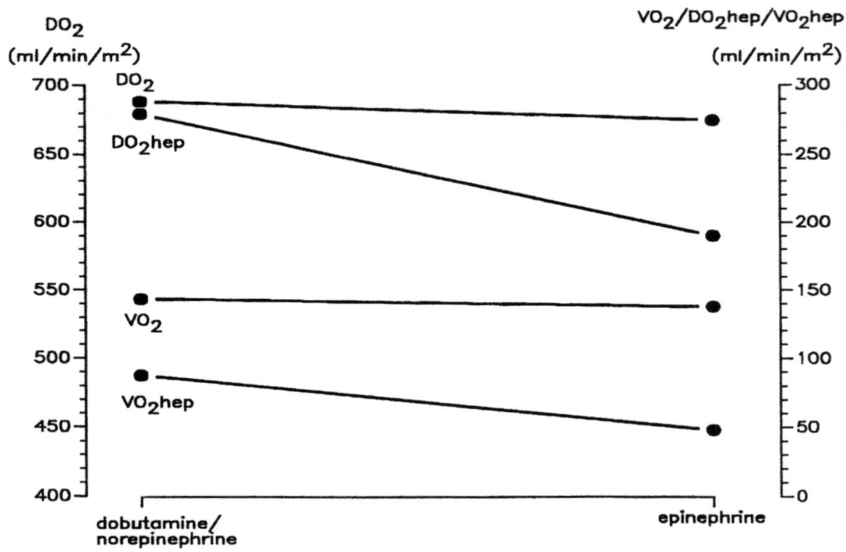

Fig. 2. Change in catecholamine treatment from dobutamine with norepinephrine to epinephrine alone. Effects on oxygen delivery (*DO_2*), oxygen consumption (*$\dot{V}O_2$*), splanchnic oxygen delivery (*DO_2hep*), and splanchnic oxygen consumption (*$\dot{V}O_2hep$*)

an unchanged CO. The decreased splanchnic DO_2 lead to a decreased splanchnic $\dot{V}O_2$. These extreme changes in splanchnic oxygenation were not detected by whole body DO_2 and $\dot{V}O_2$, underlying the importance of measuring DO_2 and $\dot{V}O_2$ in specific regions. Furthermore, the increase in lactate levels and the decrease in pHi indicates tissue hypoxia in the splanchnic region (Fig. 3).

Due to the lack of information regarding epinephrine in the treatment of septic shock a closing statement is not possible. Our investigation with preliminary results has demonstrated a decrease in splanchnic perfusion and oxygenation accompanied by signs of severe tissue hypoxia. If further investigations also demonstrate these negative effects, the use of epinephrine in patients with septic shock cannot be recommended.

Dopamine

Dopamine has effects on α, β and dopaminergic receptors. The dopaminergic receptors can be divided into presynaptic (DA1) and postsynaptic (DA2) receptors. Stimulation of DA1 receptors causes renal and splanchnic vasodilation. Stimulation of DA2 receptors blocks norepinephrine output from sympathetic nerves [67].

Dopaminergic receptors are found in renal, mesenteric and hepatic vessels [67]. The effects of dopamine are dose dependent. In doses up to 3 μg/kg/min, dopamine selectively stimulates the dopaminergic receptors. In doses up to

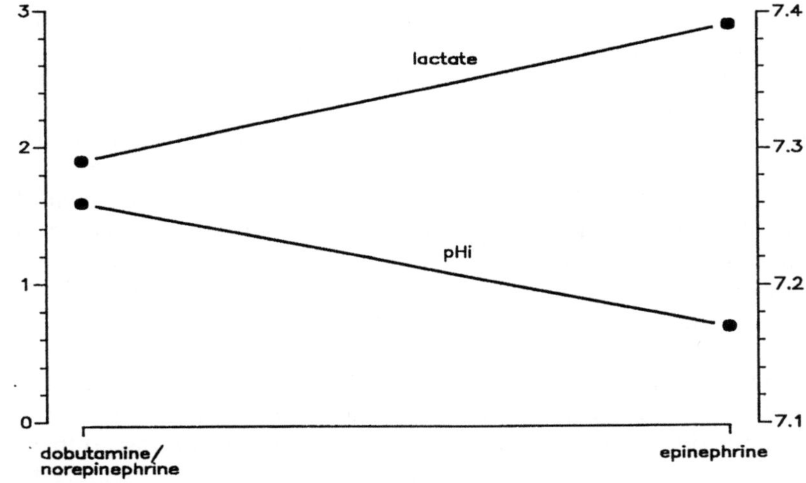

Fig. 3. Change in catecholamine treatment from dobutamine with norepinephrine to epinephrine alone. Effects on lactate and gastric mucosal pH (*pHi*)

5 μg/kg/min there is stimulation of β receptors and in doses greater than 5 μg/kg/min the α receptors are also stimulated.

Vincent and Preiser [68] advocate dopamine as the drug of choice in the primary management of decreased MAP, present in patients in septic shock. It is the opinion of other authors that the α mimetic effects of dopamine are a disadvantage because a previously disturbed microcirculation could be further compromised [26, 27]. In 437 critical care patients Shoemaker et al. [35] more fequently induced an increase of DO_2 and $\dot{V}O_2$ with dobutamine than with dopamine. In brain dead patients treatment with dopamine to elevate MAP to within a normal range caused a lower mitochondrial redox state in liver cells than in patients with a lower MAP who were not treated with dopamine [69]. This effect of dopamine can be interpreted as a hypoxia mediated organ failure.

Dopamine in low doses is often recommended as an additional drug for the improvement of renal function and splanchnic perfusion. Nevertheless it is not proven that treatment with low dose dopamine is beneficial to patients in septic shock.

In animals and healthy humans an increase is demonstrated in the inulin clearance, renal plasma flow and sodium excretion after dopamine infusion [67]. Mousdale et al. [32] demonstrated that dopamine in doses of 2.5, 5.0 and 10.0 μg/kg/min induced a significantly higher renal plasma flow than dobutamine in a similar dose and dopexamine in doses of 1.0, 2.0 and 4.0 μg/kg/min in healthy humans. The effects of dopamine on renal function in patients with septic shock is not completely understood. It is not known if dopamine influences the incidence of renal failure in septic shock patients.

Dopamine improved a decreased hepatic blood flow in dogs ventilated with positive end-expiratory pressure [70]. In septic rats dopamine induced a selective improvement of hepatic blood flow [71]. An increase in hepatic blood flow does not guarantee improved splanchnic oxygenation because a redistribution of blood flow in the splanchnic area may lead to a deterioration in tissue oxygenation. Giraud et al. [54] infused dogs with dopamine and were able to measure an increase in blood flow in the superior mesenteric artery and in the muscularis of the gut with a decreased blood flow to the gut mucosa accompanied by a decrease in splanchnic $\dot{V}O_2$. The improvement of global blood flow measured in a major artery seems to be accompanied by a deterioration of blood flow and oxygenation in other tissues such as the gut mucosa. Pawlik et al. [72] demonstrated that intraarterial infusion of dopamine 1 μg/kg/min in dogs caused splanchnic vasoconstriction with reduction of blood flow and splanchnic $\dot{V}O_2$. In the same investigation epinephrine also led to a reduction in splanchnic blood flow but did not influence the splanchnic $\dot{V}O_2$. Therefore the authors suggested that dopamine is a drug with deleterious side effects on splanchnic oxygenation. In contrast to these findings Kullmann et al. [73] showed an increased blood flow to the intestinal organs and an improved perfusion of the mucosa and submucosa in rabbits measured by microsphere technique. Leier [31] reported in congestive heart failure patients that 3 μg/kg/min dopamine significantly increased renal blood flow and did not change splanchnic blood flow. In nonseptic pigs Roytblat et al. [74] measured a dose independent increase in splanchnic DO_2 and a dose dependent increase in splanchnic $\dot{V}O_2$ after dopamin infusion. Since higher doses of dopamin increase splanchnic $\dot{V}O_2$ to a greater extent than splanchnic DO_2 the authors conclude that dopamine did not improve splanchnic oxygenation and explained the increased splanchnic $\dot{V}O_2$ as a calorigenic effect of dopamine [75–77].

In our studies the addition of 2.8–3.0 μg/kg/min dopamine to norepinephrine increased $Sh\bar{v}O_2$ more than $S\bar{v}O_2$. The difference between the two became smaller after dopamine infusion. On one hand this finding correlates with the reported improvement of splanchnic blood flow under dopamine [70, 78, 79]. On the other hand, there is no guarantee that the increased $Sh\bar{v}O_2$ is not the result of a decreased splanchnic $\dot{V}O_2$. In some individuals we observed an increase in splanchnic $\dot{V}O_2$ with low dose dopamine. This occurred if dopamine was added to norepinephrine (Fig. 4) and also if dopamine was added to dobutamine (Fig. 5). However further investigations are required to confirm the effects of dopamine.

Whether management with a higher dose of dopamine alone compared to the combination of dobutamine and norepinephrine is of advantage in the treatment of septic shock has not yet proven. The improvement of renal function is an argument for the use of low dose dopamine although under the conditions of septic shock there are only few and nonequivocal studies.

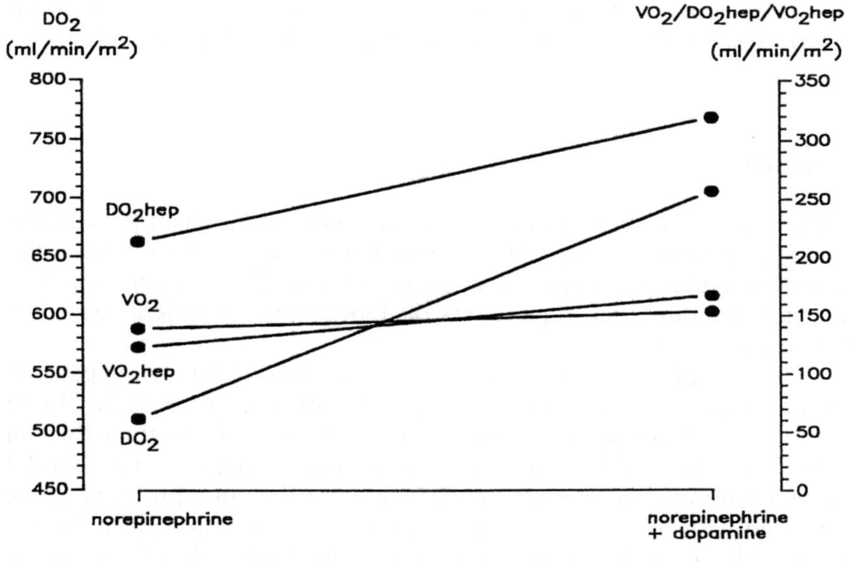

Fig. 4. Addition of low dose dopamine to norepinephrine. Effects on oxygen delivery (*DO_2*), oxygen consumption (*$\dot{V}O_2$*), splanchnic oxygen delivery (*DO_2hep*), and splanchnic oxygen consumption (*$\dot{V}O_2hep$*)

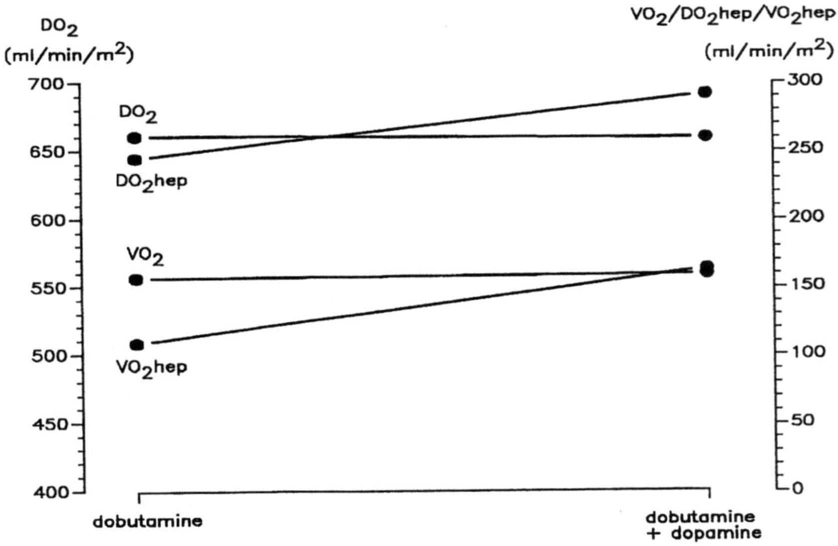

Fig. 5. Addition of low dose dopamine to dobutamine. Effects on oxygen delivery (*DO_2*), oxygen consumption (*$\dot{V}O_2$*), splanchnic oxygen delivery (*DO_2hep*), and splanchnic oxygen consumption (*$\dot{V}O_2hep$*)

Animal studies reported deleterious effects of dopamine on splanchnic oxygenation. One study demonstrated an increased splanchnic $\dot{V}O_2$ after dopamine infusion while it remained unclear if the increased $\dot{V}O_2$ is the result of improved oxygenation or only the calorigenic effect of dopamine.

Dopexamine

The relatively new catecholamine dopexamine has predominant β 2 and dopaminergic receptor activity. Many animal and human studies have described the usefulness of dopexamine in heart failure [80–83]. Tan et al. [84] demonstrated a direct inotropic effect of dopexamine in patients with low output cardiac failure.

To date, only a few studies examining the effect of dopexamine in patients with septic shock exist. Colardyn et al. [85] reported an increase in CI and heart rate and a decrease in systemic vascular resistance. Unfortunately data regarding the DO_2 and $\dot{V}O_2$ were not mentioned. Cain and Curtis [86] did not note a difference in mesenteric venous blood flow in a group of septic dogs treated with dopexamine and a control group without catecholamine treatment. The gut of the dopexamine treated animals produced less lactate and the authors concluded that dopexamine caused gut mucosa to be preferentially perfused. Biro et al. [87] measured a relatively higher skeletal muscle and gastric blood flow in nonseptic dogs with dopexamine than with dobutamine. In dogs in hemorrhagic shock Lokhandwala and Jandhyala [88] demonstrated an increase in splanchnic perfusion to 40%–50% from baseline after blood retransfusion, whereas splanchnic perfusion increased to 80%–90% of baseline if dopexamine was added to the transfusion.

In our studies the addition of 4.0 μg/kg/min dopexamine did not influence the difference between $S\bar{v}O_2$ and $Sh\bar{v}O_2$. This finding is in agreement with Leier who reported in patients with heart failure that an increase of CO accompanied an increase in splanchnic perfusion.

To date, little is known concerning the effects of dopexamine on renal blood flow in patients with septic shock. Dopexamine increased urine output in both healthy and patients with heart failure [89]. In comparison with dopamine there is no further increase in urine output in patients undergoing hepatic surgery [90]. Stephan et al. [91] demonstrated a more profound decrease in renal vascular resistance under dopamine as under dopexamine in patients with cardiac surgery. The increase in renal blood flow was to the same extent as the increase in CO. The authors therefore conclude that a selective dopaminergic effect of dopexamine is not proven. Magrini et al. [92] reported an increase in renal blood flow to a higher extent than the increased CO in patients with hypertension. Mousdale et al. [32] demonstrated that dopamine in doses of 2.5, 5.0, and 10.0 μg/kg/min increased renal plasma flow more than dopexamine in doses of 1.0, 2.0, and 4.0 μg/kg/min.

In conclusion, there are some references which recommend dopexamine to improve splanchnic oxygenation and renal function. Further studies are required to prove the usefulness of dopexamine in the treatment of septic shock patients and compare the effects with those of low dose dopamine.

Conclusion

Few controversial studies exist regarding effects of the different catecholamines on regional blood flow. Therefore a clear recommendation for a specific catecholamine regimen in septic shock is lacking. Furthermore, it is unknown whether the choice of a specific catecholamine in the treatment of septic shock influences the patient's outcome. It is suggested that an increase in DO_2 within a supranormal range is associated with an improved patient outcome [93–95].

A fundamental step in the treatment of septic shock is adequate volume substitution. In our studies we demonstrated that consequent volume treatment improves pHi [96]. Figure 6 demonstrates the change in whole body DO_2 and $\dot{V}O_2$ and splanchnic DO_2 and $\dot{V}O_2$ in a patient in septic shock after the infusion of 1800 ml colloid, this increases the pulmonary capillary wedge pressure from 12 mm Hg to 17 mm Hg. The increase in whole body and splanchnic $\dot{V}O_2$ underlines the importance of adequate volume substitution.

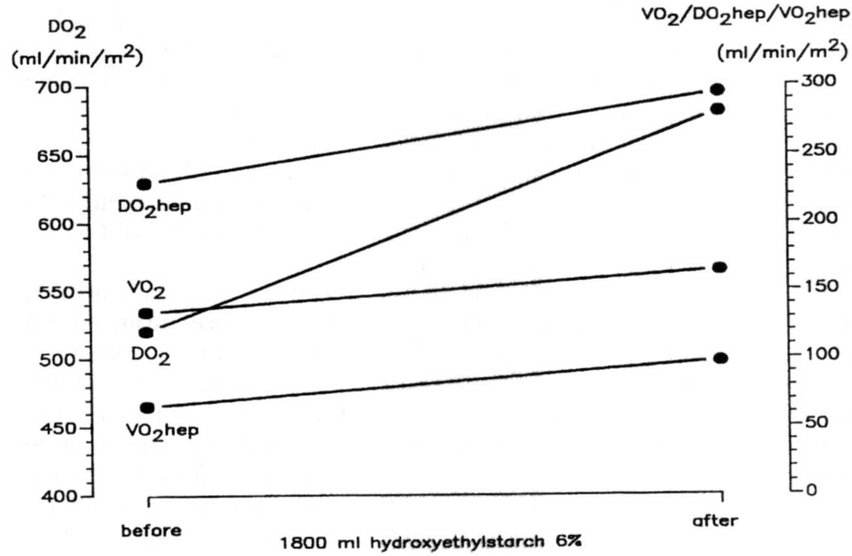

Fig. 6. Effects of volume management with 1800 ml hydroxyethylstarch (6%) on oxygen delivery (*DO_2*), oxygen consumption (*$\dot{V}O_2$*), splanchnic oxygen delivery (*DO_2hep*), and splanchnic oxygen consumption (*$\dot{V}O_2hep$*)

In most patients, the use of vasopressors is indispensable because adequate hemodynamic perfusion pressure is mandatory. The negative effects of vasopressors on splanchnic perfusion are known from studies carried out under nonseptic conditions. Norepinephrine and dopamine in doses of 10 µg/kg/min in septic animals are without negative effects on splanchnic perfusion. Preliminary results show a decrease in splanchnic oxygenation in patients with septic shock treated with epinephrine.

Catecholamines with β mimetic effects are often used to increase DO_2. The question as to whether dobutamine or dopamine should be primarily used in treatment of septic shock cannot be answered yet.

Whether treatment with low dose dopamine or dopexamine actually improves renal function and splanchnic oxygenation is the purpose of ongoing studies.

References

1. Fiddian-Green RG (1991) Role of gut in shock and resuscitation. In: Stoutenbeck CP, van Saene HKF (eds) Infection and the anesthetist, vol 5 (1). Bailliere Tindall/Saunders, London, pp 75–99
2. Schumacker P, Cain S (1987) The concept of a critical oxygen delivery. Intensive Care Med 13:223–229

3. Sibbald WJ, Bersten A, Rutledge FS (1989) The role of tissue hypoxia in multiple organ failure. In: Reinhart K, Eyrich K (eds) Clinical aspects of oxygen transport and tissue oxygenation. Springer, Berlin Heidelberg New York, pp 102–114
4. Gilbert EM, Haupt MT, Mandanas RY, Huaringa AJ, Carlson RW (1986) The effect of fluid loading, blood transfusion, and catecholamine infusion on oxygen delivery and consumption in patients with sepsis. Am Rev Respir Dis 134:873–878
5. Kaufman BS, Rackow EC, Falk JL (1984) The relationship between oxygen delivery and consumption during fluid resuscitation of hypovolemic and septic shock. Chest 85, 3:337–340
6. Parker MM, Parillo JF (1983) Septic shock. Hemodynamics and pathogenesis. JAMA 250:3324–3327
7. Fry DE, Pearlstein L, Fulton RL (1980) Multiple-system organ failure: the role of uncontrolled infection. Arch Surg 115:136–140
8. Lucas CE (1976) The renal response to acute injury and sepsis. Surg Clin North Am 56:953–975
9. Tran DD, Groeneveld ABJ, van der Meulen J et al (1990) Age, chronic disease, sepsis, organ system failure, and mortality in a medical intensive care unit. Crit Care Med 18:474–479
10. Deitch EA, Berg R, Specian R (1987) Endotoxin promotes the translocation of bacteria from the gut. Arch Surg 122:185–190
11. Marshall JC, Christou NV, Horn R et al (1988) The microbiology of multiple organ gailure: the proximal GI tract as an occult reservoir of pathogens. Arch Surg 123:309–315
12. Meakins JL, Marshall JC (1989) The gut as the motor of multiple system organ failure. In: Marston A, Bulkley GB, Fiddian Green RG et al (eds) Splanchnic ischemia and multiple organ failure. Mosby, St Louis, pp 339–348
13. Nelson DP, Samsel RW, Wood LD, Schumacker PT (1988) Pathologic supply dependence of systemic and intestinal O_2 uptake during endotoxemia. J Appl Physiol 64:2410–2419
14. Dahn MS, Lange P, Lobdell K, Hans B, Jacobs LA, Mitchel RA (1989) Hepatic blood flow and splanchnic oxygen consumption measurements in clinical sepsis. Surgery 107:295–301
15. Dahn MS, Lange P, Lobdell K, Hans B, Jacobs LA, Mitchell RA (1987) Splanchnic und total body oxygen consumption differences in septic and injured patients. Surgery 101:69–80
16. Lang CH, Bagby GJ, Ferguson JL, Spitzer JJ (1984) Cardiac output and redistribution of organ blood flow in hypermetabolic sepsis. Am J Physiol 246 R:331–337
17. Wang P, Ba ZF, Chaudry IH (1991) Hepatic extraction of indocyanine green is depressed early in sepsis despite increased hepatic blood flow and cardiac output. Arch Surg 126:219–224
18. Fong Y, Marano MA, Moldawer LL et al (1990) The acute splanchnic and peripheral tissue metabolic response to endotoxin in humans. J Clin Invest 85:1896–1904
19. Johnson GA, McNamara JJ (1981) Organ ischemia after hemorrhagic shock. Surg Forum 32:24–26
20. Leevy CM, George W, Lesko W et al (1961) Observations on hepatic oxygen metabolism in man. JAMA 178:565–567
21. Brown RS, Carey JS, Mohr PA, Monson DO, Shoemaker WC (1966) Comparative evaluation of sympathomimetic amines in clinical shock. Circulation 34:260–271
22. Sibbald WJ, Calvin JE et al (1983) Concepts in the pharmacologic and nonpharmacologic support of cardiovascular function in critically ill surgical patients. Surg Clin North Am 63:456–465
23. Dhainaut JF, Edwards JD, Grootendorst AF et al (1990) Practical aspects of oxygen transport: conclusions and recommendations of the Round Table Conference. Intensive Care Med 16:179–180
24. Reinhart K, Hannemann L, Kuss B (1990) Optimal levels of O_2 delivery in the critically ill. Intensive Care Med 16:149–154

25. Shoemaker WC, Appel PL, Kram HB, Bishop M, Abraham E (1993) Hemodynamic and oxygen transport monitoring to titrate therapy in septic shock. New Horizons 1:145–159
26. Shoemaker WC, Appel PL, Kram HB, Duarte D, Harrier D, Ocampo HA (1989) Comparison of hemodynamic and oxygen transport effects of dopamine and dobutamine in critically ill surgical patients. Chest 96:120–126
27. Vincent JL, van der Linden P, Domb M, Blecic S, Azimi G, Bernard A (1987) Dopamine compared with dobutamine in experimental septic shock: relevance to fluid administration. Anesth Analg 66:565–571
28. Vincent JL, Roman A, Kahn RJ (1990) Dobutamine administration in septic shock: addition to a standard protocol. Crit Care Med 18:689–693
29. Silverman HJ, Tuma P (1992) Gastric tonometry in patients with sepsis. Effects of dobutamine infusions and packed red blood cell transfusions. Chest 102:184–188
30. Schneider AJ, Groeneveld ABJ, Teule GJJ, Nauta J, Heidendal GAK, Thijs LG (1987) Volume expansion, dobutamine and noradrenaline for treatment of right ventrikular dysfunction in porcine septic shock: a combined invasive and radionuclide study. Circ Shock 23:93–106
31. Leier CV (1988) Regional blood flow responses to vasodilators and inotropes in congestive heart failure. Am J Cardiol 62:86E–93E
32. Mousdale S, Clyburn PA, Mackie AM, Groves ND, Rosen M (1988) Comparison of the effects of dopamine, dobutamine, and dopexamine upon renal blood flow: a study in normal healthy volunteers. Br J Clin Pharmacol 25:555–560
33. Granger DN, Richardson PDI, Kvietys PR, Mortillaro NA (1980) Intestinal blood flow. Gastroenterology 78:837–863
34. Mills LC, Moyer JH, Handley CA (1960) Effects of various sympathicomimetic drugs on renal hemodynamics in normotensive and hypotensive dogs. Am J Physiol 198:1279
35. Shoemaker WC, Appel PL, Kram HB (1991) Oxygen transport measurements to evaluate tissue perfusion and titrate therapy: dobutamine and dopamine effects. Crit Care Med 19:672–688
36. Melchior JC, Pinaud M, Blanloeil Y, Bourreli B, Potel G, Souron R (1987) Hemodynamic effects of continuous norepinephrine infusion in dog with and without hyperkinetic endotoxic shock. Crit Care Med 15:687–691
37. Bakker J, Vincent JL (1993) Effects of norepinephrine and dobutamine on oxygen transport and consumption in a dog model of endotoxic shock. Crit Care Med 21:425–432
38. Schreuder WO, Schneider AJ, Groeneveld ABJ, Thijs LG (1989) Effect of dopamine vs norepinephrine on hemodynamics in septic shock. Emphasis on right ventricular performance. Chest 95:1282–1288
39. Meadows D, Edwards JD, Wilkins RG, Nightingale P (1988) Reversal of intractable septic shock with norepinephrine therapy. Crit Care Med 16:663–666
40. Specht M, Meier-Hellmann A, Hannemann L, Spies C, Wirbelauer Ch, Heil Th, Reinhart K (1993) Effects of dobutamine vs norepinephrine therapy on oxygen supply and oxygen consumption in septic patients. Crit Care Med 21:S276
41. Desjars P, Pinaud M, Potel G, Tasseau F, Touze MD (1987) A reappraisal of norepinephrine in human septic shock. Crit Care Med 15:134–137
42. Hesselvik JF, Brodin B (1989) Low dose norepinephrine in patients with septic shock and oliguria: effects on afterload, urine flow, and oxygen transport. Crit Care Med 17:179–180
43. Martin C, Eon B, Saux P, Aknin P, Gouin F (1990) Renal effects of norepinephrine used to treat septic shock patients. Crit Care Med 18:282–285
44. Redl-Wenzl EM, Armbruster C, Edelmann G, Fischl E, Kolacny M, Wechsler-Fördös A, Sporn P (1993) The effects of norepinephrine on hemodynamics and renal function in severe septic shock states. Intensive Care Med 19:151–154
45. Fukuoka T, Nishimura M, Imanaka H, Taenaka N, Yoshiya I, Takezawa J (1989) Effects of norepinephrine on renal function in septic patients with normal and elevated lactate levels. Crit Care Med 17:1104–1107

46. Bersten AD, Hersch M. Cheung H, Rutledge FS, Sibbald WJ (1992) The effect of various sympathomimetics on the regional circulations in hyperdynamic sepsis. Surgery 112:549–561
47. Baker CH, Wilmoth FR (1984) Microvascular responses to E. coli endotoxin with altered adrenergic activity. Circ Shock 12:165–176
48. Gray GA, Furman BL, Parratt JR (1990) Endotoxin-induced impairment of vascular reactivity in the pithed rat: role of arachidonic acid metabolites. Circ Shock 31:395–406
49. Hollenberg SM, Cunnion RE, Parrillo JE (1992) Effect of septic serum on vascular smooth muscle: In vitro studies using rat aortic rings. Crit Care Med 20:993–998
50. Kato T, Hayashi K, Takamizawa K (1988) Response of femoral arteries to norepinephrine following endotoxicosis. Circ Shock 26:383–390
51. Seaman KL, Greenway CV (1984) Loss of hepatic venous responsiveness after endotoxin in anesthetized cats. Am J Physiol 246:H658–H663
52. Breslow MJ, Miller CF, Parker SD, Walman AT, Traystman RJ (1987) Effect of vasopressors on organ blood flow during endotoxin shock in pigs. Am J Physiol 252:H291–H300
53. Meier-Hellmann A, Hannemann L, Specht M. Schaffartzik W, Spies C, Reinhart K (1993) The relationship between mixed venous and hepatic venous O_2 saturation in patients with septic shock. Adv Exp Med Biol, Oxygen Transport to Tissue (in press)
54. Giraud GD, MacCannell KL (1984) Decreased nutrient blood flow during dopamine- and epinephrine-induced intestinal vasodilatation. J Pharmacol Exp Ther 230:214–220
55. Reilly FD, McCuskey RS, von Cilento E (1981) Hepatic microvascular regulatory mechanisms. I. Adrenergic mechanisms. Microvasc Res 21:103–116
56. Bollaert PE, Bauer Ph, Audibert G, Lambert H, Larcan A (1990) Effects of epinephrine on hemodynamics and oxygen metabolism in dopamine-resistant septic shock. Chest 98:949–953
57. Lipman J, Roux A, Kraus P (1991) Vasoconstrictor effects of adrenaline in human septic shock. Anaesth Intens Care 19:61–65
58. Mackenzie SJ, Kapadia F, Nimmo GR, Armstrong IR, Grant IS (1991) Adrenaline in treatment of septic shock: effects on hemodynamics and oxygen transport. Intensive Care Med 17:36–39
59. Innes IR, Nickerson M (1975) Norepinephrine, epinephrine and the sympathomimetic amines. In: Goodman LD, Gilman A (eds) The pharmalogical basis of therapeutics. MacMillan, New York, pp 483–504
60. Moran JL, O'Fathartaigh MS, Peisach AR, Chapman MJ, Leppard Ph (1993) Epinephrine as an inotropic agent in septic shock: a dose-profile analysis. Crit Care Med 21:70–77
61. Haddy FJ, Chou CC, Scott JB et al (1967) Intestinal vascular responses to naturally occurring vasoactive substances. Gastroenterology 52:444–451
62. Haddy FJ, Molnar JI, Borden CW et al (1962) Comparison of direct effects of angiotensin, and other vasoactive agents on small and large blood vessels in several vascular beds. Circulation 25:239–246
63. Pawlik W, Shepherd AP, Jacobson ED (1975) Effects of vasoactive agents on intestinal oxygen consumption and blood flow in dogs. J Clin Invest 56:484–490
64. Greenway CV, Lawson A (1966) The effects of adrenaline and noradrenaline on venous return and regional blood flow in the anesthetized cat with special reference to intestinal blood flow. J Physiol (Lond) 187:579–595
65. Dahn MS, Lange P, Jacobs LA (1988) Central mixed and splanchnic venous oxygen saturation monitoring. Intensive Care Med 14:373–378
66. Kainuma M, Fujiwara Y, Kimura N, Shitaokoshi A, Nakashima K, Shimado Y (1991) Monitoring hepatic venous hemoglobin oxygen saturation in patients undergoing liver surgery. Anesthesiology 74:49–52
67. Goldberg LI (1972) Cardiovascular and renal actions of dopamine. Potential clinical applications. Pharmacol Rev 24:1–29

68. Vincent JL, Preiser JC (1993) Inotropic agents. New Horizons 1:137–144
69. Nakatani T, Isihkawa Y et al (1991) Hepatic mitochondrial redox state in hypotensive brain-dead patients and an effect of dopamine administration. Intensive Care Med 17:103–107
70. Johnson DJ, Johannigman JA, Branson RD, Davis K, Hurst JM (1991) The effect of low dose dopamine on gut hemodynamics during PEEP ventilation for acute lung injury. J Surg Res 50:344–349
71. Townsend MC, Schirmer WJ, Schirmer JM, Fry DE (1987) Low-dose dopamine improves effective hepatic blood flow in murine peritonitis. Circ Shock 21:149–153
72. Pawlik W, Shepherd AP, Mailman D, Shanbour LL, Jacobson ED (1976) Effects of dopamine and epinephrine on intestinal blood flow and oxygen uptake. In: Grote J, Reneau D, Thews G (eds) Oxygen transport to the tissue II. Plenum, New York, pp 511–516
73. Kullmann R, Breull WR, Reinsberg J, Wassermann K, Konopatzki A (1983) Dopamine produces vasodilation in specific regions and layers of the rabbit gastrointestinal tract. Life Sci 32:2115–2122
74. Roytblat L, Gelman S, Bradley EL, Henderson T, Parks D (1990) Dopamine and hepatic oxygen supply-demand relationship. Can J Physiol Pharmacol 68:1165–1169
75. Jackson LK, Key BM, Cain SM (1982) Total and hindlimb O_2 uptake and blood flow in hypoxic dogs given dopamine. Crit Care Med 10:327–331
76. Regan CJ, Duckworth R, Fairhurst JA, Maycock PF, Frayn KN, Campbell IT (1990) Metabolic effects of low-dose dopamine infusion in normal volunters. Clin Sci 79:605–611
77. Ruttimann Y, Chidero R et al (1989) Effects of dopamine on total oxygen consumption and oxygen delivery in healthy men. Am J Physiol 257:E541–546
78. Lundberg J, Lundberg D, Norgren L, Ribbe E, Thörne J, Werner O (1990) Intestinal hemodynamics during laparotomy: effects of thoracic epidural anesthesia and dopamine in humans. Anesth Analg 71:9–15
79. Winsö O, Biber B, Martner J (1985) Does dopamine suppress stress-induced intestinal and renal vasoconstriction? Acta Anaesthesiol Scand 29:508–514
80. Baumann G, Gutting M, Pfafferott C, Ningel K, Klein G (1988) Comparison of acute haemodynamic effects of dopexamine hydrochloride, dobutamine and sodium nitroprusside in chronic heart failure. Eur Heart J 9:503–512
81. De Marco T, Kwasman M, Au D, Chatterjee K (1988) Dopexamine hydrochloride in chronic congestive heart failure with improved cardiac performance without increased metabolic cost. Am J Cardiol 62:57C–62C
82. Parratt JR, Wainwright CL, Fagbemi O (1988) Effect of dopexamine hydrochloride in the early stages of experimental myocardial infarction and comparison with dopamine and dobutamine. Am J Cardiol 62:18C–23C
83. Svenson G, Strandberg LE, Lindvall B, Erhardt L (1988) Haemodynamic response to dopexamine hydrochloride in postinfarction heart failure: lack of tolerance after continuous infusion. Br Heart J 60:489–496
84. Tan LB, Littler A, Murray RG (1987) Beneficial haemodynamic effects of intravenous dopexamine in patients with low-output heart failure. J Cardiovasc Pharmacol 10:280–286
85. Colardyn FC, Vandenbogaerde JF, Vogelaers DP, Verbeke JH (1989) Use of dopexamine hydrochloride in patients with septic shock. Crit Care Med 17:999–1003
86. Cain SM, Curtis SE (1991) Systemic and regional oxygen uptake and delivery and lactate flux in endotoxic dogs infused with dopexamine. Crit Care Med 19:1552–1560
87. Biro GP, Douglas JR, Keon WJ, Taichman GC (1988) Changes in regional blood flow distribution induced by infusions of dopexamine hydrochloride or dobutamine in anesthetized dogs. Am J Cardiol 62:30C–36C
88. Lokhandwala MF, Jandhyala BS (1992) Effects of dopaminergic agonists on organ blood flow and function. Clin Intensive Care 3(1) [Suppl]:12–16

89. Baumann G, Felix SB, Filcek SAL (1990) Usefulness of dopexamine hydrochloride versus dobutamine in chronic congestive heart failure and effects on hemodynamics and urine output. Am J Cardiol 65:748–754
90. Gray PA, Bodenham AR, Park (1991) A comparison of dopexamine and dopamine to prevent renal impairment in patients undergoing orthotopic liver transplantation. Anaesthesia 46:638–641
91. Stephan H, Sonntag H, Henning H, Yoshimine K (1990) Cardiovascular and renal haemodynamic effects of dopexamine: comparison with dopamine. Br J Anaesth 65:380–387
92. Magrini F, Foulds RA, Roberts N, Macchi G, Mondadori C, Zanchetti A (1988) Renal hemodynamic effects of dopexamine hydrochloride. Am J Cardiol 62:53C–56C
93. Shoemaker WC, Appel PL, Kram HB (1988) Tissue oxygen debt as a determinant of lethal and nonlethal postoperative organ failure. Crit Care Med 16:117–120
94. Shoemaker WC, Appel PL, Kram HB, Waxman K, Lee TS (1988) Prospective trial of supranormal values of survivors as therapeutic goals in high risk surgical patients. Chest 94:1176–1186
95. Tuchschmidt J, Fried J, Swinney R et al (1989) Early hemodynamic correlations of survival in patients with septic shock. Crit Care Med 17:719–723
96. Hannemann L, Meier-Hellmann A, Specht M, Spies C, Reinhart K (1993) O_2-Angebot, O_2-Verbrauch und Mucosa pH-Wert des Magens. Anaesthesist 42:11–14

Metabolic Changes in Sepsis – Can the Host Response be Influenced Metabolically?

M. Georgieff, T. Schricker and B. Kugler

Introduction

Total parenteral nutrition (TPN) means administration of all required nutritional compounds parenterally without any need of additional enteral feeding. Of major importance in this context is the adaptation of nutritional support to the patient's individual metabolic situation (trauma, sepsis or starving).

The metabolic response to sepsis is characterized by diverse alterations in substrate turnover both systemically and at tissue levels. Peripheral skeletal muscle protein breakdown causes muscle wasting and net negative whole body nitrogen balance systemically [1]. The splanchnic region, including the intestine, the reticuloendothelial system and the liver with its macrophages, the Kupffer cells, represents the main site of sepsis-induced accelerated metabolic response with regional augmentation of oxygen consumption and turnover rates in glucose, fatty acid and amino acid metabolism [2].

Although the issues of protein sparing and energy requirement remain paramount to successful nutritional support, a new sphere of influence has materialized: nutritional modulation of the immune system. Immunomodulation, by effecting a shift in the prevailing balance of cell-cell communication, cytokine production and prostaglandin milieu can produce salutary changes in the circulation, cell-mediated immune response and the hypermetabolism syndrome.

Thus, the pharmacological aspects of different nutrients have increasingly gained attention during the last few years. This chapter will focus on such cell- and organ-specific actions of single substances and discuss their potential benefits in the treatment of septic patients.

Lipids

Lipids have a wide range of immunomodulatory potencies. These effects are thought to be mediated through modulation of eicosanoid synthesis, changes in all membrane properties, changes at receptor binding sites and finally through synthesis, release, and/or binding of various substances. The lipid composition of monocytes, macrophages and lymphocytes reflects the fatty acid composition of dietary lipids [3]. These cells can synthesize all the non-essential fatty acids of cellular lipids, but apparently acquire the essential fatty acids, linoleic acid (LA), its product arachidonic acid (AA), and linolenic acid (LNA) and its products, eicosapentaenoic acid (EPA) and docosahexaenoic acid (DHA), from the circulating blood. The mature cells lack δ-6 desaturase, which is the critical rate-limiting enzyme required for the conversion of dietary LA to AA [4]. Thus, the immune cells depend on the activity of hepatic δ-6 desaturase. Hence, factors which affect the activity of that enzyme influence the AA content of immune cells. Dietary fatty acids (amounts and types) are able to modulate the rate of AA synthesis. This is important because the eicosanoid products of AA exert potent effects on several aspects of the immune system. Eicosanoids of the 2-series prostaglandins PGE_2, PGI_2 and TXA_2, and the 4-series leukotrienes (LTB_4, LTD_4, LTE_4) are potent inflammatory mediators synthesized from AA [5].

High levels of PGE_2 produced by macrophages suppress the immune system. PGE_2 released from injured tissue may actually cause an impaired immune response of T cells [5]. After severe trauma, delayed-type hypersensitivity, allograft rejection and T-dependent antibody response are all diminished, which is typical for T cell suppression [6]. Endotoxins from infectious microbes activate monocytes to produce PGE_2 resulting in lymphocyte suppressor activity [7]. The suppressive behavior on lymphocytes is similar to that in burn patients. A reduction in cell-mediated immune responsiveness after burn injury was avoided in animals, in which PGE_2 synthesis was blocked by a cyclooxygenase inhibitor [8]. All these effects are consistent with the excess and chronic synthesis of PGE_2.

LTC_4, LTD_4 and LTE_4 are bronchial vasoconstrictors which are about four times more potent than histamine [9]. LTC_4 and LTD_4 increase microvascular permeability, contributing to a vascular leakage [10]. LTB_4 is a powerful chemoattractant and chemokinetic agent for peripheral blood mononuclear cells (PMNs) to aggregate and adhere to endothelial cells [11].

TXA_2 induces vasoconstriction and platelet aggregation [12]. In contrast, the eicosanoids of the 3-series and leukotrienes of the 5-series show different qualities. TXA_3 exhibits attenuated vasodepressor effects and will not aggregate platelets [13], and LTB_5 is much less chemotactic than LTB_4 [14]. PGI_3 possesses all the vasodilatory and antiaggregating effects of PGI_2 [15].

These facts suggest that modification of eicosanoid synthesis could have beneficial effects. Three ways exist to modify the prostaglandin milieu: (1) blockade of prostaglandin synthesis globally with nonsteroidal anti-inflammatory drugs, (2) exogenous administration of prostaglandins or their analogues, and (3) use of alternative lipids to alter arachidonate-derived metabolites. The last method will be discussed in detail.

Ω-3 Fatty Acids

Ω-3 polyunsaturated fatty acids (PUFA), either from plant oils containing LNA such as linseed oil or from marine fish oils containing EPA and DHA, are known to inhibit the metabolism of Ω-6 fatty acids (LA, AA) through their competition for δ-6 desaturase, thereby lowering the formation of the 2-series prostaglandins and the 4-series leukotrienes [16]. At the same time, fish oil yields the alternative 3-series prostaglandins and 5-series leukotrienes, which exhibit a different spectrum of activity [17]. The growing amount of evidence on the role of Ω-3 fatty acids in the control of plasma lipids, platelet aggregation and inflammation has caused speculation on the advantage of Ω-3 rich oils in stress and sepsis.

Mascioli et al. have recently shown that i.v. feeding of fish oil emulsions, when compared to safflower oil, enhanced survival of endotoxin-induced shock in guinea pigs [18]. Ingestion of 18 g of fish oil per day in healthy volunteers resulted in a lower interleukin 1 (IL-1) production in monocytes stimulated in vitro with endotoxin, a phenomenon probably mediated by LTB_5 [19]. A reduced pyrogenic effect was also noted in animals fed with fish oil [20].

Evidence indicates that several prostanoid products mediate salutary changes in tissue perfusion during sepsis. This is reflected in the improved survival of critically ill patients with a high PGI to TXA ratio [21]. Alterations in regional blood flow, particulary in the splanchnic region, are important in the pathogenesis of organ failure during endotoxemia and sepsis. A recent study demonstrated that short-term i.v. feeding with fish oil improved intestinal and portal venous blood flow, improved glucose tolerance, and increased lactate clearance in a low dose endotoxin rat model [22]. The facilitation of the release of endothelial-derived relaxing factor (EDRF) by Ω-3 fatty acids also contributes to these effects on organ perfusion [23]. Data from other studies indicate protective effects of Ω-3 fatty acids with respect to the liver exposed to septicemia. Fish oil diets could prevent the fatty infiltration of the liver, which is a common abnormality in patients suffering from gram-negative sepsis [24]. The release of TXA_2 and IL-1 from endotoxin-stimulated liver macrophages (signs of the hepatic inflammatory response) was diminished when fish oil had been administered [25].

It is becoming increasingly evident that prostaglandins play an integral role in regulating the functions of cells involved in inflammatory reactions of the lung. The leukotrienes of the 4-series have been found to induce bronchospasm, pulmonary vascular constriction, while increasing mucus secretion and vascular permeability [9–11]. A reduction of leukotriene synthesis could be expected to have an anti-inflammatory effect on the lung. The Ω-3 fatty acids have been shown to reduce leukotriene production from AA by substrate competition for the lipooxygenase enzyme [5], resulting in a lower release of oxygen free radicals from leukocytes and/or IL-1 from monocytes [26]. Additionally, leukotrienes of the 5-series are significantly less chemotactic than those of the 4-series [27].

All these experimental observations of Ω-3 fatty acids may serve as an underlining basis for their future clinical use in the treatment of sepsis.

Long Chain Triglycerides

Currently, the long chain triglycerides (LCTs) used in parenteral nutritional regimes are provided by soybean and safflower oils. The effects of these lipid emulsions on the immune system has long been controversially discussed. On the one hand, the need for LA as part of a nutritional regime is well accepted, because LA blood levels fall very rapidly; if LA is not substituted, this leads to the essential fatty acid deficiency syndrome [28]. On the other hand, high doses of LA may induce additional elaboration of the eicosanoids of the 2-series. Since reduced PGI_2 synthesis by the damaged endothelium is of particular importance in the early course of multiple organ failure, endothelial cell damage is further enhanced by TXA_2-induced platelet aggregation and LTB_4-enhanced leukocyte accumulation. The immune response, as indicated by mitogenic activity, is accentuated when intake of essential fatty acids (EFAs) is limited. This probably reflects a reduction in PGE_2 synthesis and leukotriene production from macrophages [29]. This may account for the relief of immunosuppression in EFA deficiency states due, as described above, to the various immunsuppressive actions of PGE_2. Thus, in terms of intervention strategies to minimize prostanoid and leukotriene-related pathophysiologies, limitation of EFA during various metabolic states may be desirable in certain instances [30].

One of the complications of TPN during sepsis is the fatty infiltration of the liver with cholestasis. Recently it could be shown that this alteration was prevented when a mixture of medium chain triglycerides (MCTs) and LCTs was used as the fat component instead of LCTs alone [31]. In premature infants LCT administration was associated with liver dysfunction in terms of disturbed bilirubin excretion. This was not observed when MCTs were given [32]. Reticuloendothelial system (RES) integrity measured by ^{99}Tc-sulfur colloid clearance rate also was better preserved in patients who received MCTs instead of LCTs [33].

Many studies have suggested varying degrees of apparent pulmonary dysfunction when i.v. fat emulsions are given [34]. According to the various effects of prostaglandins on inflammation and pulmonary vasomotor tone, i.v. LCTs containing high amounts of LA could have profound pharmacologic actions aside from the provision of lipid calories. It remains unclear if these changes are of sufficient magnitude to carry clinical significance. Further studies are warranted to delineate the complex role of LCTs in the septic lung.

Medium Chain Triglycerides

Medium chain triglycerides (MCTs) are 6–12 carbon atoms long and are mainly extracted from coconut oil. The lower molecular weight and higher solubility of MCTs than LCTs permit rapid plasma clearance. Furthermore, hydrolysis of MCTs is faster than that of LCTs, because less albumin and apoprotein C II is required for cleavage by lipoproteinlipase (LPL) [35]. This might be advantageous especially during sepsis, because the activity of LPL is reduced during such states [36]. The rapid removal of MCTs may explain the absence of RES dysfunction seen in MCT-fed patients. Rats given MCTs demonstrated improved uptake of injected radiolabeled bacteria in the liver, suggesting preserved RES function [37].

MCT is not a good substrate for eicosanoid formation and therefore offers an avenue for global reduction in AA-dependent inflammatory mediator synthesis. This fact is reflected in the lower AA membrane content and lower eicosanoid production in coconut oil-fed animals [38]. Compared to safflower oil (LCT)-fed animals, rats fed a diet enriched with coconut oil exhibit a diminished acute phase response to endotoxin challenge [39].

LCT requires carnitine for transport into the mitochondria, whereas MCT is not carnitine-dependent for β-oxidation. Hence, MCT provides a readily available fuel source. In burn and injury animal models, ketone bodies formed from MCT are energy substrates in the muscle, thus reducing proteolysis from branched chain amino acid breakdown [40].

Structured Lipids

In the future, patients will probably be receiving a combination of the three types of lipids described above. Whereas nutritionally supported patients usually receive a pure Ω-6 LCT lipid source or a combination of LCTs and MCTs, future lipids may comprise Ω-6 LCT for essential fatty acids, Ω-3 LCT for the immune modulating effect, and MCT as a readily available fuel source that prevents RES compromise. Incorporation of these lipid moieties into one molecule of glycerol to produce the so-called structured lipid has advantages over a physical mixture of these fats. An LCT/MCT structured lipid had superior protein-sparing qualities over LCT or a physical mixture of LCT and MCT in a burned rat model [42]. When fish oil is also incorporated into the structured lipid molecule, its protein-sparing qualities are even more accentuated in an animal burn model and lactic acidosis is reduced in an endotoxin model [41].

Carbohydrates

Hyperglycemia, increased glucose turnover together with impaired glucose utilization are characteristic metabolic findings in septic patients [2]. Glucose is the most frequently chosen energy source during intravenous nutrition. Glucose alone, however, fails to completely suppress protein catabolism even under insulin substitution and aggravates preexisting hyperglycemia [42]. Hyperglycemia is associated with deleterious consequences for the critically ill patient. Glucose concentrations above 13 mmol/L are acompanied by impaired leukocyte phagocytosis [43] and elevated mortality rates following cerebral ischemia [44], brain trauma [45] or cardiopulmonary resuscitation [46]. From an energetic point of view, hyperglycemia causes an acceleration of energy-demanding futile cycling of alanine, glutamine, glucose and free fatty acids [47]. Glucose exhibits limited oxidation when given in high doses parenterally. Consequently, a large portion enters the pathways of glycogen formation and hepatic lipogenesis possibly causing fatty infiltration of the liver [48]. The accompanying rise of insulin reduces endogenous free fatty acid release and oxidation still further [49]. Early administration of large glucose doses in septic patients who were 10 days on TPN reduced whole body protein stores by 1.5 ± 0.2 kg. At the same time, fat body mass increased by 2.2 ± 0.8 kg [50]. Although muscular nitrogen balance improved, visceral nitrogen retention declined from 13 ± 2.4 to 3.1 ± 1.6 g/m^2/day [51].

These relative disadvantages have led to a search for alternative fuels for intravenous use. One such fuel is xylitol, a five carbon polyol yielding 4.06 kcal/g. Xylitol is a normal intermediate product in the human glucuronic acid–xylulose and pentose–phosphate cycle. Metabolized primarily in the liver, where it is converted through insulin-independent pathways to glucose-6-phosphate (approximately 70% conversion to glucose), xylitol results in only modest increases of blood glucose and insulin levels in both normal and in traumatized patients [48]. Early studies have revealed that the maximal disposal rate of i.v. xylitol increases substantially during postinjury metabolism, whereas the disposal rate of glucose declines [52].

Gluconeogenesis, which requires 50% of hepatic oxygen consumption in the postabsorptive state [53], is typically increased during septicemia. The use of xylitol during such states can reduce hepatic glucose production and simultaneously increase fatty acid oxidation thereby augmenting the contribution of endogenous fat to overall resting energy expenditure [48]. Since fatty acids are the primary hepatic energy source and gluconeogenesis is a highly energy consuming process, these effects of xylitol seem to be beneficial especially for the septic liver. These observations have been confirmed by a new study by Ardawi, who demonstrated improved positive nitrogen balance, increased protein synthesis and RNA content in the liver of septic rats treated with xylitol [54].

Amino Acids

The sequelae of the defensive response to sepsis and infection are characterized by profound changes in the pattern of visceral protein synthesis, an increased whole body protein turnover, and, especially during the hypermetabolic phase, a pronounced catabolism of peripheral protein. The increased amino acid demand of the liver and proliferating cells results in a redistribution of interorgan amino acid flow. Subsequently, muscles become a net producer of precursors, predominantely lactate, glutamine and alanine, for acute phase protein synthesis, gluconeogenesis and mitosis. The branched chain amino acids arising from muscle degradation are transaminated to their ketoacids within the myocyte and serve as important oxidative fuels for muscle during the catabolic phase. This glucose-sparing effect is further enhanced by the relative insulin resistance of muscle cells during sepsis. Thus, glucose produced through gluconeogenesis at a high energetic and structural cost is preserved to feed glucose-dependent tissues like wound tissue, immune cells, visceral organs and the nervous system [55].

The therapeutic goals of amino acid supplementation during sepsis are, on one hand, to ensure the adequate supply of precursors for visceral protein synthesis, structural metabolism of immune cells and gluconeogenesis and, on the other hand, to minimize peripheral protein wasting to avoid general protein depletion. Failure of the host to meet these specific metabolic demands during the early phase of sepsis results in a higher mortality.

Growth Factors

Among new protein-sparing therapy concepts, the recent availability of growth factors has become an interesting option. Recombinant human growth factor and insulin-like growth factor are potent natural anabolics that are able to increase protein synthesis and thereby ameliorate net protein catabolism even in the posttraumatic and septic patient. In a study in burned children, the administration of 0.2 mg/kg body weight daily reduced mortality and recovery time and improved graft healing significantly. Although results in adults are equivocal, it seems that growth hormone therapy improves outcome in children and protein-depleted cachectic patients [56]. It should be noted, however, that especially septic patients benefit only from a combination of amino acid infusion and growth hormone therapy. A sole growth hormone therapy would reduce amino acid flow to the liver and the immune system and thereby jeopardize the protein synthetic capacity of these tissues.

Glutamine

A marker of the substantial efflux of amino acids from the musculature is the decrease of intracellular glutamine content to approximately 30% of normal values in the hypermetabolic phase following sepsis [57]. Intracellular glutamine concentration regulates protein synthesis rate and has therefore an important regulatory function [58]. Present amino acid solutions are free of glutamine because of its thermal instability and poor solubility. Recent advances in biotechnology make glutamine-containing dipeptides available for medical use in sufficient quantities. Several studies revealed that glutamine-containing dipeptides, in contrast to standard amino acid solutions, prevented the postoperative decrease in intramuscular glutamine concentration and improved cumulative nitrogen balance. In severely catabolic and septic patients these effects were less pronounced [59]. In addition to its effects on protein synthesis, glutamine serves as an important fuel for rapidly proliferating cells of the gut and the immune system. In bone marrow transplant recipients, glutamine-enriched parenteral nutrition was able to reduce infection rate and length of hospital stay [60]. As translocation of endotoxin and bacteria from the physiological gut flora is currently looked upon as a key mechanism in the development of multiple organ failure, feeding the gut specifically to preserve its barrier function is a promising therapeutic approach. In fact, many investigators were able to confirm a reduction of bacterial translocation after glutamine feeding in animal studies. In general, glutamine seems to be an effective nutrient to improve the functional integrity of the gut when administered via the enteral route [61]. The efficacy of intravenous glutamine-containing dipeptides on gut function, however, seems to be far less [62]. Especially for parenteral administration in severely ill patients, the use of glutamine analogues like a-ketoglutarate (AKG) or ornithine-a-ketoglutarate (OKG) are promising alternatives to glutamine-containing dipeptides. As already mentioned, the protein-sparing effect of dipeptides is less pronounced in this patient group. Some authors therefore suggest giving higher doses of glutamine-containing dipeptides to overcome this problem. However, critically ill patients often face renal insufficiency and might not tolerate the proposed enormous nitrogen load. Therefore, delivering the carbon skeleton of glutamine as the α-ketoacid salts AKG or OKG may be more appropriate for these patients since the excessive nitrogen from the amino groups can be avoided. In a study in postoperative patients, Vinnars et al. were able to show that AKG and OKG were equipotent to alanine-glutamine in preserving the intracellular glutamine pool and in improving nitrogen balance [63]. Similar to glutamine, AKG and OKG seem to exert specific anabolic effects [64].

Arginine

There is a growing interest in the metabolism of arginine, as it is the substrate of the enzyme nitric oxide synthase. The multiple properties of nitric oxide (NO) in the regulation of vascular tone, regional perfusion, neuronal signaling and immune defense revealed a series of revolutionary new discoveries and has particularly changed our understanding of cardiovascular physiology. A series of studies suggest a central role of NO derived from the inducible form of NO synthase of macrophages in the generalized vasodilatation during septic shock. NO synthesis can be competitively inhibited by arginine analogues like N^G-methyl-L-arginine, and these NO antagonists are able to reverse septic shock in animal studies. Thus, the role of arginine in parenteral nutrition of septic patients needs to be clarified. In a normal posttraumatic situation arginine enriched formulas exert a beneficial immunostimulatory effect and an improvement in wound healing [65]. In contrast, Gonce et al. observed an increased mortality of pigs with chronic abdominal sepsis treated with arginine enriched amino acid infusions [66]. In conclusion, an increased arginine supply in patients with severe inflammatory disease may be detrimental. Probably the opposite approach, the use of arginine analogues, may be the therapeutic future.

Branched Chain Amino Acids

During the catabolic phase, branched chain amino acids are important oxidative substrates of myocytes and are used in preference to glucose. Many investigators therefore have tried to reduce protein breakdown by increasing the supply of branched chain amino acids in their parenteral infusion regime. The results of the clinical studies undertaken have been conflicting, thus a clinically relevant advantage of solutions enriched in branched chain amino acids must be questioned [67].

Micronutrients

Since oxygen free radicals are released throughout the course of the inflammatory process, it is especially desirable to maximize the oxygen-scavenging potential of the plasma with adequate zinc, copper, selenium, and vitamin E. Addition of these substances to feeding regimens can prevent microsomal, microchondrial, and membrane lipid damage. A potential hazardous property of fish oil is its propensity to peroxidation. This leads to rapid perishability *in vitro* and can be measured *in vivo* by ethane excretion. In rats fed with cod liver oil, membrane peroxidation induced by CCL_4 was five times that of lard-fed rats; mortality was also greater, but, with the administration of antioxidants, was restored to control levels [68]. The addition of antioxidants, such as vitamin E and *ter*-butyldydrochinone, in any dietary preparation containing long chain PUFA such as fish oil is therefore vital to prevent lipid peroxidation [69].

Trace elements and essential minerals, including zinc, copper, chromium, selenium, and iron, are required for important coenzymes in nucleic acid metabolism and for protein synthesis [70]. Zinc deficiency has been associated with impaired antibody-mediated responses to T lymphocytes, impaired natural killer cell activity, defective chemotaxis of leukocytes, and delayed wound healing [71]. The importance of these factors cannot be overemphasized if the optimum environment for cellular and immunologic function is to be achieved. However, care must be taken when administering iron into the patient who also has low levels of plasma protein, since increased levels of free iron in conjunction with low concentrations of serum transferrin can increase susceptibility to bacterial pathogens [72].

Summary

A major goal of this review article is to show that nutritional physiology in normal individuals is rather different from patients bearing an inflammatory response. Known nutrients and a variety of energy sources reveal pharmacologic actions during such metabolic circumstances. An understanding of the pathophysiologic state of sepsis is essential for adequate nutritional support especially in this patient population.

References

1. Bower RH (1990) Nutritional and metabolic support of critically ill patients. J Parenter Enteral Nutr 14:257S
2. Wilmore WD (1983) Alterations in protein, carbohydrate, and fat metabolism in injured and septic patiens. J Am Coll Nutr 2:3
3. Johnston PV, Marshall LA (1984) Dietary fat, prostaglandins and the immune response. Prog Food Nutr Sci 8:3
4. Johnston PV (1985) Dietary fat, eicosanoids and immunity. Adv Lipid Res 21:103
5. Green DR, Faist E (1988) Trauma and the immune response. Immunol Today 9:253
6. Kinsella JE (1990) Lipids, membrane receptors, and enzymes: effects of dietary fatty acids. J Parenter Enteral Nutr 14:200S
7. Ninneman JL, Stockland AE, Condie JT (1983) Reduction of prostaglandin E synthesis-dependent suppressor cells with endotoxin. J Clin Immunol 3:142
8. Freeman TR, Shelby J (1988) Effects of anti-PGE antibody on cell mediated immune response in thermally injured mice. J Trauma 28:190
9. Adelroth E, Morris MM, Hargreave FE (1986) Airway responsiveness to leukotrienes C_4 and D_4 and to methacholine in patients with asthma and normal controls. N Engl J Med 315:480
10. Drazen JM, Austen KF, Lewis RA (1980) Comparative airway and vascular activities of leukotrienes C-1 and D in vivo and in vitro. Proc Natl Acad Sci USA 77:4354
11. Samuelsson B (1983) Leukotrienes: mediators of immediate hypersensitivity reactions and inflammation. Science 220:258
12. Moncada TH, Vane J (1985) Arachidonic acid metabolites and the interactions between platelets and blood vessels walls. N Engl J Med 312:1142
13. Fischer S, Weber PC (1983) Thromboxane A_3 is found in human platelets after dietary eicosapentaenoic acid. Biochem Biophys Res Commun 116:1091
14. Lee TH (1989) Pharmocological modulation of leukotriene and platelet activating factor biosynthesis and activities by alternative dietary fatty acids. Clin Exp Allergy 19:15
15. Dyerberg J, Bang HO, Stofferson E, Moncada S, Vane JR (1978) Eicosapentaenoic acid and prevention of thrombosis and atherosclerosis. Lancet 15:117
16. Bagley JS, Wan J, Georgieff M, Forse A, Blackburn G (1991) Cellular nutrition in support of early multiple organ failure. Chest 100:182S
17. Lee TH, Hoover RL, Williams JD (1985) Effect of dietary enrichment with eicosapentaenoic acids on in vitro neutrophil and monocyte leukotriene generation and neutrophile function. N Engl J Med 312:1217

18. Mascioli E, Leader L, Flores E, Trimbo S, Bistrian BR, Blackburn GL (1988) Enhanced survival to endotoxin in guinea pigs fed IV fish oil emulsion. Lipids 213:623
19. Endres S, Ghorbani R, Kelly VE, Georgilis K, Lonnemann G, van der Meer JWM (1989) The effect of dietary supplementation with Ω-3 polyunsaturated fatty acids on the synthesis of interleukin-1 and tumor necrosis factor by mononuclear cells. N Engl J Med 320:265
20. Pomposelli JJ, Mascioli E, Bistrian BR, Lopes SM, Blackburn GL (1989) Attenuation of the febrile response in guinea pigs by fish oil enriched diets. J Parenter Enteral Nutr 13:136
21. Oettinger W, Peskar BA, Begar HG (1987) Profiles of endogenous prostaglandin F2a, thromboxane A2 and prostacyclin with regard to cardiovascular and organ functions in early septic shock in man. Eur Surg Res 19:65
22. Pscheidl E, Wan JM, Blackburn GL, Bistriain BR, Istfan NW (1992) Influence of Ω-3 fatty acids on splanchnic blood flow and lactate metabolism in an endotoxemic rat model. Metabolism 41:698
23. Vanhoutte PM (1990) Fish oil and endothelium-dependent relaxations (abstract). In: 2nd international conference on the health effects of omega-3 polyunsaturated fatty acids in seafoods
24. Lanza-Jacoby S, Smythe C, Phetteplace H, Tabares A (1992) Adaption to a fish oil diet before inducing sepsis in rats prevents fatty infiltration of the liver. J Parenter Enteral Nutr 16:353
25. Biliar TR, Bankey PE, Svingen BA (1988) Fatty acid intake and Kupffer cell function: fish oil alters eicosanoid and monokine production to endotoxin stimulation. Surgery 104:343
26. Lee TH, Hoover RL, Williams JD (1985) Effect of dietary enrichment with eicosapentaenoic acids on in vitro neutrophil and monocyte leukotriene generation and neutrophile function. N Engl J Med 312:1217
27. Lee TH, Mencia-Huerta JM, Shil C, Corey EJ, Lewis AR, Austen KF (1984) Characterization and biologic properties of 5,12-dihydroxy derivatives of eicosapentaenoic acid including leukotriene B5 and the double lipoxygenase product. J Biol Chem 259:2383
28. Wolfram G (1987) Essentielle Fettsäuren in der parenteralen Ernährung. Infusionstherapie 14 [Suppl 3]:20
29. Lefkowith JB, Jakchik BA, Stahl P (1987) Metabolic and functional alterations in macrophages induced by essential fatty acid deficiancy. J Biol Chem 262:6668
30. Kinsella JE, Lokesh B (1990) Dietary lipids, eicosanoids, and the immune system. Crit Care Med 18:S94
31. Baldermann H, Wicklmayr M, Rett K, Banholzer P, Dietze G, Mehnert H (1991) Changes of hepatic morphology during parenteral nutrition with lipid emulsions containing LCT or MCT/LCT quantified by ultrasound. J Parenter Enteral Nutr 15:601
32. Rubin M, Herell D, Naor N, Moser A, Wielunsky E, Merlob P, Lichtenberg D (1991) Lipid infusion with different triglyceride cores (long-chain vs medium-chain/long-chain triglycerides): effect on plasma lipids and bilirubin binding in premature infants. J Parenter Enteral Nutr 15:642
33. Jensen GL, Mascioli EA, Seidner DL et al (1990) Parenteral infusion of long- and medium-chain triglycerides and reticuloendothelial system function in man. J Parenter Enteral Nutr 14:467
34. Hageman J, Hunt C (1986) Fat emulsions and lung function. Clin Chest Med 7:69
35. Deckelbaum RJ, Carpentier Y, Olivecrona T, Moser A (1986) Hydrolysis of medium vs long chain triglycerides in pure and mixed intravenous lipid emulsions by purified lipoprotein lipases in vitro. Clin Nutr 5[Suppl]:54
36. Bagby GJ, Corll CB, Thompson JJ, Wilson LA (1986) Lipoproteinlipase-suppressing mediators in serum of endotoxin-treated rats. Am J Physiol (Endocrinol Metab 14) 251:E470
37. Sobrado J, Moldawer LL, Pomposelli JJ, Mascioli EA, Babayan VK, Bistrian BR

(1985) Lipid emulsions and reticuloendothelial system function in healthy and burned guinea pigs. Am J Clin Nutr 42:855
38. Croft KD, Beilin LJ, Vandongen R, Mathews E (1984) Dietary modification of fatty acid and prostaglandin synthesis in rats. Biochim Biophys Acta 795:195
39. Wan J, Grimble RF (1987) Effect of dietary linoleate content on the metabolic response of rats to Escherichia coli endotoxin. Clin Sci 72:383
40. Mok KT, Maiz A, Sobrado J, Yamazaki K, Sorado J, Babayan VK (1984) Structured medium chain and long chain triglyceride emulsions are superior to physical mixtures in sparing body protein in the burned rat. Metabolism 10:910
41. Babayan VK (1987) Medium chain triglycerides and structured lipids. Lipids 22:417
42. Wolfe RR, Allsop JR, Burke JF (1979) Glucose metabolism in man: response to intravenous glucose infusion. Metabolism 28:210
43. Bagdade J, Root R, Bulger R (1971) Impaired leukocyte function in patients with poorly controlled diabetes. Diabetes 23:9
44. Lanier WL, Stangland KJ, Scheithauer BW (1987) The effects of dextrose infusion and head position on neurologic outcome after complete cerebral ischemia in primates: examination of a model. Anesthesiology 66:39
45. Longstreth WT, Inui TS (1985) High blood glucose level on hospital admission and poor neurological recovery after cardiac arrest. Ann Surg 198:59
46. Sieber FE, Smith DS, Traystman RJ (1987) Glucose: a reevaluation of its intraoperative use. Anesthesiology 67:72
47. Shaw JHF, Wolfe RR (1989) An integrated analysis of glucose, fat, and protein metabolism in severely traumatized patients. Ann Surg 209:63
48. Georgieff M, Moldawer L, Bistrian BR, Blackburn GL (1985) Xylitol, an energy source for intravenous nutrition after trauma. J Parenter Enteral Nutr 9:199
49. Georgieff M, Pscheidl E, Moldawer LL, Bistrian BR, Blackburn GK (1991) Mechanism of protein conservation during xylitol infusion after burn injury in rats: isotope kinetics and indirect calorometry. Eur J Clin Inv 21:249
50. Streat SJ, Beddoe AH, Hill GL (1987) Aggressive nutritional support does not prevent protein loss despite fat gain in septic intensive patients. J Trauma 27:262
51. Radrizzani D, Iapichino G, Cambisano M (1988) Peripheral, visceral and body nitrogen balance of catabolic patients, without and with parenteral nutrition. Intensive Care Med 14:212
52. Ackermann RH (1980) Bestimmung des Xylitumsatzes unter der Geburt und nach Operationen bei parenteraler Zufuhr. Infusionstherapie 7:113
53. Jungas RL, Halperin ML, Brosnan JT (1992) Quantitative analysis of amino acid oxidation and related gluconeogenesis in humans. Physiol Rev 72:419
54. Ardawi MSM (1992) Effects of xylitol- and/or glutamine-supplemented parenteral nutrition on septic rats. Clin Sci 82:419
55. Wilmore WD (1983) Alterations in protein, carbohydrate, and fat metabolism in injured and septic patients. J Am Coll Nutr 2:3
56. Herndon DN, Barrow RE, Kunkel KR, Broemeling L, Ruran RL (1990) Effects of recombinant human growth hormone on donor site healing in severely burned children. Ann Surg 218:424
57. Roth E, Funovics J, Mühlbacher F (1982) Metabolic disorders in severe abdominal sepsis: glutamine deficiency in skeletal muscle. Clin Nutr 1:25
58. Jepson MM, Bates PC, Broadbent P (1988) Relationship between glutamine concentration and protein synthesis in rat skeletal muscle. Am J Physiol 255:E166
59. Fürst P, Albers S, Stehle P (1990) Glutamine-containing dipeptides in parenteral nutrition. J Parenter Enteral Nutr 14:118S
60. Ziegler TR, Young LS, Benfell K et al (1992) Clinical and metabolic efficacy of glutamine-supplemented parenteral nutrition after bone marrow transplantation. A randomized, doubleblind, controlled study. Ann Intern Med 116:821
61. Klimberg VS, Souba WW, Dolson DJ (1989) Oral glutamine supports crypt cell turnover and accelerates intestinal healing following abdominal radiation. J Parenter Enteral Nutr 13[Suppl 1]:35A

62. Burke DJ, Alverdy JC, Aoys W, Moss GS (1990) Effect of route of glutamine administration on mortality following experimental enterocolitis. J Parenter Enteral Nutr 14:8S (abstract)
63. Vinnars E, Hammarqvist F, von der Decken A, Wernermann J (1990) Role of glutamine and its analogues in posttraumatic muscle protein and amino acid metabolism. J Parenter Enteral Nutr 14:125S
64. Wernermann J, Hammarqvist F, von der Decken A, Vinnars E (1987) Ornithine-alpha-ketoglutarate improves skeletal muscle protein synthesis as assessed by ribosome analysis and nitrogen use after surgery. Ann Surg 206:674
65. Daly JM, Reynolds J, Sigal RK, Shou J, Liberman MD (1990) Effect of dietary protein and amino acids on immune function. Crit Care Med 18:86S
66. Gonce SJ, Peck MD, Alexander JW, Miskell PW (1990) Arginine supplementation and its effect on established peritonitis in guinea pigs. J Parenter Enteral Nutr 14:237
67. Sax HC, Talamini MA, Fischer JE (1986) Clinical use of branched-chain amino acids in liver disease, sepsis, trauma and burns. Arch Surg 121:338
68. Hafeman DG, Hoekstra WG (1977) Protection against carbon tetrachloride-induced lipid peroxidation in the rat by dietary vitamin E, selenium and methionine as measured by ethane evolution. J Nutr 107:656
69. Combs GF, Noguchi T, Scott ML (1975) Mechanism of action of selenium and vitamin E in protection of biological membrane. Fed Proc 34:2090
70. Fernandez-Madrid F, Prasad AS, Oberleas D (1973) Effect of zinc deficiency on nucleic acids, collagen and non-collagenous protein of the connective tissue. J Lab Clin Med 82:951
71. Fernandes G, Nair M, Onoe K, Tanaka T, Floyd R, Good RA (1979) Impairment of cell-mediated immunity functions by dietary zinc deficiency in mice. Proc Natl Acad Sci USA 76:457
72. Bullen JJ (1981) The significance of iron in infection. Rev Infect Dis 3:1127

VI. New Therapeutic Approaches

Is there a Place for Monoclonal Antibodies Against Endotoxin in the Therapy of Sepsis?

L. Eidelman and C. L. Sprung

Introduction

Sepsis remains the leading cause of mortality in critically ill patients. The naive belief that the introduction of new, more potent antibiotics will be sufficient to deal with the problem of infections has been discarded. Gram-negative sepsis is associated with a particularly high morbidity and mortality estimated between 20% and 75% [1–3]. Some characteristic features of gram-negative bacteria are believed to be reponsible for the not infrequent development of multiple organ failure and death despite the use of potent antibacterial compounds to sensitive microorganisms. The intravenous injection of endotoxin causing the typical clinical manifestations of gram-negative bacteremia including fever, shock; leukopenia and/or leukocytosis and disseminated intravascular coagulation was revealed as far back as 1942 [4]. Endotoxin has been proposed as a major causal factor in the development of gram-negative sepsis [5]. Bacteremia and septic shock are associated with the release of endotoxin into the circulation which is believed to activate the biologic cascade involving tumor necrosis factor (TNF) and other cytokines such as interleukin-1 (IL-1) and interleukin-6 (IL-6). As the development of many systemic septic responses can be explained by the action of these substances, immunotherapy directed against endotoxin has been suggested as a possible method to decrease morbidity and mortality in patients with sepsis.

Pathophysiology

Endotoxin is the lipopolysaccharide component of the cell walls of gram-negative bacteria that triggers many of the adverse systemic reactions and serious sequellae in patients with sepsis. Lipopolysaccharide is a complex molecule consisting of three distinct regions: lipid A, the core polysaccharide, and the oligosaccharide (O)specific side chains. The core polysaccharide region is identical, or nearly identical for many strains of bacteria. Although the polysaccharide components possess biologic activity, lipid A is responsible for the majority of the biologic effects of lipopolysaccharide. Presently, there are significant data to suggest that lipopolysaccharide is important in the pathophysiology of many cases of the sepsis syndrome. Normal volunteers given small intravenous doses of endotoxin reproduce many of the clinical features of the sepsis syndrome including fever, tachycardia, leukocytosis, lymphopenia, decreased left ventricular ejection fraction, low systemic vascular resistance, and increased levels of cortisol, ACTH, TNF, and epinephrine [6–8]. Detectable blood levels of endotoxin are present in patients with sepsis and shock whereas endotoxin is usually not present in patients with fever or shock from other etiologies [9–11]. The presence of circulating endotoxin in patients with sepsis correlates with the development of complications such as shock, adult respiratory distress syndrome (ARDS), acute renal failure and death [10, 12, 13].

Polyclonal or Monoclonal Antibodies

Polyclonal or monoclonal antibodies directed against the O-antigenic determinants of the lipopolysaccharide have been demonstrated to provide serotype-specific protection [14, 15]. Unfortunately, because of the wide differences in O-specific serotypes, the use of serotype-specific antibodies is not very practical as their spectrum is too narrow. A more useful approach has been the development of antibodies directed at the highly conserved lipid A and the core polysaccharide regions of the lipopolysaccharide which are believed to confer a much wider protection against different bacteria. Passive immunization with polyclonal antisera to mutant *Salmonella minnesota* and *Escherichia coli (J5)* have been shown to protect animals from the lethal effects of endotoxin and live bacteria [16, 17]. Following the positive results of antibodies against J5 demonstrated in animals, Ziegler et al. [18] showed, in a randomized controlled study, that human antiserum was effective in decreasing mortality in humans from 38% in the control patients to 24% in the *anti-J5* treated patients with gram-negative bacteremia ($p<0.05$). The treatment effect of *anti-J5* was especially prominent in patients with profound shock in whom mortality was decreased from 77% to 44% ($p<0.05$) [18]. In a subsequent prospective study, Baumgartner et al. [19] demonstrated that the prophylactic use of polyclonal anti-J5 antibodies in high risk surgical patients did not decrease the incidence of gram-negative infections but did decrease the incidence of septic shock and mortality, especially in patients undergoing abdominal surgery ($p<0.05$). Calandra et al. [20] could not demonstrate a decrease in the mortality of patients with gram-negative bacteremia and shock treated with human IgG polyclonal anti-J5 antibodies. These latter conflicting results may be related to the use of IgG rather than IgM antibodies as IgM antibodies appear to possess the beneficial effects of polyclonal antisera [16].

If polyclonal J5 antiserum was shown to be so effective, why are we not using it clinically today? Antiserum has not turned out to be clinically feasible because of the mild vaccine toxicity to donors, the lack of a booster response making more than one donation unlikely, and variations in antibody content in different antiserum preparations [21]. The most important reason, however, is that human serum is associated with the serious risk of transmission of such viral illnesses as hepatitis and the acquired immunodeficiency syndrome (AIDS) [21]. The use of monoclonal antibody technology circumvents these problems and allows for the production of large quantities of antibodies of known epitope specificity [21].

Murine and human anti-core monoclonal antibodies have been demonstrated to provide protection in animal models of gram-negative sepsis [22, 23]. Following the impressive results with polyclonal antiserum to J5 [18, 19], Ziegler et al.[21], conducted a multicenter, randomized, double-blind, placebo-controlled study of a human monoclonal IgM antibody to the lipid A domain of endotoxin (HA-1A). HA-1A is produced by a stable heteromyeloma cell line A6 (H4C5) developed by Teng et al. [23]. The same *E. coli* (J5) vaccine that was used to develop the polyclonal J5 antiserum was used to develop this cell line. As anti-J5 seemed efficacious in patients with gram-negative bacteremia and as it was expected that the greatest benefit of an anti-endotoxin antibody would be in patients who had the greatest likelihood of endotoxin, patients with gram-negative bacteremia, the HA-1A trial prospectively defined the group of patients with gram-negative bacteremia as the group of primary interest. Of 543 patients with sepsis that were randomly allocated to receive either a single 100 mg intravenous dose of HA-1A or placebo, 200 patients had gram-negative bacteremia [21]. In the group of patients with gram-negative bacteremia, monoclonal antibody therapy decreased 28 day mortality from 49% to 30% ($p<0.05$) [21]. HA-1A therapy was especially effective in patients with gram-negative bacteremia and shock, decreasing 28 day mortality from 57% to 33% ($p<0.05$) [21]. The reduction in mortality was evident within the first days after treatment and was sustained throughout the observation period. When patients were stratified according to severity of illness at entry, HA-1A decreased 28 day mortality of patients with APACHE II scores >25 or ≤ 25. There was no difference in mortality in the total 543 group of septic patients (39% vs 43%) enrolled into the study. Of the patients without gram-negative bacteremia, the 28 day mortality was 68 (45%) of 150 HA-1A treated patients and 73 (40%) of 184 placebo treated patients (NS). There were no serious adverse reactions in the patients who received HA-1A and none developed human antibodies against HA-1A [21].

In a substudy of 82 septic patients enrolled in the above mentioned, larger multicenter study, levels of endotoxin, TNF and IL-6 were obtained before infusion of HA-1A and 1 h and 24 h after infusion [11]. Of the 82 patients, 32 (39%) had gram-negative bacteremia. Endotoxemia was detected in 27 (33%) of the 82 patients, in 18 (56%) of the 32 patients with gram-negative bacteremia, and in nine (18%) of the 50 patients who did not have gram-negative bacteremia ($p<0.05$). Of the patients with endotoxemia, the mortality rate was 73% in the placebo group compared with 31% in the HA-1A group ($p<0.05$). HA-1A, however, did not significantly reduce mortality in the group of patients without endotoxemia. TNF levels decreased in both groups of patients 1 h and 24 h after study drug infusion. The decrease in TNF was significantly greater in HA-1A treated patients at 24 h after infusion. In addition, this study, as others, demonstrated a strong correlation between TNF and IL-6 levels and mortality.

Several concerns related to the HA-1A trial and monoclonal antibodies have been suggested. Questions concerning the epitopic specificity, binding characteristics, and biologic effects of the antibodies remain unanswered with some negative animal studies [15, 24, 25]. In addition, the beneficial effect of HA-1A [21] was found in only one of the three subgroups in the efficacy analysis, the statistical result was marginal, and the beneficial results may be secondary to more patients in the placebo group than the HA-1A group having end organ failure, receiving inadequate antibiotics, and having *Pseudomonas* bacteremia [24]. These concerns have been addressed [26]. The HA-1A trial prospectively defined the patients with gram-negative bacteremia as the group of primary interest [26]. The beneficial results of HA-1A were robust and did not change substantially after adjusting for age, APACHE II score, presence of shock, site of infection, adequacy of antibiotics, infecting organism, and neutropenia [26]. Critics of the study do not mention that there were more patients with malignancy and polymicrobial bacteremia in the HA-1A group than in the placebo group as well as a longer time from the diagnosis of sepsis until the infusion of the study drug in the HA-1A group.

Negative animal studies may be related to several factors [16, 26, 27]. Animal species vary in their sensitivity to endotoxin. Rats and mice typically require much higher doses of endotoxin to produce mortality than other species. Therefore, anti-core antibodies must bind and inactivate much larger amounts of endotoxin to demonstrate efficacy. Most of the studies that have failed to show protection of the antibody have used large inocula of infecting organisms. The extent of side chain substitution can effect the accessibility of the core to anti-core antibodies. Finally, the action of some antibodies may involve different mechanisms in humans than in animals. HA-1A, for instance, mediates the complement-dependent immune adherence of antibody-endotoxin complexes to CR1 receptors on human red blood cells and neutrophils [28]. After the results of the Ziegler study [21] became available, HA-1A was licensed and released for use in several European countries and was available for compassionate use as an open-label trial in the United States. The licensure application for HA-1A was not approved by the US Federal Drug Administration (FDA) because Centocor's claim of efficacy was based on an analysis of the gram-negative bacteremia patients, there was no statistically significant effect of HA-1A on the primary end point of survival of gram-negative patients at 14 days as stated in the original protocol, and the revised analytical plan by Centocor to study survival over 28 days was submitted after certain Centocor staff learned about the interim-analysis results [29]. Due to the potential for the introduction of bias, analyses based on the revised analytic plan were not accepted [29]. The original authors [21], however, had decided that the primary end point of survival of gram-negative bacteremic patients should be over 28 days and they did not have access to the interim-analysis results [30]. Because of the lack of approval by the FDA, Centocor performed a second trial of effectiveness of HA-1A. The initial results have not been published but what information has been released indicates that HA-1A in the second trial did not decrease mortality in patients with gram-negative bacteremia. In addition, because of an excess mortality in patients without gram-negative bacteremia, Centocor voluntarily withdrew HA-1A from the European market [31].

Recently, Quezado et al. [32] demonstrated that HA-1A did not alter levels of bacteremia or endotoxemia and actually decreased survival in a canine model of *E. coli* sepsis. Only 2 (15%) of 13 animals in the HA-1A group, compared with 8 (57%) of 14 control animals, survived 28 days ($p = 0.05$) [32]. These data, together with the increased although not significant mortality noted in the trials of patients without gram-negative bacteremia [21, 31] receiving HA-1A, prompted the authors to call for further study of the conditions under which HA-1A has beneficial, neutral, or deleterious effects before its widespread clinical use. As noted above, animal models are very different than the clinical situation. In addition, there are many differences between this particular canine model and the human experience. Animals received a five to ten times higher dose of HA-1A than in the clinical trials, antibiotics were given 6 h after HA-1A whereas patients were typically treated with antibiotics prior to HA-1A, and cardiac function was depressed in animals whereas there was no change in patients [32, 33]. The timing of antibiotic treatment may be extremely important as antibiotics enhance the binding of HA-1A to smooth gram-negative bacteria [34]. Despite the potential danger of HA-1A in patients without gram-negative bacteremia, the clinical prospective and open-label trials have demonstrated HA-1A to be safe.

The present chapter has focused on HA-1A. There have also been clinical trials with E5 murine monoclonal IgM antibody to endotoxin in the treatment of gram-negative sepsis [35, 36]. The reader is referred to recent reviews of those trials [37–39]. Interestingly, as opposed to the beneficial effect of HA-1A in patients with gram-negative bacteremia and shock, beneficial effects of E5 were seen in patients with gram-negative sepsis (bacteremic and nonbacteremic) who were not in shock [35, 36].

Although recent questions have arisen concerning the efficacy of HA-1A and a second efficacy trial may be required, it is important to note that there are differences between efficacy and effectiveness trials. HA-1A is probably most effective in patients with gram-negative bacteremia, shock and endotoxemia [11, 21]. Part of the problem with HA-1A is that of diagnosis. The problem of early identification of patients likely to benefit from HA-1A treatment may be solved if a reliable, clinically useful, rapid endotoxin or gram-negative bacteremia test becomes available. HA-1A is not a magic bullet but it seems to have given us new insights into the pathophysiology of sepsis.

References

1. Sprung CL, Caralis PV, Marcial EH et al (1984) The effects of high-dose corticosteroids in patients with septic shock. N Engl J Med 311:1137–1143
2. Bone RC, Fisher CJ Jr, Clemmer TP et al (1987) A controlled clinical trial of high-dose methylprednisolone in the treatment of severe sepsis and septic shock. N Engl J Med 317:653–658
3. The Veterans Administration Systemic Sepsis Cooperative Study Group (1987) Effects of high-dose glucocorticoid therapy on mortality in patients with clinical signs of systemic sepsis. N Eng J Med 317:659–665
4. Favorite GO, Morgan HR (1942) Effects produced by intravenous injection in man of a toxic antigenic material derived from Eberthella typhosa: clinical hematological, chemical and serological studies. J Clin Invest 21:589-599
5. Hamill RJ, Maki DG (1986) Endotoxin shock in man caused by gram-negative bacilli. Etiology, clinical features, diagnosis, natural history and prevention In: Proctor RA (ed) Handbook of endotoxin. Elsevier, Amsterdam, pp 55–126
6. Michie HR, Manogue KR, Spriggs DR et al (1988) Detection of circulating tumor necrosis factor after endotoxin administration. N Engl J Med 318:1481–1486
7. Revhaug A, Michie HR, Manson J McK et al (1988) Inhibition of cyclooxygenase attenuates the metabolic response to endotoxin in humans. Arch Surg 123:162–170
8. Suffredini AF, Fromm RE, Parker MM et al (1989) The cardiovascular response of normal humans to the administration of endotoxin. N Engl J Med 321:280–287
9. van Deventer SJH, Buller HR, ten Cate JW et al (1988) Endotoxaemia: an early predictor of septicaemia in febrile patients. Lancet 1:605–608
10. Danner RL, Elin RJ, Hosseini JM et al (1991) Endotoxemia in human septic shock. Chest 99:169–175
11. Wortel CH, von der Mohlen MAM, van Deventer SJH et al (1992) Effectiveness of a human monoclonal anti-endotoxin antibody (HA-1A) in gram-negative sepsis. Relationship to endotoxin and cytokine levels. J Infect Dis 166:1367–1374
12. Parsons PE, Worthen GS, Moore EE, et al (1989) The association of circulating endotoxin with the development of the adult respiratory distress syndrome. Am Rev Respir Dis 140:294–301
13. Brandtzaeg P, Kierulf P, Gaustad P et al (1989) Plasma endotoxin as a predictor of multiple organ failure and death in systemic meningococcal disease. J Infect Dis 159:195–204
14. Kirkland TN, Ziegler EJ (1984) An immunoprotective monoclonal antibody to lipopolysaccharide. J Immunol 132:2590–2592
15. Baumgartner JD, Heumann D, Gerain J et al (1990) Association between protective efficacy of anti-lipopolysaccharide (LPS) antibodies and suppression of LPS-induced tumor necrosis factor alpha and interleukin-6: comparison of O side chain specific antibodies with core LPS antibodies. J Exp Med 171:889–896
16. McCabe WR, DeMaria A Jr, Berberich H et al (1988) Immunization with rough mutants of Salmonella minnesota: protective activity of IgM and IgG antibody to the R595 (Re Chemotype) mutant. J Infect Dis 158:291–300
17. Ziegler EJ, Douglas H, Sherman JE et al (1973) Treatment of E. coli and Klebsiella bacteremia in agranulocytopenic animals with antiserum to a UDP-Gal epimerase-deficient mutant. J Immunol 111:433–438
18. Ziegler EJ, McCutchan JA, Fierer J et al (1982) Treatment of gram-negative bacteremia and shock with human antiserum to a mutant Escherichia coli. N Engl J Med 307:1225–1230
19. Baumgartner JD, Glauser MP, McCutchan JA et al (1985) Prevention of gram-negative shock and death in surgical patients by antibody to endotoxin core glycolipid. Lancet ii:59–63
20. Calandra T, Glauser MP, Schellekens J et al (1988) Treatment of gram-negative septic

shock with human IgG antibody to Escherichia coli J5: a prospective, doubleblind, randomized trial. J Infect Dis 158:312–319
21. Ziegler EJ, Fisher CJ, Sprung CL et al (1991) Treatment of gram-negative bacteremia and septic shock with HA-1A human monoclonal antibody against endotoxin. A randomized, double-blind, placebo-controlled trial. N Engl J Med 324:429–436
22. Dunn Dl, Ewald DC, Chandan N et al (1986) Immunotherapy of gram-negative bacterial sepsis: a single murine monoclonal antibody provides cross-genera protection. Arch Surg 121:58–62
23. Teng NNH, Kaplan HS, Herbert JM et al (1985) Protection against gram-negative bacteremia and endotoxemia with human monoclonal IgM antibodies. Proc Natl Acad Sci USA 82:1790–1794
24. Warren HS, Danner Rl, Munford RS (1992) Anti-endotoxin monoclonal antibodies. N Engl J Med 326:1153–1157
25. Baumgartner JD, Heumann D, Glauser MP (1991) The HA-1A monoclonal antibody for gram-negative sepsis. N Engl J Med 325:281–282
26. Ziegler EJ, Smith CR (1992) Anti-endotoxin monoclonal antibodies. N Engl J Med 326:1165
27. Ziegler EJ (1988) Protective antibody to endotoxin core: the emperor's new clothes? J Infect Dis 158:286–290
28. Krieger JI, Fletcher RC, Siegel SA et al (1992) HA-1A (Centoxin TM), a human monoclonal IgM anti-endotoxin antibody, mediates immune adherence of endotoxin via CR1 of human RBCs and neutrophils. Clin Res 40:286A (abstract)
29. Siegel JP, Stein KE, Zoon KC (1992) Anti-endotoxin monoclonal antibodies. N Engl J Med 327:890–891
30. Sprung CL, Eidelman LA (1993) Monoclonal antibodies, new technologies and critical care medicine (editorial). Crit Care Med (in press)
31. Inglis TJJ, Lacey RW, Kay E et al (1993) Monoclonal antiendotoxin agent HA-1A (Centoxin). Lancet 341:303
32. Quezado ZMN, Natanson C, Alling DW et al (1993) A controlled trial of HA-1A in a canine model of gram-negative bacteremia. JAMA 269:2221–2227
33. Kett DH, Quartin AA, Pena MA et al (1992) Hemodynamic effects of HA-1A monoclonal antibody to endotoxin. Crit Care Med 20:S100 (abstract)
34. Siegel SA, Evans ME, Pollack M et al (1993) Antibiotics enhance binding by human lipid A-reactive monoclonal antibody HA-1A to smooth gram-negative bacteria. Infect Immun 61:512–519
35. Greenman RL, Schein RMH, Martin MA et al (1991) A controlled clinical trial of E5 murine monoclonal IgM antibody to endotoxin in the treatment of gram-negative sepsis. JAMA 266:1097–1102
36. Wenzel R, Bone R, Fein A et al (1991) Results of a second double-blinded, randomized, controlled trial of antiendotoxin antibody E5 in gram-negative sepsis. In: Program and abstracts of the 31st interscience conference on antimicrobial agents and chemotherapy. 29 Sept–2 Oct, Chicago, IL, p294
37. Barriere SL, Gugleilmo BJ (1992) Gram-negative sepsis, the sepsis syndrome, and the role of antiendotoxin monoclonal antibodies. Clin Pharm 11:223–235
38. Fink MP (1993) Adoptive immunotherapy of gram-negative sepsis: use of monoclonal antibodies to lipopolysaccharide. Crit Care Med 21:S32–S39
39. Caplan ES (1993) Role of immunomodulator therapy in sepsis. Am J Surg 165:20S–25S

Endotoxin in Septic Shock*

Z. M. N. Quezado, C. Natanson and W. D. Hoffmann

Introduction

Endotoxin is a lipopolysaccharide located on the outer membrane of gram-negative bacteria. Over the last 60 years, researchers have given endotoxin to animals and human volunteers to induce septic shock and investigated the pathophysiologic events associated with this syndrome [1, 2]. Recently, researchers evaluated the effects of antibody therapies directed against endotoxin in septic patients [3, 4]. The inconclusive results of these studies have raised new questions about the rôle of endotoxin in live bacterial infections [5]. To help answer questions about endotoxin, we review its biochemistry, its possible role in human disease, and its relationship to clinical antibody therapies.

Structure of Endotoxin

Exposed on the outside surface of gram-negative bacteria is the O-polysaccharide chain [6] (Fig. 1). This structure, when injected into animals, is relatively nontoxic. However, the O-polysaccharide chain is considered a virulence factor, because it forms a capsule that interferes with opsonization and killing of bacteria [6]. The molecular structure of O-polysaccharide chains vary within and among bacterial species, so infected hosts often develop a delayed serotype-specific opsonizing antibody response to the O-side chain antigens [6].

Endotoxin is also comprised of a core oligosaccharide and a lipophilic fatty acid moiety called lipid A (Fig. 1). These structures are less well exposed than the O-polysaccharide chain. Animals injected with lipid A develop symptoms of sepsis, indicating that lipid A mediates the toxic effects of endotoxin [7]. Furthermore, the structure of lipid A component and core sugars, in contrast to the O-polysaccharide chain, are relatively similar among gram-negative bacteria [8]. Researchers have developed monoclonal antibodies directed against the core and lipid A regions of endotoxin in an attempt to develop therapeutic antibodies for treating infections caused by diverse gram-negative organisms [8].

---

* Modified and Updated from Hoffman, WD and Natanson, C (1993) The role of endotoxin in bacterial septic shock. In: Vincent, J.-L. (ed) Yearbook of intensive care and emergency medicine. Springer, Berlin Heidelberg New York, pp 49–63

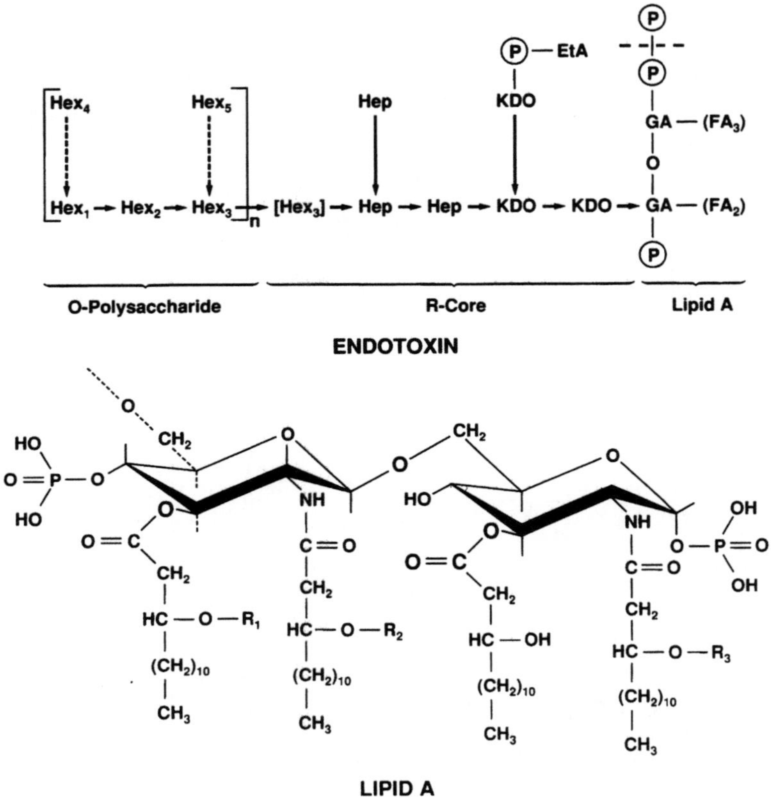

Fig. 1. The chemical structures of endotoxin and lipid A. (From [110])

Endotoxin Challenge

More than 60 years ago, Schwartzman showed that endotoxin injections produced abnormal coagulation and necrotic skin lesions in experimental animals [9]. More recently, endotoxin challenges have been shown to cause lung injury in sheep [10, 11], intestinal mucosal injury in pigs [12], and renal dysfunction in rats [13–15]. Thus, researchers have found that endotoxin challenges in many species produce the type of organ failure frequently associated with septic shock in humans.

At the National Institutes of Health (NIH), we have studied the effects of endotoxin challenge in a canine model of septic shock [16]. In these experiments, purpose-bred dogs are surgically implanted with a standard dose of endotoxin in an intraperitoneal fibrin-thrombin clot. Unlike an intravenous challenge, the clot releases endotoxin over an extended period of time. To study the effects of endotoxin challenge, we measure hemodynamic and laboratory values and endotoxin levels before and 10–28 days after challenge

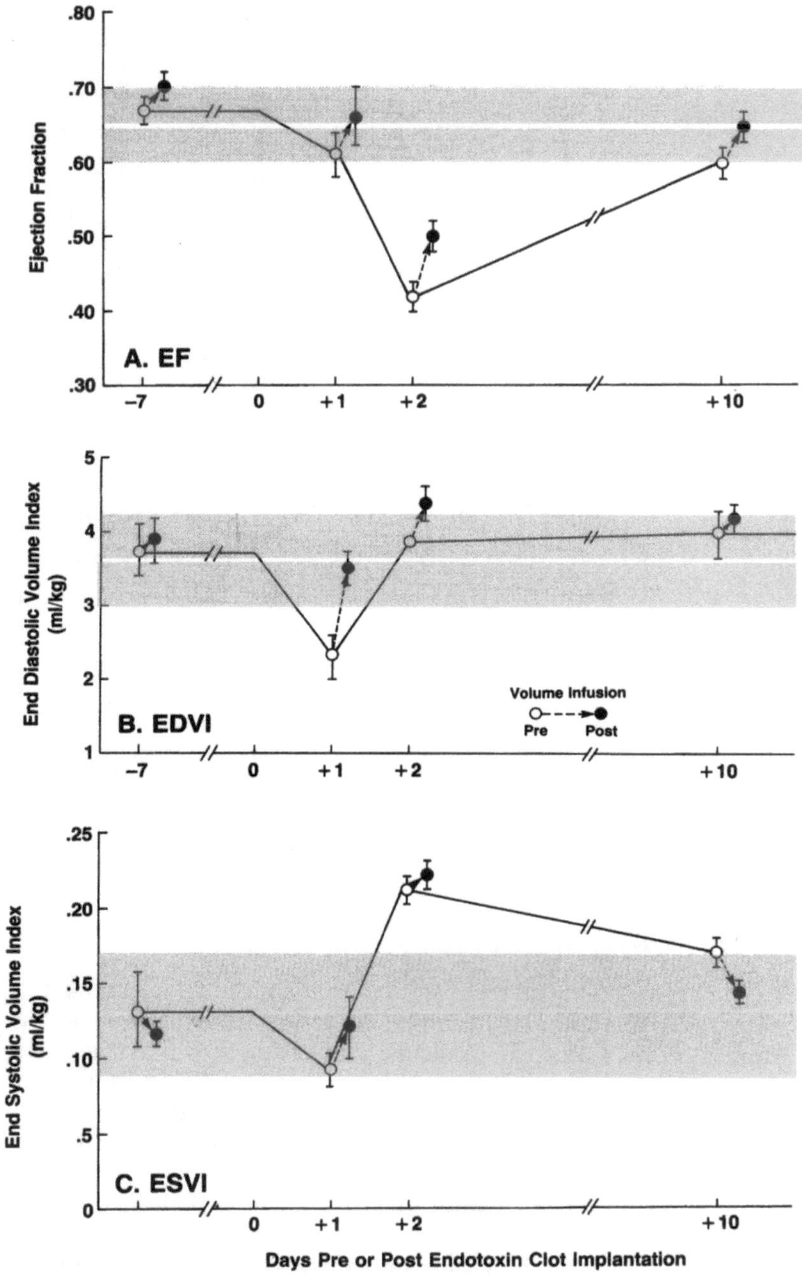

Fig. 2. A–C. Serial (over 10 days) **A** left ventricular ejection fraction (*EF*), **B** end diastolic volume index (*EDVI*), and **C** end systolic volume index (*ESVI*) for canines given an intraperitoneal clot (day 0) containing endotoxin. Baseline (pre-clot) values are shown at day −7. *Hollow circles* and *filled circles* (connected by *dashed arrows*) represent values (mean ± SE) obtained before and after fluid challenge, respectively. Similar to animals and humans with bacterial septic shock, 2 days after clot implantation, endotoxin challenge produced a decrease in EF with increases in EDVI (after volume challenge) and ESVI that returned to baseline values in 10 days. (From [16])

(Fig. 2). Although animals have sterile blood cultures, they show the same characteristic pattern of hemodynamic dysfunction seen in humans with septic shock and canines challenged with live bacterial infected clots.

In healthy human volunteers, an intravenous bolus of endotoxin (2–4 ng/kg) produces transient circulating levels of endotoxin and reversible physiologic dysfunction over 3–24 h [17]. In volume-resuscitated humans, cardiac index and heart rate increases, and systemic vascular resistance index and left ventricular ejection fraction decreases 3–5 h after endotoxin infusion [17]. Other studies of human volunteers have shown that endotoxin challenge induces the release of tissue plasminogen activator and plasminogen activator inhibitor [18, 19] and increases intestinal permeability to lactulose and mannitol [20]. Thus, low doses of endotoxin produce reversible abnormalities in cardiovascular function, coagulation, and intestinal function which are qualitatively similar to, but not as intense or prolonged as, those seen in humans with septic shock.

C3H/HeJ mice have a genetic abnormality that makes them less responsive to endotoxin [21, 22]. After stimulation by endotoxin, macrophages from these mice produce abnormally low amounts of tumor necrosis factor (TNF), a host protein that may mediate many of the manifestations of septic shock [23]. Interestingly, these C3H/HeJ mice are more susceptible to bacterial challenge than normal mice [24, 25]. These findings show that sensitivity to endotoxin is not essential for gram-negative bacteria to produce lethality. A normal and vigorous response to endotoxin may actually initiate protective reactions that resist bacterial invasion and lethality.

Circulating Endotoxin

Endotoxin activates a proenzyme produced by horseshoe crab amebocytes and the proenzyme forms a visible gel when combined with a lysate of amebocytes. This finding led scientists to develop a limulus amebocyte lysate (LAL) bioassay that quantifies endotoxin blood levels [26–28]. Initially, the LAL test was believed to lack sensitivity and clinical correlation, partly because lysate preparations varied in their ability to detect endotoxin and plasma samples contained inhibitors of the assay [29, 30].

Since its original development, the LAL assay has been improved by methods that remove nonspecific interfering substances and add a semiquantitative chromogenic substrate to increase the sensitivity of the assay (lower limit of the assay is 0.5 pg/ml) [31–33]. Although the improved LAL assay is thought to be relatively specific [34–36], there is no direct measure of endotoxin to validate the specificity of this bioassay.

At NIH, Danner et al. performed serial LAL plasma tests in 100 patients with septic shock [37]. Numerous samples were obtained from each patient on several days, but only 43% of patients with septic shock had LAL positivity, indicating endotoxemia. Interestingly, the presence of endotoxemia was associated with more episodes of renal failure and adult respiratory distress syndrome, although endotoxin levels did not correlate with severity of illness [37]. No other clinical reports have correlated the degree of LAL positivity with outcome in a heterogeneous population of patients with septic shock.

In the Danner study [37], LAL positivity did not correlate well with type of infecting organism. No endotoxemia was found in 8 of 18 patients with gram-negative bacteremia. Surprisingly, endotoxemia was found in 8 of 14 patients with gram-positive bacteremia, 7 of 7! patients with fungemia, and 19 of 63 patients with negative cultures. Endotoxemia in gram-positive infections, fungemia, and culture negative septic shock may represent undetected gram-negative bacteremia, leakage of endotoxin into the blood stream from an isolated gram-negative bacterial infection, or leakage of endotoxin across the intestinal mucosa. In patients with gram-negative bacteremia and no endotoxemia, the level of endotoxin in the blood could be below the sensitivity of the LAL assay. Other investigators have also found that LAL positivity correlates poorly with the presence of gram-negative bacteremia [38, 39]. These observations have raised questions about the relationship of LAL levels and pathophysiologic events in septic shock.

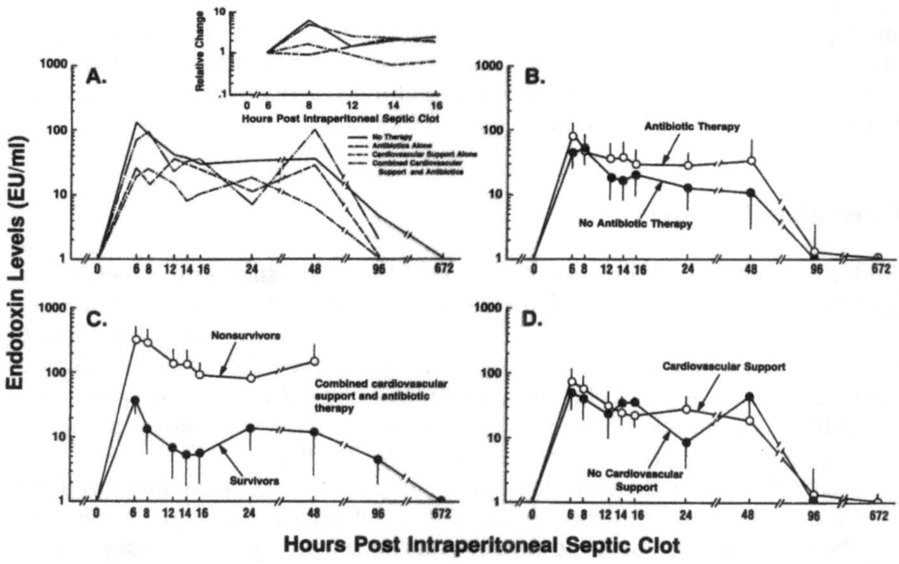

Fig. 3. A–D. Serial (over 28 days) mean endotoxin levels for canines receiving an *E. coli* infected intraperitoneal clot (hour 0). In this study four treatment groups were defined: animals received no therapy, antibiotics alone, cardiovascular support (fluids and pressors) alone, or combined antibiotics and cardiovascular support. **A** Serial endotoxin levels were similar in these four treatment groups. **B** Antibiotic therapy had no significant effect on endotoxin levels. **C** When considering animals given combined antibiotics and cardiovascular support, endotoxin levels were greater in nonsurvivors and greater levels at 6 h predicted decreased survival time. **D** Cardiovascular support had no significant effect on endotoxin levels. (From [40])

We examined LAL activity in canines infected with an intraperitoneal clot containing live *Escherichia coli* [40]. LAL levels were correlated with cardiovascular abnormalities and lethality. Compared with surviving animals, nonsurviving animals had higher levels of endotoxemia which predicted a decrease in survival time. Antibiotics and cardiovascular support improved outcome but did not affect the level of endotoxemia (Fig. 3). In another experiment, two monoclonal antibodies directed against endotoxin also improved outcome, but the ability of the antibody to reduce endotoxemia depended on the specificity of the antibody [41]. These results suggest that under certain circumstances the level of endotoxemia may indicate severity of illness [41, 42]. However, these results also suggest that therapies can improve outcome without decreasing endotoxemia, indicating that endotoxin levels may not be an appropriate measure of therapeutic success.

Using our canine model of septic shock, we compared different infecting organisms and determined their effects on LAL positivity and septic shock. Compared with animals given intraperitoneal challenges of *E. coli*, those given *Pseudomonas aeruginosa* (comparable numbers of colony forming units) had lower levels of endotoxemia [43] (Table 1). However, animals given *P. aeruginosa* demonstrated greater cardiovascular dysfunction and lethality. In another study, we compared a virulent *E. coli* strain (with an antiphagocytic capsule, serum resistance, and the ability to produce hemolysins) to a nonvirulent *E. coli* strain (without these properties) [44, 45]. The virulent *E. coli* produced less endotoxemia but greater cardiovascular dysfunction and lethality suggesting that bacterial virulence may be more important than endotoxemia in determining cardiovascular changes and lethality [44]. These results suggest that, in studies of subjects infected with different microorganisms, levels of circulating endotoxin do not predict clinical outcomes.

We also examined whether endotoxemia exists during non-gram-negative infection. In separate studies we challenged animals with *Staphylococcus aureus* (an organism without endotoxin) or a heat-treated *E. coli* (a nonviable product that had minimal endotoxin) [44, 46]. *S. aureus* produced all of the cardiovascular changes and lethality of septic shock but without endotoxemia (Table 1, Fig. 4). Compared with *E. coli, S. aureus* at lower doses

Table 1. Median values (and range) for endotoxemia during septic shock

	Sterile clots (controls)	*S. aureus* (viable)	*E. coli* (viable)	*P. aeruginosa* (viable)
Endotoxin concentration (EU/ml)[a]		1×10^9 CFU/kg	14×10^9 CFU/kg	14×10^9 CFU/kg
Median	0.8	0.0	45.5	2.4
Range	(0–1.7)	(0–0.64)	(3.72–74.8)	(0.05–77.4)

CFU, colony forming units.
[a] One endotoxin unit (EU) is equal to the activity of 100 pg of U.S. standard endotoxin.

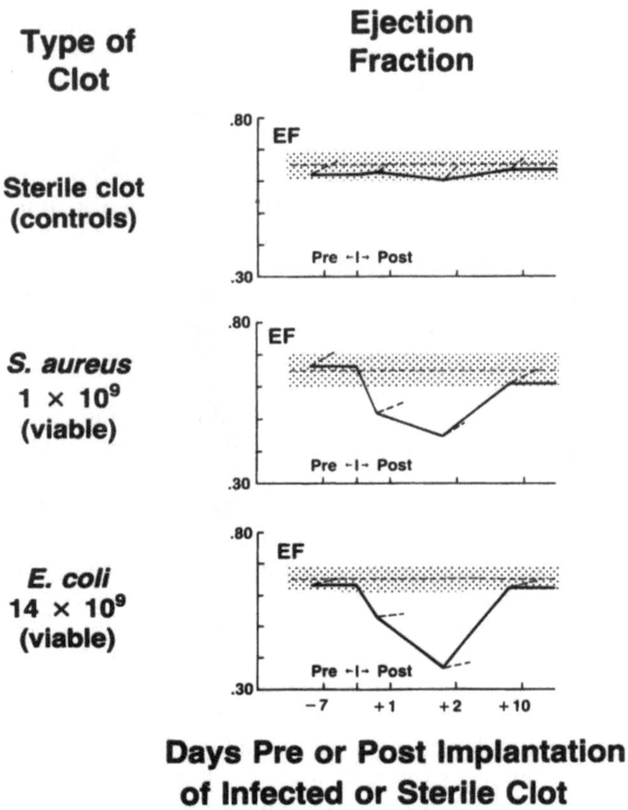

Fig. 4. Serial (over 10 days) mean left ventricular ejection fractions (*EF*) for animals receiving intraperitoneal clots (day 0) containing no bacteria (sterile), *S. aureus,* and *E. coli.* The baseline (pre-clot) time is designated day −7. *Dashed lines* represent the effect of fluid therapy on days −7, 1, 2, and 10. Comapred with *E. coli* (an organism with endotoxin), *S. aureus* (an organism without endotoxin) produced similar decreases in EF but was more potent. (From [46])

produced greater morbidity and mortality. Animals given the heat-treated *E. coli* had minimal levels of endotoxemia but marked cardiovascular changes and lethality. These data show that severe septic shock can occur without endotoxin or high circulating levels of endotoxin.

These findings show a lack of correlation between level of endotoxemia and clinical outcome, which suggests that the development of endotoxemia after infection may be an epiphenomenon. Thus, endotoxemia may be one marker of the disease but not necessarily a persistent mediator of toxicity.

The Host Response to Endotoxin

Human serum and cell membranes contain proteins and receptors that specifically bind endotoxin (Fig. 5). These molecules may regulate the host complex immunologic response to this exogenous bacterial toxin. A more detailed understanding of these host proteins and receptors may lead to pharmacological agents that diminish the toxic effects of endotoxin while maintaining the beneficial aspects of the host response.

Endotoxin Binding Proteins

Human lipoproteins bind and transport endotoxin in plasma and may be part of the natural host defense against endotoxin. Among these, high densi-

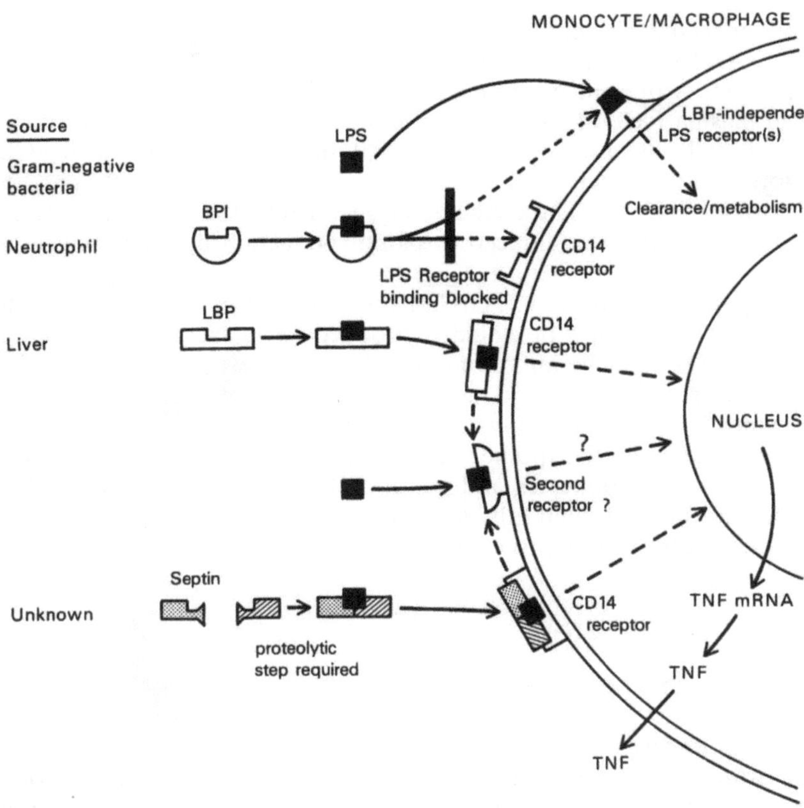

Fig. 5. Endotoxin binding proteins and endotoxin cellular receptors. *LPS*, lipopolysaccharide; *BPI*, bactericidal permeability increasing protein; *LBP*, lipopolysaccharide binding protein; *TNF*, tumor necrosis factor. (From [111])

ty lipoproteins have been shown to decrease toxicity of endotoxin and to increase its plasma clearance [47–49]. In addition, a 55 kDa molecule found in neutrophil granules, bactericidal/permeability increasing protein (BPI), has bactericidal effects and antiendotoxin activities [50–53]. Lipopolysaccharide binding protein (LBP), a 60 kDa lipoprotein produced by the liver, binds with high affinity to the lipid A component of endotoxin. LBP opsonizes endotoxin for recognition of specific receptors (CD14) on neutrophils [54, 55]. These LBP-endotoxin complexes can increase production of potentially toxic mediators, such as TNF, by macrophages [56]. Septin, a term for an opsonic activity in plasma (distinct from LBP), has been recently described. Septin opsonizes endotoxin-coated particles for recognition by neutrophils and macrophages via CD14 receptors [57].

Endotoxin Receptors

Several endotoxin receptors have been identified on white blood cells (CD14, CD11/CD18, the scavenger receptor, etc.). CD14 [55], a 55 kDa glycoprotein, is present on monocytes, tissue macrophages, and in soluble form in plasma (sCD14). Occupation of cell associated CD14 receptors by LBP bacteria leads to secretion of TNF [55]. Interestingly, cells lacking CD14 receptors can still be activated by endotoxin-LBP-sCD14 complexes and produce cytokines [55, 58]. These results, suggest that CD14 is not necessary, but may facilitate endotoxin-induced cytokine production by macrophages [54, 55].

Binding of endotoxin to CD11/CD18 receptor on macrophages [59] does not result in stimulation of cytokine production. In fact, there is evidence that CD11/CD18 may be important in endotoxin clearance mechanisms [59]. The scavenger receptor, a 95 kDa molecule, was recently identified as acetyl-LDL, which is present on many cells of myeloid lineage [60], but its function is not well understood. Another 73 kDa endotoxin receptor has been described in human monocytes and neutrophils. Although the role of the 73 kDa receptor has not been fully understood, monoclonal antibodies against this 73 kDa receptor have protected mice against endotoxin-induced lethality [61, 62].

Anti-endotoxin Therapies

Multiple approaches to block endotoxin effects have been developed as therapeutic strategies for treatment of septic shock. These include anti-endotoxin antibodies (Tables 2 and 3), nonantibody agents that bind endotoxin, and analogues of lipid A that either induce tolerance to endotoxin or act as its direct antagonist (Table 4). Although no anti-endotoxin therapy has been approved by the U.S.A Food and Drug Administration (FDA) for clinical

Table 2. Clinical trials with endotoxin core-directed antiserum or plasma

Therapy	Reference	Reported efficacy	Reported *p* value (survival)	Methodological concerns about reported results	Target group	*p* value (survival)
J5 antiserum	[76]	GNB + (GNI and appropriate antibiotic therapy)	0.01	High mortality in controls	GNS	Not reported
J5 antiserum	[112]	None	None	None	Prophylaxis of GNS in patients with prolonged neutropenia	NS
J5 immune plasma	[78]	GNS (shock)	0.046	One-tailed test for efficacy	Prophylaxis of GNS in high-risk surgical patients	NS
J5 immune plasma	[113]	None	None	None	Infectious purpura in children (shock)	NS
J5 IVIG	[114]	None	None	None	GNS (shock)	NS
J5 IVIG	[115]	None	None	None	Prophylaxis of high-risk surgical patients	NS

GNB, gram-negative bacteremia; GNI, gram-negative infection; GNS, gram-negative sepsis; IVIG, intravenous immunoglobulin; NS, not significant.

use, antibodies directed against endotoxin have undergone several multicenter clinical trials.

Therapy with Anti-endotoxin Antibodies

Comparison of O-side Chain and Core/Lipid A Antibodies

Antibodies directed against the O-polysaccharide component of endotoxin have antibacterial (complement-dependent bactericidal and opsonophagocytic activities) and protective effects in gram-negative infections [63–71]. Since the O-polysaccharide antigen is structurally different for each strain of gram-negative bacteria, antibodies directed at this antigen only protect against infection from the homologous strain of bacteria. Antibodies directed against core/lipid A antigens are thought to neutralize toxic effects or enhance clearance of endotoxin [72–76]. Furthermore, core and lipid A an

Table 3. Clinical trials with endotoxin core-directed monoclonal antibodies

Therapy	Reference	Reported efficacy	Reported *p* value (survival)	Methodological concerns about reported results	Target group	*p* value (survival)
E5	[4]	GNS (no shock)	0.01	Retrospective	GNS	NS
E5	[88]	None	None	None	GNS (no shock)	NS
HA-1A	[3]	GNB (shock, 28 day all cause mortality)	0.017	Revised analytical plan rejected	GNS (14 day mortality)	NS
HA-1A[a]	[93]					

GNS, gram-negative sepsis; GNB, gram-negative bacteremia; NS, not significant.
[a] Early stopping criteria met for excess mortality in the HA-1A treatment group.

Table 4. Approaches to anti-endotoxin therapies for septic shock

Type of agent	Possible effect	Examples
Anti-endotoxin antibodies	Enhance clearance of endotoxin Augment bactericidal activity	Core/lipid A reactive antibodies O-side chain antibodies
Peptides and lipoproteins that bind endotoxin	Neutralize or enhance clearance of endotoxin	Cationic polypeptides (polymyxin B, colistin) Bactericidal/permeability increasing protein High density lipoproteins
Lipid A derivatives	Induce tolerance to endotoxin Direct antagonism of endotoxin	Deacylated endotoxins Lipid X Monophosphorylated lipid A

tigens are more phylogenetically conserved than O-polysaccharide antigen, and antibodies directed against core structures may protect against diverse gram-negative bacteria [77–81]. However, because these core/lipid A antigens are not well exposed in gram-negative bacteria, they may be less available for binding with antibodies.

Using our canine model of septic shock, we investigated *in vivo* effects of murine IgG anti-endotoxin monoclonal antibodies directed at the O-polysaccharide and at the core/lipid A regions of endotoxin [41, 42]. The O-polysaccharide monoclonal antibody reduced bacteremia before antibiotic treatment, lowered plasma endotoxin levels, and enhanced survival. When combined with antibiotic therapy, the core/lipid A monoclonal antibody had a borderline ($p < 0.07$) effect on survival and caused a more rapid recovery of mean arterial pressure, but had no effect on bacteremia or endotoxemia. Thus, in our canine model of septic shock, we found core/lipid A reactive antibodies to have distinct functions and more modest effects than O-polysaccharide reactive antibody.

Polyclonal Antibodies Directed at Core and Lipid A Antigens

Six clinical trials of core-directed antiserum or core-specific intravenous immunoglobulin have been conducted as treatment or prophylaxis of gram-negative sepsis (Table 2).

In preparation for the first clinical trial, human volunteers were challenged with a heat-killed "rough" mutant *E. coli* J5, comprised of core and lipid A structures but no O-polysaccharide chain [76]. Plasma obtained after challenge was expected to contain polyclonal antibodies directed at core structures of endotoxin. In a double-blind multicenter trial of patients with presumed gram-negative infection, researchers compared serum obtained after immunization (J5 antiserum) with that obtained before immunization (control serum). All-cause mortality and the mortality of the group with gram-negative infection were not reported. J5 antiserum treatment decreased mortality in an assembled group of patients with gram-negative bacteremia and patients with gram-negative infection on appropriate antibiotics (22% vs 39%). J5 antiserum was most beneficial in the subset of patients who were in shock before randomization (44% vs 77%) [76]. However, the high mortality rate of the control group with shock (77%) has suggested that randomization of patients may have resulted in imbalances [70, 82, 83]. In addition, investigators subsequently found no relationship between anti-J5 antibody levels and improved outcome. Thus, differences between the J5 antiserum group and controls may have been caused by factors other than "cross-protective" anti-endotoxin antibodies.

In another clinical trial, investigators prophylactically gave J5 immune plasma or control therapy to surgical patients at high risk for gram-negative infections [78]. Patients given J5 immune plasma did not have lower rates of gram-negative infections but showed a (nonsignificant) trend toward reductions in gram-negative septic shock (5% vs 11%) and death rates from gram-negative septic shock (2% vs 7%).

Four other clinical trials failed to demonstrate any therapeutic efficacy of core-directed antiserum or immunoglobulin for the prophylaxis or treatment of patients with gram-negative sepsis (Table 2). These studies raise doubts about whether therapies directed at core/lipid A structures of endotoxin will cross-protect against infections with heterologous gram-negative bacteria. Nevertheless, many investigators still believe that anti-J5 antiserum contains protective core-directed anti-endotoxin antibodies. Thus, researchers have developed monoclonal antibodies against core and lipid A antigens with the hope of finding a more specific and therefore efficacious therapy for gram-negative sepsis.

Monoclonal Antibodies Directed at Core and Lipid A Antigens

Data on the use of monoclonal antibodies against endotoxin have clinical originated from the use of two IgM monoclonal antibodies, the murine monoclonal antibody (E5) (XOMA, Berkeley, CA, USA) and the human monoclonal antibody (HA-1A) (Centocor Inc., Malvern, PA, USA). E5 had been found to diminish the effects of endotoxin challenge in sheep and to protect mice challenged with live bacterial infections [85, 86]. HA-1A had been reported to protect mice from lethal bacteremia and to protect rabbits from the dermal Schwartzman reaction, although other investigators were not able to confirm these results [46, 87].

Partially because of the positive results in some of these animals experiments, E5 and HA-1A were both studied in two clinical trials of patients with sepsis (Table 3).

In the first E5 trial [4], a total of 486 patients with signs of gram-negative sepsis were enrolled. Of these, 316 patients had confirmed gram-negative infections. In this study, E5 did not affect survival in patients with gram-negative infection or patients with gram-negative infection and shock. However, E5 significantly increased survival (70% vs 57%) and improved organ function in a retrospectively defined subgroup of patients ($n=137$) with gram-negative infections who were not in refractory shock. A second trial of E5 was prospectively conducted to confirm these results. There were 847 patients who were enrolled in the second E5 trial, 530 of which had gram-negative infections without refractory shock. This second E5 trial did not show a beneficial effect in survival in patients without refractory shock [88].

The human monoclonal antibody HA-1A has been tested in a randomized placebo-controlled trial of 543 patients with presumed gram-negative sepsis [3]. Investigators reported that HA-1A significantly increased 28 day survival in a subgroup of patients with gram-negative bacteremia (30% vs 49%). However, since its publication, the study has been the focus of much debate in the scientific community [5]. Since sicker patients and patients not given effective antibiotic therapy were assigned more often to the control group, the randomization of patients may have produced imbalances. In addition, the analytical plan submitted to the FDA described three overlapping patient subgroups, two categories of mortality (septic and all-cause), and two survival endpoints (14 and 28 day). There is no standard procedure to adjust p values derived from these multiple comparisons. Nevertheless, FDA reviewers concluded that HA-1A had, at best, a borderline beneficial effect in some subgroups.

During this time, we conducted a blinded, controlled study of HA-1A in a canine model of septic shock [89]. In this study, animals were infected with an intraperitoneal clot containing *E. coli* 0111:B4, the native form of the mutant *E. coli* J5 (the organism used to develop the heteromyeloma cell line that produces HA-1A), and treated with fluid and antibiotics. Unexpectedly, HA-1A increased lethality; only 2 of 13 animals in the HA-1A group, as compared with 8 of 14 controls, survived 28 days (Fig. 6). In addition, HA-1A did not alter levels of bacteremia or endotoxemia (Fig. 7). Moreover, compared to septic controls, the HA-1A group had lower mean arterial

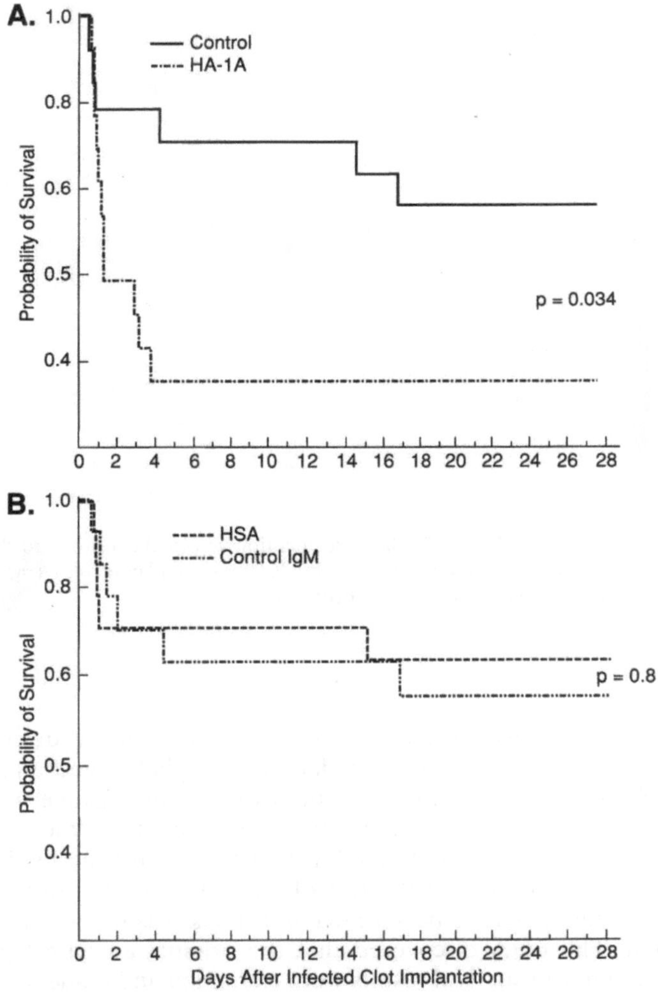

Fig. 6. A, B. Probability of survival after infected clot (containing *E. coli*) implantation for **A** animals given HA-1A ($n = 13$) or control therapy, consisting of combined control human IgM antibody and control human serum albumin (*HSA*, $n = 14$), and **B** infected animals given control human IgM antibody ($n = 11$) or control HSA therapy ($n = 11$). (From [89])

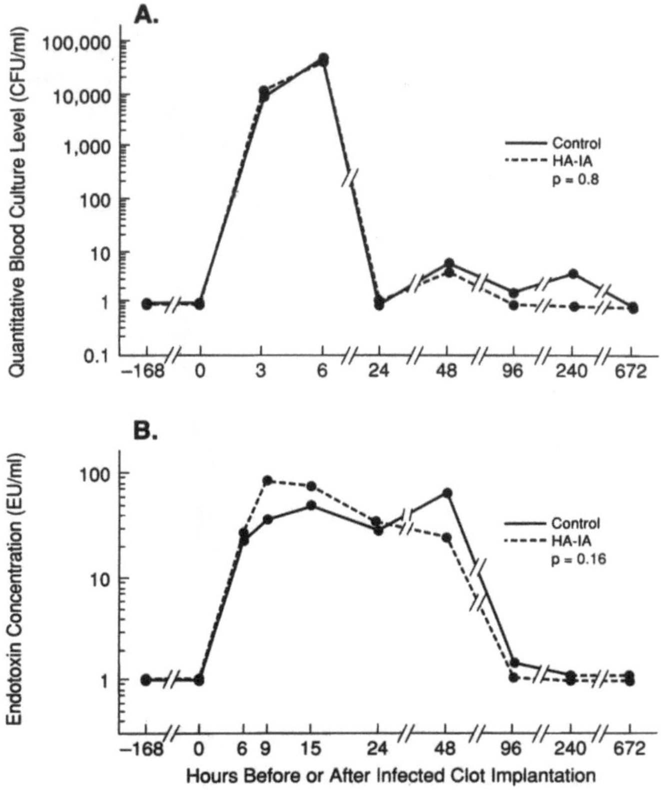

Fig. 7. A, B. Serial (over 28 days) **A** quantitative blood cultures and **B** endotoxin concentrations for infected HA-1A-treated animals ($n=13$) and controls ($n=14$). *CFU*, colony forming units; *EU*, endotoxin units. (From [89])

pressure and worse lactic acidosis and cardiac injury, during sepsis. Thus, the results of this study strongly demonstrate that a mechanism exists by which HA-1A can be harmful to animals with gram-negative septic shock.

Subsequent to our canine study, reviewers from the FDA concluded that the first clinical trial of HA-1A did not demonstrate its therapeutic efficacy. The reported beneficial effect of HA-1A in 28 day survival rate of patients with gram-negative bacteremia and shock was based on a revised analytical plan. The FDA discovered that the original analytical plan was amended after interim survival results were examined and made available to Centocor [90–92]. Accordingly, FDA reviewers rejected the revised analytical plan because this interim examination may have biased the results. When reviewers analyzed the study using the original analytical plan 14 day mortality endpoint, they found that there was no survival benefit from HA-1A in patients with gram-negative bacteremia. Consequently, the use of HA-1A was not approved for clinical use.

Subsequently, investigators at Centocor undertook a second multicenter clinical trial of HA-1A to determine the safety and efficacy of HA-1A in patients with gram-negative bacteremia. More than 1 year after the results of the HA-1A canine study were reported, the second clinical trial of HA-1A was stopped because an interim analysis of the accrued survival data showed that patients receiving HA-1A had excess mortality [93].

In summary, there is no convincing data at this time to support the use of antibodies against the core region of endotoxin for the treatment of septic patients. Importantly, the detrimental effects of one monoclonal antibody (HA-1A) in animals [89] and humans [93] underscore the need to investigate the conditions under which these agents have beneficial, neutral, or deleterious effects [94].

Other Therapies Directed at Endotoxin in Septic Shock

The results of clinical trials with therapies directed against core structures of endotoxin are disappointing; however, other agents that actually neutralize endotoxin have been developed. These therapies (Table 4) are currently under investigation and hopefully, results of these investigations will help to clarify the role of endotoxin in septic shock.

Peptides and Lipoproteins That Bind to Endotoxin

Polymyxin B and colistin (polymyxin E) are two polycationic antibiotics that bind to the lipid A region of endotoxin by ionic and hydrophobic interactions and neutralize some of its biologic effects [95–98]. In mice, polymyxin B reduced endotoxin-induced lethality [95], and in rabbits prevented the generalized Schwartzman reaction [96]. However, these polycationic antibiotics produce many side effects, such as nephrotoxicity and neurotoxicity. In an attempt to prevent these toxic effects and at the same time maintain beneficial properties, polymyxin B has been immobilized on filters and used to remove endotoxin via extracorporeal circulation [99].

BPI, a cationic protein, is being actively investigated because of its ability to bind the lipid A component of various gram-negative bacteria and neutralize the biologic effects of endotoxin. In particular, BPI has been shown to inhibit endotoxin-induced CR1 and CR3 expression in human neutrophils, production of TNF by macrophages, neutrophil priming, LAL assay activity, and pyrogenicity in rabbits [51, 53].

Reconstituted lipoproteins have been evaluated for the treatment of sepsis and septic shock. In small animals, reconstituted high density lipoprotein (R-HDL) is protective against the lethal effects of endotoxin challenge [100]. R-HDL, in our canine model of gram-negative sepsis and septic shock, decreased endotoxemia and serum levels of TNF. However, R-HDL produced hepatotoxicity and neurotoxicity and increased lethality. If these toxic effects of R-HDL can be diminished by an improved preparation or better modes of administration, the observed anti-endotoxin effects of R-HDL could potentially improve outcome in sepsis.

Lipid A Derivatives

Deacylated endotoxins, derived from the hydrolysis of acyloxyacyl bonds in lipid A [101, 102], inhibit some proinflammatory effects of endotoxin (endothelial cell-neutrophil adhesion, prostaglandin production, plasminogen activator-1 expression) [103] and maintain some immunostimulatory properties of endotoxin [102]. The role of deacylated proteins in animal models of sepsis have yet to be evaluated.

Lipid X is a monosaccharide precursor of lipid A [104, 105]. Data from animal studies suggest that lipid X has anti-endotoxin activity and protective effects in animal models using endotoxin challenge [106]. However, such beneficial effects were not seen in animals models with live bacterial infection [105].

Monophosphorylated lipid A, another lipid A derivative, has been isolated from a mutant strain of *Salmonella* [107]. This agent has been shown *in vitro* to inhibit endotoxin-induced neutrophil superoxide production [108]. In addition, in animal models of endotoxin challenge, monophosphorylated lipid A attenuated detrimental cardiovascular effects and increased survival [107, 109]. Further studies to determine toxicity and therapeutic efficacy of monophosphorylated lipid A in live bacterial infections are ongoing.

Summary

In normal animals, endotoxin challenge can initiate a complex host response that can produce the multiple organ failure characteristic of human septic shock. Since gram-positive infections produce a similar syndrome, endotoxin may be only one of many molecules or "signals" that can initiate this reaction. Thus, endotoxin is sufficient but not necessary to produce the physiologic dysfunction typical of septic shock.

When given without bacterial infection, endotoxin is rapidly cleared from the circulation, and the host response, which is prolonged and produces multiple organ dysfunction, is of no apparent benefit. In gram-negative bacterial infection, however, the relationship among endotoxin, other bacterial toxins and components, host mediators, and the ability of gram-negative organisms to produce invasive disease and lethality has not been fully defined.

The presence of circulating endotoxin has been associated with severe illness in infected humans. However, the LAL bioassay for endotoxin has not been standardized, and results between centers have not been consistent. In addition, patients without documented gram-negative infection frequently have endotoxemia. In animal studies, the importance of the level of endotoxemia seems to depend on the infecting organism, as organisms producing little or no endotoxemia can produce more severe disease than those producing substantial endotoxemia. Thus, the cause-effect ralationship between circulating levels of endotoxin and outcome of bacterial septic shock may not be generalizable to the full range of clinical infections.

In four multicenter trials of patients with sepsis and presumed gram-negative infection, monoclonal antibodies against the core region of endotoxin had no significant beneficial effect on survival or were harmful [3, 4, 88, 93]. Despite these discouraging results, other agents that may actually neutralize endotoxin are under investigation. Results of studies using these agents may clarify whether endotoxin is an appropriate therapeutic target for septic shock.

Acknowledgements: The authors would like to thank Robert L. Danner, M.D. for his careful review of this manuscript and Lee Hoffman for her considerable editorial contributions.

References

1. Caridis DT, Reinhold RB, Woodruff PWH, Fine J (1972) Endotoxaemia in man. Lancet 1:1381–1386
2. Danner RL, Suffredini AF, Natanson C, Parrillo JE (1989) Microbial toxins: role in the pathogenesis of septic shock and multiple organ failure. In: Bihary DJ, Cerra FB (eds) New horizons: multiple organ failure. Fullerton, Society of Critical Care Medicine, pp 151–192
3. Ziegler EJ, Fisher CJ Jr, Sprung CL et al (1991) Treatment of gram-negative bacteremia and septic shock with HA-1A human monoclonal antibody against endotoxin. N Engl J Med 324:429–436
4. Greenman RL, Schein RM, Martin MA et al (1991) A controlled clinical trial of E 5 murine monoclonal IgM antibody to Endotoxin in the treatment of gram-negative sepsis. JAMA 266:1097–1102
5. Warren SH, Danner RL, Munford RS (1992) Anti-endotoxin monoclonal antibodies. N Engl J Med 326:1153–1157
6. Westphal O, Hann K, Himmelspach K (1983) Chemistry and immunochemistry of bacterial lipopolysaccharide as cell wall antigens and endotoxin. Prog Allergy 33:9–39
7. Galanos C, Luderitz O, Reitchel E et al (1985) Synthetic and natural Escherichia coli free lipid A express identical endotoxin activities. Eur J Biochem 148:1–5
8. Brade H, Brade L, Schade U et al (1988) Structure, endotoxicity, immunogenicity and antigenicity of bacterial lipopolysaccharides (endotoxins, O-antigens). Prog Clin Biol Res 272:17–45
9. Schwartzman G (1928) Studies on Bacillus typhosus substance. I. Phenomenon of local skin reactivity to B. typhosus culture filtrate. J Exp Med 38:247–268
10. Esbenshade AM, Newman JH, Lams PM, Jolles H, Bringham KL (1982) Respiratory failure after endotoxin infusion in sheep: Lung mechanics and lung fluid balance. J Appl Physiol 53:967–976
11. Bringham KL, Bowewrs RE, Haynes J (1979) Increased sheep lung vascular permeabiliy caused by Escherichia coli endotoxin. Circ Res 45:292–297
12. Fink MP, Antonsson JB, Wang HL, Rothschild HR (1991) Increased intestinal per-

meability in endotoxic pigs. Mesenteric hypoperfusion as an etiologic factor. Arch Surg 126:211–218
13. Kikery D, Pennell JP, Hwang KH, Jacob AI, Richman AV, Bourgoignie JJ (1986) Endotoxemic acute renal failure in awake rats. Am J Physiol 250:1098–1106
14. Zager RA (1986) Escherichia coli endotoxin injections potentiate experimental ischemic renal injury. Am J Physiol 251:988–994
15. Zager RA, Prior RB (1986) Gentamicin and gram-negative bacteremia. A synergism for the development of experimental nephrotoxic acute renal failure. J Clin Invest 78:196–206
16. Natanson C, Eichenholz PW, Danner RL et al (1989) Endotoxin and tumor necrosis factor challenges in dogs simulate the cardiovascular profile of human septic shock. J Exp Med 169:823–832
17. Suffredini AF, Fromm RE, Parker MM et al (1989) The cardiovascular response of normal humans to the administration of endotoxin. N Engl J Med 321:280–287
18. Suffredini AF, Harpel PC, Parrillo JE (1989) Promotion and subsequent inhibition of plasminogen activation after administration of intravenous endotoxin to normal subjects. N Engl J Med 320:1165–1172
19. Gralnick HR, McKeown LP, Wilson OM, Williams SB, Elin RJ (1989) Von Willebrand factor release induced by endotoxin. J Lab Clin Med 113:118–122
20. Odweyer ST, Michie HR, Ziegler TR, Revhaug A, Smith RJ, Wilmore DW (1988) A single dose of endotoxin increases intestinal permeability in healthy humans. Arch Surg 123:1459–1464
21. Weinstein DL, Lissner CR, Swanson RN, O'Brien AD (1986) Macrophage defect and inflammatory cell recruitment dysfunction in Salmonella susceptible C3H/HeJ mice. Cell Immunol 102:68–77
22. Ayala A, Kisala JM, Felt JA, Perrin MM, Chaudry IH (1992) Does endotoxin tolerance prevents the release of inflammatory monokines (interleukin 1, interleukin 6, or tumor necrosis factor) during sepsis? Arch Surg 127:191–196
23. Beutler B, Krochin N, Milsark IW, Luedke C, Cerami A (1986) Control of cachectin (tumor necrosis factor) synthesis. Mechanisms of resistance. Science 232:977–980
24. Adi S, Pollock AS, Shigenaga JK, Moser AH, Feingold KR, Grunfeld C (1992) Role for monokines in the metabolic effects of endotoxin. J Clin Invest 89:1603–1609
25. De SK, McMaster MT, Andrews GK (1990) Endotoxin induction of murine metallothionein gene expression. J Biol Chem 2265:15267–15274
26. Levin J, Bang F (1965) The role of endotoxin in the extracellular coagulation of Limulus blood. Johns Hopkins Med J 115:265–274
27. Levin J, Poore TE, Zauber NP, Oser RS (1970) Detection of endotoxin in the blood of patients with sepsis due to gram-negative bacteria. N Engl J Med 283:1313–1316
28. Reinhold R, Fine JA (1971) Technique for quantitative measurement of endotoxin in human plasma. Proc Soc Exp Biol Med 137:334–340
29. Elin RJ, Robinson RA, Levine AS, Wolff SM (1975) Lack of clinical usefulness of the Limulus test int the diagnosis of endotoxemia. N Engl J Med 293:521–523
30. Jorgensen JH, Carvajal HF, Chipps BE, Smith RJ (1973) Rapid detection of gram-negative bacteriuria by the use of the Limulus endotoxin assay. Appl Microbiol 26:38–43
31. Thomas LL, Sturk A, Buller HR, Ten Cate JW, Spijker RE, Ten Cate H (1984) Comparative investigation of a quantitative chromogenic endotoxin assay and blood cultures. Am J Clin Pathol 82:203–206
32. Iwanaga S, Morita T, Harada T (1978) Chromogenic substrate for horse shoe crab clotting enzyme: its application for the assay of bacterial endotoxins. Haemostasis 7183:183–188
33. Thomas LLM, Sturk A, Kahle LH, Ten Cate JW (1981) Quantitative endotoxin determination in blood with chromogenic substrate. Clin Chem Acta 116:63–68
34. Jorgensen JH (1986) Clinical applications of the Limulus amebocyte lysate test. In: Proctor RA (ed) Clinical aspects of endotoxin shock. Handbook of endotoxin. Elsevier, Amsterdam, pp 127–160

35. Elin RJ, Wolf SM (1973) Nonspecificity of the Limulus amebocyte lysate test: positive relations with polynucleotides and proteins. J Infect Dis 128:349
36. Elin RJ, Sandberg AL, Rosenstreich DL (1976) Comparison of the pyrogenicity, Limulus activity, mitogenicity, and complement reactivity of several bacterial endotoxins and related compounds. J Immunol 117:1238–1242
37. Danner RL, Elin RJ, Hosseini JM, Wesley RA, Reilly JM, Parrillo JE (1991) Endotoxemia in human septic shock. Chest 99:169–175
38. McCartney AC, Robertson MRI, Piotrowicz BI, Lucie NP (1987) Endotoxemia, fever, and clinical status in immunosuppressed patients: a preliminary study. J Infect Dis 15:201–206
39. Elin RJ (1979) Clinical utility of the Limulus test with blood, CSF, and synovial fluid. In: Cohen E (ed) Biomedical applications of the horseshoe crab (Limulidae). Liss, New York, pp 279–292
40. Natanson C, Danner RL, Reilly JM et al (1990) Antibiotics versus cardiovascular support in a canine model of human septic shock. Am J Physiol 259:H1440–H1446
41. Hoffman WD, Pollack M, Banks S et al (1990) Monoclonal anti-endotoxin antibodies as therapy in a canine model of human septic shock. Clin Res 38:454A (abstract)
42. Hoffman WD, Pollack M, Banks S et al (1991) A controlled trial of IgG monoclonal anti-endotoxin antibodies in a canine model of human septic shock. Clin Res 39:164A (abstract)
43. Danner RL, Natanson C, Elin RJ et al (1990) Pseudomonas aeruginosa compared with Escherichia coli produces less endotoxemia but more cardiovascular dysfunction and mortality in a canine model of septic shock. Chest 98:1480–1487
44. Hoffman WD, Danner RL, Koev CA et al (1990) Ability of endotoxin and heat stable components of two strains of E. coli to produce lethality in canine septic shock. Clin Res 38:454 (abstract)
45. Hoffmann WD, Natanson C, Danner RL et al (1989) Bacterial organisms virulence factors may be more important in determining cardiovascular (CV) dysfunction and mortality in canine septic shock. Clin Res 37:344 (abstract)
46. Baumgartner JD, Heumann D, Gerain J, Weinbreck P, Grau GE, Gkauser MP (1990) Association between protective efficacy of anti-lipopolysaccharide (LPS) antibodies and suppression of LPS-induced tumor necrosis factor alfa and interleukin 6. J Exp Med 171:889–896
47. Warren HS, Riveau GR, DeDeckker FA, Chedid LA (1988) Control of endotoxin activity and interleukin-1 production through regulation of lipopolysaccharide-lipoprotein binding by a macrophage factor. Infect Immun 56:204–212
48. Ulevitch RJ, Johnston AR, Weinstein DB (1981) New function for high density lipoproteins. Isolaation and characterization of a bacterial lipopolysaccharide-high density lipoprotein complex formed in rabbit plasma. J Clin Invest 67:827–837
49. Harris HW, Grunfeld C, Feingold KR, Rapp JH (1990) Human very low density lipoproteins and chylomicrons can protect against endotoxin-induced death in mice. J Clin Invest 86:696–702
50. Weiss J, Muello K, Victor M, Elsbach P (1984) The role of lipopolysaccharide in the action of the bactericidal/permeability-increasing protein on the bacterial envelope. J Immunol 132:3109–3115
51. Marra MN, Wilde CG, Collins MS, Snable JL, Thornton MB, Scott RW (1992) The role of bactericidal/permeability-increasing protein as a natural inhibitor of bacterial endotoxin. J Immunol 148:532–537
52. Weersink AJL, van Kessel KPM, van der Tol ME et al (1992) Human granulocytes express a 55-Kd lipopolysaccharide-binding protein on the cell surface that is identical to the bactericidal/permeability increasing protein. J Immunol 150:253–263
53. Marra MN, Wilde CG, Griffith JE, Snable JL, Scott RW (1990) Bactericidal/permeability-increasing protein has endotoxin-neutralizing activity. J Immunol 144:662–666
54. Raetz CRH, Ulevitch RJ, Wright SD, Sibley CH, Ding A, Nathan CF (1991) Gram-negative endotoxin: an extraordinary lipid with profound effects on eukaryotic signal transduction. FASEB J 5:2652–2660

55. Wright SD, Ramos RA, Tobias PS, Ulevitch RJ, Mathison JC (1990) CD14, a receptor for complexes of lipopolysaccharide and LPS binding protein. Science 249:1431–1433
56. Schumann RR, Leong SR, Flaggs GW et al. (1990) Structure and function of lipopolysaccharide binding protein. Science 249:1429–1433
57. Wright SD, Ramos RA, Patel M, Miller DS (1992) Septin: a factor in plasma that opsonizes lipopolysaccharide-bearing particles for recognition by CD14 on phagocytes. J Exp Med 176:719–727
58. Frey EA, Miller DS, Jahr TG et al. (1992) Soluble CD14 participated in the response of cells to lipopolysaccharide. J Exp Med 176:1665–1671
59. Wright SD (1991) Multiple receptors for endotoxin. Curr Opin Immunol 3:83–90
60. Hampton RY, Golenbock DT, Penman M, Krieger M, Raetz CRH (1991) Recognition and plasma clearance of endotoxin by scavenger receptors. Nature 352:342–344
61. Halling JL, Hamill DR, Lei MG, Morrison DC (1992) Identification and characterization of lipopolysaccharide-biding proteins on humans peripheral blood cell populations. Infect Immun 60:845–852
62. Bright S, Chen T, Flebbe L, Lei M, Morrison D (1990) Generation and characterization of hamster–mouse hybridomas secreting monoclonal antibodies with specificity for lipopolysaccharide receptor. J Immunol 145:1–7
63. Croo AS, Gemski P, Sadoff JC, Orskov F, Orskov I (1984) The importance of the K1 capsule in invasive infection caused by E. coli. J Infect Dis 149:184–193
64. Sadoff JC, Wright DC, Futrovsky S, Sidberry H, Collins H, Kaufmann B (1985) Characterization of mouse monoclonal antibodies directed against Pseudomonas aeruginosa lipopolysaccharides. Antibiot Chemother 36:134–146
65. Sagawa T, Hitsumoto Y, Kaanoh M, Utsumi S, Kimura S (1990) Mechanisms of neutralization of endotoxin by monoclonal antibodies to O and R determinants of lipopolysaccharide. Adv Exp Med Biol 256:341–344
66. Pollack M, Oishi K, Chia J, Evans M, Guelde G, Koles N (1990) Specificity and function of monoclonal antibodies reactive with discrete structural elements of bacterial lipopolysaccharide. Adv Exp Med Biol 256:331–340
67. Johns M, Skehill A, McCabe WR (1983) Immunization with rough mutants of Salmonella minnesota. IV. Protection by antisera to O and rough antigens against endotoxin. J Infect Dis 147:57–87
68. Kaufman BM, Cross AS, Futrovsky S, Sidberry HF, Sadoff JC (1986) Monoclonal antibodies reactive with K1-encapsulated Escherichia coli lipopolysaccharide are opsonic and protect mice against lethal challenge. Infect Immun 52:617–619
69. Stoll BJ, Pollack M, Young LS, Koles N, Gascon R, Pier GB (1986) Functionally active monoclonal antibody that recognizes an epitope on the O side chain of Pseudomonas aeruginosa immunotype-1 lipopolysaccharide. Infect Immun 53:656–662
70. Pennington JE (1988) Impact of molecular biology on Pseudomonas aeruginosa immunization. J Hosp Infect 11 [Suppl]:96–102
71. Hector RF, Collins MS, Pennington JE (1989) Treatment of experimental Pseudomonas aeruginosa pneumonia with a human IgM monoclonal antibody. J Infect Dis 160:483–489
72. Ziegler EJ, Douglas H, Sherman JE, Davis CE, Braude AI (1983) Treatment of E. coli and Klebsiella bacteremia in agranulocytic animals with antiserum to a UDP-Gal epimerase deficient mutant. J Immunol 111:443–448
73. Mayoral JL, Schewich CJ, Dunn DL (1990) Decreased tumor necrosis factor production during the initial stages of infection correlates with survival during murine gram-negative sepsis. Arch Surg 215:24–27
74. Young LS, Stevens P, Ingram J (1975) Functional role of antibody against "core" glycolipid of Enterobacteriaceae. J Clin Invest 56:850–861
75. Marks MI, Ziegler EJ, Douglas H, Corbeil LB, Braude AI (1982) Induction of immunity against lethal Haemophilus influenzae type b infection Escherichia coli lipopolysaccharide. J Clin Invest 69:742–749

76. Ziegler EJ, McCutchan JA, Fiere J et al (1982) Treatment of gram-negative bacteremia and shock with human antiserum to a mutant Escherichia coli. N Engl J Med 307:1225–1230
77. Bruins SC, Stumacher R, Johns MA, McCabe WR (1977) Immunization with R mutants of Salmonella minnesota. II. Comparison of the protective effect of immunization with lipid A and the Re mutant. Infect Immun 17:16–20
78. Baumgartner JD, McCutchan JA, Melle G et al (1985) Prevention of gram-negative shock and death in surgical patients by antibody to endotoxin core glucolipid. Lancet 2:59–63
79. Baumgartner JD, Obrien TX, Kirkland TN, Glauser MP, Ziegler EJ (1987) Demonstration of cross-reactive antibodies to smooth gram-negative bacteria in antiserum to Escherichia coli J5. J Infect Dis 156:136–143
80. Corss AS, Sidberry H, Sadoff JC (1989) The human antibody response during natural bacteremic infection with gram-negative bacilli against lipopolysaccharide core determinants. J Infect Dis 160:225–236
81. Heumann D, Baumgartner JD, Jacot-Guillarmond H, Glauser MP (1991) Antibodies to core lipopolysaccharide determinants: absence of cross-reactivity with heterologous lipopolysaccharides. J Infect Dis 163:762–768
82. Baumgartner JD, Glauser MP (1990) Immunotherapy of gram-negative septic shock. In: Vincent JL (ed) Update in intensive care and emergency medicine. Springer, Berlin Heidelberg New York, pp 107–120
83. Baumgartner JD (1990) Monoclonal anti-endotoxin antibody for the treatment of gram-negative bacteremia and septic shock. Eur J Microbiol Infect Dis 9:711–716
84. Vinnicombe J, Stamey TA (1969) The relative nephrotoxicities of polymyxin B sulfate, sodium sulfomethyl polymyxin B, sodium sulfomethyl colistin, and neomycin sulfate. Invest Urol 6:505–509
85. Wheeler AP, Hardie WD, Bernard G (1990) Studies of an antiendotoxin antibody in preventing the physiologic changes of endotoxemia in awake sheep. Am Rev Respir Dis 142:775–781
86. Young LS, Gascon R, Alam S, Bermudez LEM (1989) Monoclonal antibodies for treatment of gram-negative infections. Rev Infect Dis 11 [Suppl 7]:S1564–S1571
87. Teng NNH, Kaplan HS, Hebert JM et al (1985) Protection against gram-negative bacteremia and endotoxemia with human monoclonal IgM antibodies. Proc Natl Acad Sci USA 82:1790–1794
88. Wenzel RP, Bone RC, Fein A et al (1991) Results of a second double-blind randomized, controlled trial of antiendotoxin antibody. E5 in gram-negative sepsis. Interscience conference on antimicrobial agents and chemotherapy, 19. Sept–2. Oct, p 294 (abstract)
89. Quezado ZMN, Natanson C, Alling DW et al (1993) A controlled trial of HA-1A in a canine model of gram-negative septic shock. JAMA 269:2221–2227
90. Siegel JP (1990) Editorial review of protocols for clinical trials. N Engl J Med 323:1355
91. Relman AS (1990) Editorial review of protocols for clinical trials. N Engl J Med 323:1355 (editor's reply)
92. Siegel JP, Stein KE, Zoon KC (1992) Anti-endotoxin monoclonal antibodies. N Engl J Med 327:890–891
93. Pierce L (1993) HA-1A has a checkered past. Biol World Financial Watch 25:1–2
94. Quezado ZMN, Hoffman WD (1993) Therapies against endotoxin: has the time come? West J Med 158:424–425
95. Rifkind D (1967) Prevention by polymyxin B of endotoxin lethality in mice. J Bacteriol 93:1463–1467
96. Craig WA, Turner JH, Kunin CM (1974) Prevention of the generalized Shwartzman reaction and endotoxin lethality by polymyxin B localized in tissues. Infect Immun 10:287
97. Danner RL, Joiner KA, Rubin M et al (1989) Purification, toxicity, and antiendotoxin activity of polymixin B nonapeptide. Antimicrob Agents Chemother 33:1428–1434

98. Stokes DC, Shenep JL, Fishman M, Hildner WK, Bysani GK, Rufus K (1989) Polymyxin B prevents lipopolysaccharide-induced release of tumor necrosis factor-alpha from alveolar macrophages. J Infect Dis 160:52–58
99. Hanasawa K, Tani T, Oka T et al (1988) Selective removal of endotoxin from the blood by extracorporeal perfusion with polymixin B immobilized fiber. Prog Clin Biol Res 264:337
100. Quezado ZMN, Hoffman WD, Banks S et al (1993) Therapeutic trial of reconstituted human high density lipoprotein in a dog model of gram-negative septic shock: preliminary results. Clin Res 41:175A (abstract)
101. Munford RS, Hall CL (1985) Uptake and decollation of bacterial lipopolysaccharide by macrophages from normal and endotoxin-hyporesponsive mice. Infect Immun 48:464
102. Munford RS, Hall CL (1986) Detoxification of bacterial lipopolysaccharide (endotoxins) by a human neutrophil enzyme. Science 234:203–205
103. Pohlman TH, Munford RS, Harlan JM (1987) Deacylated lipopolysaccharide inhibits neutrophil adherence to endothelium induced by lipopolysaccharide in vitro. J Exp Med 165:1393–1402
104. Takayama K, Qureshi N, Mascagni P, Nashed MA, Anderson L, Raetz CR (1983) Fatty acyl derivatives of glucosamine-1-phosphate in Escherichia coli and their relation to lipid A. Biol Chem 258:7379
105. Danner RL, Joiner KA, Parrillo JE (1990) Inhibition of endotoxin-induced priming of human neutrophils by lipid X and 3-aza-lipid X. J Clin Invest 80:605–612
106. Lam C, Hildebrandt J, Schutze E et al (1991) Immunostimulatory, but not endotoxin, activity of lipid X is due to small amounts of contaminating N,O-acylated disaccharide-1-phosphate: in vitro and in vivo reevaluation of the biological activity of synthetic lipid X. Infect Immun 59:2351–2358
107. Rackow EC, Astiz ME, Kim YB, Wil MH (1989) Monophosphoryl lipid A blocks hemodynamic effects of lethal endotoxemia. J Lab Clin Med 113:112–120
108. Heiman DF, Astiz ME, Rackow EC, Rhein D, Kim YB, Weil MH (1990) Monophosphoryl lipid A inhibits priming by lipopolysaccharide. J Lab Clin Med 116:237
109. Carpati C, Astiz ME, Rackow EC, Kim JW, Kim YB, Weil MH (1990) Monophosphoryl lipid A attenuates septic shock in pigs. Crit Care Med 18:S260 (abstract)
110. Parrillo JE, Parker MM, Natanson C et al (1990) Septic shock in humans: advances in the understanding of pathogenesis, cardiovascular dysfunction, and therapy. Ann Intern Med 113:227–242
111. Couriveau CC, Danner RL (1993) Endotoxin as a therapeutic target in septic shock. Infect Agents Dis 2:35–43
112. McCutchan JA, Wolf JL, Ziegler EJ, Braude AI (1983) Ineffectiveness of single-dose human antiserum to core glycolipid (Escherichia coli J5) for prophylaxis of bacteremic gram-negative infection in patients with prolonged neutropenia. Schweiz Med Wochenschr 113 [Suppl 14]:40–55
113. The J5 Study Group (1992) Treatment of severe infectious purpura in children with human plasma from donors immunized with Escherichia coli J5: a prospective, double-blind study. J Infect Dis 165:695–701
114. Calandra T, Glauser MP, Schellekens J, Verhoef J, Swiss-Dutch J 5 Immunoglobulin Study Group (1988) Treatment of gram-negative septic shock with human IgG antibody to Escherichia coli J5: A prospective, double-blind, randomized study. J Infect Dis 158:312–319
115. The Intravenous Immunoglobulin Collaborative Study Group (1992) Prophylactic intravenous administration of standard immune globulin as compared with corelipopolysaccharide immune globulin in patients at high risk of postsurgical infection. N Engl J Med 327:234–240

Tumour Necrosis Factor as a Therapeutic Target in Sepsis

S. Sriskandan and J. Cohen

Introduction

Tumour necrosis factor (TNF) is an essential mediator in the pathogenesis of septic shock due to lipopolysaccharide (LPS) from gram-negative organisms, and its significance in gram-positive infections and malaria is now receiving more attention [1–3]. For these reasons, there was considerable expectation that modulation of the TNF-response would be of benefit to patients suffering the consequences of severe infection. Much experimental work has been done in the last 10 years to identify potential stages in the TNF response which could be targeted therapeutically. This would have important consequences not just in the field of septic shock but also in graft versus host disease, rheumatoid arthritis, autoimmune disorders and other diseases mediated partly by TNF [4–6].

Active TNF exists in two forms: TNFα (157 amino acids, 17 kDa), which is produced mainly by monocytes and TNFβ (171 amino acids, 25 kDa), which is produced largely by lymphoid cells. The genes for both forms of TNF are located on chromosome 6 and are subject to a number of controls both at the level of transcription and translation. TNF is cleaved from a precursor transmembrane molecule and is then secreted as a trimer. It exerts its effects on target cells in virtually all parts of the body by interaction with TNF receptors, located on target cell membranes [7, 8].

Whilst both forms of TNF share the same receptors, there are two types of TNF receptor, of 55 kDa and 75 kDa size, respectively. Many of the deleterious effects of TNF, such as induction of cytokine synthesis and cytotoxicity, are mediated via the 55 kDa receptor. The role of the 75 kDa receptor is far from clear, although it exists in greatest density on cells of lymphoid origin, and may trigger specialized responses such as thymocyte proliferation. The extracellular domains of the two TNF receptors exhibit only 28% sequence homology at the amino acid level, despite both having the ability to bind either form of TNF. There is no significant homology between the cytoplasmic domains of the two receptor types. This is in keeping with the observation that the two receptors trigger differing cellular events, presumably because different types of signal are generated [9, 10].

Hence, the TNF pathway is complex and pleiotropic; antagonism at any single stage may not be protective in all infections. It should also be remembered that TNF has a beneficial role during infection. It is of particular importance in resistance to intracellular organisms such as *Listeria monocytogenes* and also to candidiasis, parasitic and mycobacterial infections [6, 10, 11].

The approach to therapy in TNF-mediated sepsis will be considered in the following stages (Fig. 1):

1) Modulation of TNF gene transcription and translation
2) Control of TNF release
3) Direct inhibition of free TNF
4) Antagonism at the TNF receptor level
5) Modulation of signal transduction in target cells

Modulation of Tumour Necrosis Factor Gene Transcription and Translation

Strieter et al. demonstrated that the methylxanthine *pentoxifylline (POF)* was able to inhibit the formation of TNF mRNA by over 50% in macrophage cell culture [12]. Similar results were obtained using other methylxanthines such as theobromine and theophylline, in addition to dibutyryl cAMP. The methylxanthines lead to elevation of intracellular cAMP by inhibiting phosphodiesterase, and this is thought to impede transcription of the TNF gene. Since then, others have attempted to use POF in both animal and human studies to see if a beneficial outcome in sepsis could be observed.

Favourable effects of POF at doses of 20–50 mg/kg have been observed in animal models of sepsis, particularly in prevention of endotoxin-induced acute lung injury [13, 14], although the therapeutic range is narrow; toxicity is evident at concentrations over 50 mg/kg [15]. Gibson et al. have shown that POF can inhibit TNF production *in vivo* in an animal (piglet) model of group B streptococcal infection and that some parameters of haemodynamic stability, such as pulmonary vascular resistance and arterial oxygenation, were improved [16].

Human experiments have been performed on healthy volunteers who were given an endotoxin challenge [17]. It was found that POF could block endotoxin-induced TNF production in the volunteers although there was no difference in clinical responses between POF-treated subjects and controls.

Naturally occurring cytokines such as *interleukin-4 (IL-4)* and *interleukin-10 (IL-10)* are able to inhibit TNF production at the transcriptional and translational level. IL-4 is a potent anti-inflammatory cytokine and can suppress production of TNFα, at the transcriptional level, and interleukin-1 (IL-1) [18–20]. Whilst IL-4 can inhibit TNF synthesis in human monocytes *in vitro*, monocytes from patients receiving IL-4 in cancer therapy trials do not exhibit this inhibition *in vitro*. This suggests that human monocytes can

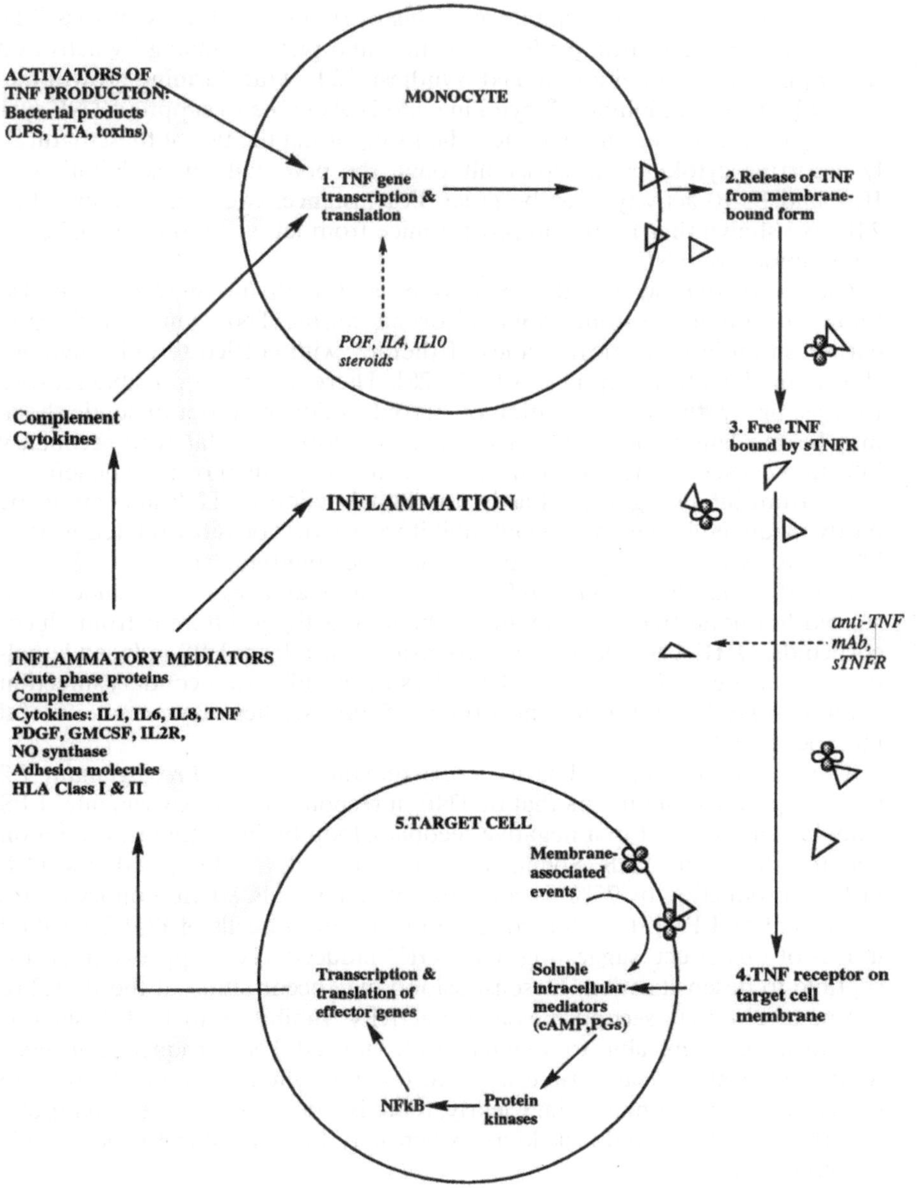

Fig. 1. The TNF biosynthetic pathway: Stages for intervention.
→ TNF synthetic pathway
⇢ Inhibitory effects on TNF biosynthesis
▷ TNF trimer
✤ TNF receptor
Abbreviations not otherwise mentioned in text:
LTA, lipoteichoic acid; PDGF, platelet-derived growth factor; IL2R, interleukin-2 receptor; NO synthase, nitric oxide synthase; PG, prostaglandins

become refractory to the inhibitory effects of IL-4 on TNF biosynthesis [21]. IL-10 can suppress nitric oxide production and parasite killing by activated macrophages via inhibition of TNF synthesis [20]. Transforming growth factor-β (TGFβ) is an inhibitory cytokine and is also able to suppress TNF synthesis [20, 22]. As yet, there are few data supporting the use of these naturally occurring cytokines in sepsis, although the potential for exploitation of IL-4 and IL-10 activity must be great. For instance, two recent reports [23, 24] have shown that IL-10 can protect mice from lethal endotoxin challenge by inhibition of TNF.

Glucocorticoids such as dexamethasone and methylprednisolone are also known to inhibit posttranscriptional events during TNF synthesis. Despite earlier enthusiasm, clinical studies of therapy with corticosteroids have not shown any benefit in septic shock [25–28]. There are many possible reasons for this: firstly, the administration of steroids following onset of septic shock may be too late to be of use. Secondly, the mortality related to secondary infection caused by steroid therapy may counteract any mortality benefit accrued from inhibiting TNF. Lastly, the lethal action of TNF appears to be partly mediated by glucocorticoid inhibitory activity, possibly related to IL-1 [29]. Any exogenous steroid may therefore be counteracted.

Dehydroepiandrosterone (DHEA) is a weakly androgenic, adrenocortical steroid hormone that has immunomodulating activity different from glucocorticoids. DHEA has been shown to protect mice from LPS-induced lethality by reducing TNF production [30]. As susceptibility to secondary infection is not observed with this adrenocorticoid, future studies may reveal a useful therapeutic role.

The role of prostaglandins in sepsis remains unclear. *Prostaglandin E2* (PGE2) production mirrors that of TNF in response to an experimental LPS stimulus and may act in a negative feedback loop by inhibiting transcription and translation of TNF. Spengler et al. showed that PGE2 reduces TNF mRNA production by 75% as compared with controls, when monocytes are stimulated by LPS [31]. Interestingly, preexposure of cells of PGE2 resulted in loss of this effect, suggesting that PGE2-induced TNF suppression is susceptible to desensitization. Desensitization may occur either at the PGE2 re ceptor level or via second messenger activity. Inhibitors to PGE2, such as *indomethacin*, were able to augment LPS-induced TNF production *in vitro* when added at the same time as LPS, but not when the monocytes were pretreated with indomethacin. Clearly, there is a delicate balance in naturally occurring cytokine feedback loops which may be amenable to therapeutic invervention.

Human studies in this area have centred on the effects of other cyclooxygenase inhibitors, such as *ibuprofen,* in experimental sepsis [32, 33]. These show that ibuprofen augments the production of TNF in response to LPS challenge. Despite this, ibuprofen can blunt some of the clinical responses to endotoxin, such as fever, headache and myalgia. There is therefore an apparent dichotomy between the observed and predicted clinical responses to changes in TNF levels. This no doubt reflects the importance of other cytokines involved in the pathogenesis of septic shock, such as IL-1 and interleukin-6 (IL-6).

Other drugs such as *lactulose, ethanol* and *chloroquine* have been shown to have inhibitory actions on TNF gene transcription and translation though none are thought to have a clinical role to play [22]. *Thalidomide* also appears to have a selective inhibitory effect on TNF biosynthesis, based upon *in vitro* evidence, by enhancing TNF mRNA degradation [34, 35]. This may explain some of the anti-inflammatory actions of thalidomide observed in the type II lepra reaction and perhaps also its use in graft versus host disease.

Control of Tumour Necrosis Factor Release

Once manufactured, TNF is anchored to the cell membrane as a large precursor molecule (26 kDa in the case of TNFα). It is released by proteolytic cleavage into its bioactive form by serine protease enzymes. Niehorster et al. have demonstrated that the serine protease inhibitor *α1-antitrypsin* can protect against LPS-induced (TNF-mediated) hepatotoxicity in D-galactosamine sensitized mice [36]. However, it cannot protect against hepatotoxicity induced by exogenous TNF. TNF levels in the protected mice were very low, and they concluded that α1-antitrypsin protected the mice by inhibiting the production of TNF, most probably by preventing cleavage.

Granulocyte colony-stimulating factor (G-CSF) is normally used to improve granulocyte proliferation in neutropenic patients. It also appears that neutropenic patients receiving G-CSF are less susceptible to septic shock than those not receiving G-CSF. Whilst the exact mechanism is unclear, G-CSF is able to protect D-galactosamine sensitized mice from LPS-induced hepatitis and LPS-induced lethality by somehow preventing the release of TNF [37]. In contrast with these *in vivo* experiments, G-CSF was not able to prevent TNF release by LPS-stimulated monocytes *in vitro*. This suggests that G-CSF does not exert its inhibitory effects on monocytes directly, but acts via other target cells which in turn signal to monocytes and thereby reduce TNF release.

Cyclosporin A (CsA) is a potent immunosuppressive drug used extensively in human organ transplantation to prevent graft rejection and to treat some inflammatory diseases. Whilst CsA is known to inhibit T cell events, reducing interleukin-2 (IL-2) and interferon-γ (IFNγ) biosynthesis at the mRNA level, it has been shown more recently to reduce LPS-induced TNF production both *in vivo* and *in vitro* [38]. No reductions in TNF mRNA or cell-associated TNF were seen, although levels of released TNF were reduced, both *in vitro* and *in vivo*.

Direct Inhibition of Free Tumour Necrosis Factor

The inhibition of freely circulating TNF might seem an attractive way of blocking an already established cascade of lethal cytokines. It is important to remember that, at least experimentally, the $t_{1/2}$ of TNF is very short, suggesting that bioavailability for binding may be poor once TNF is released. TNF is measurable in serum 30 min after an experimental bolus of endotoxin and reaches peak levels at 90 min [1]. Previous studies [39] had suggested that TNF levels could remain elevated for several hours or even days later; much of this measurable TNF may in fact be bound to soluble receptors, detectable by immunoassay but not bioactive [40]. The clinical significance of this is uncertain and needs to be studied with some urgency.

Monoclonal Antibody to Tumour Necrosis Factor

Neutralizing monoclonal antibody (mAb) to TNF has been shown to be protective in several animal models of gram-negative sepsis [41, 42]. Serum levels of TNF were reduced concurrent with reductions in mortality and histopathological evidence of multiorgan failure. Although mAb to TNF protects animals from gram-negative sepsis if administered prophylactically or within 30 min of bacterial challenge, delay of 2.5 h leads to loss of protection, an observation of considerable importance in the clinical setting [43]. In this study, the protection by TNFmAb afforded to an *E. coli* model of bacteraemic sepsis was not seen when other gram-negative infections were studied, such as *Pseudomonas aeruginosa* and *Klebsiella pneumoniae*. This suggests that there are several factors of importance in the host immune response and susceptibility to gram-negative infection, of which TNF production is just one.

The protection conferred by TNFmAb varies also with the route of experimental infection. Several studies have shown that TNFmAb protects animals given intravenous gram-negative bacterial challenge but does not protect those given intraperitoneal challenge, even when the anti-TNF monoclonal is given via the intraperitoneal route [44, 45]. This could be of clinical relevance, as the intraperitoneal (i.p.) challenge may represent a more realistic model of clinical sepsis than the intravenous (i.v.) challenge. TNF levels in serum rise more slowly after i.p. than i.v. challenge, despite the fact that both models are bacteraemic. Unlike the i.v.-challenged models, serum levels of IL-1 and IL-6 remain elevated in the i.p.-challenged models despite treatment with TNFmAb. High levels of peritoneal TNF can be measured in the i.p.-challenged models and the difference in protection conferred by TNFmAb may reflect this local production of cytokines.

It is striking that comparatively few studies of anti-TNF in gram-positive sepsis exist, in spite of the fact that gram-positive infections account for at least half of community-acquired bacteraemias [46] and are known to induce TNF production on a scale similar to gram-negative infections [28]. There have been reports that mAb to TNF protects against experimental gram-positive sepsis [2, 47] though our own experiments using a murine model of lethal streptococcal shock have failed to show any benefit [48]. The reasons for this are unclear but may well reflect the number of diverse immunological pathways stimulated by toxins and cell wall products of gram-positive bacteria. Animal studies suggesting that TNFmAb could prevent the cerebral complications of malaria, though not the parasitaemia, have been followed by pilot studies in humans with encouraging results [3, 49].

The main clinical studies of mAb to TNF have, however, been undertaken in the field of bacterial septic shock. Early pilot studies demonstrated the safety of murine monoclonals in patients with the sepsis syndrome [50] although the criteria applied for entry were stringent. Hence, the drug was only given to patients with established septic shock and multiorgan failure. No conclusions as to efficacy could be drawn as a result of this study, though a further pilot study showed that TNFmAb can transiently improve myocardial function if administered within the first 24 h of onset of septic shock [51]. A phase II study of 80 patients with sepsis has not shown any overall benefit from use of mAb to TNF, although there was a subgroup of patients with high TNF levels at entry to the trial (>50 pg/ml) who did appear to derive some clinical benefit from mAb to TNF at a dose of 10 mg/kg [52]. Large, multicenter, prospective, double-blind randomized trials are clearly needed to evaluate the clinical use of this drug and such studies are now underway. It is anticipated that human monoclonals will also enter the market and may replace the murine monoclonals used previously [53].

Soluble Tumour Necrosis Factor Receptors

Seckinger et al. discovered naturally occurring inhibitors of TNF in the urine of five patients suffering from a variety of malignant and inflammatory diseases [54]. So-called TNF binding proteins (TNF-BP) have since been identified in the urine and serum of many such patients and are now known to be fragments from soluble TNF receptors (sTNFR).

Van Zee et al. showed that sTNFR circulate during human inflammation *in vivo* and that they can protect against excessive TNF activity *in vitro*, presumably by binding TNF and rendering it inactive. They went on to show that sTNFR could delay the appearance of TNF in the serum and also improve haemodynamic stability in a baboon model of gram-negative sepsis [55]. Recombinant "immunoadhesins", created from genetic chimeras of TNF receptor and the human IgG heavy chain, show even greater affinity for TNF and may be of clinical use [56, 57]. One of the reasons for using such immunoadhesins is that the binding of a native receptor to the Fc portion of IgG may prolong the half-life of the molecule. Furthermore, twice as many binding sites can be created if two receptor molecules are bound to the IgG heavy chain [58]. TNF elicits a biological response by cross-linking three receptor monomers on the cell surface; the TNF trimer then holds the monomers tightly together [7, 8]. It may be that these recombinant molecules are able to bind the TNF trimer with greater affinity. Preliminary *in vitro* and animal studies suggest that there may be a difference in efficacy between the biosynthetic 55 kDa and 75 kDa sTNFRs. A phase II/III clinical trial with sTNFR p75-IgG suggested that treated patients had a higher mortality than controls (J. Agosti, Immunex Corp., personal communication).

Antagonism at the Tumor Necrosis Factor Receptor Level

The TNF receptor cDNAs have been cloned and the two receptors are now known to belong to a family of related receptor proteins, including the receptor for nerve growth factor [59]. Unlike the IL-1 receptor, no clinically useful antagonist acting on TNF receptors has yet been developed. Monoclonal antibodies directed against TNF receptors are, however, available and have varying agonist and antagonist actions [60, 61]. Recent research suggests that antagonism of the 55 kDa TNF receptor would protect against endotoxic shock. In an elegant study, Pfeffer et al. developed a TNFRp55-deficient mouse strain; these mice were resistant to endotoxin and superantigen-induced shock, but succumbed easily to listeriosis [10]. This confirms the importance of the 55 kDa receptor and also underscores the potential risks when ablating an entire cytokine pathway such as that of TNF.

It is likely that the two TNF receptors on the target cell membrane must undergo internalization prior to signal transduction. Tiegs et al. made the interesting observation that colchicine can prevent LPS-induced TNF-mediated hepatitis and lethality without inhibiting TNF production or reducing TNF levels. *Colchicine* was also able to prevent directly induced TNF toxicity, suggesting that it was acting at the target cell level [62]. Colchicine is an alkaloid with the ability to affect leucocyte mobility. It is also an inhibitor of microtubular function and thus may prevent internalization of the TNF receptor.

Modulation of Signal Transduction in Target Cells

To date, no inhibitor of TNF-triggered signal transduction has been developed. The receptor itself has no intrinsic protein kinase activity and therefore a series of complex events must occur, culminating in the transcription of a wide variety of lethal and not so lethal genes, coding for cytokines, growth factors, adhesion molecules and other enzymes such as nitric oxide synthase [6, 8]. Within seconds of TNF binding to its receptor, a number of membrane associated biochemical events occur, generating intracellular mediators such as cAMP, diacylglycerol and prostaglandins. These mediators are crucial to several other biochemical pathways essential to life and it would be a remarkable (if not impossible) feat to selectively ablate TNF-triggered events alone. Protein kinases, such as PKA, PKC and a novel serine kinase are then activated, which in turn induce or activate transcription factors. NFKB, a major transcription factor activated by TNF [10], is largely preformed and therefore activation can occur without protein synthesis, in a relatively rapid and direct fashion, allowing little leeway for therapeutic intervention.

Summary

Several potential stages exist at which TNF can be therapeutically targeted. To date, no TNF inhibitor has been shown convincingly to offer definite therapeutic advantage in the clinical setting of human septic shock. The use of such agents remains, therefore, experimental. Agents likely to prove successful include pentoxifylline analogues, cytokines such as IL-4 and IL-10, monoclonal antibody to TNF and the recombinant sTNFR.

The goal of TNF inhibition was created at a time when TNF was considered to be the final step in a cytokine cascade leading to shock and, ultimately, death. We now know that a whole library of cytokines and inflammatory mediators, including nitric oxide, act as joint mediators of vasodilatation, hypotension and multiorgan failure in gram-negative and, probably, gram-positive septic shock. The development of novel nitric oxide inhibitors and other cytokine antagonists must run in parallel with the development of TNF antagonists. Combination therapy, using different inhibitors of inflammation together, may also prove useful.

References

1. Fong Y, Lowry SF (1990) Tumour necrosis factor in the pathophysiology of infection and sepsis. Clin Immunol Immunopathol 55:157–170
2. Freudenberg MA, Galanos C (1991) Tumor necrosis factor alpha mediates lethal activity of killed gram-negative and gram-positive bacteria in D-galactosamine-treated mice. Infect Immun 59:2110–2115
3. Grau GE, Fajardo LF, Piguet PF, Allet B, Lambert PH, Vassalli P (1987) Tumor necrosis factor (cachectin) as an essential mediator in murine cerebral malaria. Science 237:1210–1212
4. Piguet PF, Grau GE, Allet B, Vassalli P (1987) Tumor necrosis factor/cachectin is an effector of skin and gut lesions of the acute phase of graft-vs-host disease. J Exp Med 166:1280–1289
5. Pujol-Borrell R, Todd I, Doshi M et al (1987) HLA class II induction in human islet cells by interferon-g plus tumour necrosis factor or lymphotoxin. Nature 326:304–306
6. Vassalli P (1992) The pathophysiology of tumor necrosis factors. Annu Rev Immunol 10:411–452
7. Semenzato G (1990) Tumour necrosis factor: a cytokine with multiple biological activities. Br J Cancer 61:354–361
8. Vilcek J, Lee TH (1991) Tumor necrosis factor: new insights into the molecular mechanisms of its multiple actions. J Biol Chem 266:7313–7316
9. Beutler B (1992) Cytokines in shock: 1992. In: Lamy M, Thijs LG (eds) Update in intensive care and emergency medicine: mediators of sepsis. Springer, Berlin Heidelberg New York, pp 51–67
10. Pfeffer K, Matsuyama T, Kundig TM et al (1993) Mice deficient for the 55kd tumor necrosis factor receptor are resistant to endotoxic shock, yet succumb to L. monocytogenes infection. Cell 73:457–467

11. Desiderio JV, Kiener PA, Lin PF, Warr GA (1989) Protection of mice against Listeria monocytogenes infection by recombinant human tumor necrosis factor alpha. Infect Immun 57:1615–1617
12. Strieter RM, Remick DG, Ward PA et al (1988) Cellular and molecular regulation of tumor necrosis factor-alpha production by pentoxifylline. Biochem Biophys Res Commun 155:1230–1236
13. Hoffmann H, Hatherill JR, Crowley J et al (1991) Early post-treatment with pentoxifylline or dibutyryl cAMP attenuates Escherichia coli-induced acute lung injury in guinea pigs. Am Rev Respir Dis 143:289–293
14. Harada H, Ishizaka A, Yonemaru M et al (1989) The effects of aminophylline and pentoxifylline on multiple organ damage after Escherichia coli sepsis. Am Rev Respir Dis 140:974–980
15. Maderazzo EG, Breaux S, Woronick CL, Krause PJ (1990) Efficacy, toxicity and pharmacokinetics of pentoxifylline and its analogs in experimental Staphylococcus aureus infections. Antimirob Agents Chemother 34:1100–1106
16. Gibson RL, Redding GJ, Henderson WR, Truog WE (1991) Group B Streptococcus induces tumor necrosis factor in neonatal piglets. Am Rev Respir Dis 143:598–604
17. Zabel P, Schonharting MM, Wolter DT, Schade UF (1989) Oxpentifylline in endotoxemia. Lancet 2:1474–1477
18. Hart PH, Vitti GF, Burgess DR, Whitty GA, Piccoli SD, Hamilton JA (1989) Potential anti-inflammatory effects of interleukin-4: suppression of human monocyte tumor necrosis factor alpha, interleukin-1 and prostaglandin E2. Proc Natl Acad Sci USA 86:3803–3807
19. Dofferhof ASM, Vellenga E, Limburg PC, van Zanten A, Mulder POM, Weits J (1991) Tumour necrosis factor (cachectin) and other cytokines in septic shock: a review of the literature. Neth J Med 39:45–62
20. Sher A, Gazzinelli RT, Oswald IP et al (1992) Role of T-cell derived cytokines in the downregulation of immune responses in parasitic and retroviral infection. Immunol Rev 127:183–204
21. Wong HL, Lotze MT, Wahl LM, Wahl SM (1992) Administration of recombinant IL-4 to humans regulates gene expression, phenotype and function in circulating monocytes. J Immunol 148:2118–2125
22. Wardle N (1991) Tumour necrosis factor and its control. Clin Intensive Care 2:282–287
23. Howard M, Muchamuel T, Andrade S, Menon S (1993) Interleukin 10 protects mice from lethal endotoxemia. J Exp Med 177:1205–1208
24. Gerard C, Bruyns C, Marchant A et al (1993) Interleukin 10 reduces the release of tumor necrosis factor and prevents lethality in experimental endotoxemia. J Exp Med 177:547–550
25. Cohen J, Glauser MP (1991) Septic shock: treatment. Lancet 338:736–739
26. Hinshaw LB, Peduzzi P, Young E et al (1987) Effect of high-dose glucocorticoid therapy on mortality in patients with clinical signs of sepsis. N Engl J Med 317:659–665
27. Bone RC, Fisher CJ, Clemmer TP, Slotman JG, Metz CA, Balk RA (1987) A controlled clinical trial of high-dose methylprednisolone in the treatment of severe sepsis and septic shock. N Engl J Med 317:653–658
28. Marks JD, Berman Marks C, Luce JM et al (1990) Plasma tumor necrosis factor in patients with septic shock. Am Rev Respir Dis 141:94–97
29. Brouckaert P, Everaerdt B, Fiers W (1992) The glucocorticoid antagonist RU38486 mimics interleukin-1 in its sensitization to the lethal and interleukin-6-inducing properties of tumor necrosis factor. Eur J Immunol 22:981–986
30. Danenberg HD, Alpert G, Lustig S, Ben-Nathan D (1992) Dehydroepiandrosterone protects mice from endotoxin toxicity and reduces tumor necrosis factor production. Antimicrob Agents Chemother 36:2275–2279
31. Spengler RN, Spengler ML, Strieter RM, Remick DG, Larrick JW, Kunkel SL (1989) Modulation of tumor necrosis factor-a gene expression: desensitization of prostaglandin E2-induced suppression. J Immunol 142:4346–4350

32. Martich GD, Danner RL, Ceska M, Suffredini AF (1991) Detection of interleukin-8 and tumor necrosis factor in normal humans after intravenous endotoxin: the effect of antiinflammatory agents. J Exp Med 173:1021–1024
33. Spinas GA, Bloesch D, Keller U, Zimmerli W, Cammisuli S (1991) Pretreatment with ibuprofen augments circulating tumor necrosis factor-a, interleukin-6 and elastase during endotoxinemia. J Infect Dis 163:89–95
34. Sampaio EP, Sarno EN, Galilly R, Cohn ZA, Kaplan G (1991) Thalidomide selectively inhibits tumor necrosis factor-a production by stimulated human monocytes. J Exp Med 173:699–703
35. Moreira AL, Sampaio E, Zmuidzinas A, Frindt P, Smith KA, Kaplan G (1993) Thalidomide exerts its inhibitory action on tumor necrosis factor a by enhancing mRNA degradation. J Exp Med 177:1675–1680
36. Niehorster M, Tiegs G, Schade UF, Wendel A (1990) In vivo evidence for protease-catalysed mechanism providing bioactive tumor necrosis factor-a. Biochem Pharmacol 40:1601–1603
37. Gorgen I, Hartung T, Leist M et al (1992) Granulocyte colony-stimulating factor treatment protects rodents against lipopolysaccharide-induced toxicity via suppression of systemic tumor necrosis factor-a. J Immunol 149:918–924
38. Nguyen DT, Eskandari MK, DeForge LE et al (1990) Cyclosporin A modulation of tumor necrosis factor gene expression and effects in vitro and in vivo. J Immunol 144:3822–3828
39. Calandra T, Baumgartner JD, Grau GE et al (1990) Prognostic values of tumor necrosis factor/cachectin, interleukin-1, interferon-alpha, and interferon-gamma in the serum of patients with septic shock. J Infect Dis 161:982–987
40. Engelberts I, Stephens S, Francot GJM, Van der Linden CJ, Buurman WA (1991) Evidence for different effects of soluble TNF-receptors on various TNF measurements in human biological fluids. Lancet 338:515–516
41. Opal SM, Cross AS, Sadoff JC et al (1991) Efficacy of antilipopolysaccharide and anti-tumor necrosis factor monoclonal antibodies in a neutropenic rat model of Pseudomonas sepsis. J Clin Invest 88:885–890
42. Fiedler VB, Loof I, Sander E, Voehringer V, Galanos C, Fournel MA (1992) Monoclonal antibody to tumor necrosis factor-a prevents lethal endotoxin sepsis in adult rhesus monkeys. J Lab Clin Med 120:574–588
43. Silva AT, Bayston KF, Cohen J (1990) Prophylactic and therapeutic effects of a monoclonal antibody to tumor necrosis factor-a in experimental Gram-negative shock. J Infect Dis 162:421–427
44. Zanetti G, Heumann D, Gerain J et al (1992) Cytokine production after intravenous or peritoneal Gram-negative bacterial challenge in mice. J Immunol 148:1890–1897
45. Bagby GJ, Plessala KJ, Wilson LA, Thompson JJ, Nelson S (1991) Divergent efficacy of antibody to tumor necrosis factor-a in intravascular and peritonitis models of sepsis. J Infect Dis 163:83–88
46. Rayner BL, Willcox PA (1988) Community-acquired bacteraemia: a prospective survey of 239 cases. Q J Med 259:907–919
47. Saukkonen K, Sande S, Cioffe C et al (1990) The role of cytokines in the generation of inflammation and tissue damage in experimental Gram-positive meningitis. J Exp Med 171:439–448
48. Wayte J, Silva AT, Krausz T, Cohen J (1993) Observations on the role of TNF-a in a murine model of shock due to Streptococcus pyogenes. Crit Care Med 21:1207–1212
49. Grau GE, Piguet PF (1993) Tumor necrosis factor in cerebral and non-cerebral malaria. In: Fiers W, Buurman WA (eds) Tumor necrosis factor: molecular and cellular biology and clinical relevance. Karger, Basel, pp 162–171
50. Exley AR, Cohen J, Buurman W et al (1990) Monoclonal antibody to TNF in severe septic shock. Lancet 353:1275–1277
51. Vincent JL, Bakker J, Marecaux G, Schandene L, Kahn RJ, Dupont E (1992) Administration of anti-TNF antibody improves left ventricular function in septic shock patients. Results of a pilot study. Chest 101:810–815

52. Fisher CJ, Opal SM, Dhainaut JF et al (1993) Influence of an anti-tumor necrosis factor monoclonal antibody on cytokine levels in patients with sepsis. Crit Care Med 21:318–327
53. Stephens S, Athwal D, Chaplin L et al (1993) Pharmacokinetics of CDP571, an anti-TNFa engineered human antibody, in the cynomolgus monkey and man. Circ Shock [Suppl] 1:60
54. Seckinger P, Isaaz S, Dayer JM (1988) A human inhibitor of tumor necrosis factor-a. J Exp Med 167:1511–1516
55. Van Zee KJ, Kohno T, Fischer E, Rock CS, Moldawer LL, Lowry SF (1992) Tumor necrosis factor soluble receptors circulate during experimental and clinical inflammation and can protect against excessive tumor necrosis factor-a in vitro and in vivo. Proc Natl Acad Sci USA 89:4845–4849
56. Lesslauer W, Tabuchi H, Gentz R et al (1991) Recombinant soluble tumor necrosis factor receptor proteins protect mice from lipopolysaccharide-induced lethality. Eur J Immunol 21:2883–2886
57. Ashkenazi A, Marsters SA, Capon D et al (1991) Protection against endotoxic shock by a tumor necrosis factor receptor immunoadhesin. Proc Natl Acad Sci USA 88:10535–10539
58. Mayforth RD, Quintans J (1990) Designer and catalytic antibodies. N Engl J Med 323:173–177
59. Smith CA, Davis T, Anderson D et al (1990) A receptor for tumor necrosis factor defines an unusual family of cellular and viral proteins. Science 248:1019–1023
60. Espevik T, Brockhaus M, Loetscher H, Nonstad U, Shalaby R (1990) Characterization of binding and biological effects of monoclonal antibodies against a human tumor necrosis factor receptor. J Exp Med 171:415–426
61. Thoma B, Grell M, Pfizenmaier K, Scheurich P (1990) Identification of a 60-kD tumor necrosis factor receptor as the major signal transducing component in TNF responses. J Exp Med 172:1019–1023
62. Tiegs G, Freudenberg MA, Galanos C, Wendel A (1992) Colchicine prevents tumor necrosis factor-induced toxicity in vivo. Infect Immun 60:1941–1945

Tumor Necrosis Factor-Neutralization with a Specific Monoclonal Antibody

M. Kluge and M. Kaul

Introduction

Sepsis is a clinical condition which represents a systemic response to infection. It has been described for more than 40 years [1]. In spite of significant advances in antimicrobial therapy, lethality of this disease is still high, and septic shock is still estimated to account for about 100000 deaths in the USA annually [2]. During recent years the involvement of both humoral pathways and the cytokine network of the host and their interaction with cellular mechanisms in the induction of the clinical symptoms and consequences of sepsis have gained major scientific attention [3]. The interruption of the endogenous inflammatory cascade has become a novel approach for the treatment of sepsis and septic shock [4].

Several experimental studies have suggested that tumor necrosis factor (TNF), as a host factor, seems to play a crucial role as a mediator of sepsis [5]. High TNF levels were demonstrated to correlate with clinical outcome in meningitis and septicemia in patients [6, 7]. Besides interleukin-1 (IL-1), TNF is considered to be one of the central endogenous cytokines for the initiation of the mediator cascade leading to the clinical consequences of sepsis or the systemic inflammatory response syndrome (SIRS) [4]. Thus, blocking or neutralizing TNF with a specific antibody may have considerable therapeutic potential [8].

Preparation of the Antibody Fragment MAK 195F

In order to neutralize the toxic effects of TNF-α, highly specific monoclonal antibodies were developed. A monoclonal antibody with the code name MAK 195 was finally chosen for clinical development from a panel of different murine monoclonal antibodies. MAK 195 has been described earlier [9] and is characterized by binding human TNF-α with an affinity constant of 3.5×10^9 l/mol. It does not show any cross-reactivity to the related cytokine lymphotoxin (TNF-β) nor to other human serum components. The antibody is of the IgG3 isotype with κ light chains. MAK 195 is very particular in its cross-reactivity to TNFs of different animal species. It is highly species-specific for human TNF-α and, apart from binding to chimpanzee TNF,

MAK 195 does not show any cross-reactivity to TNF from other animal species including other primates. Thus, this antibody defines an epitope not described for previously published antibodies [10–14]. For clinical development, the $F(ab')_2$ fragment MAK 195F, which has a molecular weight of about 95 kDa, was derived from the complete antibody MAK 195 by pepsin cleavage. The fragment rather than the complete antibody was chosen in order to reduce the potential immunogenicity of the murine protein and to facilitate tissue penetration of the compound. In several *in vitro* and *in vivo* studies the antibody fragment has been demonstrated to be similarly active in reducing the biological effects of recombinant human TNF (rhuTNF) compared to the complete antibody.

Animal Experiments with MAK 195F

Testing the efficacy of MAK 195F in animal experiments is hampered by the fact that MAK 195F is highly species-specific for TNF derived from humans and chimpanzees but does not cross-react with TNF from other species. Therefore testing MAK 195F in animal models of sepsis requires induction of such conditions with rhuTNF. This is justifiable by the fact that an animal model of sepsis syndrome is not only inducible by exogenous stimulants, such as lipopolysaccharides (LPSs) from gram-negative bacteria, but LPS has also been demonstrated to be a potent stimulator of TNF production [15]. Indeed, TNF alone is able to initiate the same complex cardiovascular changes as those seen in sepsis when administered intravenously in animals [16]. Thus, it may be concluded that LPS or other exogenous mediators exert their effects mainly through early endogenous mediators like TNF.

Prophylactic Administration of MAK 195F in a Pyrogenic Rabbit Model

A series of experiments was carried out to investigate whether intravenous administration of MAK 195F is able to suppress the pyrogenic activity of rhuTNF in rabbits. Body temperature of the animals was recorded rectally and compared to a control group which received a sham treatment with solvents only.

Intravenous injection of rhuTNF induces a dose-dependent increase of body temperature in rabbits (Fig. 1). The rise in temperature is maximal after about 6 h and returns to baseline values within 24 h. Maximal relative increased body temperature after rhuTNF was 2.8°C observed with a single rhuTNF dose of 1000 μg/kg i.v. A semimaximal effect with an increased body temperature of about 1.5°C was observed with a single rhu/TNF dose of 10 μg/kg.

Administration of MAK 195F prior to 10 μg/kg rhuTNF resulted in a dose-dependent prophylactic effect (Fig. 2). The pyrogenic effect of 10 μg/kg

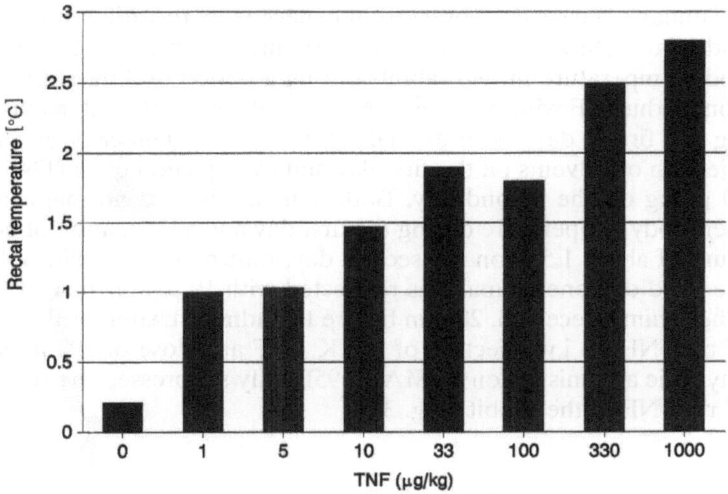

Fig. 1. Pyrogenic effect of various doses of recombinant human tumor necrosis factor (*TNF*) in rabbits: maximal relative changes from baseline

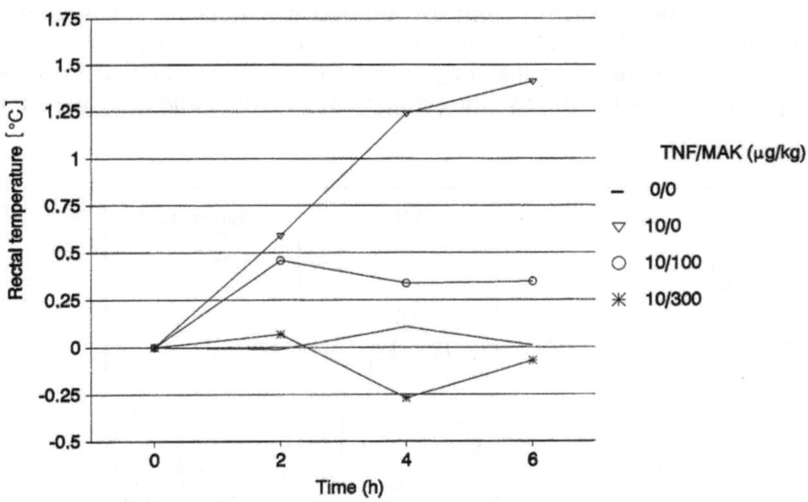

Fig. 2. Prophylactic effect of MAK 195F (*MAK*) in various doses on the pyrogenic effect of a constant dose of recombinant human tumor necrosis factor (*TNF*) in rabbits

rhuTNF in rabbits was attenuated significantly ($p<0.01$) by pretreatment with MAK 195F at a dose of 100 μg/kg (about twofold molar surplus) and was completely abolished ($p<0.01$) by increasing the dose of MAK 195F to 300 μg/kg.

Similar effects were observed in experiments recording body temperature and heart rate in rabbits by telemetric means. In Fig. 3 the time course of body temperature in two rabbits during a period of 3 days after administration of rhuTNF with or without MAK 195F pretreatment is illustrated. During the first 2 days both animals were treated identically and received i.v. injection of solvents on the first day and i.v. injection of rhuTNF at a dose of 10 μg/kg on the second day. Both animals showed no major alteration of their body temperature during the first day and an elevation of body temperature of about 1.5°C on the second day, returning to baseline 24 h later. On the third day one animal was reinjected with 10 μg/kg rhuTNF whereas the other animal received, 20 min before the administration of the same amount of rhuTNF, an i.v. injection of MAK 195F at a dose of 100 μg/kg. The prophylactic administration of MAK 195F fully suppressed the pyrogenic effect of rhuTNF in the rabbit (Fig. 3).

Administration of MAK 195F in a Rat Sepsis Model

Serial measurements of TNF levels in septic patients have demonstrated that TNF was elevated in these patients over a time period of several days [17]. In order to imitate such a clinical condition in animals a small osmotic minipump filled with rhuTNF was implanted into rats. After the implantation the animals were infused constantly over 10 days with rhuTNF at a dose of 65μg/kg per hour. After 10 days the pump was explanted and the rhuTNF infusion

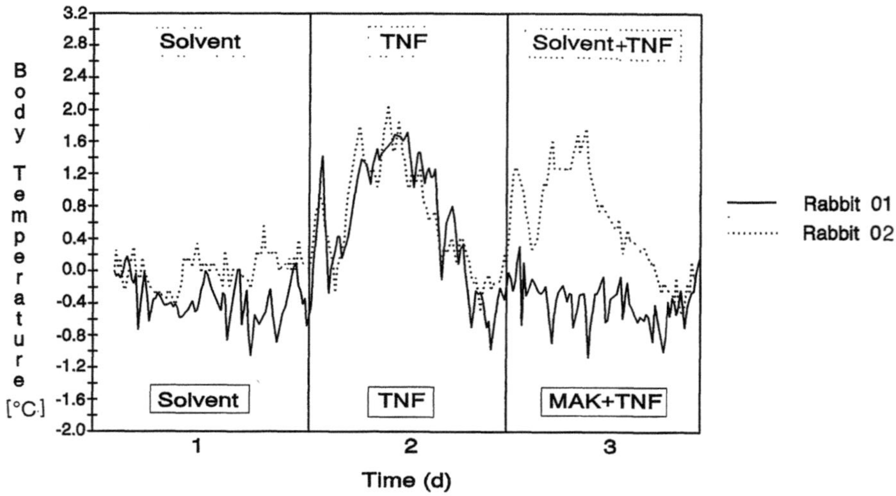

Fig. 3. Time course of body temperature in two rabbits after administration of solvents (day 1), recombinant human tumor necrosis factor 10 μg/kg (*TNF*) (day 2) and TNF 10 μg/kg preceded by MAK 195F 100 μg/kg (*MAK*) (*solid line*) or solvents (*dotted line*) (day 3)

was stopped. Rats receiving TNF in this way without any antibody administration demonstrated a constant decline in body weight and finally died after 5–8 days.

In order to investigate the efficacy of MAK 195F in this animal model four different treatment regimens of the monoclonal antibody were tested in the rhuTNF-infused animals. In regimen 1, a single i.v. dose of MAK 195F was administered 24 h after the onset of rhuTNF infusion. In regimen 2, MAK 195F was administered for 3 days as a twice daily i.v. injection, starting 24 h after the onset of continuous rhuTNF infusion. In regimen 3, the same scheme was used as in regimen 2, but an additional early injection of MAK 195F was added 8 h after the onset of rhuTNF infusion. Finally, in regimen 4, MAK 195F was administered over 10 days once daily, i.e., during the whole administration period of rhuTNF infusion, starting 24 h after the onset of rhuTNF infusion. The four treatment regimens are summarized in Table 1.

In treatment regimens 1–3, single doses of MAK 195F varied between 8 mg/kg and 40 mg/kg, whereas in treatment regimen 4, single doses between 2 mg/kg and 16 mg/kg were used.

Except for the single administration of MAK 195F in any dose (regimen 1) a statistically significant prolongation of the median survival times of the animals was observed in regimens 2–4 (Fig. 4 and 5). Administration of MAK 195F over the complete time period in which rhuTNF was administered (regimen 4) led to a complete reduction of mortality even in the lowest dose tested (Fig. 5). On the other hand, one single administration of MAK 195F 24 h after the initiation of TNF infusion (regimen 1) was not able to significantly reduce the decline in body weight of the rats compared to sham treatment with solvents. This is in contrast to the other treatment regimens (regimens 2–3) using an administration of MAK 195F over a time period of several days (Fig. 6).

Recently a beneficial effect of MAK 195F on LPS-induced pathophysiological changes in anesthesized chimpanzees was demonstrated (T. van der Poll, unpublished). MAK 195F administered 30 min after LPS counteracted the rise of endogenous cytokines and other physiological changes induced by LPS.

Table 1. Treatment regimens of MAK 195F in rats constantly infused with recombinant human tumor necrosis factor (rhuTNF) 65 μg/kg/h over 10 days

	rhuTNF infusion days	MAK195F Single injection	
		Treatment days	Number of doses/day
Regimen 1	1–10	2	1
Regimen 2	1–10	2–4	2
Regimen 3	1–10	1	1
		2–4	2
Regimen 4	1–10	2–10	1

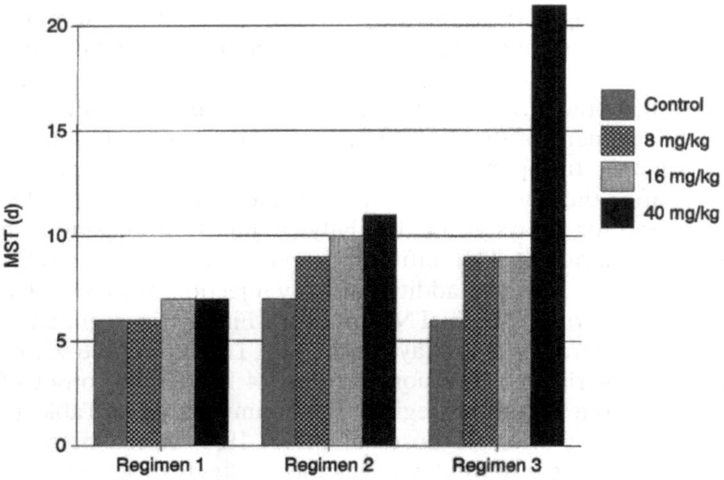

Fig. 4. Median survival time in days (*MST*) of rats receiving a continuous infusion of recombinant human tumor necrosis factor (65 μg/kg per hour over 10 days) and treated with different regimens of MAK 195F (see Table 1; regimens 1–3) in single doses between 8 and 40 mg/kg

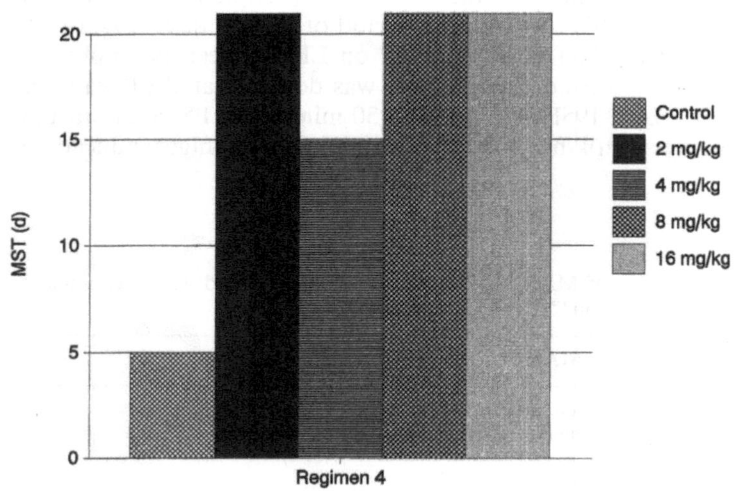

Fig. 5. Median survival time in days (*MST*) of rats receiving a continuous infusion of recombinant human tumor necrosis factor (65 μg/kg per hour over 10 days) and treated with MAK 195F in single daily doses between 2 and 16 mg/kg for 9 days, starting 24 h after the onset of rhuTNF infusion (regimen 4)

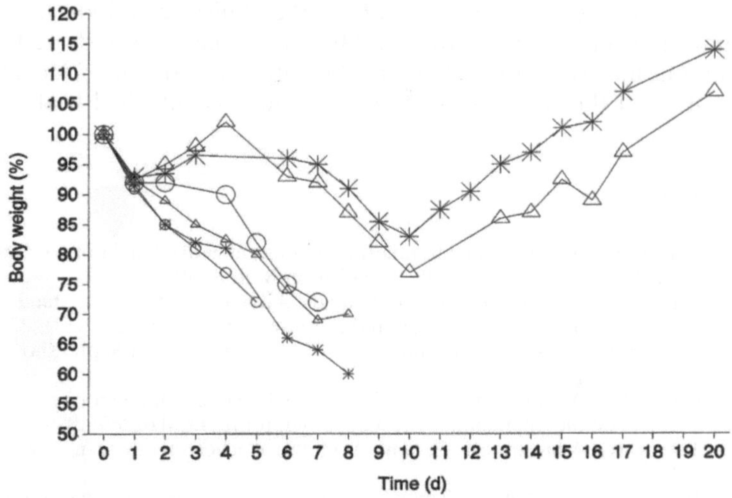

Fig. 6. Effect of three different treatment regimens of MAK 195F (see Table 1; regimens 1–3) on body weight and survival of rats receiving a continuous infusion of recombinant human tumor necrosis factor (65 μg/kg per hour over 10 days). *Circles,* regimen 1; *triangles,* regimen 2; *asterisks,* regimen 3; *large symbols,* verum treatment (MAK 195F); *small symbols,* sham treatment (solvents). Cessation of weight curve prior to day 20 indicates death of animal

Conclusions

The prominent role of endogenous cytokines such as TNF and IL-1 in the pathophysiology of sepsis and SIRS is well established. Recent laboratory investigations and animal experiments suggest that TNF and IL-1 are the main promotors of the biochemical changes and the clinical characteristics of such diseases.

Interrupting the inflammatory cascade in sepsis by neutralization of an early mediator such as TNF with monoclonal antibodies could be of great clinical importance [18]. The biochemical characteristics of MAK 195F, the $F(ab')_2$ fragment of a neutralizing murine monoclonal antibody against TNF, as well as animal experiments in sepsis models either induced in rodents with rhuTNF or in chimpanzees with LPS have demonstrated the beneficial effects of this compound. The animal experiments have demonstrated that MAK 195F is still active after the cytokine cascade has already been initiated. They also suggest that MAK 195F should be used in the clinical setting as early as possible after the initiation of the mediator cascade and to administer it over a prolonged time period.

Nevertheless it has to be pointed out that positive results with anti-TNF antibodies in animal models of sepsis depend on the kind of model chosen for the experimental setting [19]. Furthermore due to the pleiotropic effects of TNF the neutralization of this important mediator with antibodies in sepsis has to be considered carefully in the clinical condition [20]. Preliminary clinical experience with MAK 195F in sepsis has demonstrated its safety and the pharmacokinetics in humans. Detailed assessment of its clinical efficacy must await the results of large scale, placebo-controlled trials.

References

1. Waisbren BA (1951) Bacteremia due to gram-negative bacilli other than salmonella: a clinical and therapeutic study. Arch Intern Med 88:467
2. Parillo JE (1990) Septic shock in humans. Advances in the understanding of pathogenesis, cardiovascular dysfunction and therapy. Ann Intern Med 113:227
3. Glauser MP, Zanetti G, Baumgartner JD, Cohen J (1991) Septic shock: pathogenesis. Lancet 338:732
4. Dinarello CA, Gelfand JA, Wolff SM (1993) Anticytokine strategies in the treatment of the systemic inflammatory response syndrome. JAMA 269:1829
5. Tracey KJ, Vlassara H, Cerami A (1989) Cachectin tumor necrosis factor. Lancet ii:1122
6. Waage A, Halstensen A, Espevik T (1987) Association between tumour necrosis factor in severe and fatal outcome in patients with meningococcal disease. Lancet i:355
7. Debets JMH, Kampmeijer R, van der Linden PMH et al (1989) Plasma tumour necrosis factor and mortality in critically ill septic patients. Crit Care Med 17:489
8. Cohen J, Glauser MP (1991) Septic shock treatment. Lancet 338:736
9. Möller A, Emling F, Blohm D et al (1990) Monoclonal antibodies to tumour necrosis factor alpha: in vitro and in vivo application. Cytokine 2:162
10. Hirai M, Okamura N, Terano Y et al (1987) Production and characterisation of monoclonal antibodies to human tumor necrosis factor. J Immunol Methods 96:57
11. Meager A, Parti S, Leung H et al (1987) Preparation and characterisation of monoclonal antibodies directed against antigenic determinants of recombinant human tumour necrosis factor. Hybridoma 6:305
12. Liang CM, Liang SM, Jost T et al (1986) Production and characterisation of monoclonal antibodies against recombinant human tumor necrosis factor/cachectin. Biochem Biophys Res Commun 137:847
13. Fendly BM, Toy KJ, Creasey AA et al (1987) Murine monoclonal antibodies defining neutralizing epitopes on tumor necrosis factor. Hybridoma 6:359
14. Shimamoto Y, Chen RI, Bollon A et al (1988) Monoclonal antibodies against human recombinant tumor necrosis factor. Immunol Lett 17:311
15. Beutler BA, Milsark IW, Cerami A (1985) Cachectin/tumor necrosis factor: production, distribution and metabolic fate in vivo. J Immunol 135:3972
16. Natanson C, Eichenholz PW, Danner RL et al (1989) Endotoxin and tumour necrosis factor challenges in dogs simulate the cardiovascular profile of human septic shock. J Exp Med 169:823
17. Calandra T, Baumgartner JD, Grau GE et al (1990) Prognostic values of tumour necrosis factor/cachectin, interleukin-1, alpha-interferon and gamma-interferon in the serum of patients with septic shock. J Infect Dis 161:982
18. Saravolatz LD, Pokriefka RA, Markowitz N (1993) Monoclonal antibodies against TNF: a non-antibiotic strategy for the treatment of sepsis. In: Vincent JL (ed) Yearbook of intensive care and emergency medicine. Springer, Berlin–Heidelberg–New York, pp 100
19. Eskandari MK, Bolgos G, Miller C et al (1992) Anti-tumor necrosis factor antibody therapy fails to prevent lethality after cecal ligation and puncture or endotoxemia. J Immunol 148:2724
20. Bone RC (1993) Monoclonal antibodies to tumor necrosis factor in sepsis: help or harm? Crit Care Med 21:311

Cardiovascular Effects of Repeated Administration of the F(ab′)$_2$ Fragment of an Anti-tumor Necrosis Factor-α Monoclonal Antibody in Patients with Severe Sepsis

P. Boekstegers, S. Weidenhöfer, R. Zell, G. Pilz, E. Holler, T. Kapsner, M. Kaul, J. Kempeni and K. Werdan

Introduction

Tumor necrosis factor-α (TNF-α) is a principal mediator in sepsis and induces cardiovascular impairment either by direct effects on vascular and heart cells [1–6] or by liberating and synergizing with other cytokines such as interleukin-1, interleukin-6 and interferon-γ [2, 7, 8]. Intravenous administration of recombinant human TNF-α in experimental models mimics the hypotension and hyperdynamic state [1, 9, 10] and the cardiac dysfunction [5, 11] which is seen in human sepsis [12, 13]. When anti-TNF-α antibodies were administered prior to or shortly after induction of septic shock in animals, they have counteracted cardiovascular impairment [9] and protected against lethal bacteremia [9], endotoxemia [14, 15] and TNF-α cytotoxicity [16, 17]. The potential value of anti-TNF-α antibodies in human sepsis, however, remains to be established.

The efficacy of anti-TNF-α antibody administration in patients with sepsis may depend on its onset, dosage and duration [18]. Furthermore, different types of anti-TNF-α monoclonal antibodies such as F(ab′)$_2$ fragments, in contrast to complete murine antibodies, are likely to differ in their pharmacokinetics, antigeneity, TNF-α affinity and tissue penetration, factors which may alter the efficacy of each particular anti-TNF-α antibody.

Pilot studies in patients with septic shock indicated that the administration of a complete murine anti-TNF-α antibody might improve hypotension and left ventricular function even in the late stage of sepsis [19–21]. The improvement of left ventricular function, however, was only transient with a high variability in response and was not sustained 24 h after administration of the anti-TNF-α antibody [20].

The aim of the present trial was to study the effects of multiple dose administration of the F(ab′)$_2$ fragment of a murine monoclonal anti-TNF-α antibody during several days on the cardiovascular system in patients with severe sepsis. Furthermore, the influence of two different dosages of the F(ab′)$_2$ fragment of a murine-anti-TNF-α antibody is discussed in the light of recently published data from a phase II trial using a complete murine anti-TNF-α antibody [18].

Patients and Methods

Patients

After approval of the study protocol by the ethics committee of the University of Munich, 20 patients with severe sepsis were included after they met the following criteria:

1) Sepsis criteria score $\geq$ 4 of 8 points (according to [22, 23]),
2) systemic vascular resistance (SVR) <800 dyn $\times$ s $\times$ cm^{-5},
3) Elebute score [24] ≥ 12 points,
4) APACHE II score [25] ≥ 20 and ≤ 35 points and
5) written informed consent from a responsible relative.

Clinical data are summarized in Table 1.

Before inclusion into the study all patients had adequate fluid replacement. The right atrial pressure (RAP) was ≥ 10 and ≤ 20 mm Hg and pulmonary capillary wedge pressure (PCWP) was ≥ 10 and ≤ 20 mm Hg for at least 24 h. Vasopressors were delivered if required to maintain systolic arterial pressure (SAP) >90 mm Hg. The amount of vasopressors was determined each day in every patient and used to calculate a vasopressor score with the following scale: 1, dopamine ≤ 10 μg/kg per minute; 2, dopamine ≥ 10 μg/kg per minute; 3, dopamine and dobutamine ≥ 10 μg/kg per minute; 4, epinephrine or norepinephrine ≤ 10 μg/kg per minute; 5, epinephrine or norepinephrine ≥ 10 μg/kg per minute; 6, epinephrine and norepinephrine ≥ 10 μg/kg per minute; and 7, epinephrine and norepinephrine ≥ 50 μg/kg per minute. All patients received standard supportive care and antibiotic treatment. Inclusion into the study did not depend on proven bacterial cultures.

Methods

After inclusion into the study (day 0), intravenous administration of the anti-TNF-α antibody was started on the morning of day 1 (single administration lasting 15 min). From day 2, it was administered every 8 h until the morning of day 5, resulting in a total number of 11 single doses per patient. The anti-TNF-α antibody used was a F(ab′)$_2$ fragment of a murine monoclonal antibody against human TNF-α (MAK 195 F, Knoll AG, FRG) [16]. The patients received either 1 mg/kg ($n=10$) or 3 mg/kg ($n=10$) anti-TNF-α antibody per dose.

Serum levels of the F(ab′)$_2$ fragments of the murine monoclonal anti-TNF-α antibody were measured by an enzyme-linked immunosorbent assay (ELISA). Briefly, recombinant human TNF-α was coated onto the wells of microtiter plates and dilutions of patients' sera were added and incubated for 16–18 h at 4°C. After washing of the wells, a biotinylated anti-mouse immu-

Table 1. Clinical data of 20 patients with severe sepsis

Patient	Sex	Age	Underlying disease	Source of sepsis	Microorganism	Dose of anti-TNF-α/ antibody	Outcome (days after first administration of anti-TNF-α antibody)
1	F	65	Endocarditis	Heart	*Mycoplasma pneumoniae*	1 mg/kg	Died after 17 days
2	M	56	Endocarditis	Heart	*Staphylococcus aureus*[a]	1 mg/kg	Survived[b]
3	M	69	Aortic stenosis	Lung	*Enterococcus faecalis, Candida albicans*	1 mg/kg	Survived[b]
4	M	70	Coronary artery disease, aspiration pneumonia	Lung	*Enterococcus faecalis*	1 mg/kg	Survived[b]
5	M	63	Mallory-Weiss syndrome, abdominal surgery	Lung	*Klebsiella oxytoca, Proteus mirabilis*[a]	3 mg/kg	Died after 38 days
6	M	32	Pneumonia	Lung	*Pseudomonas aeruginosa*	3 mg/kg	Survived[b]
7	F	62	Pulmonary embolism	Lung	*Staphylococcus epidermidis, Candida glabrata*	3 mg/kg	Survived[b]
8	F	38	COPD, hysterectomy	Lung	*Candida albicans*	3 mg/kg	Survived[b]
9	M	56	Endocarditis, aortic and mitral valve replacement	Heart	*Streptococcus bovis*[a]	1 mg/kg	Died after 38 days
10	F	47	Coronary artery disease	Lung	*Staphylococcus aureus*	1 mg/kg	Survived[b]
11	M	53	Pneumonia	Lung	*Candida albicans*	1 mg/kg	Died after 17 days
12	F	68	Aortic stenosis	Lung	*Staphylococcus aureus, Serratia marcescens*	1 mg/kg	Died after 1 day

Table 1. Continued Clinical data of 20 patients with severe sepsis

Patient	Sex	Age	Underlying disease	Source of sepsis	Microorganism	Dose of anti-TNF-α/antibody	Outcome (days after first administration of anti-TNF-α antibody)
13	M	54	Coronary artery disease	Lung	*Haemophilus influenca*	1mg/kg	Survived[b]
14	F	66	Endocarditis, aortic valve replacement	Heart	*Staphylococcus aureus, Staphylococcus epidermidis*	3 mg/kg	Died after 2 days
15	M	59	Tricuspid regurgitation, valve replacement	Lung	*Pseudomonas aeruginosa, Candida albicans*	3 mg/kg	Died after 2 days
16	M	43	Endocarditis, aortic valve replacement	Lung	*Staphylococcus epidermidis*	3 mg/kg	Died after 37 days
17	M	55	Renal insufficiency, coronary artery disease	Urosepsis		3 mg/kg	Died after 9 days
18	M	66	Renal insufficiency, coronary artery disease	Lung		3 mg/kg	Died after 11 days
19	M	50	Aortic aneurysma, aortic prosthesis	Lung, catheter	*Staphylococcus epidermidis*	3 mg/kg	Died after 2 days
20	M	49	Renal adenocarcinoma, nephrectomy	Lung	*Pseudomonas aeruginosa, Klebsiella pneumoniae, Staphylococcus aureus*	1 mg/kg	Died after 28 days

F, female; M, male; COPD, chronic obstructive pulmonary disease.
[a] Positive blood cultures.
[b] Patient was discharged from the intensive care unit.

noglobulin specific antibody was added. The wells were washed again to eliminate the unbound labeled antibody and incubated for 4–5 h. After incubation for 1 h with a streptavidin-peroxidase conjugate, a peroxidase substrate was added and the reaction was determined spectrophotometrically (450 nm).

In addition to clinical observation of the patients, possible signs of toxicity related to the administration of anti-TNF-α antibody were analyzed using the WHO toxicity scale [26].

All patients were monitored using a pulmonary artery catheter (93A-431-7,5F Baxter, Irvine, CA) and an arterial catheter. Hemodynamic measurements were performed 12–24 h before (day 0/1), just prior to (day 0/2) and 4–6 h after (day 1) the first administration of anti-TNF-α antibody. From days 2–7 they were repeated every 24 h. Cardiac output (CO) was measured by thermodilution using five injections of 10 ml cold (<6°C) 0.9% saline solution. Right ventricular end diastolic volume (RVEDV), end systolic volume (RVESV) and ejection fraction (RVEF) were derived from the thermodilution curve with the use of a REF-1 system (Baxter, Irvine, CA). Arterial pressure, pulmonary artery pressure (PAP) and PCWP were obtained at end-expiration. From the above data cardiac index (CI), left ventricular stroke work index (LVSWI), systemic vascular resistance index (SVRI), pulmonary vascular resistance index (PVRI), right ventricular end diastolic volume index (RVEDVI) and end systolic volume index (RVESVI) were calculated.

APACHE II [25] and Elebute [24] scores were determined as described earlier in detail [22] on each day taking into account all data from 9 A.M. to 9 A.M. of the following day.

Statistics

Data were analyzed with the use of BMDP (BMDP Statistical Software, Los Angeles, CA) on a UNIX workstation. Serial measurements for each patient were reduced to three time points: before the administration of anti-TNF-α antibody (day 0/2), 24 h after the first administration of anti-TNF-α antibody (day 1), and by taking the mean from days 2–7 [27]. Thus, patients who died between day 2 and 7 were included into analysis.

Differences between the two groups of patients treated either with 1 mg/kg ($n=10$) or with 3 mg/kg ($n=10$) anti-TNF-α antibody per dose were assessed by using Hotelling T^2 test. For analysis of differences between the three time points in all patients ($n=20$), a nonparametric two way ANOVA (Friedman) was used. If this test was statistically significant, pairwise comparisons between individual time points were done using the Wilcoxon test. Two-tailed p values are given. A p value <0.05 was considered to be statistically significant. No adjustments for multiple testing were done. All data are shown as mean ± SD unless otherwise indicated.

Results

The $F(ab')_2$ fragment of the murine monoclonal antibody was well tolerated in all patients. No signs of toxicity were observed clinically or revealed by analysis of toxicity data. In one patient treated with 1 mg/kg per dose of anti-TNF-α antibody, a skin exanthem occurred 5 days after the first treatment and a relationship to the administration of anti-TNF-α antibody cannot be ruled out. None of the patients who could be followed up 28 days or longer after the first administration of anti-TNF-α antibody ($n=9$) developed anti-murine antibodies.

At study entry, demographic data, APACHE II scores, Elebute scores and sepsis criteria scores were similar in both dose groups (Table 2). Furthermore, time between admission of the patients to the intensive care unit and the first anti-TNF-α antibody administration was similar in both dose groups (Table 2). The overall average 28 day mortality rate after administration of anti-TNF-α antibody was 45% ($n=20$), being 40% in the 1 mg/kg group ($n=10$) and 50% in the 3 mg/kg group ($n=10$).

A complete profile of serum concentrations of anti-TNF-α antibody (MAK 195F) over time (168 h) was assessed and analyzed in eight patients of the 1 mg/kg group and in five patients of the 3 mg/kg group. As expected, peak concentrations and the area under the curve (day 1 and day 5) were about three times higher in the 3 mg/kg group than in the 1 mg/kg group. The pharmacokinetic data fit a two compartment model best, with the first serum half-life being 3.0±0.7 h in the 1 mg/kg group (2.2±0.7 h in the 3 mg/kg group) and the second serum half-life being 33±7.4 h (20.1±6.6 h).

Table 2. Demographic data and scores at study entry

Treatment groups (dose of anti-TNF-α antibody)	1 mg/kg ($n=10$)	3 mg/kg ($n=10$)
Age	58.7±8.6	53.4±12.2
Sex (female/male)	3/7	3/7
APACHE II score (points)	32.8±3.9	33.0±3.3
ELEBUTE score (points)	14.6±2.4	15.8±2.6
Sepsis criteria score (points)	6.5±0.9	6.5±0.5
Days at ICU before inclusion	5.3±3.8	3.7±3.7

The volume of distribution (V^c) was estimated at 67 ± 10.5 ml/kg (78.9 ± 33 ml/kg) and the clearance at 10.9 ± 3.6 ml/h per kilogram (16.9 ± 10.9 ml/h per kilogram).

Hemodynamic Measurements (Table 3)

Repeated administration of anti-TNF-α antibody from day 1 to day 5 was associated with an increase of mean arterial pressure (MAP) (Fig. 1). This increase from 63 mm Hg (baseline) to 72 mm Hg occurred within 4–6 h after

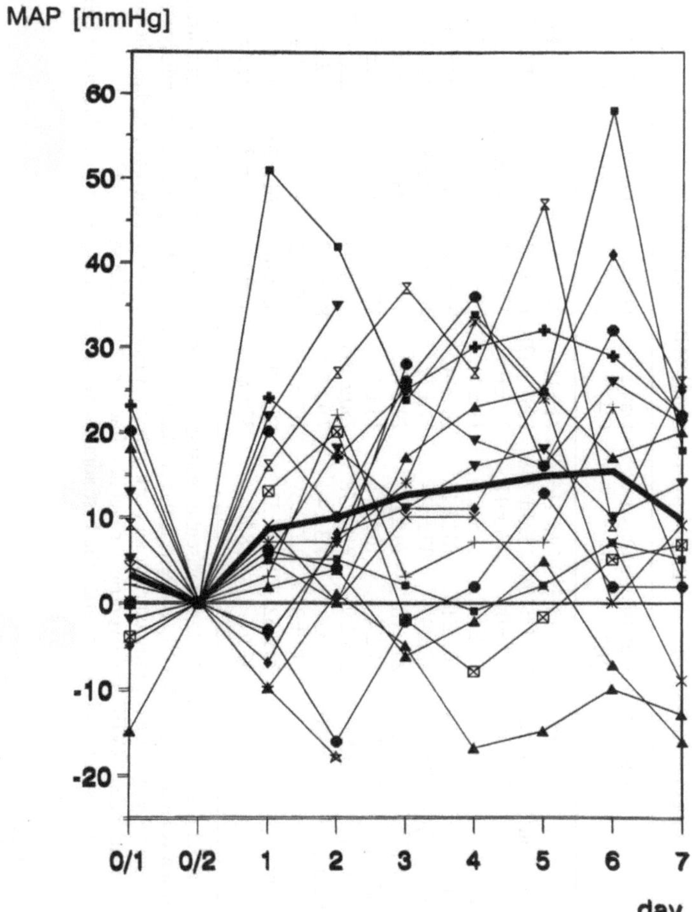

Fig. 1. Change of mean arterial pressure (*MAP*) after repeated administration of F(ab′)$_2$ fragments of the anti-TNF-α antibody. Development in individual patients (*symbols*) and mean (*bold line*) of all patients ($n = 20$) are given

Table 3. Hemodynamics before and after the administration of anti-TNF-α antibody

Parameter	Day 0/1 (−24)[a]	Day 0/2 (0)[a]	Day 1 (4)[a]	Day 2 (24)[a]	Day 3 (48)[a]	Day 4 (72)[a]	Day 5 (96)[a]	Day 6 (120)[a]	Day 7 (144)[a]	Days 2–7
MAP (mm Hg)	67±10	63±10	72±11*	74±11	77±10	79±12	80±13	80±13	74±9	77±9*
SVRI (dyn·s/cm^5·m^2)	1202±227	1107±158	1393±248*	1583±421	1405±294	1466±274	1400±317	1552±318	1459±365	1515±325*
CI (l/min/m^2)	3.7±0.5	3.7±0.6	3.6±0.8	3.4±0.9	3.7±0.7	3.7±0.6	4.0±0.8	3.7±0.8	3.6±0.8	3.5±0.7
RAP (mm Hg)	12±4	12±4	11±4	11±4	13±6	12±5	12±5	11±6	12±4	12±5
HR (beats/min)	102±14	101±16	102±16	96±14	97±19	96±19	99±18	95±17	97±19	96±14
LVSVI (ml/beat/m^2)	37±8	38±9	37±11	37±12	40±10	39±8	41±9	40±12	39±12	39±11
LVSWI (g·m/m^2)	25±8	25±10	29±13	29±12	33±12	33±9	36±11	35±11	32±11	32±9
PCWP (mm Hg)	17±5	17±4	16±5	16±5	17±6	16±6	16±5	17±7	15±5	17±5
PVRI (dyn·s/cm^5·m^2)	245±108	218±91	218±78	250±105	223±99	240±91	220±77	238±116	240±119	240±73
RVSWI (g·m/m^2)	8.0±4.0	7.5±4.2	7.3±4.1	7.9±5.4	8.1±3.3	8.7±4.5	8.2±5.5	9.1±5.7	7.2±4.8	8.3±4.9
RVEDVI (ml/m^2)	—	112±39	107±39	107±38	102±23	101±24	101±20	106±24	99±27	105±36
RVESVI (ml/m^2)	—	73±32	68±32	68±30	62±18	61±20	59±16	65±15	60±19	66±28
RVEF (%)	—	37±6	38±7	37±8	39±9	40±8	42±8	39±7	40±9	39±7

MAP, mean arterial pressure; SVRI, systemic vascular resistance index; CI, cardiac index; RAP, right atrial pressure; HR, heart rate; LVSVI, left ventricular stroke volume index; LVSWI, left ventricular stroke work index; PCWP, pulmonary capillary wedge pressure; PVRI, pulmonary vascular resistance index; RVSWI, right ventricular stroke work index; RVEDVI, right ventricular end diastolic volume index; RVESVI, right ventricular end systolic volume index; RVEF, right ventricular ejection fraction; *, $p < 0.05$ vs day 0/2.

[a] Numbers in parentheses indicate hours after the first administration of anti-tumor necrosis factor-α (TNFα) antibody.

the first administration of anti-TNF-α antibody ($p=0.051$) and sustained from day 2 to day 7 ($p=0.001$). The concomitant increase of SVRI mainly resulted from the increase in MAP, since CI and RAP did not change (Table 3). During administration of anti-TNF-α antibody the amount of catecholamines necessary to maintain systolic arterial blood pressure (SAP) higher than 90 mm Hg was reduced, as indicated by a decrease of catecholamine score (see methods) from 4.2 ± 1.9 points (day 0) to 2.9 ± 2.2 points (days 2–7) ($p=0.006$). The increase of MAP and SVRI as well as the reduction of catecholamine score were similar in both dose groups.

Mean LVSWI of all patients ($n=20$) increased from $24.6 \pm 8\ g \times m/m^2$ (day 0/2) to $36.6 \pm 11\ g \times m/m^2$ (day 5). However, this increase during the 7 days was not statistically significant and resulted from an inhomogenous change of LVSWI in individual patients after the administration of anti-TNF-α antibody (Fig. 2). In ten patients a sustained increase of LVSWI from day 0 to day 7 was observed, whereas in the other ten patients LVSWI remained at the baseline level or decreased. The change of LVSWI was not influenced by the individual dose of anti-TNF-α antibody (1 mg/kg vs 3 mg/kg).

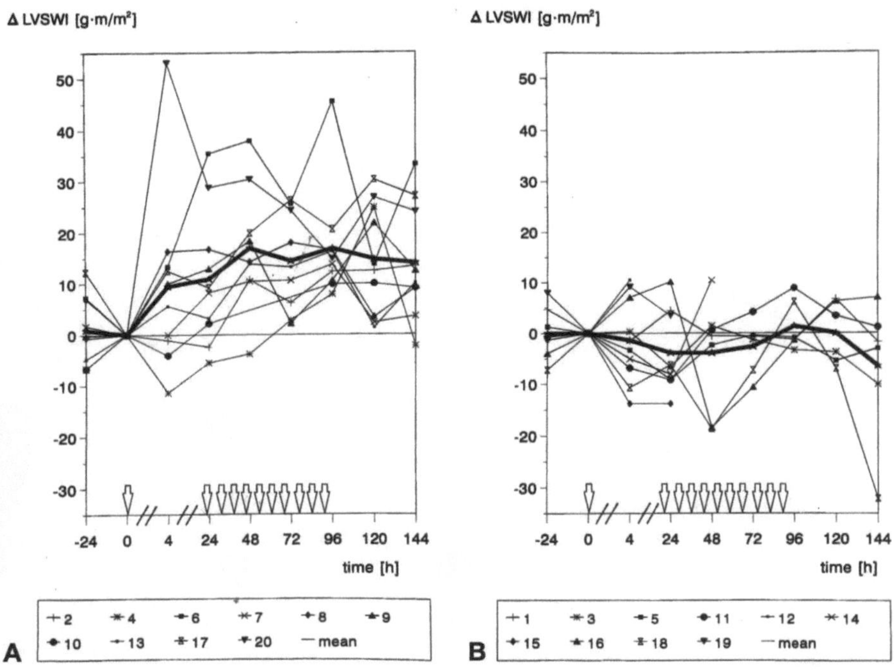

Fig. 2. A, B. Change of left ventricular stroke work index (Δ*LVSWI*) after repeated administration of $F(ab')_2$ fragments of the anti-TNF-α antibody (*arrows*). Development in individual patients (*symbols*) and mean (*bold line*) of patients with ($n=10$; **A**) or without ($n=10$; **B**) an increase in LVSWI are given

Right ventricular function as assessed by RVEF, RVSWI and right ventricular volume indices did not change significantly after the administration of anti-TNF-α antibody (Table 3) in the whole group and in both dose groups. There was a concomitant sustained increase of RVEF in the ten patients who showed an increase in LVSWI (Figs. 2, 3).

Discussion

The aims of the trial were to assess safety and pharmacokinetics of repeated administration of the $F(ab')_2$ fragment of a murine monoclonal anti-TNF-α antibody (MAK 195F) during several days, and to study the effects on the cardiovascular system in patients with severe sepsis.

In patients with severe sepsis and septic shock, the characteristic pattern of cardiovascular abnormalities is hypotension despite normal or elevated CO resulting in a decrease of SVR [28]. All patients included into this study had a SVR below 800 $dyn \times s \times cm^{-5}$ suggesting severe vascular impairment,

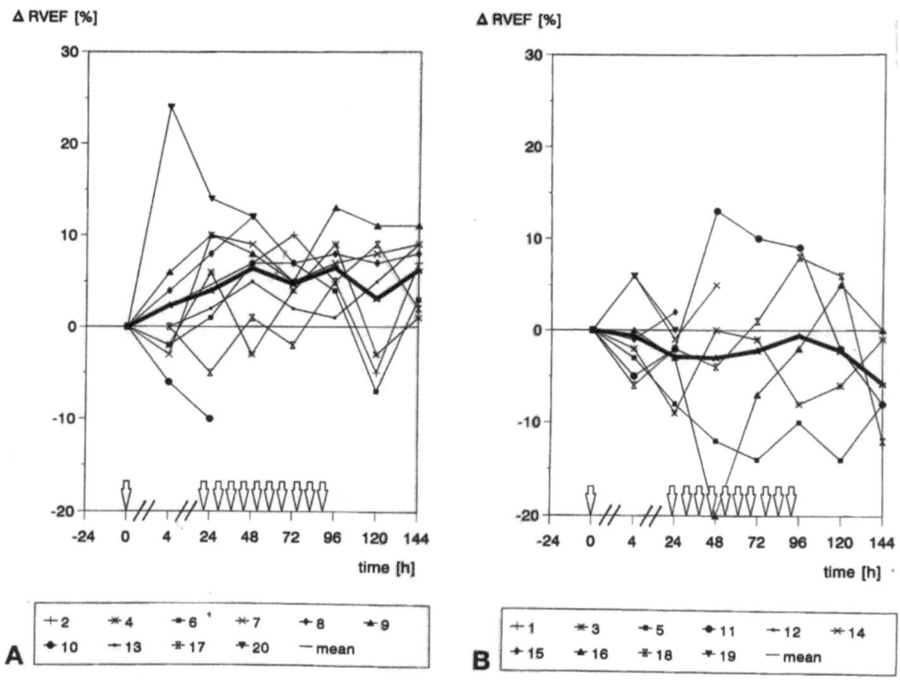

Fig. 3. A, B. Change of right ventricular ejection fraction (Δ*RVEF*) after repeated administration of $F(ab')_2$ fragments of the anti-TNF-α antibody (*arrows*). Development in individual patients (*symbols*) and mean (*bold line*) of patients with ($n=10$; **A**) or without ($n=10$; **B**) an increase in RVEF are given

which was also indicated by the requirement of vasopressor treatment in 16 of 20 patients.

Simultaneous depression of myocardial function involving both the left and right ventricle was indicated by a decreased LVSWI of 25 ± 8 g $\times$ m/m^2 [20, 29, 30] and a decreased RVEF of 37% $\pm$6% associated with an increase in end diastolic and end systolic volume indices [13, 31–33] (Table 3).

A combination of inclusion criteria was used to achieve a high sensitivity in the diagnosis of sepsis [22, 23]. Furthermore, including only patients within a certain range of APACHE II "severity of disease" score [25], a subgroup of patients with severe sepsis and an expected mortality higher than 30% and below 70% was probably selected [23]. Mortality was not an end point of this trial. Therefore, the following observations must be regarded as preliminary. In our patients included into the study with a pretreatment mean APACHE II score of 33 ± 3.5 points the overall average 28 day mortality rate of 45% was in the same range as in a group of patients treated with immunoglobulins (48%, pretreatment mean APACHE II score of 29.4 ± 4.1 points, $n = 23$) who were analyzed retrospectively using the same inclusion criteria [34]. Comparison between different studies is troublesome particularly in patients with sepsis. Nevertheless, it is interesting that the overall 28 day mortality rate of 45% in our patients was similar to the 28 day mortality rate of 41% reported from a study in 80 patients using a complete murine monoclonal anti-TNF-α antibody [18] despite a higher pretreatment mean APACHE II score in our patients (33 ± 3.5 points vs 23.5 ± 8.1 points). Whether mortality of patients with severe sepsis can be reduced by repeated administration of the $F(ab')_2$ fragments of the anit-TNF-α antibody, however, awaits the results of ongoing, larger placebo-controlled trials.

Effects on the Cardiovasuclar System

Since this clinical trial was not placebo-controlled and was restricted to a small number of patients, the effects on the cardiovascular system are reported as preliminary observations and are discussed in the light of recent data from studies that have used a different, complete monoclonal murine anti-TNF antibody [19–21].

Potential effects of the F(ab'2) fragments of the murine monoclonal anti-TNF-α antibody on the vascular system were determined using systemic parameters such as MAP and SVRI. These parameters seem to be adequate criteria to indicate response of the vascular system to anti-TNF-α antibody administration in experimental models and in clinical sepsis [9, 19].

An interesting finding of the present study was that 4–6 h after the first administration of anti-TNF-α antibody MAP increased and remained at a higher level during the observation period of 7 days (Fig. 1). Since cardiac filling pressures and CI did not change (Table 3), the rapid increase of MAP suggests that the vascular system was already influenced by the first administration of anti-TNF-α antibody within a few hours. The higher dose of anti-

TNF-α antibody did not further improve this effect. Similar increases in blood pressure after administration of anti-TNF-α antibody have been described in other phase I/II studies using a complete murine anti-TNF-α antibody [19, 20]. In these studies, however, the increase was either transient [20] or not documented beyond 72 h [19]. Though there was a considerable variability in the time course of blood pressure, in the majority of patients repeated administration of anti-TNF-α antibody seemed to induce a sustained increase in MAP (Fig. 1) accompanied by a decrease in the amount of vasopressors required.

In dogs, improvement of TNF-α-induced established hypotension was observed within minutes after administration of N^G-methyl-L-arginine suggesting effective competitive antagonism to an overproduction of nitric oxide by endothelial cells [1] or vascular smooth muscle cells [1, 2]. Administration of anti-TNF-α antibodies after induction of sepsis, however, did not protect against hypotension in animal models [9]. Therefore, it appears to be unlikely that an increase of MAP after the administration of anti-TNF-α antibody in the patients with sepsis (Fig. 1) results from counteracting the effects induced by TNF-α, which had already bound to target cells. This leads to the assumption that increasing the neutralization capacity of serum for TNF-α by administration of anti-TNF-α antibody in the patients with sepsis might have protected against the effects of "de novo"-synthesis of TNF-α.

Assessment of left and right ventricular function in association with anti-TNF-α antibody treatment showed no statistically significant changes considering all patients (Figs. 2, 3). Due to the lack of a control group, the observation of a nonsignificant increase in mean LVSWI does not rule out that left ventricular function might have been stabilized or improved by the administration of anti-TNF-α antibody. The mean increase in LVSWI of $4\ g \times m/m^2$ within 4 and 24 h after the first administration of anti-TNF-α antibody in our patients was similar to the results observed in studies using the complete murine anti-TNF-α antibody [20, 21].

Analysis of individual patients showed that in only about half of our patients treated by anti-TNF-α antibody was a sustained increase in LVSWI and RVEF observed (Figs. 2, 3). This might reflect either the natural improvement of disease independent from the administration of anti-TNF-α antibody or a response rate of only about 50% in our patients with severe sepsis.

Conclusions

Repeated administration of the $F(ab')_2$ fragments of a murine monoclonal anti-TNF-α antibody (MAK 195F) was well tolerated in all patients without signs of toxicity and without development of murine antibodies. As assessed by hemodynamics there was no evidence that the higher dose of anti-TNF-α antibody (3 mg/kg) was more effective than the lower dose (1 mg/kg). Comparison of our data with recent data from phase I/II trials using a complete murine monoclonal anti-TNF-α antibody [18–21] suggests that the $F(ab')_2$ fragments of the murine monoclonal anti-TNF-α antibody may be of similar efficacy. Definitive conclusions, however, with respect to improvement of mortality and improvement of the cardiovascular system await the results of larger, ongoing placebo-controlled trials.

References

1. Kilbourn RG, Gross SS, Jubran A, Adams J, Griffith OW, Levi R, Rodato RF (1990) N^G-methyl-L-arginine inhibits tumor necrosis factor-induced hypotension: implications for the involvement of nitric oxide. Proc Natl Adac Sci USA 87:3629–3632
2. Geng Y, Hansson GK, Holme E (1992) Interferon-γ and tumor necrosis factor synergize to induce nitric oxide production and inhibit mitochondrial respiration in vascular smooth muscle cells. Circ Res 71:1268–1276
3. Gulick T, Chung MK, Pieper SJ, Lange LG, Schreiner GF (1989) Interleukin 1 and tumor necrosis factor inhibit cardiac myocyte β-adrenergic responsiveness. Proc Natl Acad Sci USA 86:6753–6757
4. Reithmann C, Gierschik P, Werdan K, Jakobs KH (1991) Tumor necrosis factor α up-regulates $G_{i\alpha}$ and G_β proteins and adenylyl cyclase responsiveness in rat cardiomyocytes. Eur J Pharmacol 206:53–60
5. DeMeules JE, Pigula FA, Mueller M, Raymond SJ, Gamelli RL (1992) Tumor necrosis factor and cardiac function. J Trauma 32:686–692
6. Finkel MS, Oddis CV, Jacob TD, Watkins SC, Hattler BG, Simmons RL (1992) Negative inotropic effects of cytokines on the heart mediated by nitric oxide. Science 257:387–389
7. Tredget EE, Yu YM, Zhong S et al (1988) Role of interleukin 1 and tumor necrosis factor on energy metabolism in rabbits. Am J Physiol 255:E760–E768
8. Finkel MS, Hoffman RA, Shen L, Oddis CV, Simmons RL, Hattler BG (1993) Interleukin-6 (IL-6) as a mediator of stunned myocardium. Am J Cardiol 71:1231–1232
9. Tracey KJ, Fong Y, Hesse DG et al (1987) Anti-cachectin/TNF monoclonal antibodies prevent septic shock during lethal bacteraemia. Nature 330:662–664
10. Schirmer JW, Schirmer JM, Fry DE (1989) Recombinant human tumor necrosis factor produces hemodynamic changes characteristic of sepsis and endotoxemia. Arch Surg 124:445–448
11. Natanson C, Eichenholz PW, Danner RL et al (1989) Endotoxin and tumor necrosis factor challenges in dogs simulate the cardiovascular profile of human septic shock. J Exp Med 169:823–832
12. Parrillo JE (1990) Septic shock in humans. Ann Intern Med 113:227–242
13. Kimchi A, Ellrodt G, Berman DS, Riedinger MS, Swan HJC, Murata GH (1984) Right ventricular performance in septic shock: a combined radionuclide and hemodynamic study. J Am Coll Cardiol 4:945–951
14. Beutler B, Milsark IW, Cerami AC (1985) Passive immunization against cachectin/tumor necrosis factor protects mice from lethal effect of endotoxin. Science 229:869–871
15. Bagby GJ, Plessala KJ, Wilson LA, Thompson JJ, Nelson S (1991) Divergent efficacy of antibody to tumor necrosis factor-α in intravascular and peritonitis models of sepsis. J Infect Dis 163:83–88
16. Möller A, Emling F, Blohm D (1990) Monoclonal antibodies to human tumour necrosis factor alpha: in vitro and in vivo application. Cytokine 2:162–169
17. Galloway CJ, Madanat MS, Mitra G (1991) Monoclonal anti-tumor necrosis factor (TNF) antibodies protect mouse and human cells from TNF cytotoxicity. J Immunol Methods 140:37–43

18. Fisher CJ, Opal SM, Dhainaut JF, Stephens S, Zimmermann JL, Nightingale P, Harris SJ, Schein RM, Panacek EA, Vincent JL, Foulke GE, Warren EL, Garrard C, Park G, Bodmer MW, Cohen J, van der Linden C, Gross AL, Sadoff JC and the CB0006 Sepsis Syndrome Study Group (1993) Influence of an anti-tumor necrosis factor monoclonal antibody on cytokine levels in patients with sepsis. Crit Care Med 21:318–327
19. Exley AR, Cohen J, Buurman W et al (1990) Monoclonal antibody to TNF in severe septic shock. Lancet 2:1275–1277
20. Vincent JL, Bakker J, Marecaux G, Schandene L, Kahn RJ, Dupon E (1992) Administration of anti-TNF antibody improves left ventricular function in septic shock patients. Results of a pilot study. Chest 101:810–815
21. Lanore JJ, Dhainaut JF, Fisher JC, Opal SM, Zimmerman J, Nightingale P, Stephens S, Schein RL, Panacek EA, Vincent JL, Foulke GE, Warren EL, Garrard C, Park G, Bodmer MW, Cohen J, van der Linden C, Sadoff JC, Pochard F and the CB0006 Study Group (1992) Effects of an anti-TNF IgG monoclonal antibody on left ventricular performance in septic patients (Abstr). Intensive Care Med 18:S49
22. Pilz G, Gurniak T, Bujdoso O, Werdan K (1991) A basic program for calculation of APACHE II and Elebute scores and sepsis evaluation in intensive care medicine. Comput Biol Med 21:143–159
23. Pilz G, Fateh-Moghadam S, Viell B et al (1993) Supplemental immunoglobin therapy in sepsis and septic shock – comparison of mortality under treatment with polyvalent i.v. immunoglobin versus placebo: protocol of a multicenter, randomized, prospective, double-blind trial. Theor Surg 8:61–83
24. Elebute EA, Stoner HB (1983) The grading of sepsis. Br J Surg 70:29–31
25. Knaus WA, Draper EA, Wagner DP, Zimmermann JE (1985) APACHE II: a severity of disease classification system. Crit Care Med 13:818–829
26. WHO (1979) Handbook for reporting results of cancer treatment. WHO, Geneva
27. Matthews JN, Altman DG, Campbell MJ, Royston P (1990) Analysis of serial measurements in medical research. Br Med J 300:230–235
28. Parker ME, Shelhamer JH, Natanson C, Alling DW, Parrillo JE (1987) Serial cardiovascular variables in survivors and nonsurvivors of human septic shock: heart rate as an early predictor of prognosis. Crit Care Med 15:923–929
29. Rackow EC, Kaufman BS, Falk JL, Astiz ME, Weil MH (1987) Hemodynamic response to fluid repletion in patients with septic shock: evidence for early depression of cardiac performance. Circ Shock 22:11–22
30. Ellrodt AG, Riedinger MS, Kimchi A, Berman DS, Maddahi J, Swan HJ, Murata GH (1985) Left ventricular performance in septic shock. Reversible segmental and global abnormalities. Am Heart J 110:402–409
31. Dhainaut JF, Lanore JJ, deGournay JM, Huyghebaert MF, Brunet F, Villemant D, Monsallier JF (1988) Right ventricular dysfunction in patients with septic shock. Intensive Care Med 14:488–491
32. Zellner JE, Spinale FG, Crawford FA, Cook JA (1991) Right ventricular pump dysfunction with acute experimental septic shock. J Surg Res 50:93–99
33. Brunet F, Dhainaut JF, Devaux JY, Huyghebaert MF, Villemant D, Monsallier JF (1988) Right ventricular performance in patients with acute respiratory failure. Intensive Care Med 14:474–477
34. Boekstegers P, Weidenhöfer S, Pilz G, Holler E, Kempeni J (1992) Response to TNF-antibody therapy (MAK 195F) in patients with severe sepsis: comparison to polyvalent IgG-therapy (Abstr). Eur Cytokine Netw 3:215

Modulating Effects of Pentoxifylline on Cytokine Release Syndromes

F. U. Schade and P. Zabel

Introduction

Tumor necrosis factor-α (TNF) has been identified as the most important mediator of septic shock and cachexia in animals and humans. Moreover, TNF plays a major role in the pathophysiological events of many other infectious and immunological diseases. Therefore, drugs interfering with the formation of TNF may have beneficial effects in these clinical circumstances.

Among the various compounds elaborated by macrophages in response to endotoxins, prostaglandins have been recognized to contribute to the regulation of cytokine biosynthesis [1, 2]. TNF synthesis is negatively controlled by prostaglandin E (PGE), most probably by increases in intracellular cAMP. This finding has led to the hypothesis that endogenously formed PGE limits the extent of TNF synthesis by macrophages. In agreement with this, it has been found that inhibition of prostaglandin synthesis by indomethacin or aspirin results in increased TNF production [3]. Based on the above results, the assumption seemed reasonable that intracellular increases in cAMP by inhibition of phosphodiesterases (PDEs) would also lead to attenuation of TNF synthesis and, hence, should be of benefit in the syndromes described above. In our laboratories and clinic, a PDE inhibitor which is clinically in wide use, pentoxifylline (3,7-dimethyl-1-(5-oxo-hexyl)-xanthine, POF), has been tested with regard to its effects on cytokine production and endotoxin lethality. Pentoxifylline is a drug of known hemorrheological activity. Its effects were supposed to be based on its ability to increase erythrocyte flexibility, to reduce blood viscosity and filterability, and to increase capillary flow in several diseases. It has been used clinically for therapy of patients with various types of vascular insufficiency particularly intermittent claudication [4].

Pentoxifylline Inhibits Tumor Necrosis Factor Synthesis in Macrophage Cultures and in Lipopolysaccharide-Treated Mice

The putative TNF inhibitory activity of POF was first tested in macrophage cultures stimulated with endotoxin (lipopolysaccharide, LPS; 100 ng/ml) in the presence of POF. The results shown in Fig. 1 provide evidence that POF, over the whole concentration range of 3.1–50 μg/ml, provided significant inhibition on the formation of TNF by macrophages [5]. This finding is in agreement with the reported evidence of others that POF inhibited the formation of TNF mRNA in mouse peritoneal macrophages [6] and TNF released by human monocytes [7]. In order to further characterize the action of POF on TNF synthesis, its inhibitory activity was studied in mice [5]. TNF determinations were done in sera of D-galactosamine-sensitized mice challenged with endotoxin (LPS; 10 μg/animal). The sera were sampled 1 h after LPS injection and TNF was quantified in an L-cell cytolysis assay. The values for TNF activity in serum are shown in Fig. 2. POF, at a dose of 50 mg/kg suppressed TNF formation completely and 10 mg/kg had pronounced inhibitory effects on the appearance of TNF in serum.

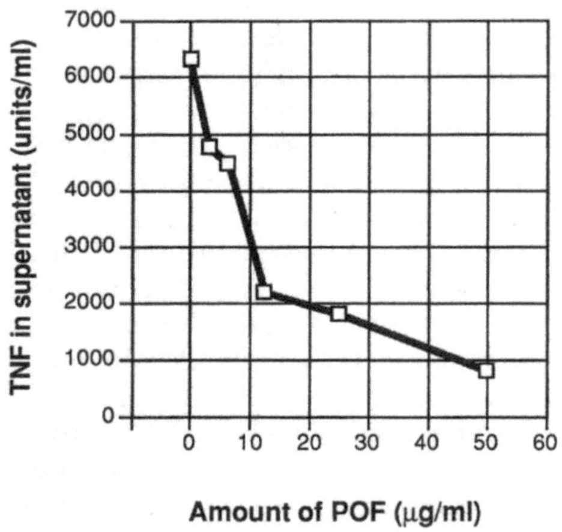

Fig. 1. Inhibition of endotoxin (LPS)-induced tumor necrosis factor (*TNF*) synthesis in mouse peritoneal macrophages by pentoxifylline (*POF*). Values obtained with more than 10 μg/ml POF were significantly ($p < 0.05$) different from controls without POF

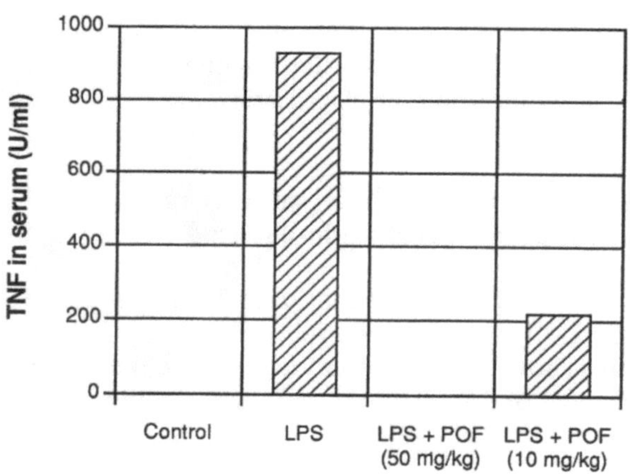

Fig. 2. Inhibition of endotoxin (LPS)-induced tumor necrosis factor (*TNF*) synthesis in mice by pentoxifylline (*POF*)

Effects of Pentoxifylline on Endotoxin Lethal Toxicity

Since the above data showed that POF was able to inhibit TNF synthesis *in vitro* and *in vivo,* it was suggested that xanthine derivatives potentially could be of benefit in endotoxin shock. Therefore, the effect of POF was investigated in several models of endotoxin shock [5, 8–10].

Pretreatment of normal mice with POF (50 mg/kg) 1 h before the challenge with LPS (500 μg/mouse, equivalent to a LD_{50}) led to a significant increase in the survival rate compared to mice challenged with LPS alone. The overall survival rate increased from 50% to 90% (Fig. 3). Mice were rendered hypersensitive against endotoxin by a pretreatment with endotoxin 14 h before the challenge injection. Injection of 200 μg LPS corresponded in LPS-hypersensitive mice to a LD_{80}. Pretreatment of LPS-hypersensitive mice with POF (50 mg/kg) led to a survival rate of 90% (Fig. 3). Mice were rendered tolerant by a pretreatment with endotoxin (80 μg) 4 day prechallenge. When these mice were challenged with a dose of LPS, otherwise corresponding to a LD_{50}, and POF (50 mg/kg), a survival rate of 90% was observed (Fig. 3). As shown in Fig. 3, POF interferes with the lethal effects of LPS in normal, LPS-hypersensitive, and LPS-tolerant mice.

Pentoxifylline Inhibits Endogenous Tumor Necrosis Factor Formation in Endotoxemia in Human Volunteers

Based on the promising findings obtained in experimental animals we sought to approach the question as to the possibility that POF could be of benefit in humans too. A study, therefore, was designed to investigate the effects of

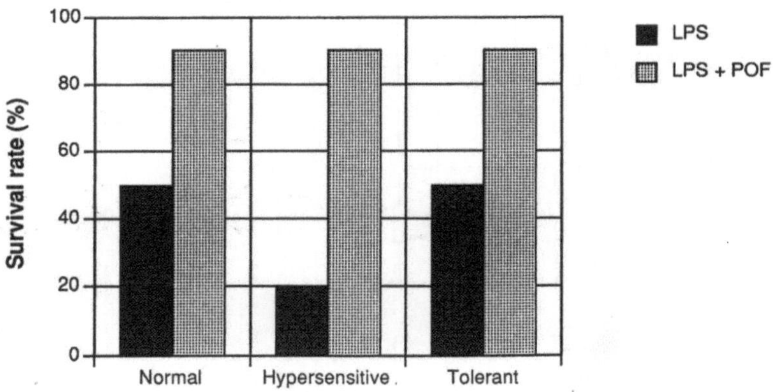

Fig. 3. Protective effect of pentoxifylline (*POF*; 50 mg/kg) on endotoxin (lipopolysaccharide, *LPS*)-induced lethality in normal (15 mg/kg) LPS-hypersensitive (6 mg/kg), and LPS-tolerant (90 mg/kg) mice

POF in human volunteers under conditions of controlled endotoxemia [11].

Ten male volunteers (26–38 years old), each of whom had given informed consent before joining the study, were treated with endotoxin and examined on two occasions separated by at least 21 days: endotoxin preparation (sodium salt of LPS from *Salmonella abortus equi*) was dissolved in isotonic saline and given as a bolus injection (100 ng) intravenously at 8.00 a.m. An intravenous infusion of isotonic saline (125 ml/h) on the first occasion or POF (500 mg in 500 ml isotonic saline) on the second occasion was started 30 min before endotoxin administration and continued for 4 h.

In nine of ten subjects there was a rise in body temperature of at least 1.0 °C, paralleled by an increase in heart rate. The only subject who did not respond to endotoxin weighed more than 95 kg; the endotoxin dose of 100 ng may not have been high enough to induce the typical symptoms. Eight of the remaining nine subjects responded to endotoxin with symptoms such as myalgia and headache, which started 70–100 min after the injection. Two subjects also had nausea (120 min after endotoxin). Systolic and diastolic blood pressure were not affected. None of the clinical responses to endotoxin were affected by POF.

Circulating TNF levels were determined in sera sampled over short time intervals. It was found that a maximum serum level was reached 2 h postendotoxin (Fig. 4). This increase was statistically significant. At no other time could significant increases in TNF levels be determined. When POF was infused, no increase in TNF levels was observed (Fig. 4). Interleukin-6 (IL-6) serum levels showed a significant increase with its maximum 3 h after endo-

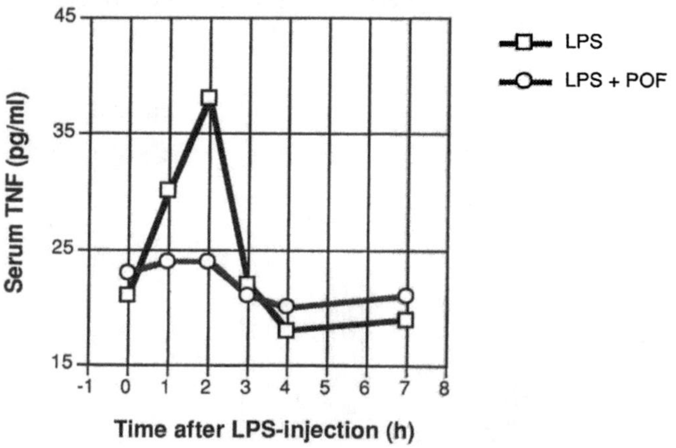

Fig. 4. Effect of pentoxifylline (*POF*; 500 mg/4 h) on circulating tumor necrosis factor (*TNF*) levels in humans after injection of lipopolysaccharide (*LPS*; 100 ng). TNF levels 2 h after LPS administration were significantly different between treatment with and without POF

toxin in comparison to baseline levels. The rise of IL-6 was strictly correlated with the rise of body temperature and appeared 1 h after TNF peak levels. POF treatment did not affect IL-6 levels after endotoxin administration.

In all subjects the cortisol levels before endotoxin injection were in the normal range. In contrast to the expected slight fall due to the known circadian rhythm, cortisol levels 1 h after endotoxin were much lower than baseline. This fall was followed by an apparent rise with a peak 4 h after endotoxin injection, but the levels had reached the normal range of afternoon cortisol levels 7 h after endotoxin injection. POF treatment did not affect the changes in cortisol levels induced by endotoxin.

In conclusion, we have confirmed the findings of Michie et al. [12] that endotoxin injection in humans leads to a short-term rise in circulating TNF levels. Infusion of POF totally abolished the endotoxin-induced rise in TNF levels. We conclude, therefore, that the lower levels of TNF are due to suppression of its formation by POF. This inhibition was selective for TNF without affecting IL-6 levels. This finding supports the hypothesis that endotoxin-induced IL-6 synthesis occurs independently from the preceding TNF synthesis. Also, clinical signs of endotoxemia, such as fever and myalgia as well as high cortisol levels, which are all thought to be provoked by interleukins [13], are not affected by POF treatment. This result suggested distinct regulatory pathways for different cytokines. It is also in agreement with the earlier finding that increases in cellular cAMP selectively suppressed endotoxin-induced gene expression in macrophages [14]. This study showed that the positive effects of POF determined in animal models may also apply to the human situation. Although controlled endotoxemia in volunteers differs from septic shock and related clinical conditions, our data provide evidence that POF may also have beneficial effects in these clinical situations.

Pentoxifylline Suppresses OKT3-Induced Tumor Necrosis Factor Formation in Renal Transplant Recipients

Treatment of allograft transplant recipients with the murine anti-CD3 monoclonal antibody OKT3 leads to a systemic reaction, characterized by chills, fever, nausea, vomiting, diarrhea and sometimes lung edema. Several reports strongly suggested that these side effects are related to the release of cytokines. In particular, TNF seems to play a pivotal role in the pathophysiology of OKT3-induced systemic reactions. It was demonstrated that passive immunization against TNF attenuated the severe side effects of OKT3 in experimental mice [15]. Furthermore, a strong correlation between OKT3 first dose reaction and serum levels of TNF was shown in humans [16]. We, therefore, investigated the efficacy of POF in inhibiting TNF formation and, thus, preventing the severe side effects of OKT3 first dose administration in renal transplant recipients [17].

We studied 16 recipients of a renal allograft during steroid-resistent rejection episodes. The diagnosis of rejection was based on clinical and laboratory data and histological findings from fine-needle biopsy. Acute rejection episodes were initially treated with methylprednisolone (MP): 500 mg/day on 4 consecutive days. In the cases where treatment with corticosteroids failed, OKT3 was administered as a daily bolus injection of 5 mg intravenously on at least 5 consecutive days. As recommended by the manufacturer, a single dose of hydrocortisone (100 mg) was administered immediately after the OKT3 first dose injection. Eight patients (controls) were treated with MP (1 mg/kg) 30 min prior to OKT3. Another group of eight patients (POF group) received an intravenous infusion of POF (400 mg in 500 ml isotonic saline) which was started 30 min before the OKT3 first dose and continued for 3 h.

TNF serum levels increases significantly 2 h after OKT3 administration in the controls as compared to baseline levels and POF treatment suppressed OKT3-induced TNF formation (Fig. 5). A significant increase of IL-6 levels

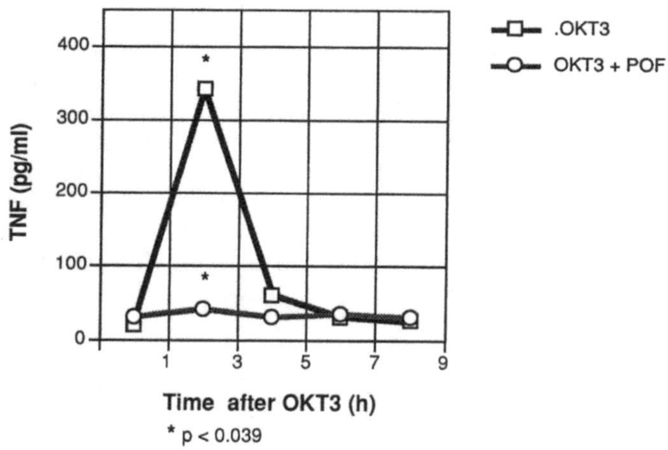

Fig. 5. Effect of pentoxifylline (*POF*; 1.2 g/day) on endogenous tumor necrosis factor (*TNF*) formation in renal transplant recipients after OKT3 first dose injection (5 mg)

Table 1. Clinical response to OKT3 first dose administration in renal transplant recipients: effect of pentoxifylline (POF)

	Controls	POF-treated
Fever >39°C	5/8	2/8
Vomiting/diarrhea	4/8	0/8
Dyspnea	2/8	0/8
Headache	4/8	0/8

as compared to baseline levels was found in all patients 4 and 6 h after OKT3 injection. There were slight but no significant differences in maximal IL-6 values at 6 h post-OKT3 between controls and POF-treated patients. The same was true for circulating interleukin-8 (IL-8) levels, which reached maximal levels 2 h after OKT3 injection in all patients, and which also remained unaffected by POF treatment. With respect to the clinical symptoms (Table 1), POF did not abolish the febrile response, although the number of patients developing high grade temperature seemed to be lower in the POF group. Severe side effects of OKT3 first dose, such as gastrointestinal symptoms, headache and dyspnea, were not observed in any patient in the POF group, whereas nearly all of the controls showed at least one of these symptoms. Most importantly, the OKT3-induced reduction of CD3-positive peripheral blood lymphocytes was not influenced by POF, suggesting that POF did not alter the efficacy of the OKT3 therapy.

In conclusion, this pilot trial demonstrated that POF is of potential benefit in OKT3 treatment based on its ability to suppress TNF formation, thus preventing severe clinical side effects. The data of this trial are encouraging and have been confirmed by others [18, 19].

Effects of Pentoxifylline on Circulating Cytokines in Severe Pulmonary Tuberculosis

Tumor necrosis factor has been identified as an important mediator of chronic cachexia in animals and humans [20]. After having shown that POF can reduce both endotoxin and OKT3-induced endogenous TNF formation in humans, we were also interested in its effects on diseases related to cachexia possibly due to chronic release of TNF. Severe pulmonary tuberculosis is associated with systemic reactions, including cachexia, fever and night sweat. These symptoms may be caused by a chronic cytokine release syndrome, in particular, the release of TNF.

Therefore, circulating cytokines were determined in patients with severe pulmonary tuberculosis and systemic reactions under treatment with tuberculostatic agents, and these patients were treated with POF. Patients with a low disease activity and without systemic symptoms served as controls [21].

As shown in Fig. 6, patients with severe pulmonary tuberculosis including systemic reactions (group 1) showed significantly elevated serum TNF levels in comparison to patients with low disease activity without any systemic reaction (group 2). In patients of group 2 serum TNF levels were found at the detection limit of the assay. TNF levels were strictly correlated with the severity of the disease. POF treatment (1.2 g orally/day) of patients in group 1 resulted in an immediate decrease of circulating TNF levels to baseline inducing well-being and a stop of weight loss. IL-6 levels were also significantly increased in patients of group 1 as compared to patients without clinical symptoms (group 2). Patients of group 2 also showed IL-6 levels at the

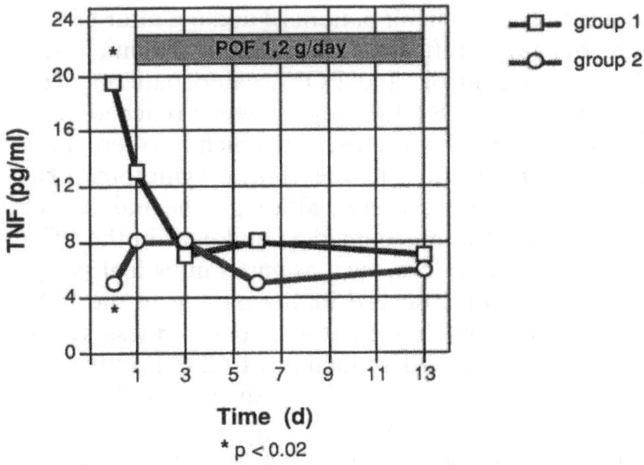

Fig. 6. Modulating effect of pentoxifylline (*POF*; 1.2 g/day) on elevated circulating tumor necrosis factor (*TNF*) levels in patients with severe pulmonary tuberculosis and systemic reactions (group 1; *squares*). Patients with low disease activity without systemic symptoms served as controls (group 2; *circles*)

detection limit of the assay. POF treatment failed to influence the elevated serum IL-6 levels or the febrile response in patients of group 1.

In conclusion, it was found that severe pulmonary tuberculosis is associated with elevated levels of circulating cytokines (TNF and IL-6). Furthermore, POF treatment inhibited chronic TNF formation selectively, and thus reduced TNF-dependent cachexia without affecting chronic IL-6 formation and related symptoms, such as the febrile response and night sweat.

Table 2. Inhibition of endogenous tumor necrosis factor formation by pentoxifylline: new therapeutic strategies

Indication	Efficacy
Transplantation	
Bone marrow transplant	GVH reaction, vascular leakage syndrome, pneumonitis
Renal transplant	OKT3 side effects, acute renal failure
Septic syndrome	ARDS, multiple organ failure
AIDS	Cachexia, virus replication
Tumors	Cachexia
CNS	
Cerebral malaria	Clinical outcome
Multiple sclerosis	Disease activity

Perspectives

As shown above, POF is able to attenuate endogenous TNF formation in humans both in experimental and clinical conditions and thus may improve therapeutic strategies in various diseases in which TNF is identified as a pivotal pathophysiological factor (Table 2). Some of these indications have been examined or will be investigated in further clinical studies.

1) In allogenic bone marrow transplantation increased serum levels of TNF precede major complications such as graft-vs-host (GVH) reaction, vascular leakage syndrome and pneumonitis [22]. Preliminary data of a clinical study performed in Seattle (Washington, USA) in patients undergoing allogenic bone marrow transplantation showed that prophylactic administration of POF can prevent major complications and significantly decreases mortality after 1 year of follow-up [23]. In renal transplantation, POF treatment may improve OKT3 therapy as shown above. Furthermore, there is evidence that POF may prevent hypoxia-related changes in the renal function of transplanted kidneys [24].
2) *In vivo,* POF protected against increased pulmonary vascular permeability and sequestration of neutrophils in the lung of different animal models of acute lung injury [25]. Consequently, as a general outcome, POF was found to improve survival in different models of hemorrhagic [26] and endotoxic shock [8, 27]. Our data show that these findings from animal models may also apply to human beings [28].
3) Increased TNF levels have been observed in cachectic patients with the acquired immunodeficiency syndrome (AIDS), and TNF is known to increase expression of the human immunodeficiency virus type 1 (HIV-1) by acting on its long terminal repeat. Moreover, TNF was found to decrease the therapeutic efficacy of zidovudine (AZT). POF is able to decrease the replication of HIV-1 in human peripheral blood mononuclear cells and in cultured T cells [29]. Thus, patients with AIDS may benefit from POF treatment because it blocks TNF-mediated HIV-1 up-regulation, potentially increases the efficacy of AZT, and may prevent TNF-induced cachexia.
4) TNF has been implicated as mediator of the severe wasting seen in terminal cancer patients, from which its name cachectin is derived [30]. Recently, it was shown that POF-treated cancer patients experienced an improvement in general well-being accompanied by significant decreases in TNF mRNA levels of peripheral blood monocytes [31].
5) In some diseases of the central nervous system such as cerebral malaria [32] and multiple sclerosis [33], elevated TNF levels in the serum and cerebrospinal fluid correlate with fatal outcome and disease progression, respectively. POF was able to prevent cerebral malaria in *Plasmodium berghei*-infected mice [34]. In POF-treated mice, TNF in serum was non-detectable, whereas control mice had high TNF levels on day 6 after infec-

tion. These findings make POF a potential candidate as a supportive agent in human cerebral malaria.

In conclusion, POF is an established drug with no severe side effects and a wide therapeutic range. It may improve therapeutic strategies in cases of acute and chronic cytokine release syndromes by acting as a selective inhibitor of TNF synthesis.

References

1. Dinarello C (1989) Interleukin 1 and its biologically related cytokines. Adv Immunol 44:153–162
2. Schade FU, Burmeister I, Elekes E, Egel R, Wolter DT (1989) Mononuclear phagocytes and eicosanoids: aspects of their synthesis and biological activities. Blut 59:475–479
3. Spengler RN, Spengler ML, Lincoln P, Remick DG, Strieter RM, Kunkel SL (1989) Dynamics of dibutyryl cyclic AMP and prostaglandin E2-mediated suppression of lipopolysaccharide-induced tumor necrosis factor alpha gene expression. Infect Immun 57:2837–2844
4. Porter JM, Cutler BS, Lee BY (1982) Pentoxifylline efficacy in the treatment of intermittant claudication: multicenter controlled double-blind trial with objective assessment of chronic occlusive arterial disease patients. Am Heart J 104:66–72
5. Schade FU (1990) Pentoxifylline increases survival in endotoxin shock and decreases TNF formation. Circ Shock 31:171–181
6. Strieter RM, Remick DG, Ward PA, Spengler RN, Lynch JP, Larrick J, Kunkel SL (1988) Cellular and molecular regulation of tumor necrosis factor-alpha production by pentoxifylline. Biochem Biophys Res Commun 155:1230–1236
7. Waage A, Sorensen M, Stordal B (1990) Differential effect of oxpentyfylline on tumor necrosis factor and interleukin-6 production. Lancet 335:543
8. Schade FU, Schönharting MM (1986) Effect of pentoxifylline on the endotoxin-induced shock reaction. Clin Hemorheol 6:462–468
9. Schade FU, von der Bosch J, Schönharting MM (1988) Increase of survival rate by pentoxifylline in endotoxin shock. In: Mandell GL, Nowick WJ (eds) Pentoxifylline and leukocyte function. Hoechst Roussel Pharmaceuticals, Somerville, pp 175–183
10. Schade FU, von der Bosch J, Schönharting MM (1989) Pentoxifylline increases survival of mice in endotoxin shock. In: Schrör K, Sinzinger H (eds) Prostaglandins in clinical research. Liss, New York, pp 223–227
11. Zabel P, Wolter DT, Schönharting MM, Schade UF (1989) Oxpentifylline in endotoxaemia. Lancet 1334:1474–1477
12. Michie HR, Manogue KR, Spriggs DR et al (1988) Detection of circulating tumor necrosis factor after endotoxin administration. N Engl J Med 318:1418–1426
13. Dinarello CA (1987) The biology of interleukin-1 and comparison to tumor necrosis factor. Immunol Lett 16:227–232
14. Tannenbaum CS, Hamilton TA (1989) Lipopolysaccharide-induced gene expression in murine peritoneal macrophages is selectively suppressed by agents that elevate intracellular cAMP. J Immunol 142:1274–1280
15. Ferran C, Sheehan K, Schreiber R, Bach JF, Chatenoud L (1991) Anti-TNF abrogates the cytokine-related anti-CD-3 induced syndrome. Transplant Proc 23:849–854
16. Gaston SG, Deierhoi MH, Patterson T (1991) OKT3 first dose reaction: association with T cell subsets and cytokine release. Kidney Int 39:141–146
17. Zabel P, Leimenstoll G, Schröder P, Elfeldt R, Schlaak M, Niedermayer W (1991)

Pentoxifylline suppresses OKT3-induced tumor necrosis factor alpha formation in renal transplant recipients. Z Tx Med 3:62–65
18. Schandene P, Vandenbussche P, Crusiaux A et al (1992) Differential effects of pentoxyfylline on the production of tumor necrosis factor-alpha and interleukin-6 by monocytes and T-cells. Immunology 76:30–34
19. Alegre ML, Gastaldello K, Abromowicz D et al (1991) Pentoxyfylline reduces anti-CD3 monoclonal antibodies-induced cytokine release syndrome. Transplantation 52:674–690
20. Tracey JK, Lowry SF, Cerami A (1988) Cachectin: a hormone that triggers acute shock and chronic cachexia. J Infect Dis 157:413–420
21. Zabel P, Greinert U, Entzian P, Schlaak M (1992) Effects of pentoxifylline on circulating cytokines (TNF and IL-6) in severe pulmonary tuberculosis. Eur Cytokine Network 3:248A
22. Holler E, Kolb HJ, Möller A et al (1990) Increased serum levels of tumor necrosis factor α precede major complications of bone marrow transplantation. Blood 75:1011–1016
23. Bianco AJ, Appelbaum FR, Nemunaitis J et al (1991) Phase I-II trial of pentoxyfylline for the prevention of transplant-related toxicities following bone marrow transplantation. Blood 78:1205–1211
24. Berens KL, Luke DR (1990) Pentoxifylline in the isolated perfused rat kidney. Transplantation 49:876–879
25. Welsh CH, Lien D, Wothen GS, Weil JV (1988) Pentoxifylline decreases endotoxin-induced pulmonary neutrophil sequestration and extravascular protein accumulation in the dog. Am Rev Respir Dis 138:1106–1114
26. Coccia MT, Waxman K, Soliman MH, Tominaga G. Pinderski L (1989) Pentoxifylline improves survival following hemorrhagic shock. Crit Care Med 17:36–38
27. Schönharting MM, Schade FU (1989) The effect of pentoxifylline in septic shock – new pharmacological aspects of an established drug. J Med 20:97–105
28. Zabel P, Schönharting MM, Schade FU, Schlaak M (1991) Effects of pentoxifylline in endotoxaemia in human volunteers. In: Sturck A (ed) Bacterial endotoxins, cytokine mediators and new therapies for sepsis. Wiley-Liss, New York, pp 207–213
29. Fazely F, Dezube BJ, Allen-Ryan J, Pardee AB, Ruprecht RM (1991) Pentoxifylline (Trental) decreases the replication of the human immunodeficiency virus type 1 in human peripheral blood mononuclear cells and in cultured T-cells. Blood 77:1653–1656
30. Beutler B, Cerami A (1987) Cachectin: more than a tumor necrosis factor. N Engl J Med 316:379–382
31. Dezube BJ, Fridovich-Keil JL, Bouvard I, Lange RF, Pardee AB (1990) Oxpentifylline and well being in patients with cancer. Lancet 335:662
32. Kern P, Hemmer CJ, von Damme J, Gruss HJ, Dietrich M (1989) Elevated tumor necrosis factor alpha and interleukin-6 serum levels as markers for complicated Plasmodium falciparum malaria. Am J Med 87:139–143
33. Sharief MK, Hentges R (1991) Association between tumor necrosis factor alpha and disease progression in patients with multiple sclerosis. N Engl J Med 325:467–472
34. Kremsner PG, Grundmann H, Neifer S, Sliwa K, Sahlmüller G, Hegenscheid B, Blenzie U (1991) Pentoxyfylline prevents murine cerebral malaria. J Infect Dis 164:605–608

The Treatment of Sepsis with Interleukin-1 Receptor Antagonist

S. M. Opal, C. J. Fisher, Jr. and J. Pribble

Introduction

Compelling experimental evidence and considerable clinical experience indicate that the proinflammatory cytokines are central to the pathogenesis of septic shock [1, 2]. Interleukin-1 (IL-1) and tumor necrosis factor-α (TNF) play an essential protective role in the priming and initiation of the host innate and acquired immune response to localized infection and inflammatory stimuli. However, excess systemic activation of these monocyte/macrophage-derived cytokines is clearly detrimental to the host and participate in the diffuse endothelial injury and disordered hemodynamic sequelae of sepsis [3]. In addition to their own intrinsic inflammatory actions, IL-1 and TNF stimulate the synthesis of additional host-derived inflammatory mediators such as platelet activating factor, eicosanoid compounds, interleukin-8 (IL-8), and other mediators which act in concert to produce septic shock. It has now become evident that activation of the cytokine-dependent nitric oxide synthase system by IL-1 and TNF is primarily responsible for the hypotension observed in septic shock [4].

For these reasons, both IL-1 and TNF have become targets for immunotherapeutic agents in the treatment of septic shock. While IL-1 and TNF are derived from separate genetic loci on different chromosomes and bind to structurally dissimilar tissue receptors, the actions of these two cytokines are remarkably similar. Both cytokines are pleotrophic and have overlapping activities which affect a myriad of metabolic processes throughout the human body [3]. Infusions of either cytokine reproduces many of the pathophysiologic consequences of septic shock in animal models. There is experimental evidence that IL-1 and TNF function in a synergistic manner upon the mammalian cardiovascular system. Okusawa et al. [5] have demonstrated that an infusion of IL-1 or TNF at levels which are insufficient to produce hypotension alone will produce severe hypotension and shock when administered simultaneously in a rabbit model. These findings suggest that IL-1 potentiates the systemic effects of TNF and indicate that blockade of either TNF or IL-1 might provide a survival benefit in septic shock. Initial clinical experience with infusions of either of these proinflammatory cytokines confirm their potent ability to induce metabolic and hemodynamic derangements in humans.

Since IL-1 may be deleterious when present in excess quantities in the systemic circulation, its synthesis and release is a highly controlled and regulated process. The control of IL-1 synthesis and release occurs at the translational, transcriptional, and posttranscriptional levels [3, 6]. Control of IL-1 action also occurs in the systemic circulation and at peripheral tissue sites. A variety of serum proteins and lipids act as nonspecific inhibitors of IL-1 activity. In addition, soluble IL-1 receptors bind to IL-1 and subsequently clear the cytokine from the systemic circulation. An increasing number of counterregulatory, anti-inflammatory cytokines are now recognized, such as interleukin-4 (IL-4), interleukin-6 (IL-6), and IL-10 (IL-10), which modulate the physiologic effects of IL-1 and TNF. IL-1 has an additional control mechanism which is apparently unique to cytokine biology. A natural inhibitor of IL-1 action exists which functions at the tissue receptor level. This IL-1 inhibitor, known as interleukin-1 receptor antagonist (IL-1ra), has become the focus of considerable research investigation as a potential therapeutic agent in the control of IL-1 action in septic shock and in other inflammatory and infectious states.

The Biology of Interleukin-1 Receptor Antagonist

The discovery of IL-1ra is attributed to the work of Secklinger and Dayer [7] and Arend et al [8]. Unlike previously described soluble cytokine receptors, this natural inhibitor of IL-1 does not bind to IL-1 itself. IL-1ra binds to the functional receptors for IL-1 at the tissue level. There are two recognized tissue receptors for IL-1. The type I receptor (IL-1 RtI) is 80 kDa in size and is primarily found on the cell surfaces of T cells, endothelial cells, and hepatocytes. The second tissue receptor has a molecular weight of 68 kDa and is known as the type II receptor (IL-1 RtII). Type II receptors are found primarily on B cells, neutrophils, and bone marrow precursor cells. Both type I and type II receptors have high affinity extracellular binding domains for their natural ligands, IL-1 α or IL-1 β. Both receptors have a transmembrane domain and an intracytoplasmic tail. The intracytoplasmic tail of type II receptors is short and it is unclear as to the extent to which type II receptors induce signal transduction and an intracellular message. It has been speculated that type II receptors primarily function as a source for the generation of soluble IL-1 receptors in the circulation and perhaps as a "molecular sponge" for binding at the tissue level of excess quantities of IL-1 α or IL-1 β [9]. The apparent disassociation constant (K_d) for type I and type II IL-1 receptors is in the range of 0.1–20 nM, and the receptors are expressed on cell surfaces from several hundred to several thousand receptor sites per cell.

IL-1ra binds with similar avidity to type I and type II receptors at a level that approximates that of IL-1 α or IL-1 β on a molar basis. However, on some cell lines, IL-1ra binds less avidly than does IL-1 α for type II receptors and requires up to 200-fold excess of IL-1ra to effectively block the action of IL-1 α at the receptor level [3, 9].

IL-1ra binds to either type I or type II receptors but has no intrinsic agonist activity. Once a given receptor binding site is occupied by IL-1ra, IL-1 α and IL-1 β are sterically inhibited from binding to that receptor. If sufficient quantities of IL-1ra are available, an essentially complete blockade of IL-1 action can be generated. Since as little as 5% receptor occupancy by IL-1 is sufficient to completely induce signal transduction and activation of IL-1 action, the IL-1ra needs to be present in substantially greater quantity than IL-1 to fully induce IL-1 blockade. It has been found that up to a 10000-fold excess of IL-1ra may be necessary to create IL-1 blockade in highly sensitive tissues. Following the binding of IL-1ra to type I or type II receptors, no receptor internalization or signal transduction occurs. This is in marked contrast to the events which follow receptor binding for the natural ligands, IL-1 α or IL-1 β. IL-1 binding results in internalization of the receptor-ligand complex with signal transduction through a protein kinase-mediated mechanism. The precise molecular events which activate the nuclear signals for IL-1 action are currently unknown. It appears that IL-1ra binding to IL-1 receptors is a reversible process and that IL-1ra may leave the receptor on the cell surface over time. There is no evidence of up-regulation or down-regulation of receptor density induced by IL-ra itself [10].

IL-1ra has been successfully cloned and sequenced by Eisenberg et al. [11]. The protein exists as a single 152 amino acid peptide which shares 26% amino acid sequence homology with IL-1 β and 19% sequence homology with IL-1 α. Presumably, these areas of homology result in the ability of these molecules to bind to IL-1 receptors. The genes for IL-1ra and IL-1 α and β are located on human chromosome 2. It is speculated that all three proteins were derived from a single ancestral gene which diverged during mammalian evolution and now mediate separate physiologic effects. A critical amino acid substitution exists in IL-1ra at position 145. Naturally occurring IL-1ra has a lysine at position 145 while IL-1 α and IL-1 β both have an aspartic acid in this position. Replacement of the lysine on IL-1ra with aspartic acid by site-specific mutagenesis results in a protein which has regained agonist activity. The presence of lysine at this position in naturally occurring IL-1ra apparently removes essentially all agonist activity from IL-1ra [12]. It may be possible to generate truncated versions of IL-1ra or genetic constructs of IL-1ra with differing pharmacokinetics and binding avidities to IL-1 receptors.

IL-1ra exists in the human circulation both as a 17.4 kDa nonglycosylated protein and as a glycosylated molecule which may range in size from 22 to 25 kDa. Human recombinant IL-1ra has been successfully cloned and produced by *Escherichia coli* fermentation. The recombinant protein is identical in structure and function to the natural nonglycosylated molecule with the exception of an additional methionine at the NH_2-terminal of the molecule. This additional amino acid does not appear to affect the function or immunogenicity of the molecule. This recombinant human protein has been shown to have potent IL-1 inhibitory effects *in vitro* and in animal models of inflammation and septic shock. This recombinant protein is now undergoing clinical trials in a variety of infectious and inflammatory states. Considerable clinical information is becoming available with the use of IL-1ra in treating human sepsis.

Experimental Basis for the Use of Interleukin-1 Receptor Antagonist

IL-1ra has been shown to inhibit endotoxin-induced neutrophil accumulation in the peritoneal cavity in an experimental mouse model [13]. It has also been shown to reduce the acute inflammatory response with neutrophil infiltration in the rat lung following intratracheal administration of bacterial endotoxin [14]. IL-1ra has been shown to be capable of providing a 50% protection in an otherwise lethal challenge of *E. coli* endotoxin following intraperitoneal injection in mice [15]. IL-1ra has also been shown to protect rabbits given a dose of *E. coli* endotoxin which is lethal in eight out of ten placebo treated control animals. A dose-response effect was observed in this model in which 100 mg/kg of IL-1ra produced 90% survival whereas 30 mg/kg resulted in an intermediate level of mortality and 10 mg/kg led to no improvement survival over the placebo control group [16].

Injection of heat-killed *E. coli* at 2.0×10^9 colony forming units (CFU)/kg results in profound hypotension, tachycardia, leukopenia, thrombocytopenia and high mortality in anaesthetized rabbits. Injection of IL-1ra at 10 mg/kg prior to the *E. coli* challenge greatly reduced hypotension, leukopenia and prevented death in this experimental model [17]. Intravenous inoculation of approximately 10^{11} CFU of live *E. coli* in baboons resulted in severe hypotension and death in the majority of animals within 24 h. Seven animals treated with this otherwise lethal challenge of intravenous *E. coli* were protected from lethality and had less severe hypotension following IL-1ra therapy [18]. Analysis of the cytokine profiles observed in this experimental model revealed interesting findings. IL-1ra had no effect on circulating levels of TNFα which rose and fell precipitously following the *E. coli* injection. Circulating levels of IL-1, however, were significantly reduced by the administration of IL-1ra. This may reflect the finding of IL-1 receptors on the cell surface of mononuclear cells which produce IL-1. IL-1ra blocks the autocrine activation of IL-1 synthesis during endotoxemia and this may account for the attenuation of IL-1 levels observed in these animals. While no consistent effect was observed on circulating IL-8 levels, IL-6 levels were significantly reduced by the administration of IL-1ra in this primate model of *E. coli* sepsis [18].

There is also experimental evidence that IL-1ra may be beneficial in an animal model of gram-positive bacterial sepsis. The administration of heat-killed *Staphylococcus epidermidis* (approximately 10^{11} CFU/kg) to anaesthetized rabbits resulted in profound hypotension. These animals had elevated serum levels of both IL-1 β and TNF following infusion of this gram-positive organism. Pretreatment with human recombinant IL-1ra prevented hypotensive shock in this animal model of gram-positive sepsis [19].

Clinical Experience with Interleukin-1 Receptor Antagonist in the Treatment of Sepsis

The safety and pharmacokinetics of an intravenous administration of IL-1ra in human volunteers was first analyzed in a phase 1 trial in preparation for the use of IL-1ra as a potential therapeutic modality in the treatment of human sepsis [20]. A total of 25 normal volunteers received an intravenous dose of IL-1ra as a continuous infusion in an escalating dose clinical trial. Subjects received IL-1ra at a dose from 1 mg/kg to up to 10 mg/kg over 3 h without any hemodynamic sequelae. It was anticipated that IL-1ra would be well tolerated in that it is a naturally occurring human protein which is known to be in the systemic circulation in a variety of infectious and inflammatory states in humans. In fact, injection of small amounts of endotoxin in human volunteers resulted in a greater than 100-fold excess of IL-1ra levels in the systemic circulation when compared to IL-1 β levels [21].

The pharmacokinetics of IL-1ra in normal human volunteers demonstrate an apparent volume of distribution of the molecule of approximately 0.16 l/kg. The α serum half-life is approximately 20 min and the β elimination phase reveals a serum half-life of approximately 1.8 h which is dependent upon normal renal function. The pharmacokinetics are similar over a large range of intravenous doses of IL-1ra. The peak serum levels reached 29 μg/ml in the high dose group of this study. The infusion was well tolerated without evidence of systemic toxicity, hematologic abnormalities, cytokine abnormalities, or biochemical abnormalities. No anti-IL-1ra antibodies were detected in these subjects following IL-1ra infusion. IL-1ra treatment resulted in an attenuation of IL-6 levels when subject's peripheral blood mononuclear cells were stimulated with endotoxin *ex vivo*.

It is remarkable that no toxicity was observed in this clinical study. Previous experiments with human recombinant IL-1 suggested that the highest tolerated dose would be approximately 10 ng/kg intravenously [22]. At this dose, subjects experienced myalgia, headache and malaise. IL-1ra, by contrast, can be given at up to 1 million times this dose (10 mg/kg) without any apparent systemic toxicity. This would indicate that human recombinant IL-1ra is essentially devoid of any intrinsic agonist activity and should prove safe to administer to septic patients [21].

A phase II trial in patients with sepsis syndrome was conducted in the United States in 1991. This was an open label, randomized, placebo-controlled, multicenter trial designed to assess the safety, pharmacokinetics, efficacy, and cost effectiveness of IL-1ra in patients who met the sepsis syndrome criteria [23]. The study consisted of 99 patients who were randomized into a placebo group or one of three treatment groups, with IL-1ra given at the following doses: 17 mg/h (low dose); 67 mg/h (mid-dose); 133 mg/h (high dose). Each patient randomized to the IL1ra treatment group received an initial 100 mg bolus over 60 s followed by a continuous infusion of one of the three doses of IL-1ra over the next 72 h. Patients were then monitored for 28 days for evidence of drug toxicity, organ dysfunction, and ultimate outcome in this septic population. At study entry, patients had a mean APACHE II score of 22.3. Of the 99 patients enrolled in this trial, two thirds were hypotensive at study entry and 30% were bacteremic. By an intention-to-treat analysis, a dose-dependent survival advantage was observed with IL-1ra therapy ($p=0.015$). The 28 day all cause mortality rate in the placebo group was 44%; the low dose IL-1ra group had a 32% mortality; the mid-dose treatment group had a 25% mortality; while the high dose IL-1ra treatment group had only a 16% mortality rate [24].

Elevated plasma IL-6 levels at study entry predicted a fatal outcome with nonsurvivors having a mean plasma IL-6 level of 8.5 ± 23.1 ng/ml while survivors had a mean IL-6 level at study entry of 0.6 ± 1.4 ng/ml ($p=0.006$). Treatment with IL-1ra resulted in a more rapid decrement of IL-6 levels over the first 24 h than found in the placebo group [25]. These results are similar to data obtained in experimental models of sepsis in which IL-1ra was shown to attenuate the IL-6 response in septic animals [18].

A cost effectiveness analysis was also performed with this phase II trial. It was observed that survivors who were treated with IL-1ra spent less time in the intensive care unit and had a shorter duration of total hospital stay than survivors in the placebo-treated control group. If this sort of analysis can be duplicated in a large prospective clinical trial, it may prove that anticytokine therapy will indeed be cost effective in the treatment of septic patients. It is hoped that this form of immunotherapy should hasten recovery of organ dysfunction and prevent secondary organ failure thereby shortening hospital stays in addition to improving patient outcome [26].

Based on the favorable results of the phase I and phase II trials of IL-1ra in septic patients, a multicenter phase III trial was conducted in 1992 in North America and Europe. This trial was a randomized, double-blind, placebo-controlled trial in 900 patients with sepsis syndrome. Patients were randomized into one of three treatment arms: (1) placebo; (2) 1 mg/kg per hour IL-1ra; (3) 2 mg/kg per hour IL-1ra. The 1 mg/kg per hour dose approximated to mid-dose (67 mg/h) of the phase II trial and the 2 mg/kg per hour dose of IL-1ra approximated the previous high dose (133 mg/h). The study drug was preceded by a 100 mg intravenous bolus of IL-1ra in the two patient groups that received IL-1ra. The patients received test article for a 72 h continuous infusion and then were followed for a total of 28 days. A total of 893 patients received the actual test article following randomization. There was no significant differences in survival time among the three treatment groups ($p=0.22$, generalized Wilcoxon test). The point mortality at 28 days was as follows: placebo, 34%; 1 mg/kg IL-1ra, 31%; and 2 mg/kg per hour IL-1ra, 29%. A comparison of mortality rates in the phase II and phase III trials is presented in Fig. 1. A total of 713 patients randomized in this trial

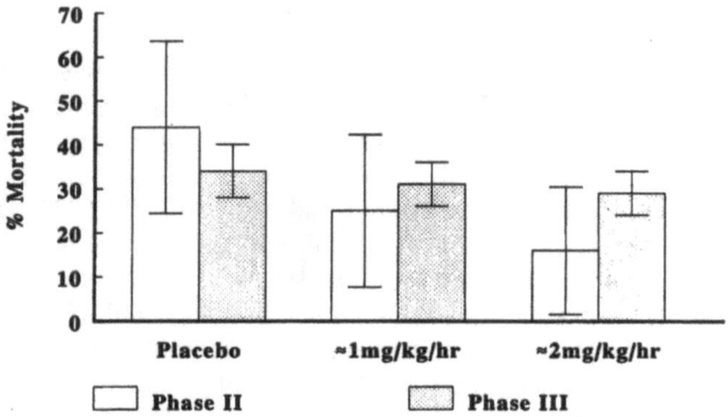

Fig. 1. Comparison of the 28 day all cause mortality rate for patients enrolled in the phase II and phase III IL-1 receptor antagonist sepsis trials. Results are presented as the point mortality rate at 28 days with 95% confidence intervals for each study group. Patients in the phase II trial received 67 mg/h which approximates the 1 mg/kg per hour dose in the phase III trial. Patients in the phase II trial received 133 mg/h in the high dose group which approximates the 2 mg/kg per hour dose in the phase III trial

were characterized as being in shock at study entry. Analysis of this subgroup of patients also failed to show a statistically significant increase in survival time with IL-1ra therapy ($p=0.23$) [27, 28].

A retrospective analysis of outcome in this trial as a function of predicted risk of mortality suggested a survival benefit with IL-1ra treatment in patients with increasing severity of illness [29]. In patients who had a predicted risk of mortality of 24% or greater at study entry ($n=595$), a statistically significant increase in survival time was detected ($p=0.03$; generalized Wilcoxon statistic). A 22% reduction in point mortality at 28 days was observed with IL-1ra therapy in this group of patients (placebo, 45%; 1 mg/kg per hour IL-1ra, 37%; and 2 mg/kg per hour IL-1ra, 35%). An extensive analysis of clinical, microbiologic and cytokine data from this clinical trial is currently ongoing.

The currently available clinical data indicate that systemic administration of IL-1ra may be of value in severely ill patients with sepsis. An additional multicenter clinical trial of IL-1 in severe sepsis is planned which will focus upon those patients with a predicted risk of mortality of 24% or greater in an effort to confirm the results of the first phase III trial.

References

1. Bone RC (1991) Pathogenesis of Sepsis. Ann Intern Med 115:457–465
2. Parrillo JE (1993) Pathogenetic mechanisms of septic shock. N Engl J Med 328:1471–1477
3. Dinarello CA (1991) The proinflammatory cytokines: Il-1 and TNF in the treatment of septic shock syndrome. J Infect Dis 136:1177–1184

4. Kilbourn RG, Gross SS, Jubran A et al (1990) N^G-methyl-L-arginine inhibits TNF-induced hypotension: implications for the involvement of nitric oxide. Proc Natl Acad Sci USA 87:3622–3632
5. Okusawa S, Gelfand JA, Ikejima T, Connolly RJ, Dinarello CA (1988) IL-1 induces a shock-like state in rabbits. Synergism with TNF and the effect of cyclooxygenase inhibition. J Clin Invest 81:1162–1172
6. Dinarello CA (1988) Biology of IL-1. FASEB J 2:108–115
7. Secklinger P, Dayer JM (1987) IL-1 inhibitors. Ann Inst Pasteur/Immunol 138:461–516
8. Arend WP, Joslin FG, Thompson RC, Hannum CH (1989) An IL-1 inhibitor from human monocytes. Production and characterization by logic properties. J Immunol 143:1851–1858
9. Dinarello CA, Thompson RC (1991) Blocking IL-1: IL-1ra in vivo and in vitro. Immunol Today 12:404–410
10. Dripps DJ, Brandhuber BJ, Thompson RC, Eisenberg SP (1991) IL-1ra binds to the 80 kDa IL-1 receptor but does not initiate IL-1 signal transduction. Biol Chem 266:10331–10336
11. Eisenberg SP, Evans RJ, Arend WP et al (1990) Primary structure and functional expression from complimentary DNA of a human IL-1ra. Nature 343:141–146
12. Ju G, Labriola-Tompkins E, Campen CA et al (1991) Conversion of the IL-1ra into an agonist by site-specific mutagenesis. Proc Natl Acad Sci USA 88:2658–2662
13. McIntyre KW, Stepan GJ, Kolinsky JD et al (1991) Inhibition of IL-1 binding and bioactivity in vitro and modulation of acute inflammation in vivo by IL-1ra and anti-IL-1 receptor monoclonal antibody. J Exp Med 173:931–939
14. Ulich TR, Yin S, DelCastillo J, Eisenberg SP, Thompson RC (1991) The intratracheal administration of endotoxin and cytokines. III. The IL-1ra inhibits endotoxin and IL-1 induced acute inflammation. Am J Pathol 138:521–524
15. Alexander HR, Doherty GM, Buresh CM, Venzon DJ, Norton JA (1991) A recombinant human receptor antagonist to IL-1 improves survival after lethal endotoxemia in mice. J Exp Med 173:1029–1032
16. Ohlsson K, Bjork P, Bergenfeldt M, Hageman R, Thompson RC (1990) IL-1ra reduces mortality from endotoxin shock. Nature 348:550–552
17. Wakabayashi G, Gelfand JA, Burke JF, Thompson RC, Dinarello CA (1991) A specific receptor antagonist for IL-1 prevents E. coli induced shock in rabbits. FASEB J 5:338–343
18. Fischer E, Marano MA, VanZee JK et al (1992) IL-1 receptor blockade improves survival in hemodynamic performance in Escherichia coli septic shock, but fails to alter host responses to sub-lethal endotoxemia. Clin Invest 89:1551–1557
19. Aiura K, Gelfand JA, Wakabayashi G et al (1991) IL-1ra blocks hypotension in a rabbit model of gram-positive septic shock. Cytokine 3:498
20. Granowitz EV, Porat R, Mier JW et al (1992) Pharmacokinetics, safety and immunomodulatory effects of human recombinant IL-1ra in healthy humans. Cytokine 4:353–360
21. Granowitz EV, Santos AA, Poutsiaka DD et al (1991) Production of IL-1ra during experimental endotoxaemia. Lancet 33A:1423–1424
22. Walsh CE, Liu JM, Anderson SM, Russio JL, Nienhuis AS, Young MS (1992) A trial of recombinant IL-1 in patients with severe refractory aplastic anemia. Br J Haematol 80:106–110
23. Bone RC, Fisher CJ, Clemmer TP et al (1989) Sepsis syndrome: a valid clinical entity. Crit Care Med 17:389–393
24. Fisher CJ, Slotman G, Opal S, Pribble J, Catalano M, IL-1ra Sepsis Study Group (1991) Results of a phase II study of IL-1ra in the treatment of sepsis syndrome. American College of Chest Physicians, 57th annual meeting, San Francisco, California
25. Opal SM, Fisher CJ, Slotman GJ et al and the IL-1ra Sepsis Study Group (1992) Phase II IL-1ra sepsis syndrome trial: analysis of clinical, cytokine, and microbial features

with outcome. 32nd annual meeting of the interscience conference of antimicrobial agents and chemotherapy, Anaheim, California (abstract 1570)
26. Gordon G, Fisher CJ, Opal SM, Pribble J, Catalano M (1992) Cost-effectiveness of IL-1ra in sepsis. Clin Res 40:254-A (abstract)
27. Fisher CJ, Dhainaut J-F, Pribble JP, Knause WA, IL-1ra Study Group (1993) A study evaluating the safety and efficacy of human recombinant IL-1ra in the treatment of patients with sepsis syndrome. Presented at the 13th international symposium on intensive care and emergency medicine, Brussels, Belgium
28. Dinarello CA, Gelfand JA, Wolff SM (1993) Anticytokine strategies in the treatment of the systemic inflammatory response syndrome. JAMA 269:1829–1835
29. Knaus WA, Harrell FE, Fisher CJ et al (1993) The clinical evaluation of new drugs for sepsis: a prospective study design based on survival analysis. JAMA 270:1233–1241

The Function and Potential Therapeutic Value of Lipopolysaccharide Binding Protein During Gram-Negative Sepsis: Recombinant Expression and Promoter Studies

R. R. Schuman, N. Lamping, C. Kirschning, H. P. Knopf and F. Herrmann

Introduction

Endotoxin is a complex molecule found in almost all gram-negative bacteria in the outer cell wall. Once bacteria have invaded, toxic effects towards the host are transmitted by exotoxins that are secreted, or by endotoxin (lipopolysaccharide, LPS), which can act directly or by release from bacteria either after lysis or antibiotic treatment. The chemical structure of LPS was elucidated recently and an important component of LPS, namely lipid A, a part of the molecule that carries all the "endotoxic" capacity, was found [1]. LPS was found to consist of three substructures: (1) the polysaccharides that form the O-specific chain, which has great variability among different bacterial strains; (2) the two-part core, which is more constant throughout the strains; and (3) the lipid A component which is attached to the core, is very constant within different strains, and appears to be the active center of the molecule [2]. Many investigators have studied the events triggered in the host by the appearance of endotoxin. It became clear that LPS is able to induce a stimulation cascade in immune cells, mediated by different soluble factors. Binding proteins and receptors for LPS were postulated and discovered that recognize endotoxin, bind it and subsequently regulate the cellular secretory response induced by LPS. LPS that enters the bloodstream will be bound unspecifically by serum lipoproteins, mainly of the high density class (HDL), which inhibit its effects [3]. Apolipoproteins also have been shown to bind LPS and inhibit its endotoxic potential [4] and low density class lipoproteins (LDL) can bind endotoxin and transport it through endothelial cell layers [5]. Specific binding of LPS in serum occurs by a protein which is called lipopolysaccharide binding protein (LBP) [6–10]. Complexes of LBP and LPS initiate cellular secretory responses that are much stronger than LPS alone. The data obtained so far can be summarized in that LBP enhances LPS-mediated effects on responsive cells without having activation potential of its own.

The Lipopolysaccharide Binding Protein

The lipopolysaccharide binding protein (LBP) is synthesized in the liver as a glycosylated 58 kDa protein and is constitutively secreted into the bloodstream [8, 11]. The protein concentration rises in the acute phase with a maximum after 24 h, as was found in a rabbit sepsis model. Constitutively the animals secrete 0.5 μg/ml and during acute phase induction concentrations rise within the first 10 h to maximum levels of up to 50 μg/ml LBP. In humans constitutively synthesized levels of LBP appear to be higher and the rise of LBP during the acute phase, as newer data confirm, is weaker than in rabbits. LBP transcript levels also rise during the acute phase as was revealed by northern blot experiments. Here liver mRNA of acute phase rabbit was analyzed and a dramatic increase in LBP transcript could be seen. Also, an in vitro model using a hepatoma cell line was used to analyze the induceability of LBP message. The induction pattern of LBP transcripts in Hep-G2 cells showed that levels of LBP-mRNA rise with a maximum also at 24 h, when the cells were stimulated with interleukin (IL)-1β, IL-6 and dexamethasone. Thus it appears that LBP acts like a class I acute phase protein.

Function of Lipopolysaccharide Binding Protein

Lipopolysaccharide binding protein does not block, but enhances, the effects of LPS and induces cellular responses at subthreshhold LPS levels. LPS-induced cytokine production and cytokine mRNA expression in macrophages is enhanced strongly when LPS is complexed to LBP [9–13]. Rabbit peritoneal macrophages that are in an adapted state regarding LPS stimulation (by previous administration of low dose LPS) can be restored in their ability to produce tumor necrosis factor (TNF) after LPS stimulation by the addition of LBP [14]. Also LBP acts as an opsonin for gram-negative bacteria, and macrophages detect and bind LPS faster and easier when it is complexed with LBP [15]. Also the LPS-induced response in neutrophilic granulocytes can be enhanced by the addition of LBP to the system [16]. The effects LBP has on myeloid cells thus can be summarized as complexing to LPS and subsequently triggering the defense cascade in a stronger way than LPS alone. Blocking experiments using antibodies to LBP revealed that pretreatment of serum with these antibodies, depleting it of LBP, resulted in a much weaker response to LPS stimulation than found with LBP containing serum [9].

Recombinant Expression of Lipopolysaccharide Binding Protein

After isolating and sequencing of the LBP cDNA [9] the full length cDNA was cloned into different expression vectors for recombinant expression of a functional protein. Several different expression systems were set up that differed in yield and functional activity of the protein substantially, as shown in Table 1. Intracellular expression in *Escherichia coli* gave rise to high quantities of a 50 kDa, apparently not glycosylated, protein that was immunoreactive in western blot. After purification and solubilization of the cellular inclu-

Table 1. Recombinant expression of LBP in different expression systems

System	Size (kDa)	Glycosylation	Yield	Activity
E. coli	50	No	High	No
293 cells	58/60	Full	Low	nd
Baculovirus	55	Partial	High	Yes

LBP, lipopolysaccharide binding protein; nd, not tested

sion bodies containing the protein it was found that the protein, however, was not active at all in LPS binding assays. Transient expression was achieved in an expression system using the mammalian cell line 293. A protein was expressed that showed exactly the same size as the native protein, namely, a doublet of 58/60 kDa. This immunoreactive protein was found in the cells and it was secreted into the supernatant in small amounts. Total protein yield was too low for purification and activity tests and a stable transfection was not achieved. A third expression system was established using Baculovirus and the insect cell line SF-9. High levels of a partially glysosylated 55 kDa protein were expressed which was immunoreactive and biologically active. This system is now used for the expression of mutated forms of LBP that apparently differ in their ability to bind to LPS and to present LPS to the CD14 receptor.

The Lipopolysaccharide Binding Protein Promoter

As synthesis of LBP and levels of LBP transcripts in the liver during the acute phase rise substantially, we were interested in analyzing the promoter region of LBP to study transcriptional activation of LBP during sepsis. By screening a human genomic library, we were able to isolate, subclone and sequence a clone containing the LBP promoter. The analysis of 1 kb upstream revealed several CAAT boxes, the IL-6 responsive element H-APF-1 RS, and the liver-specific transcription factor HNF-5 and HSTF-hsp 70.5 at -150 to -170. Also, the glucocorticoid-responsive elements Oct-2-D and GCRE were found, which correlates with the induction pattern of LBP mRNA in Hep-G2 cells by IL-6, IL-1 and dexamethasone. Several transcription factors, apparently important in immune regulation, also were found, namely Ig-κ.2, IgNF-A-Igκ and several of the IgHC group. Reporter gene construct experiments elucidating the functional importance of these structures are underway to determine the parts of the promoter that regulate expression of LBP.

The Cellular Lipopolysaccharide Receptor CD14

Recognition of LPS on the cell surface and the specific cellular responses most likely are mediated by a LPS receptor. Several cellular structures have been postulated as being the LPS receptor [17–20]. The majority of these compounds, like the scavenger receptor or CD11/CD18, most likely are involved in binding LPS for detoxification without being involved in secretorial cellular responses. One molecule that binds LPS-LBP complexes but also seems to be responsible for cell activation is CD14. It binds LPS/LBP complexes on the cell surface and mediates effects such as TNF production or the opsonic function of macrophages [21]. New studies show that soluble CD14 can replace cellular CD14 by regulating LPS responses in CD14-negative cells [22, 23]. CD14 is anchored on the cell surface via a phosphatidyl inositol (PI) anchor, which is unlikely to be able to induce signal transduction alone. Thus and additional compound is probably needed to build the LPS receptor, and experiments are underway to define this additional structure.

Therapeutic Intervention Strategies in Gram-Negative Sepsis

Elucidating the complex mechanisms of endotoxin recognition hopefully will lead to new therapeutic approaches in treating gram-negative sepsis. Some approaches, such as the LBP-related protein BPI, are in clinical trials already and new ones are in preclinical evaluation. In gram-negative sepsis antibiotics do not work because they usually act too slow and may enhance LPS release from bacteria. Newer therapeutic approaches have used targets at all levels of the development of septic shock. Antibodies to different portions of LPS have been tested and clinical results have been reported with an antiserum directed against the core part of LPS [24]. A problem is the variability in this region of endotoxin and the lack of cross-reactivity of such antibodies, so that controversies on the usefulness of such antibodies have arisen [25]. Soluble CD14 (sCD14) seems to augment the effects of LPS in the organism [22, 23]. Thus blocking the function of sCD14, i.e., by antibodies, could be of clinical value too, and TNF production *in vitro* successfully was suppressed by anti-CD14 antibodies [21]. Once the monocyte/macrophage is activated, key mediators like IL-1, TNF and IL-6 are targets for therapeutical intervention too. Cytokine antibodies or blocking of their receptors are strategies in antagonizing their effects in sepsis. The IL-1 receptor antagonist (IL-1 RA) was discovered recently as a natural antagonist of the potent proinflammatory cytokine IL-1; it has homology to IL-1 and binds to its receptor, but does not induce cell activation [26]. Using this molecule as an intervention strategy could be of special interest, as a strong synergism between IL-1 and TNF-α was reported, that could be blocked by addition of IL-1 RA [27].

Exploiting our findings regarding LBP, experiments using whole blood were performed, pretreating the blood with anti-LBP antibodies. TNF secretion in response to LPS could be shifted approximately two logs [9]. Assuming LBP plays a major role in binding LPS in the bloodstream and directing it to the target cell, antibodies or mutated forms of LBP that still bind LPS but cannot present it to CD14, or vice versa, would be interesting objects to study in prevention of sepsis. Mutations of LBP at the LPS binding site were performed and the mutants that were expressed in the Baculovirus system are now being tested both *in vitro* and in animal models regarding their ability to block cellular LPS recognition and uptake. Peptides synthesized according to the putative LPS binding sites of LBP, BPI and a third LPS binding protein were synthesized by Dr. Hoess (Munich). These may also be valuable tools for blocking endotoxin recognition and the fatal overreaction of the host.

References

1. Gmeiner J, Luderitz O, Westphal O (1969) Biochemical studies on lipopolysaccharides of Salmonella R mutants. VI. Investigations on the structure of the lipid A component. Eur J Biochem 7:370–379
2. Rietschel ET, Galanos C, Luderitz O (1982) Chemical structure, physiological function and biological activity of lipopolysaccharides and their lipid A component. In: Webb D (ed) Immunopharmacology and the refulation of leukocyte function. Dekker, New York, p 182
3. Ulevitch RJ, Johnston AR, Weinstein DB (1979) New function for high density lipoproteins: their participation in intravascular reactions of bacterial lipopolysaccharides (LPS). J Clin Invest 64:1516–1524
4. Flegel WA, Wolpl A, Mannel DN (1989) Inhibition of endotoxin-induced activation of human monocytes by human lipoproteins. Infect Immun 57:2237–2245
5. Navab M, Hough GP, van Lenten JA (1988) Low density lipoproteins transfer bacterial lipopolysaccharides across endothelial monolayers in a biologically active form. J Clin Invest 81:601–605
6. Tobias PS, Soldau K, Ulevitch RJ (1986) Isolation of a lipopolysaccharide binding acute phase reactant from rabbit serum. J Exp Med 164:777–793
7. Tobias PS, Mathison JC, Ulevitch RJ (1988) A family of lipopolysaccharide binding proteins involved in responses to gram-negative sepsis. J Biol Chem 263:13479–13781
8. Tobias PS, Soldau K, Ulevitch RJ (1989) Identification of a lipid A binding site in the acute phase reactant lipopolysaccharide binding protein. J Biol Chem 64:10867–10871
9. Schumann RR, Leong SR, Flaggs GW et al (1990) Structure and function of lipopolysaccharide binding protein. Science 249:1429–1431
10. Schumann RR (1992) Function of lipopolysaccharide binding protein and CD14, the receptor for LPS/LBP complexes: a short review. Res Immunol 143:11–15
11. Schumann RR, Tobias PS, Mathison JC, Ulevitch RJ (1993) Molecular mechanisms of lipopolysaccharide (LPS) induced cytokine production by monocytes. In: Faist E (ed) Host defense dysfunctions in trauma, shock and sepsis. Springer, Berlin Heidelberg New York, pp 767–772
12. Ulevitch RJ, Schumann RR, Mathison JC et al (1990) Endogenous anti-endotoxin mechanisms. In: Baumgartner J-D, Calandra T, Carlet J (eds) Endotoxin, from pathophysiology to therapeutic approaches. Flammarion, Paris, pp 31–41
13. Ulevitch RJ, Mathison JC, Schumann RR, Tobias PS (1990) A new model of macrophage stimulation by bacterial lipopolysaccharide. J Trauma 30:S190–S192

14. Mathison JC, Virca GD, Wolfson N, Tobias PS, Glaser K, Ulevitch RJ (1990) Adaptation to bacterial lipopolysaccharide (LPS) controls LPS-induced tumor necrosis factor production in rabbit macrophages. J Clin Invest 85:1108–1118
15. Wright SD, Tobias PS, Ulevitch RJ, Ramos RA (1989) Lipopolysaccharide (LPS) binding protein opsonizes LBP-bearing particles for recognition by a novel receptor on macrophages. J Exp Med 170:1231–1241
16. Vosbeck K, Tobias PS, Mueller H, Allen RA, Arfors K-E, Ulevitch RJ, Sklar LA (1990) Priming of polymorphonuclear granulocytes by lipopolysaccharides and its complexes with lipopolysaccharide binding protein and high density lipoprotein. J Leukocyte Biol 47:97–104
17. Hampton RY, Golenbock DT, Penman M, Krieger M, Raetz CRH (1990) Recognition and plasma clearance of endotoxin by scavenger receptors. Nature 352:342–344
18. Kirkland TN, Virca GD, Kuus-Reichel T, Multer FK, Kim SY, Ulevitch RJ, Tobias PS (1990) Identification of lipopolysaccharide-binding proteins in 70Z/3 cells by photoaffinity cross-linking. J Biol Chem 265:9520–9525
19. Lei M-G, Stimpson SA, Morrison DC (1991) Specific endotoxic lipopolysaccharide-binding receptors on murine splenocytes. III. Binding specificity and characterization. J Immunol 147:1925–1932
20. Couturier C, Haeffner-Cavaillon N, Caroff M, Kazatchkine M (1991) Binding sites for endotoxin (lipopolysaccharides) on human monocytes. J Immunol 147:1899–1904
21. Wright SD, Ramos RA, Tobias PS, Ulevitch RJ, Mathison JC (1990) CD14, a receptor for complexes of lipopolysaccharide (LPS) and LPS binding protein. Science 249:1431–1433
22. Frey EA, Miller DS, Jahr TG (1992) Soluble CD14 participates in the response of cells to lipopolysaccharide. J Exp Med 176:1665–1671
23. Pugin J, Schurer-Maly C-C, Leturcq D, Moriarty A, Ulevitch RJ, Tobias PS (1993) Lipopolysaccharide activation of human endothelial and epithelial cells is mediated by lipopolysaccharide binding protein and soluble CD14. Proc Natl Acad Sci USA 90:2744–2748
24. Ziegler EJ, Fisher CJ, Sprung CL and the HA-1A Sepsis Study Group (1991) Treatment of gram-negative bacteremia and septic shock with HA-1A human monoclonal antibody against endotoxin, a randomized, double-blind, placebo-controlled trial. N Engl J Med 324:429–436
25. Baumgartner JD, Heumann D, Gerain J, Weinbreck P, Grau GE, Glauser MP (1990) Association between protective efficiacy of antilipopolysaccharide (LPS) antibodies and suppression of LPS-induced tumor necrosis factor-a and interleukin 6. Comparison of O side chain-specific antibodies with core LPS antibodies. J Exp Med 171:889–896
26. Arend WP, Welgus HG, Thompson RC, Eisenberg SP (1990) Biological properties of recombinant human monocyte-derived interleukin-1 receptor antagonist. J Clin Invest 85:1694
27. Ohlson K, Bjork P, Bergenfeldt M, Hagenau R (1990) Interleukin-1 receptor antagonist reduces mortality from endotoxin shock. Nature 348:550–552

Platelet-Activating Factor: Pathophysiological Changes and Therapeutic Implications in Sepsis

J.-F. Dhainaut, J.-P. Mira and L. Fiérobe

Introduction

Platelet-activating factor (PAF) is a potent phospholipid autacoid implicated as mediator in diverse inflammatory pathologies [1–4] including the systemic inflammatory response to sepsis [5]. PAF has been identified as an important trigger of cell-to-cell interaction, leading to the release of other inflammatory mediators [1, 4]. This suggestion is based on a large body of evidence.

First, it is well documented that an infusion of exogenous PAF is able to mimic many of the hemodynamic effects and the multiple organ dysfunction syndrome observed during the course of sepsis. Indeed, PAF infusion produces the two major direct effects universal to all species: increased microvascular systemic and pulmonary circulation [6–14] and systemic hypotension usually associated with pulmonary hypertension [7, 15–19]. These major effects of PAF are accompanied by a variety of organ dysfunctions [20, 21]. The organ dysfunctions depend on the platelets' sensitivity to PAF and are largely species-specific. The infusion of PAF into the sensitive species guinea pig, rabbit, baboon, and humans [22–24] results in thrombocytopenia and leukopenia, pulmonary edema [10, 25], myocardial depression [26, 27], reduced glomerular filtration rate and sodium excretion [28], gastric ulcer [29], necrotizing enterocolitis [30], and a number of actions on the metabolism of both carbohydrates and lipids [3].

Moreover, PAF is produced during sepsis in animals and humans by a variety of cells: platelets, neutrophils, monocytes/macrophages, and endothelial cells [31], leading to increased levels of PAF in the serum and in different organs, especially lungs and kidney.

Finally, studies on the pathophysiological role of PAF have been facilitated by a variety of compounds which can specifically inhibit the binding of PAF to its receptors in various cells and tissues [20, 32]. These several, structurally different PAF antagonists have been reported to inhibit sepsis-induced hypotension, organ injury, and mortality [1, 33–37].

This brief review is intended to summarize recent knowledge on the role of PAF production and release in the pathogenesis of inflammatory response to sepsis, and the potential therapeutic use of PAF antagonists in this process.

PAF Production and Release in Sepsis

PAF Production and Release by Endotoxin-Stimulated Cells

Tissue damage mediated by activated cells is of considerable importance in sepsis. Release of large quantities of PAF is believed to result from activation of monocytes/macrophages and neutrophils during different stimuli including endotoxin [38]. Numerous in vitro studies have then used these cell types.

In rat, Salari et al [39] found that PAF was essentially synthesized by macrophages in response to endotoxin. Endotoxin required at least 30 min to cause generation of PAF by these cells. Its most striking action was found to be its priming of the macrophages to respond to another inflammatory agent, such as zymosan. This effect was also observed in the neutrophils, which were less responsive to endotoxin. In adherent guinea-pig macrophages, Stewart and Philips [40] showed that intracellular PAF levels increased following endotoxin administration, while amounts of PAF were detectable in the extracellular medium. Conversely, Worthen et al. [41] were unable to detect PAF release from endotoxin-stimulated neutrophils, despite a small but significant increase in intracellular PAF levels. Endotoxin and exogenous PAF increased prostacyclin (PGI_2) generation in resident macrophages. Fitzgerald et al. [42] also found that stimulated adherent guinea-pig alveolar macrophages released PAF and various eicosanoids. Indomethacin suppressed thromboxane B_2 (TXB_2) generation, and a selective lipoxygenase inhibitor (BW A137C) abolished leukotriene B_4 (LTB_4) secretion, but none of these drugs influenced PAF release, indicating that PAF release is independent of eicosanoid generation. The formation of eicosanoids may be an important route through which PAF exerts effects after endotoxin administration.

In guinea-pigs exposed to aerosolized endotoxin, Rylander and Beijer [43] analyzed the production of PAF alveolar macrophages and neutrophils from bronchoalveolar lavage. Measuring serotonin release from rabbit platelet to estimate the amount of cell-associated PAF, the authors demonstrated a dose-related production in alveolar macrophages for as long as 2 h after a 40-min exposure. No production appeared after 4 h, and increasing exposure time did not modify the response. No PAF production was detectable until the interval between two exposures reached 3 days.

In endotoxin-stimulated human monocyte derived macrophages, Leslie and Detty [44] examined the [^{3}H]arachidonic acid turnover, and confirmed the evidence that endotoxin enhanced PAF production. There was a dose-dependent loss of [^{3}H]arachidonic acid from phosphatidylcholine and especially phosphatidylinositol which reached a maximum (35%) between 1 to 3 h after exposure to endotoxin. Leaver et al. [36] reported that human mononuclear cells responded to endotoxin by releasing PAF during short (60-min) incubations in a dose-dependent manner. A paracrine action of PAF released from monocytes is supported by Salari and Walker's experiments [45], in which the perfusion medium from endotoxin-challenged monocytes produced greater cardiac effects than the addition of endotoxin-stimulated monocytes into the heart.

Numerous recent studies attempted to elucidate the mechanisms involved in PAF release from neutrophils and monocytes/macrophages. In human neutrophils, Reinhold et al. [46] found that ionophore A23187 stimulated phospholipase A_2 and fatty acyl-Co-A acetyltransferase, resulting in a stimulated deacylation/reacylation cycle, leading to PAF synthesis. Gomez-Cambronero et al. [47] demonstrated that PAF itself was able to enhance the release of newly synthesized PAF as measured by [^{3}H]acetate incorporation in human neutrophils. This process was enhanced by the nonmetabolizable bioactive PAF analogue C-PAF and inhibited by PAF antagonists. Moreover, several studies recently reviewed [48] support the evidence that the production and action of PAF interact with protein kinase C and Ca^{2+} transmembrane mobilization. Marquis et al. [49] reported that pertussis toxin inhibited PAF release, suggesting that functional pertussis toxin-sensitive guanine nucleotide regulatory protein is necessary for this process. In fact, PAF release is a more complicated phenomenon, requiring a coordinated action of receptor-coupled G-proteins, Ca^{2+}, and other variables. Furthermore, PAF release was potentiated by granulocyte-monocyte colony stimulating factor (GM-CSF), which was recently implicated as transmembrane signaling factor [50].

These findings support the previous reports, showing that neutrophils and monocytes/macrophages are the principal target cells of endotoxin action [38]. In addition, it is very important to remember that the PAF then released is a potent chemotactic factor for neutrophils, leading to an increase in superoxide production, aggregation, and lysomal enzyme release [51]. Enhanced release of PAF from spleen lymphocytes taken from rats exposed to bacterial peritonitis was also reported [52].

Finally, endothelial cells are also responsible for a rapid and transient PAF production and release in response to various stimuli [53]. Bussolino et al. [54] reported a new pathway which required protein synthesis and was primed by interleukin-1 (IL-1) and tumor necrosis factor (TNF). In this pathway, PAF is synthesized de novo in endothelial cells with a maximum occurring a few hours after the addition of the two cytokines. On the other hand, while the PAF then produced is able to induce endothelial alterations, interactions with cytokines may be crucial in initiating and amplifying vascular damage in sepsis.

PAF-Cytokine Interactions on Endotoxin-Activated Cells

While it is important to consider the influence of endotoxin in PAF production and release, it is also essential to understand the interactions between PAF and other mediators in modulating cell activation induced by endotoxin.

Like PAF, TNF enhances neutrophil superoxide production and adherence [55]. In addition to directly modulating neutrophil activity, at very high concentrations both TNF and PAF are able to prime neutrophils to markedly respond to subsequent agonistic stimuli that would otherwise be ineffectual. Vercellotti et al. [56] reported amplified neutrophil responses including aggregation, adhesiveness, superoxide production, and elastase release to stimuli following priming with PAF. Paubert-Braquet et al. [57] demonstrated that PAF markedly amplified superoxide production by TNF-stimulated human neutrophils. PAF antagonists not only inhibited the PAF amplification, but also partially decreased superoxide production elicited only by TNF, suggesting the involvement of endogenous PAF in this process. Pretreatment with pertussis toxin reduced the PAF amplification of superoxide production in TNF-stimulated neutrophils, implicating pertussis toxin-sensitive G-proteins in the amplification process.

Poubelle and Rola-Pleszczynski [58] recently demonstrated that TNF production by human platelet-free monocytes following stimulation with endotoxin was enhanced with PAF administration. Bonavida et al [59] also found that the addition of PAF to freshly isolated monocytes triggered a rapid, concentration-dependent TNF secretion in the absence of induction of macrophage-mediated toxicity. Monocytes primed with PAF responded by secreting TNF to both pokeweed mitogen and concanavalin A, representing unspecific stimuli, but responded poorly to specific stimulation by PAF and endotoxin. There findings suggest that PAF mediates part of the biological activity of macrophages and, further, monocyte secretion of PAF can in turn regulate monocyte function during the inflammatory response to sepsis.

An increase of IL-1 production by PAF in human monocytes treated with endotoxin was shown by Barthelson et al. [60]. In these cells, PAF and endotoxin synergetically increased intracellular IL-1 precursors and consequently the levels of this cytokine by facilitating its synthesis. In rats, long-term parenteral treatment with PAF dose-dependently stimulated IL-1 and interleukin-2 (IL-2) production in isolated spleen mononuclear cells [61]. The amplifying effect on IL-1 production was abolished by pertussis toxin, again implicating pertussis toxin-sensitive G-proteins in the priming process.

GM-CSF is known primarily for its role in regulating growth of hematopoietic progenitor cells. Recently, it has also been found to prime neutrophils to PAF which led to respiratory burst and increased LTB_4 synthesis [62].

These results clearly indicate that cells primed by endotoxin, PAF, or cytokines produce excess amounts of inflammatory mediators including PAF, 5′-lipoxygenase products, and toxic oxygen radicals.When activated by endotoxin, macrophages produce TNF and IL-1, which then induce PAF synthesis by endothelial cells, neutrophils, and macrophages [54]. Conversely, treatment with PAF has been shown to increase cytokine production.

In activated cells, mediator release can be regulated not only by priming or amplification, but also through downregulation. The balance between these processes is fundamental for protecting the cells from overstimulation and death [1, 63]. For example, eicosanoids, particularly prostacyclin, have been shown to elevate intracellular cyclic adenosine monophosphate levels, which in turn can effectively decrease eicosanoid production in platelets and vascular endothelium. TNF is known to stimulate macrophages, neutrophils, and endothelial cells to synthesize and release PAF, which then facilitates prostacyclin production and then downregulates the release of TNF.

Metabolism of PAF in Vivo

Although PAF was shown to be produced and released by many cells, there is little information on PAF metabolism in vivo during pathophysiological processes [21]. The instability of PAF in the circulation, together with some problems in the development of specific and sensitive assays for the measurement of PAF, has limited knowledge about the effect of endotoxin in PAF release. Salari et al. [39] have partly resolved this issue. Using high-pressure liquid chromatography analysis, the authors studied the murine metabolism of PAF in vivo. Titrated PAF was metabolized over 60 min into lyso-PAF (~30%), acyl-PAF (~10%), and some degraded products (~10%), and the remainder was found in the form of PAF. This study showed that most of the administered PAF remained in the circulation as PAF and not lyso-PAF, suggesting that, if PAF is generated after administration of endotoxin, it should be possible to detect it using bioassay techniques.

Blood PAF Levels in Sepsis

Strong evidence suggests that PAF is produced in sepsis, since elevated plasma levels of PAF were found during *E. coli* [64] and *S. enteritidis* [34, 65] endotoxemia in rats. Salari et al. [39] found that intravenous administration of endotoxin was accompanied by a rapid increase in blood PAF level. This level began to decrease after 5 min and reached the initial value after about 20 min. Chang et al [34] reported that, after intraperitoneal injection of *S. enteritidis* in rats, the increase in blood PAF level was quantitatively similar, but delayed to 20 min. Moreover, the high level of PAF persisted throughout the 2-h period of observation, suggesting either a high level of continued production or a marked depression in the activity of the plasma acethylhydrolase that normally degrades PAF [66].

An increase in the concentration of circulating PAF has also been reported in patients with sepsis [35, 52]. Bussolino et al. [54] reported an elevated intravascular release of this mediator with sepsis. Lopez-Diez et al. [35] showed that the high concentrations of PAF in patients with septicemia were accompanied by a reduced number of free accessible PAF receptors on platelets. This study may indicate that platelets from these septic patients had reacted with endogenous PAF and this had caused downregulation of the receptors and enhanced internalization of PAF or even trapping of PAF into another compartment. PAF was also assayed in whole-blood samples and found at high concentrations in septic patients.

Sequential Release of PAF and Cytokines in Sepsis

Several cytokines are involved in intercellular crosstalk. Mozes et al. [67, 68] found that intramesenteric infusion of endotoxin in pigs resulted in 50% early deaths. The main changes observed in the pigs that did not survive the endotoxin infusion were a marked fall in blood pressure and cardiac output associated with rapid production of TNF but release of no other mediators. This speaks for a primary role for TNF as the mediator of lethal endotoxin shock. However, endomethacin was able to rapidly normalize blood pressure and caused the moribund pigs to survive this most critical phase of shock, while TNF levels remained uninfluenced. This finding suggests that the markedly elevated TNF release observed may not be the cause, but rather a sensitive marker of lethal endotoxin shock. More interestingly, the survivor pigs remained in a severe state of shock up to the end of the 3-h observation period (2 h after termination of endotoxin infusion); they showed a release of PAF, TNF, and eicosanoids, but the increase in TNF was much less than in the nonsurvivors. When the animals received the most critical half-hour of endotoxin infusion or received a nonlethal dose of endotoxin, PAF release always preceded the peak of TNF. The sequential release of different mediators during endotoxin shock indicates an important relationship between TNF, PAF, and eicosanoids.

PAF-Mediated Organ Dysfunction in Sepsis

In guinea-pigs, Rylander and Beijer [43] showed that inhalation of endotoxin produced a dose-dependent production of PAF by alveolar macrophages, while Fitzgerald et al. [42] noted that sensitized, isolated, and perfused lungs released three times more PAF when challenged with antigen than control preparations did. In addition, Chang et al. [34] have shown that endotoxemia in rats was followed by a more impressive increase of the PAF levels in the lung than in the blood. This might suggest either that the primary source of PAF production is in the lung or that the cells that produce PAF are sequestered in the lung after endotoxemia. Although neutrophils were sequestered in the lung after endotoxin administration [69], neutropenia did not reduce the endotoxin-stimulated increase in the PAF concentrations in the lung, suggesting that neutrophils were not necessary for lung PAF synthesis. The pulmonary endothelial cells appear to be probable sources of PAF, since Camussi et al. [53, 70] have reported both in vitro and in vivo release of PAF from injured pulmonary endothelial cells, and since pulmonary endothelial injury is a prominent finding in endotoxemia. Furthermore, the recovery of PAF in pulmonary lavage fluid has been reported [71, 72], but an inflammatory alveolitis seems not detectable until 24 h after endotoxin injection [73, 74], and the lung lavage concentrations did not reflect lung tissue concentrations [34].

Using isolated, buffer-perfused rabbit lungs, free of plasma and circulating blood cells, Salzer and McCall [75] demonstrated that endotoxin synergized with PAF to injure the lung. PAF alone produced transient pulmonary hypertension and minimal edema. Lungs perfused for 2 h with endotoxin had slight pulmonary hypertension and no pulmonary edema. In contrast, lungs exposed to both endotoxin and PAF had severe pulmonary hypertension and edema. Endotoxin-primed, PAF-stimulated lungs had increased production of TXB_2. These studies suggest that endotoxin primes the lung for enhanced injury in response to PAF by amplifying the synthesis and release of TXB_2 in lung tissue.

Pirotsky et al. [76] demonstrated that the kidney may also synthesize PAF. However, in Chang et al.'s study [34] both the baseline and post-endotoxin values of renal PAF were markedly lower than those found in the lung, although the degree of enhancement by endotoxin was similar in the two organs. Tolins et al. [77] have shown that, even in the absence of systemic hypotension in the rat, both intrarenal PAF infusion and intravenous administration of endotoxin produced a significant decrease in renal blood flow and glomerular filtration rate by marked afferent arteriolar vasoconstriction. Endotoxin administration in rats results in a rapid increase in phospholipase A_2 activity in plasma, liver, and renal and intestinal tissues. Activation of this enzyme would be expected to result in increased release of lyso-PAF and arachidonic acid from membrane phospholipids [31]. Then, PAF and vasoactive arachidonic acid metabolites are cogenerated and coparticipate in the endotoxin-induced acute renal failure.

Inarrea et al. [52] also reported the appearance of PAF in the peritoneal exsudate and spleen of rats undergoing peritonitis following the inoculation of living *E. coli.* These animals developed severe septicemia with massive extravasation and a high mortality rate when they received more than 2.10^7 CFU. Under these conditions, PAF formation also preceded protein-rich plasma extravasation and hemoconcentration. Pons et al. [78] have also reported that intraperitoneal administration of endotoxin to fasted rats disrupted the cyclic occurrence of migrating myoelectronic complexes, which were replaced by an irregular spiking activity at both duodenal and jejunal levels. The authors concluded that endogenous release of PAF is partially responsible for the intestinal motor alterations induced by endotoxin, but the release of prostaglandins also participates in this dyfunction. Similar findings have also been reported by both Hsueh et al. [30] and Lagente et al. [79], showing markedly elevated levels of PAF production in an animal model where endotoxin was used to induce intestinal lesions. Lastly, Buxton et al [80], using in situ perfused rat livers challenged with soluble IgG aggregates, detected a PAF activity in the effluent following IgG challenge.

Recently, Ariditi et al. [81] detected TNF and PAF in the cerebrospinal fluid of children with bacterial meningitis, but not those with viral meningitis. Cerebrospinal PAF concentrations correlated with bacterial density, and endotoxin and TNF levels. Elevated cerebrospinal fluid levels of TNF and PAF were often present in children with bacterial meningitis, and were associated with seizures and severity of disease.

The above studies demonstrate increased blood and tissue concentrations of PAF in animal and human sepsis, and indicate that these elevated levels correlate with the outcome of the condition.

Protection by PAF Antagonists in Sepsis

The finding of increased levels of PAF in endotoxemia suggests that PAF antagonists may be effective in counteracting this pathology.

PAF Receptor Antagonists

PAF antagonists can be broadly divided into two groups: synthetic structural analogues and natural compounds.

The first PAF structural analogue described was CV-3988 [82], which blocks PAF-induced hypotension in the rat [17, 82] and hemoconcentration in the rat, guinea pig, and primate [14, 19, 83, 84]. Among the group of quaternary salt PAF antagonists, ONO-6240 inhibits PAF-induced hypotension in the rat and dermal vascular permeability in the guinea pig [85].

Several PAF antagonists related to the first two described have been developed. SRI 63–441 is the most potent of the SRI series, inhibiting all major PAF responses in several species [86]. Among a series of PAF antagonists with a heterocyclic group, RO 19-3704 seems the most potent, blocking PAF-induced aggregation and in vivo platelet thrombi [87, 88]. RP 48740 is a specific antagonist that inhibits PAF-induced hypotension, hemoconcentration, and bronchoconstriction [89, 90]. Other compounds exhibit PAF antagonistic properties, including such as BN 52730, BN 50739, BN 52770, YM 461, and the triazolo-thienodiazepines, WEB 2086 and WEB 2347, which are unrelated to the PAF structure [32].

The structural analogues of PAF can act as partial agonists, and consequently high doses of these drugs may cause adverse effects related to PAF receptor activation [20].

Many natural compounds are also potent PAF antagonists. Among a series of terpenoids isolated from the Chinese tree *Ginko biloba*, BN 52021 seems the most potent and the most evaluated PAF antagonist to date. This compound inhibits not only PAF-induced responses such as platelet aggregation [32], hypotension, and increased vascular permeability [91], but also immune aggregate-induced hypotension [35], antigen-induced pulmonary anaphylaxis [92], and prolongs cardiac allograft survival [93].

Kadsurenone, a terpene from the Chinese herbal plant *Piper futokadsurae*, is a competitive receptor antagonist to PAF, inhibiting PAF-induced platelet aggregation and neutrophil degranulation [94], as well as hypotension and extravasation in the rat [85, 94, 121]. A synthetic derivative, L-652–731, has close properties [95, 96], and exhibits the best oral activity [96].

A fermentation broth product from *Streptomyces phaeofaciens*, FR-900452 blocks PAF-induced aggregation of platelets [97]. Another fermentation product of *Penicillium terlikowki* has recently been described as a PAF antagonist: FR-49175 [98].

Moreover, many substances exhibit PAF antagonistic properties: prostaglandins [99], glucocorticoids [122], thyrotropin-releasing hormones [100], and calcium channel blockers [101].

Protection by PAF Antagonists in Experimental Sepsis

The protection afforded by PAF antagonists has been confirmed by numerous experimental studies. After endotoxin challenge in rats [33] and guinea-pigs [102], a significant dose-dependent improvement of survival rate was observed with BN 52021, total protection being provided by the highest dose of the PAF antagonist. In endotoxemic dogs, Earnest et al. [103] found that pretreatment with BN 52021 dramatically improved the permanent survival rate from 0 to 100%. Using BN 50739, a new hetrapazine-derived antagonist, Rabinovici et al. [104] showed that the mortality was reduced from 100% to 60% in endotoxemic rats, while Yue et al. [105] confirmed this protection in a rabbit model. Pretreatment with this antagonist reduced the 24-h mortality from 75% to 22% and post-treatment reduced the 10-h mortality from 67% to 13%. In different species, a similar protection was also afforded by other PAF antagonists including CV-3988 [82], SRI 63-072, SRI 63-441 [19, 86], kadsurenone, L-652-731 [64, 95, 106], and WEB 2086 [107].

Protection against sepsis-induced changes in organs and functions is also provided by PAF antagonists. In endotoxemic animals, if BN 52021 had no effect on early systemic hypotension, this antagonist beneficially attenuated late systemic hypotension and circulatory dysfunction [103, 108]. Similarly, SRI 63-441 [34, 39, 86, 109] and several other antagonists [106, 110] were able to block this hemodynamic and microcirculatory response to endotoxin in several animal models. In addition, Baum et al. [111] studying the role of PAF in endotoxin-induced myocardial dysfunction, recently demonstrated that pretreatment with a PAF antagonist, SDZ 64-688, alleviated the deleterious effect of endotoxin on murine myocardial contractility.

The PAF-mediated alterations of lung parenchyma and pulmonary circulation after endotoxin challenge are well described, suggesting that PAF antagonists may counteract these alterations. Intravenous administration of endotoxin led to rapid pulmonary hypertension and a progressive increase in permeability associated with decreased lymph flow while PaO_2 fell. Protective effects of endotoxin-induced lung alterations were obtained in different animals models, especially in sheeps and guinea-pigs with BN 52021 [112, 113], SRI 63-441 [114], WEB 2086 [115], ONO-6240 [110], but also in rats with SRI 63–441 [107] and pigs with WEB 2086 [116]. The endotoxin-induced deterioration in gas exchange and increase in inspiratory airway pressure were also partially abolished by these compounds.

Acute renal failure is another classical feature of endotoxemia, a condition in which PAF seems to play a major role. Indeed, PAF antagonists (BN 52021, SRI 63-675, and L-652-731) were able to inhibit the endotoxin-induced decreased renal blood flow and glomerular filtration rate, leading to an improvement of renal function in rats [77, 117].

The mediatory role of PAF in endotoxin-induced murine gastronintestinal injury is well known [30, 118]. Accordingly, PAF antagonists including BN 52021, CV-3988, WEB 2086, WEB 2170, and RO-193704 [118] had a protective effect against such gastric and intestinal ulceration and hemorrhage.

Lastly, the alteration of cerebral blood flow following endotoxin administration seems inhibited by BN 52021 [48].

Considerable evidence was accumulated to support the concept that PAF antagonists are able to protect against endotoxin or gram-negative challenge. However, since PAF is produced by activation of macrophages during gram-positive sepsis [35], there are no available data concerning the effect of PAF antagonists on gram-positive infection.

Protection by PAF Antagonists: Clinical Studies

An open-label, prospective, clinical trial with single doses of a natural PAF antagonist, BN 52021, was recently demonstrated its safety in 22 patients with septic shock [119]. The first dose (0.5 mg/kg delivered IV over 15 min) was tested in 7 patients. Given the good tolerance of this dose, the proposed therapeutic dose of 4 mg/kg was then used in the 15 other patients. Thirteen men and 9 women [mean age 63 ± 18 years; simplified acute physiological score (SAPS) 18 ± 5; systolic blood pressure 69 ± 12 mmHg] were enrolled in the study. Intensive care mortality was 66%. Eight out of the 13 patients with documented gram-negative infections were bacteremic. Gram-positive infections occurred in 8 patients while 3 patients had mixed infections. No clinical (bronchospasm, skin rashes, etc.), hemodynamic (hypotension, cardiac failure, etc.) or laboratory evidence of BN 52021-related toxicity was observed at any dose [119]. We concluded that the PAF antagonist BN 52021 has proven to be safe in patients with septic shock.

A randomized, placebo-controlled, double-blind, multicenter clinical trial of the efficacy (mortality at day 28) and tolerance of BN 52021 (2 IV infusions of 240 mg every day for 4 days) in severe sepsis enrolled 262 patients [5]. No significant difference was observed between the two groups in the overall study population. However, BN 52021 was associated with a 42% decrease in mortality (57% in the untreated vs 33% in the treated group) in 119 patients with documented gram-negative sepsis [120]. At inclusion, among the patients with gram-negative sepsis, the treatment and placebo groups were well balanced with respect to demographic characteristics, underlying diseases, infection sites, causative organisms, SAPS, shock, and organ failures except for liver dysfunction. In those without documented gram-negative infection, no difference was observed. No problem of tolerance was reported. From this, the PAF antagonist BN 52021 would seem to be of great interest in severe gram-negative sepsis.

Conclusion

Strong evidence indicates that PAF participates in the priming, amplification, and downregulation of the immunoinflammatory cascade in sepsis. PAF antagonists appear to be effective in animal and human severe sepsis, probably via their ability to decouple deleterious PAF-generated feedback loops with other mediators.

References

1. Braquet P, Paubert-Braquet M, Bourgain RH, Bussolino F, Hosford D (1989) PAF/cytokines autoregulated feedback networks in microvascular injury: consequences in shock, ischemia and graft rejection. J Lipid Med 1:75–112
2. Feuerstein G, Hallenbeck JM (1987) Prostaglandins, leukotrienes and platelet activating factor in shock. Annu Rev Pharmacol Toxicol 27:301–313
3. Sanchez-Crespo M, Fernandez-Gallardo S (1991) Pharmacological modulation of PAF: a therapeutic approach to endotoxin shock. J Lipid Med 4:127–144
4. Koltai M, Hosford D, Braquet P (1992) Role of PAF and cytokines in microvascular tissue injury. J Lab Clin Med 119:461–466
5. Bone RC, Balk RA, Cerra FB et al (1992) Definitions for sepsis and organ failure and guidelines for the use of innovative therapies in sepsis. Chest 101:1644–1655
6. Wendmore CV, Williams TJ (1981) Platelet-activating factor (PAF), a secretory product of polymorphonuclear leukocytes, increases vascular permeability in rabbit skin. Br J Pharmacol 74:916P–918P
7. Bessin P, Bonnet J, Apffel D, Soulard C, Desgroux L, Pelas I. Benveniste J (1983) Acute circulatory collapse caused by platelet activating factor (PAF-acether) in dogs. Eur J Pharmacol 86:403–413
8. Björk J, Lindbom L, Gerdin B, Smedegård G, Arfors KE, Benveniste J (1983) PAF-acether (platelet-activating factor) increases microvascular permeability and affects endothelium-granulocyte interaction in microvascular beds. Acta Physiol Scand 119:305–308
9. Björk J, Smedegård G (1983) Acute microvascular effects of PAF-acether, as studied by intravital microscopy. Eur J Pharmacol 96:87–94
10. Mojarad M, Hamasaki Y, Said SI (1983) Platelet-activating factor increases pulmonary microvascular permeability and induced pulmonary edema. A preliminary report. Bull Eur Physiopathol Respir 19:253–256
11. Handley DA, Arbeeny CM, Lee ML, Van Valen RG, Saunders RN (1984) Effect of platelet-activating factor on endothelial permeability to plasma macromolecules. Immunopharmacology 8:137–142
12. Handley DA, Van Valen RG, Melden MK, Saunders RN (1984) Evaluation of dose and route effects of platelet-activating factor-induced extravasation in the guinea pig. Thromb Haemost 52:34–36
13. Hwang SB, Li CH, Lam MH, Shen TY (1985) Characterization of cutaneous vascular permeability induced by platelet-activating factor in guinea pigs and rats and its inhibition by a platelet-activating factor receptor antagonist. Lab Invest 52:617–630

14. Handley DA, Farley C, Deacon R, Saunders RN (1986) Evidence for distinct systemic extravasation effects of platelet-activating factor, leukotrienes B4, C4, D4 and histamine in the guinea pigs. Prostaglandines Leukot Med 21:269–277
15. Mc Manus LM, Pinckard RN, Fitzpatrick FA, O'Rourke RA, Crawford MH, Hanahan DJ (1981) Acetyl glyceryl ether phosphorylcholine (AGEPC): intravascular alterations following intravenous infusion in the baboon. Lab Invest 45:303–307
16. Sanchez-Crespo M, Alonso F, Inarrea P, Egido J (1981) Non platelet-mediated vascular actions of 1-*O*-alkyl-2-acetyl-*sn*-3-glycerol phosphorylcholine (a synthetic PAF). Agents Actions 11:566–567
17. Gillespie M, Bowdy B (1986) Impact of PAF on vascular responsiveness in isolated rat lungs. J Pharmac Exp Ther 236:396–402
18. Goldstein R, Ezra D, Laurindo F, Fuerstein G (1986) Coronary and pulmonary vascular effects of leukotrienes and PAF-acether. Pharmacol Res Commun 18:151–162
19. Handley DA, Farley C, Melden MK, Deacon RW, Van Valen RG, Saunders RN (1986) Comparative oral and parenteral activities of several PAF antagonists in the rat and guinea pig. Presented at Platelet Activating Factor, 2nd International Conference, Gatlinburg, Tennessee
20. Saunders RN, Handley DA (1987) Platelet activating factor antagonists. Annu Rev Pharmacol Toxicol 27:237–255
21. Feuerstein G, Stren AL (1988) Platelet-activating factor and shock. Prog Biochem Pharmacol 22:181–190
22. Mc Manus LM, Hanahan DJ, Demopoulos CA, Pinkard RN (1980) Pathobiology of the intravenous infusion of acetylglycerylether-phosphorylcholine (AGEPC), a synthetic platelet activating factor (PAF) in the rabbit. J Immunol 124:2919–2924
23. Vargaftig BB, Lefort J, Chignard M, Benveniste J (1980) Platelet-activating factor induces a platelet-dependent bronchoconstriction unrelated to the formation of prostaglandin derivatives. Eur J Pharmacol 65:185–192
24. Winslow CM, Andersson RC, D'Aries FJ et al (1987) Toward understanding the mechanism of action of PAF receptor antagonists. In: Winslow CM, Lee ML (eds) New horizons in platelet activating factor research. Wiley, New York, pp 153–164
25. Heffner JE, Shoemacker SA, Canham EM et al (1983) Platelet-induced pulmonary hypertension and edema. A mechanism involving acethyl glyceryl ether phosphorylcholine and thromboxane A_2. Chest 83:78–85
26. Camussi G, Alloatti G, Montrucchio G, Meda M, Emanulli G (1984) Effect of platelet-activating factor on guinea pig papillary muscle. Experientia 40:697–699
27. Saeki S, Masugi F, Ogihara T et al (1985) Effect of 1-*O*-alkyl-2-acethyl-*sn*-glycero-3-phosphorylcholine (platelet-activating factor) on cardiac function in perfused guinea pig heart. Life Sci 37:325–329
28. Schlondorff D, Neuwirth DA (1986) PAF and the kidney. Am J Physiol 251:F1–F11
29. Rosam AC, Wallace JL, Whittle BJR (1986) Potent ulcerogenic actions of PAF in the stomach. Nature 319:54–55
30. Hsueh W, Gonzalez-Cruci F, Arroyave JL (1986) PAF-induced ischemic bowel necrosis. Am J Pathol 122:231–239
31. Braquet P, Touqui L, Shen T, Vargaftig B (1987) Perspectives in platelet-activating factor. Pharmacol Rev 39:97–145
32. Braquet P, Godfroid JJ (1986) PAF-acether specific binding sites: design of specific antagonists. Trend Pharmacol Sci 7:397–403
33. Etienne A, Hecquet F, Soulard C, Spinnewyn B, Clostre F, Braquet P (1985) In vivo inhibition of plasma protein leakage and Salmonella enteridis-induced mortality in the rat by a specific PAF-acether antagonist: BN 52021. Agents Actions 17:368–370
34. Chang SW, Feddersen CO, Henson PM, Voelkel NF (1987) Platelet activating factor mediates hemodynamic changes and lung injury in endotoxin-treated rats. J Clin Invest 79:1498–1509
35. Lopez-Diez F, Nieto M, Fernandez-Gallardo S, Gijon MA, Sanchez-Crespo M (1989)

Occupancy of platelet receptors for platelet-activating factor in patients with septicemia. J Clin Invest 83:1733–1740
36. Leaver HA, Qu JM, Smith G, Howie A, Ross WB, Yap PL (1990) Endotoxin releases platelet-activating factor from human monocytes in vitro. Immunopharmacology 20:105–113
37. Myers AK, Robey JW, Price RM (1990) Relationships between tumor necrosis factor, eicosanoids and platelet-activating factor as mediators of endotoxin-induced shock in mice. Br J Pharmacol 99:499–502
38. Miller CL (1982) Endotoxin action on macrophages. In: Collins JA, Murawski K, Schafer AW (eds) Massive transfusion in surgery and trauma. Liss, New York, p 91
39. Salari H, Demos M, Wong A (1990) Comparative hemodynamics and cardiovascular effects of endotoxin and platelet-activating factor in rat. Circ Shock 32:189–207
40. Stewart AG, Phillips WA (1989) Intracellular platelet-activating factor regulates eicosanoid generation and guinea-pig resident peritoneal macrophages. Br J Pharmacol 98:141–148
41. Worthen GS, Seccombe JF, Clay KL, Guthrie LA, Johnston RB (1988) The priming of neutrophils by lipopolysaccharide for production of intracellular platelet-activating factor. J Immunol 140:3553–3559
42. Fitzgerald MF, Parente L, Whittle BJ (1989) Release of PAF-acether and eicosanoids from guinea-pig alveolar macrophages by FMLP: effect of cyclooxygenase and lipoxygenase inhibition. Eur J Pharmacol 164:539–546
43. Rylander R, Beijer L (1987) Inhalation of endotoxin stimulates alveolar macrophage production of platelet-activating factor. Am Rev Respir Dis 135:83–86
44. Leslie CC, Detty DM (1986) Arachidonic acid turnover in response to lipopoly-saccharide and opsonized zymosan in human monocyte-derived macrophages. Biochem J 236:251–259
45. Salari H, Walker MJA (1989) Cardiac dysfunction caused by factors released from endotoxin-activated macrophages. Circ Shock 27:263–272
46. Reinhold SL, Zimmermann GA, Prescott SM, McIntyre TM (1989) Phospholipid remodeling in human neutrophils: parallel activation of a deacylation/reacylation cycle and platelet-activating factor synthesis. J Biol Chem 264:21652–21659
47. Gomez-Cambronero J, Durstin M, Molski TF, Naccache PH, Sha-afi RI (1989) Calcium is necessary for the platelet-activating factor release in human neutrophils stimulated by physiological stimuli: role of G-proteins. J Biol Chem 264:12699–12704
48. Hosford D, Koltai M, Braquet P (1993) PAF in shock, sepsis and organ failure. In: Schlag G, Redl H (eds) Pathophysiology of shock, sepsis and organ failure. Springer, Berlin, Heidelberg, New York, pp 502–517
49. Marquis O, Robaut C, Cavero I (1989) Evidence for the existence and ionic modulation of platelet-activating factor receptors mediating degranulatory responses in human polymorphonuclear leukocytes. J Pharmacol Exp Ther 250:293–300
50. DiPersico JF, Golde DW, Gasson JD (1990) GM-CSF: receptor structure and transmembrane signaling. Int J Cell Cloning 8:63–74
51. Etienne et al (1987)
52. Inarrea P, Gomez-Cambronero J, Pascual J, Carmen-Ponte M, Hernando L, Sanchez-Crespo M (1985) Synthesis of PAF-acether and blood volume changes in gram negative sepsis. Immunopharmacology 9:45–52
53. Camussi G, Aglietta M, Malavasi F et al (1983) The release of platelet activating factor from human endothelial cells in culture. J Immunol 131:2397–2403
54. Bussolino F, Tetta C, Brevario F et al (1986) IL-1 stimulates PAF production in cultured human endothelial cells. J Clin Invest 77:2027–2033
55. Berkow RL, Wang D, Larrich JW (1987) Enhancement of neutrophil superoxide production by preincubation with recombinant human tumor necrosis factor. J Immunol 139:3780–3791
56. Vercelotti GM, Yin HQ, Gustafson KS (1988) Platelet activating factor primes neutrophil responses to agonists: role in promoting neutrophil-mediated endothelial damage. Blood 71:1100–1106

57. Paubert-Braquet M, Hosford D, Koltz P, Guilbaud J, Braquet P (1990) Tumor necrosis factor α primes the platelet-activating factor-induced superoxide production by human neutrophils: possible involvement of G-proteins. J Lipid Mediat 2:S1–S14
58. Poubelle P, Rola-Pleszczynski M (1990) PAF enhances the production of tumor necrosis factor alpha by human monocytes: partial antagonism by BN 52021. In: Braquet P (ed) Ginkgolides: chemistry, biology, pharmacology and clinical perspectives, vol 2. Prous, Barcelona, pp 697–706
59. Bonavida B, Mencia-Huerta JM, Braquet P (1990) Effects of platelet-activating factor on peripheral blood monocytes: induction and priming for TNF secretion. J Lipid Mediat 2:S65–S76
60. Barthelson R, Valone FH, Debs R (1988) Synergy in interleukin 1 (IL 1) release by human monocytes stimulated with platelet-activating factor (PAF) plus gamma interferon (IFN gamma) or tumor necrosis factor (TNF). FASEB J 2:1228 (abstract)
61. Pignol PE, Hename S, Sorlin B et al (1990) Effect of long-term treatment with PAF on IL-1 and IL-2 production by rat spleen cells. J Immunol 145:980–984
62. Withmueller U, de Weck AL, Dahinden CA (1990) Studies on the mechanism of PAF production in GM-CSF primed neutrophils. Biochem Biophys Res Commun 170:556–562
63. Dhainaut JF, Hamy I, Schremmer B (1990) Manipulation of the immuno-inflammatory cascade in sepsis: facts and perspectives. In: Vincent JL (ed) Update in intensive care and emergency medicine. Springer, Berlin, Heidelberg, New York, pp 100–108
64. Doebber T, Wu MS, Robbins J, Choy B, Chang M, Shen T (1985) Platelet activating factor involvement in endotoxin induced hypotension in rats; studies with PAF receptor antagonist kadsurenone. Biochem Biophys Res Commun 127:799–808
65. Braquet P, Paubert-Braquet M, Bessin P, Vargaftig BB (1987a) Platelet-activating factor: a potential mediator of shock. In: Samuelsson B, Paoletti R. Ramwell PW (eds) Advances in prostaglandin, thromboxane and leukotriene research, vol 17. Raven Press, New York
66. Grandel KE, Farr RS, Wanderer AA, Eisenstadt TC, Wasserman SJ (1985) Association of platelet-activating factor with primary acquired cold urticaria. N Engl J Med 313:405–409
67. Mozes T, Heiligers JPC, Tak CJAM et al (1991) PAF is one of the mediators involved in endotoxin shock in pigs; protective effects of indomethacin. J Lipid Med 4:309–326
68. Mozes T, Zijlstra FJ, Heiligers JPC et al (1991) Sequencial release of TNF, PAF and eicosanoids during endotoxin shock in anesthetized pigs; protective effects of indomethacin. Br J Pharmacol 104:691–699
69. Meyrick B, Brigham KL (1983) Acute effects of Escherichia coli endotoxin on the pulmonary microvascularisation of anesthetized sheep: structure, function, relationship. Lab Invest 48:458–470
70. Camussi G, Pawlowski I, Bussolino F, Caldwell PRB, Brentjens J, Andres G (1983b) Release of platelet-activating factor in rabbits with antibody-mediated injury of the lung: the role of leukocytes and of pulmonary endothelial cells. J Immunol 131:1802–1807
71. Prevost MC, Cariven C, Simon MF, Chap H, Douste-Blazy L (1984) Platelet-activating factor (PAF) is released into rat pulmonary alveolar fluid as a consequence of hypoxia. Biochem Biophys Res Commun 119:58–63
72. Fasules J, Stenmark KR, Henson PM, Voelkel NF, Tucker A, Reeves JT (1985) Platelet-activating factor in lung lavage of chronically hypoxic neonatal calves. Am Rev Respir Dis 133:A227 (abstract)
73. Rinaldo JE, Dauber JH, Christman J, Rogers RM (1984) Neutrophils alveolitis following endotoxemia: enhancement by previous exposure to hyperoxia. Am Rev Respir Dis 130:1065–1071
74. Chang JC, Lesser M (1984) Quantitation of leukocytes in bronchoalveolar lavage samples from rats after intravascular injection of endotoxin. Am Rev Respir Dis 129:72–75

75. Salzer WL, McCall CE (1990) Primed stimulation of isolated perfused rabbit lung by endotoxin and platelet activating factor induces enhanced production of thromboxane and lung injury. J Clin Invest 85:1135–1143
76. Pirotsky E, Bidault J, Burtin C, Gubler MC, Benveniste J (1984) Release of platelet-activating factor, slow-reacting substance, and vasoactive amines from isolated rat kidneys. Kidney Int 25:404–410
77. Tolins JP, Vercelloti GM, Wilkowske MHaB, Jacob HS, Raij L (1989) Role of platelet activating factor in endotoxemic acute renal failure in the male rat. J Lab Clin Med 113:316–324
78. Pons L, Droy-Lefaix MT, Braquet P, Buéno L (1989) Involvement of platelet activating factor (PAF) in endotoxin induced intestinal motor disturbances in rats. Life Sci 45:533–541
79. Lagente V, Lidbury P, Steel G, Vargaftig BB, Wallace JL, Whittle BJ (1987) Role of PAF as the mediator of endotoxin-induced gastrointestinal damage. Br J Pharmacol 90:114 (abstract)
80. Buxton D, Hanahan DJ, Olson MS (1984) Stimulation of glycogenolysis and platelet-activating factor production by heat aggregated immunoglobulin G in the perfused rat liver. J Biol Chem 259:13758–13761
81. Arditi M, Manogue KR, Caplan M, Yogev R (1990) Cerebrospinal fluid cachectin, tumor necrosis factor-alpha and platelet-activating factor concentrations and severity of bacterial meningitis in children. J Infect Dis 162:139–147
82. Terashita Z, Taushima S, Yoshioka Y, Nomura H, Inada Y, Nishikawa K (1983) CV-3988 – a specific antagonist of platelet-activating factor (PAF). Life Sci 32:1975–1981
83. Terashita Z, Imura Y, Nishikawa K, Sumida S (1985) Is platelet activating factor (PAF) a mediator of endotoxin shock? Eur J Pharmacol 109:257–263
84. Handley DA, Deacon RW, Farley C, Saunders RN, Van Valen RG (1985) Biological effects of PAF in the non-human primate Cebus apella. Fed Proc 44:1268 (abstract)
85. Miyamoto T, Ohno H, Yano T, Okada T, Hamabaka N, Kawasaki A (1985) ONO-6240: A new potent antagonist of platelet activating factor. Adv Prostaglandins Thromboxane Leukotriene Res 15:719–720
86. Handley DA, Van Valen RG, Melden MK, Flury S, Lee ML, Saunders RN (1986) Inhibition and reversal of endotoxin, aggregated IgG and PAF-induced hypotension in the rat by SRI 63-072, a PAF receptor antagonist. Immunopharmacology 12:11–17
87. Berri K, Barner R, Cassal JM, Hadvary P, Hirth G, Muller K (1985) PAF: From agonists to antagonists by synthesis. Prostaglandins 30:691 (abstract)
88. Hadvary P, Baumgartner HK (1985) Interference of PAF-acether antagonists with platelet aggregation and with the formation of platelet thrombi. Prostaglandins 30:694 (abstract)
89. Coeffier E, Borrel MC, Lefort J et al (1985) Effect of PAF-acether antagonists RP 48740 and BN 52021, on platelet activating and bronchoconstriction induced by PAF-acether and structural analogues in guinea pig. Prostaglandines 30:699 (abstract)
90. Sediry P, Caillard CG, Floch A et al (1985) 48740 RP: A specific PAF-acether antagonist. Prostaglandins 30:688 (abstract)
91. Sanchez-Crespo M, Fernandez-Gallardo S, Nieto ML, Baranes J, Braquet P (1985) Inhibition of the vascular actions of IgG aggregates by BN 52021, a highly specific antagonist of PAF-acether. Immunopharmacology 15:69–75
92. Touvay C, Etienne A, Braquet P (1985) Inhibition of antigen-induced lung anaphylaxis in the guinea pig by BN 52021 a new specific PAF-acether antagonist isolated from Ginko biloba. Agents Actions 17:371–372
93. Foegh ML, Khirabadi BS, Braquet P, Ramwell PW (1985) Platelet-activating factor antagonist BN 52021 prolongs experimental cardiac allograft survival. Prostaglandins 30:718 (abstract)
94. Shen TY, Hwang SB, Chang MN et al (1985) Characterization of a platelet-activating factor receptor antagonist isolated from haifenteng (Piper futokadsura): specific inhi-

bition of in vitro and in vivo platelet-activating factor-induced effects. Proc Natl Acad Sci USA 82:672–676

95. Doebber T, Wu M, Biftu T (1986) Platelet activating factor mediation on rat anaphylactic responses to soluble immune complexes. Studies with PAF receptor antagonist L-652 731. J Immunol 136:4659–4668
96. Handley DA, Tomesch JC, Saunders RN (1986) Inhibition of PAF-induced responses in the rat, guinea pig, dog and primate by the receptor antagonist SRI 63-441. Thromb Haemost 56:40–44
97. Okamoto M, Yoshida K, Nishikiwa M et al (1986) FR 900452, a specific inhibitor of platelet-activating factor produced by Streptomyces phalofaciens. J Antibiot 39:198–204
98. Okamoto M, Yoshida K, Uchida I, Kohsada M, Aoki H (1986) Studies of platelet-activating factor antagonists from microbial products. II. Pharmacological studies of FR-49175 in animal models. Chem Pharm Bull 34:345–348
99. Camussi G, Tetta C, Bussolino F (1983) Inhibitory effect of prostacyclin (PGI_2) on neutropenia induced by intravenous injection of platelet-activating factor (PAF) in the rabbit. Prostaglandins 25:343–349
100. Feuerstein G, Lux WE, Snyder F, Erza D, Faden AI (1984) Hypotension produced by platelet-activating factor is reversed by thyrotropin-releasing hormone. Circ Shock 13:255–260
101. Westwick J, Marks G, Powling MJ, Kakkar VV (1983) Diltiazem, the cardiac channel calcium antagonist, is a potent, selective and competitive inhibitor of platelet-activating factor on human platelets. J Pharmacol 14:62–68
102. Adnot S, Lefort J, Lagente V, Braquet P, Vargaftig BB (1986) Interference of BN 52021, a PAF-acether antagonist, with endotoxin-induced hypotension in the guinea-pig. Pharmacol Res Commun 18:197–200
103. Earnest MA, DiSimone AG, Fletcher JR (1990) The effects of BN 52021 a PAF receptor antagonist in canine endotoxemia. In: Braquet P (ed) Ginkgolides: chemistry, biology, pharmacology and clinical perspectives, vol 2. Prous, Barcelona, pp 463–470
104. Rabinovici R, Yue TL, Farhat M et al (1990) PAF and TNF interactions in endotoxemic shock: studies with BN 50739, a novel PAF antagonist. J Pharmacol Exp Ther 255:258–263
105. Yue TI, Farhat M, Rabinovivi R, Perera PU, Vogel SN, Feuerstein G (1990) Protective effect of BN 50739 a new PAF antagonist in endotoxin-treated rabbits. J Pharmacol Exp Ther 254:976–981
106. Wu M, Biftu T, Doebber T (1986) Inhibition of the platelet-activating factor (PAF) induced in vivo responses in rats by *trans*-2,5-(3,4,5-trimethoxyphenyl) tetrahydrofuran(L-652,731), a PAF receptor antagonist. J Pharmacol Exp Ther 239:841–845
107. Chang SW, Fernyak S, Voelkel NF (1990) Beneficial effect of a platelet activating factor antagonist, WEB 2086, on endotoxin-induced lung injury. Am J Physiol 257:H153–H158
108. Fletcher JF, Di Simone BS, Earnest MA (1990) Platelet-activating factor receptor antagonist improves survival and attenuates eicosanoid release in severe endotoxemia. Ann Surg 211:312–316
109. Lang CH, Dobrescu C, Hargrove DM, Bagby G, Spitzer JJ (1988) Attenuation of endotoxin-induced increase in glucose metabolism by platelet-activating factor antagonist. Circ Shock 23:179–188
110. Toyofuku T, Kubo K, Kobayashi T, Kusama S (1986) Effects of ONO-6240, a platelet activating factor antagonist, on endotoxin shock in unanesthetized sheep. Prostaglandins 31:271–280
111. Baum TD, Heard SO, Feldman HS, Latka CA, Fink MP (1990) Endotoxin-induced myocardial depression in rats: effect of ibuprofen and SDZ 64-688, a platelet activating factor receptor antagonist. J Surg Res 48:629–634
112. Barnes PJ, Chung KF, Evans TW, Rogers DF (1986) Increased airway vascular permeability induced by plateled-activating factor, effect of specific antagonism and platelet depletion. Br J Pharmacol 89:764–765

113. Redl H, Gasser H, Bahrami S et al (1990) The role of PAF in an ovine model of endotoxin shock. In: Braquet P (ed) Ginkgolides: chemistry, biology, pharmacology and clinical perspectives, vol 2. Prous, Barcelona, pp 471–480
114. Sessler CN, Glauser FL, Signal B (1987) SRI 63-441 a platelet-activating factor antagonist prevents endotoxin induced pulmonary and hypoxemia in anesthetized sheep. Am Rev Respir Dis 135:187 (abstract)
115. Purvis AW, Christman C, McPherson CD (1988) WEB 2086 a platelet activating factor receptor antagonist attenuates the response to endotoxin in awake sheep. Am Rev Respir Dis 137:99–100
116. Siebeck M, Weipert J, Jochum M, Hoffman H (1989) A new triazolodiazepine platelet-activating factor receptor antagonist reduces pulmonary dysfunction in endotoxin shock of the pig. Am Rev Respir Dis 139:20 (abstract)
117. Wang J, Dunn MJ (1987) Platelet-activating factor mediates endotoxin induced acute renal insufficiency in rats. Am J Physiol 253:1283–1289
118. Wallace JL, Whittle BJR (1986) Prevention of endotoxin-induced gastrointestinal damage by CV-3988, an antagonist of platelet-activating factor. Eur J Pharmacol 124:209–210
119. Tenaillon A, Dhainaut JF, Boiteau R (1993) Tolerance of PAF antagonist (BN 52021) in patients with septic shock. Intensive Care Med (in press)
120. Dhainaut JF, Tenaillon A, Letulzo Y et al (1993) Un antagonist du PAF (BN 52021) réduit de 42% la mortalité des infections sévères à bactéries à gram-négatif. Réanim Urg 1:1014 (abstract)
121. Hwang SB, Lam MH, Li CH, Shen TY (1986) Release of platelet-activating factor and its involvement in the first phase of carrageenin-induced rat foot edema. Eur J Pharmacol 120:33–41
122. Myers AK, Ramey E, Ranwell P (1983) Glucocorticoid protection against PAF-acether toxicity in mice. Br J Pharmacol 79:595–598

Potential of Oxyradical Scavengers in the Therapy of Sepsis

J. J. Zimmerman

Scope of the Problem

Sepsis and associated problems such as adult respiratory distress syndrome (ARDS) and multiple organ system failure represent common scenarios in all multidisciplinary critical care units. Each of these disease entities may be characterized as subsets of the systemic inflammatory response syndrome (SIRS). That is, their patogenesis involves an apparent global dysregulation of the inflammatory response. In spite of the development of powerful, broad-spectrum antibiotics, morbidity and mortality associated with sepsis remain unacceptably high. This reflects failure to address inflammatory host autoinjury as the paramount pathophysiology in sepsis. Toxic oxyradicals represent one key constituent of the inflammatory response.

This overview outlines possible oxyradical-related therapeutic interventions in the setting of clinical sepsis.

Evidence for Oxyradical Participation in Sepsis

An abundance of data gleaned from cell culture, organ explant, intact animal, and human clinical investigation support the notion that toxic oxygen species represent key elements in the inflammatory host autoinjury characteristic of sepsis. Due to the evanescent nature of most oxyradical species, most investigators have been forced to be content with examining the effects of oxyradical interaction with various macromolecules, that is the "footprints" of oxyradical involvement. However, utilizing electron spin resonance some investigators have actually been able to demonstrate real time appearance of carbon-centered radical spin adducts in both heart and liver following endotoxin administration to live animals. This technique has unequivocally demonstrated that oxygen free radical species are generated in the setting of endotoxemia, while various other techniques have indicated the structural and functional consequences of such events.

Probably the most common assays utilized in implicating oxyradicals in sepsis autoinjury include quantitation of the lipid peroxidation products, malondialdehyde and conjugated dienes. Both reflect oxidant stress towards polyunsaturated fatty acids. Conjugated dienes are formed as a result of rearrangement of double bonds following free radical abstraction of susceptible allylic hydrogens. Since conjugated dienes are detected utilizing absorbance spectroscopy at 234 nm, the specificity of such detection can be problematic, especially in complex biologic systems. Malondialdehyde results from intramolecular rearrangement and degradation of peroxidized fatty acids and may be detected directly or more conventionally by condensation with thiobarbituric acid. Resulting thiobarbituric acid reactive species (TBARS) represent a highly sensitive but also extremely nonspecific assay.

Molecular rearrangement and β scission reactions in peroxidized polyunsaturated fatty acids can also lead to the production of ethane and penthane which can be detected utilizing head space gas chromatography/mass spectroscopy. Although the real time data available by this technique are clearly advantageous, the hardware for this technique is cumbersome and complex. Oxyradical stress also leads to the generation of spontaneously fluorescent products which can be assessed with great sensitivity but again with limited specificity. Peroxyl radicals may similarly be detected with great sensitivity utilizing the observation that such compounds activate the cyclooxygenase enzyme system. Other more remote indicators of oxyradical production include the consumption of common oxyradical scavenging compounds such as α-tocopherol and glutathione.

Each of these techniques has been utilized to demonstrate the involvement of oxyradical pathophysiology in the setting of sepsis, all in various animal models and some in actual human sepsis. Continued research clarifying sensitive and specific markers of oxyradical stress ar needed to evaluate new forms of oxyradical intervention therapy in sepsis.

Sources of Oxyradicals in Sepsis

Although innumerable sources of oxyradical generation exist, four have been studied most extensively. As noted above eicosanoid metabolism can be stimulated in the presence of oxyradicals. Moreover, normal eicosanoid metabolic pathways generate additional oxyradicals. For example the conversion of prostaglandin G to prostaglandin H results in the stoichiometric production of superoxide anion. Continuous electron bleed from the mitochondrial electron transport chain has been shown to occur, particularly at the level of NADH dehydrogenase and the ubiquinone-cytochrome b complex. Increased electron bleed resulting in formation of oxyradicals from incomplete reduction of oxygen has been hypothesized to occur in the setting of sepsis although evidence supporting this notion is fragmentary. Xanthine oxidase, found in all endothelial cells, can utilize oxygen as an electron acceptor to generate superoxide anion. Conversion of xanthine dehydrogenase to xanthine oxidase occurs in the setting of ischemia/reperfusion events which may commonly be seen in sepsis. However, this conversion can also occur directly with exogenous proteases, notably neutrophil elastase. Certainly, major sources of oxyradicals in sepsis are activated neutrophils and macrophages. These phagocytes may be primed and/or activated by a variety of mediators generated during sepsis. Although key elements in denaturation of foreign antigens (e.g., bacteria), phagocyte-associated oxyradicals may be inadvertently released from the neutrophil or macrophage into the surrounding milieu to mediate host autoinjury.

Several examples of synergy between these various oxyradical sources may be proposed. Activation of phagocytes with a concomitant production and release of oxyradicals has been proposed to disrupt metabolism including elements of the mitochondrial electron transport chain. Neutrophil elastase and probably other phagocytic proteases facilitate the conversion of xanthine dehydrogenase to xanthine oxidase allowing endothelial cells to produce superoxide anion. Oxyradicals appear to be able to activate a phospholipase A_2 which releases arachidonic acid at the source of the eicosanoid metabolic pathway. In turn various eicosanoids are capable of priming and activating macrophages and polymorphonuclear leukocytes. Xanthine oxidase production of oxyradicals can mediate an initial injury which can secondarily result in neutrophil recruitment.

Oxyradical Mediated Molecular Injury

All four classes of macromolecules including carbohydrates, proteins, lipids, and nucleic acids represent targets for oxyradical stress. Structural and functional alterations of these cellular constituents result in a variety of insults to cellular physiology.

Proteins

All amino acids are susceptible to oxyradical stress, although sulfur containing amino acids are particularly susceptible. Oxidative fragmentation of α-1 protease inhibitor represents a specific example of an active site methionine residue susceptible to oxidant injury. Denaturation of proteins by oxyradicals enhances their susceptibility to proteolysis. Numerous cellular enzymes including catalase, aconitase, glycerol-3-phosphate-acetyl transferase, glyceraldehyde-3-phosphate dehydrogenase, glutamine synthetase, sodium/potassium ATPase, xanthine oxidase, and various components of the mitochondrial electron transport chain, including NADH dehydrogenase, NADH oxidase, succinate dehydrogenase, succinate oxidase and the ATPase synthetase enzyme complex, have been shown to be specific targets of oxyradical injury. Obviously all of intermediary metabolism represents a target for oxyradical injury. Oxidant stress is also associated with an increased production of activated complement fragment C5a and enhanced cytokine release from a variety of cells.

Lipids

Phospholipids represent a particularly important target for oxyradical stress as all cell membranes and intracellular organelles are primarily structurally composed of phospholipids. Autocatalytic chain propagation of lipid peroxidation can occur in polyunsaturated fatty acids so that an initial oxidative insult may be amplified via self-sustaining reactions. Cell membrane damage to the lipid bilayer can result in calcium influx and secondary activation of intracellular proteases. As has been previously noted, oxyradical activation of phospholipase A may initiate the production of various eicosanoids. Peroxidized polyunsaturated fatty acids, like proteins, are more susceptible to hydrolysis. Erythrocyte membrane alterations by oxyradicals are associated with impaired erythrocyte deformability in the setting of sepsis.

Nucleic Acids

Oxyradical adulterated nucleic acid carries the potential of both immediate and long-term alterations in cellular function. Accordingly not only can ongoing synthetic activity of the cell be changed, but in addition the potential for future cellular replication and repair can be significantly impaired. More specifically oxyradical stress towards nucleic acid has been associated not only with chromosomal breakage but also with specific nucleic acid structural modifications which have been demonstrated by mass spectroscopy.

Evidence for Therapeutic Potential of Oxyradical Scavengers

It has been emphasized that commonly used critical care resuscitative measures may represent key directives to alleviate oxyradical stress [1]. Maximizing adequate oxygen delivery to minimize tissue oxygen debt may be important in minimizing incomplete reduction of oxygen. Achieving supranormal hemodynamic endpoints may optimize resuscitative efforts in ensuring optimal microvascular substrate delivery. Augmenting oxygen delivery with erythrocyte transfusion may be beneficial not only in terms of improving oxygen carrying capacity but also in providing specific erythrocyte antioxidants such as catalase and glutathione. Although β-adrenergic agents may improve inotropy and oxygen delivery, they may also exert significant anti-inflammatory action including inhibition of oxyradical generation. Initial emphasis on ventilation and circulation to optimize oxygen and substrate delivery to ensure aerobic metabolism should predominate resuscitation of the septic patient. Additional therapy specifically directed towards oxyradicals is discussed below. It has been suggested that those oxyradical scavengers demonstrating the greatest membrane permeability may in fact function as the best oxyradical scavengers in the setting of endotoxemia [2].

It should be recalled that in the setting of sepsis a variety of important mechanisms exist for the production of oxyradicals. Aside from interventions directly involving the free radical species, it is also apparent that interventions aimed at eicosanoid metabolism, mitochondrial electron transport chain electron flow, phagocyte activation, and xanthine oxidase might demonstrate important effects relative to the production of oxyradical species.

Enzyme Oxyradical Scavengers

Superoxide dismutase subset. At least three forms of superoxide dismutase (SOD) have now been identified: a copper-zinc cytosolic enzyme with molecular weight 32 kDa, a manganese mitochondrial enzyme with molecular weight 85 kDa, and a copper containing plasma enzyme with molecular weight 134 kDa. These enzymes exhibit a rate constant near $10^9\ M^{-1} \cdot s^{-1}$, indicating a 10000-fold enhancement of dismutation of superoxide over spontaneous rates. Exogenous SOD has been shown to significantly enhance survival in lethal models of endotoxemia in mice, rats, and dogs concomitant with inhibition of the appearance of fluorescent products of lipid peroxidation in serum or TBARS in liver [3–5].

Exogenous SOD has also been examined relative to specific organ systems in the setting of sepsis. Since ARDS represents a major comorbidity in the setting of sepsis, it is not surprising that much of the investigation related to SOD involves sepsis-associated ARDS. For example recombinant human SOD has been shown to attenuate endotoxin-induced lung injury [6]. Employing a loading dose and maintenance infusion of SOD investigators were able to modulate pulmonary capillary leak reflected by a reduction in lung lymph flow. The same strategy was similarly useful in decreasing endotoxin-associated increases in pulmonary artery pressure and pulmonary vascular resistance which were correlated with a reduction in plasma thromboxane B_2 and 6-keto prostaglandin F_1-α [7]. These findings corroborate previous studies indicating that SOD probably inhibits oxyradical-dependent increases in thromboxane production [8, 9]. Polyethylene glycol-conjugated SOD has been shown to reduce diaphragmatic contractile dysfunction in the setting of hamster endotoxemia [10]. The improvement in diaphragmatic function was associated with a decrease in the accumulation of TBARS in animals administered SOD.

Similarly in a cecal ligation/puncture model of rat sepsis, investigators have demonstrated a decrease in spontaneous chemiluminescence of hind limb adductor muscle at 4–12 h following insult in animals provided with exogenous SOD [11]. Although exogenous SOD provided no protective effects on hemodynamics in a feline model of *Escherichia coli* sepsis, gastric mucosal pathology was significantly reduced [12]. In a model of experimental pneumococcal meningitis in rats, polyethylene glycoconjugated SOD was shown to prevent increases in intracranial pressure and increases in brain water content while attenuating increases in regional cerebral blood flow

[13]. Similarly polyethylene glycoconjugated SOD or catalase was demonstrated to prevent pial arteriolar vasodilation in response to administration of group B streptococci in an adult rat meningitis model employing the cranial window technique [14].

It should be appreciated that not all studies have noted a protective effect of exogenous SOD in the setting of endotoxemia. Some of this apparent lack of effect may be secondary to inadequate circulating SOD levels. For example, investigators have demonstrated a dose-response protective effect utilizing human recombinant SOD in *E. coli* endotoxin mediated pulmonary capillary leak in rats [6]. Increasing exogenous SOD resulted in diminution of increases in wet lung weight and lung permeability index and was further associated with a decrease in pulmonary neutrophil accumulation. These authors pointed out that their highest dose of SOD resulted in a five- to tenfold higher plasma SOD level as compared to many previous studies.

Catalase. Catalase, a 240 kDa protein located primarily in peroxisomes, represents the other major enzyme oxyradical scavenger investigated therapeutically. Catalase (CAT) detoxifies hydrogen peroxide but not other larger molecular weight hydroperoxides. This enzyme demonstrates a high catalytic rate but low substrate affinity and a rate constant of approximately $10^7\,M^{-1}\cdot s^{-1}$. Glutathione peroxidase, which does attack higher molecular weight lipid peroxides, has been investigated in other models of oxyradical stress but not sepsis. Exogenous CAT has been studied in detail utilizing the chronic lung lymph fistula model in adult sheep [15, 16]. Employing this animal model, endotoxin-mediated increases in lung lymph flow, lung water content, and pulmonary hypertension were significantly attenuated concomitant with decreases in plasma conjugated dienes, lung parenchymal TBARS, and thromboxane B_2. Recent investigation employing the same model has shown that lung-specific CAT activity decreased by approximately 50% in the setting of endotoxemia concurrent with a 100% increase in TBARS in the lung and liver [17]. This finding demonstrated that CAT itself is a target of the septic inflammatory response and provides credence for intervention with exogenous CAT.

Since SOD results in the production of hydrogen peroxide, it seems logical that combined administration of SOD and CAT might confer synergistic protection compared to singular use of either enzyme. Although this approach has been utilized for other types of oxidant-related injury, it has not been rigorously examined in the setting of sepsis. It should be appreciated that several cytokines commonly elevated in the setting of sepsis such as tumor necrosis factor-α (TNF-α), interleukin-1β (IL-1β), and interferon-γ (IFN-γ) may induce the transcription and translation of a variety of oxyradical scavenger enzymes including SOD and CAT [18]. Moreover, oxyradicals themselves may interact with antioxidant responsive elements on the genome to alter the organism's response to the oxidant stress. For example, hydrogen peroxide may bind to the 5′ flanking region of glutathione-S-transferase and enhance its transcription [19]. Such molecular biology considerations may allow titration of endogenous oxyradical scavengers in more sophisticated therapeutic approaches compared to the straight forward supplementation with exogenous enzymes.

Low Molecular Weight Oxyradical Scavengers

Sulfhydryls. As protein sulfur amino acids are particularly susceptible to oxidant stress, it is not surprising that investigators have examined use of exogenous sulfhydryl compounds as therapeutic interventions in sepsis-associated oxidant stress. In the setting of endotoxin infusion in the awake sheep model, *N*-acetyl cysteine was demonstrated to decrease lung lymph clearance [20]. A related investigation utilizing a porcine model of *E. coli* sepsis reported that *N*-acetyl cysteine inhibited lipid peroxidation while limiting pulmonary albumin extravasation [21]. However, no alterations in either survival or hemodynamics were appreciated. In one resonance form dimethylthiourea similarly contains a reduced sulfhydryl. It has been shown to attenuate endotoxin-induced acute respiratory failure again in a porcine model [22].

Dimethyl sulfoxide and allopurinol. Dimethyl sulfoxide is thought to directly scavenge the hydroxyl radical originating in the nonenzymatic Fenton reaction between hydrogen peroxide and superoxide anion. Dimethyl sulfoxide alone has been demonstrated to decrease endotoxemia mortality in rats [23]. In addition dimethyl sulfoxide intervention in this model was shown to block the early hypotension, prevent hypoglycemia, attenuate hyperlacticemia and eliminate the characteristic hemorrhagic intestinal pathology. These investigators have pointed out that the hydroxyl radical, like nitric oxide, can increase the production of cyclic guanidine monophosphate (c-GMP) which mediates vasodilation. Accordingly the protective effect of dimethyl sulfoxide in reducing hypotension may relate in its inhibitory role on c-GMP production. Other investigators have examined the combined use of dimethyl sulfoxide and allopurinol in various sepsis models. Allopurinol represents a pyrazolopyrimidine mimic of xanthine which is oxidized to oxypurinol and then binds tightly to xanthine oxidase inhibiting formation of superoxide anion and hydrogen peroxide. In very high doses this compound is also thought to act directly as a hydroxyl radical scavenger. In a model employing direct endotoxin injury to cultured lung endothelial cells, dimethyl sulfoxide and allopurinol have been demonstrated to reduce endotoxin-associated cytotoxicity as reflected by endothelial release of lactic dehydrogenase [24]. In addition these agents decreased spontaneous cellular fluorescence and decreased conjugated dienes released into the cell culture supraphase. Both appeared to preserve normal cell architecture otherwise distorted by the endotoxin insult. In a hamster cheek pouch model which examined the leakage of fluorescent-labeled high molecular weight dextran (150000 kDa), investigators have ascertained that both dimethyl sulfoxide and allopurinol decreased the number of leaky sites and dextran clearance induced by endotoxin infusion (25). In this controlled model of microvascular leak it was also shown that both dimethyl sulfoxide and allopurinol preserved integrity of cellular junctions.

Nitrones. Although originally utilized to detect free radicals by acting as spin trap adducts, a variety of nitrones has more recently been explored as a potential therapeutic adjunct in the setting of sepsis-related oxidant injury. In pretreated endotoxin-challenged rats, α-phenyl *N*-tertbutyl nitrone resulted in 83% survival at day 7 as compared to control animals receiving drug vehicle who all died by day 1 [26]. In a more recent investigation, nitrones of various structure were shown to reduce mortality in a lethal model of rat endotoxemia by 80%–90% [27]. Moreover this intervention resulted in a prevention of mesocecum microcirculatory derangements as assessed by transmission microscopy, in preservation of microsomal membrane fluidity as assessed by electron spin resonance, and in reduction of lipid peroxidation, as assessed by exhaled ethane. Utilization of nitrones in high doses as exemplified by this study can manifest adverse side effects such as seizures and immunosuppression. Recently α-phenyl *N*-tertbutyl nitrone was examined in another lethal model of murine endotoxemia [28]. Animals receiving the nitrone demonstrated 100% survival to 7 days whereas a 76% mortality was noted in controls on day 2 following endotoxin. Treated animals appeared better clinically and were less hypothermic. At autopsy intestinal necrosis was significantly diminished in the treatment group. Nitrone-treated animals, moreover, demonstrated a significant reduction in peak levels of TNF and in IFN-γ. Northern blot analysis revealed a down-regulation in the messenger RNA transcripts for TNF, IFN-γ, IL-6, and c-*fos*, a protooncogene important in cell repair and regeneration. These investigators reemphasized their earlier work indicating that oxyradicals can enhance phagocytic production of cytokines and that an important role of oxyradical scavengers may be inhibiting production of these sepsis-associated cytokines (29).

Coenzyme Q10. Coenzyme Q10 represents a naturally occurring electron shuttle situated in the mitochondrial electron transport chain between flavoproteins and the cytochromes. This molecule is characterized by a long isoprenoid tail and a hydroxyl-substituted ring structure which can be reduced to a semiquinone. In a canine model of *E. coli* endotoxemia, pretreatment with coenzyme Q10 has been shown to improve survival, maintain pH, decrease lactate production, reduce circulating histamine, decrease pulmonary artery pressure, and improve pulmonary compliance [30]. In a lethal model of murine endotoxemia, coenzyme Q10 was shown to significantly enhance survival while preserving hepatic ATP content and suppressing hepatic TBARS [31]. More recently investigators have examined coenzyme Q10 in a setting of lethal *E. coli* canine sepsis. In this model exogenous coenzyme Q10 pretreatment resulted in preservation of mean arterial pressure and cardiac output and prevented the increase in spontaneous plasma lipid peroxidation fluorescence products. Moreover rises in TNF and IL-6 were blunted [32].

α-Tocopherol. α-Tocopherol (vitamin E) represents the premier hydrophobic, membrane-situated antioxidant and is characterized by a long alaphatic tail soluble in the membrane lipid bilayer and a chroman ring structure which facilitates radical stabilization. One electron reduced α-tocopherol may be reoxidized back to the native structure by redox coupling with ascorbate. In a murine model of endotoxemia, exogenous α-tocopherol has been shown to reduce accumulation of hepatic TBARS concomitant with improved survival [33]. In a rat model of sepsis employing cecal ligation/puncture, pretreatment with exogenous α-tocopherol preserved peripheral oxygen utilization as demonstrated by normal mixed venous oxygen saturations and arterial-venous oxygen content differences [34]. These positive hemodynamic effects were associated with improved survival in animals receiving α-tocopherol. In addition, endotoxin-mediated decreases in erythrocyte deformability were prevented. The investigators noted that sepsis-associated oxyradicals probably alter erythrocyte membranes resulting in impaired deformability. They hypothesized that α-tocopherol preserves membrane deformability and hence microcirculatory flow. In an *E. coli/Staphylococcus aureus* peritonitis model of sepsis in guinea pigs, α-tocopherol, but not ascorbate, was demonstrated to improve survival when administered enterally prior to sepsis [35]. Although ascorbate alone appears to be ineffective in attenuating oxidant stress in sepsis, a related compound, octadecyl ascorbic acid, has been shown to reduce mortality in murine endotoxemia [36]. This effect may relate to its greater membrane permeability as compared to native ascorbate.

Oxyradical Scavengers in Human Sepsis

Aside from small encouraging trials with *N*-acetyl cysteine, investigations examining the potential benefit of oxyradicals in the setting of human sepsis have not been reported to date. A major hindrance in the potential application of such intervention involves the difficulty of early identification of the SIRS and an incomplete understanding of the dynamics of the inflammatory response, specifically those related to oxidant stress. In most of the animal studies noted above, few or no adverse effects utilizing oxyradical scavenger intervention have been reported, albeit long-term follow-up is not characteristic of most investigations. Early detection of endotoxemia may allow rational application of a variety of oxyradical scavengers as one approach to titrating oxyradical aspects of the sepsis inflammatory response.

References

1. Youn Y-K, LaLonde C, Demling R (1991) Use of antioxidant therapy in shock and trauma. Circ Shock 35:245–249
2. McKechnie K, Furman BL, Parratt JR et al (1986) Modification by oxygen free radical scavengers of the metabolic and cardiovascular effects of endotoxin infusion in conscious rats. Circ Shock 19:429–439
3. Kunimoto F, Morita T, Fujita T (1987) Inhibition of lipid peroxidation improves survival rate of endotoxemic rats. Circ Shock 21:15–22
4. Broner CW, Shenep JL, Stidham GL et al (1988) Effect of scavengers of oxygen-derived free radicals on mortality in endotoxin-challenged mice. Crit Care Med 16:848–854
5. Morgan RA, Manning PB, Coran AG et al (1988) Oxygen free radical activity during live E. coli septic shock in the dog. Circ Shock 25:319–323
6. Schneider J, Friderichs E, Heintze K et al (1990) Effects of recombinant human superoxide dismutase on increased lung vascular permeability and respiratory disorder in endotoxemic rats. Circ Shock 30:97–106
7. Koyama S, Kobayshi T, Kubo K et al (1992) Recombinant-human superoxide dismutase attenuates endotoxin-induced lung injury in awake sheep. Am Rev Respir Dis 145:1404–1409
8. Tate RM, Morris HG, Schroeder WR et al (1984) Oxygen metabolites stimulate thromboxane production and vasoconstriction in isolated saline-perfused rabbit lungs. J Clin Invest 74:608–613
9. Chakraborti S, Gurtner GH, Michael JR et al (1989) Oxidant-mediated activation of phospholipase A2 in pulmonary endothelium. Am J Physiol 257:L430–L437
10. Shindoh C, Dimarco A, Nethery D et al (1992) Effect of PEG-superoxide dismutase on the diaphragmatic response to endotoxin. Am Rev Respir Dis 145:1350–1354
11. Peralta JG, Liesuy S, Evelson P et al (1993) Oxidative stress in skeletal muscle during sepsis in rats. Circ Shock 39:153–159
12. Arvidsson S, Fält K, Marklund S et al (1985) Role of free oxygen radicals in the development of gastrointestinal mucosal damage in Escherichia coli sepsis. Circ Shock 16:383–393
13. Pfister H-W, Koedel U, Lorenzl S et al (1992) Antioxidants attenuate microvascular changes in the early phase of experimental pneumococcal meningitis in rats. Stroke 23:1798–1804
14. McKnight AA, Keyes WG, Hudak ML et al (1992) Oxygen free radicals and the cerebral arteriolar response to group B streptococci. Pediatr Res 31:640–644
15. Milligan SA, Hoeffel JM, Goldstein IM et al (1988) Effect of catalase on endotoxin-induced acute lung injury in unanesthetized sheep. Am Rev Respir Dis 137:420–428
16. Seekamp A, LaLonde C, Zhu D et al (1988) Catalase prevents prostanoid release and lung lipid peroxidation after endotoxemia in sheep. J Appl Physiol 65:1210–1216
17. Daryani R, LaLonde C, Zhu D et al (1990) Changes in catalase activity in lung and liver after endotoxemia in sheep. Circ Shock 32:273–280
18. Harris CA, Derbin KS, Hunte-McDonough B (1991) Manganese superoxide dismutase is induced by IFN-γ in multiple cell types. Synergistic induction by IFN-γ and tumor necrosis factor or IL-1. J Immunol 147:149–154
19. Rushmore TH, Morton MR, Pickett CB (1991) The antioxidant responsive element. Activation by oxidant stress and identification of the DNA consensus sequence required for functional activity. J Biol Chem 266:11632–11639
20. Bernard GR, Lucht WD, Niedermeyer ME et al (1984) Effect of N-acetyl cysteine on the pulmonary response to endotoxin in the awake sheep and upon in vitro granulocyte function. J Clin Invest 73:1772–1784
21. Groeneveld ABJ, denHollander W, Straub J et al (1990) Effects of N-acetyl cysteine and terbutaline treatment on hemodynamics and regional albumin extravasation in porcine septic shock. Circ Shock 30:185–205

22. Olson NC, Anderson DL, Grizzle MK (1987) Dimethyl thiourea attenuates endotoxin-induced acute respiratory failure in pigs. J Appl Physiol 63:2426–2432
23. Brackett DJ, Lerner MR, Wilson MF (1991) Dimethyl sulfoxide antagonizes hypotensive, metabolic, and pathologic responses induced by endotoxin. Circ Shock 33:156–163
24. Brigham KL, Meyrick B, Berry LC et al (1987) Antioxidants protect cultured bovine lung endothelial cells from injury by endotoxin. J Appl Physiol 63:840–850
25. Matsuda T, Eccleston CA, Rubinstein I et al (1991) Antioxidants attenuate endotoxin-induced microvascular leakage of macromolecules in vivo. J Appl Physiol 70:1483–1489
26. Hamburger SA, McCay PB (1989) Endotoxin-induced mortality in rats is reduced by nitrones. Circ Shock 29:329–334
27. Novelli GP (1992) Oxygen radicals in experimental shock: effects of spin-trapping nitrones in ameliorating shock pathophysiology. Crit Care Med 20:499–507
28. Pogrebniak HW, Merino J et al (1992) Spin trap salvage from endotoxemia: The role of cytokine down-regulation. Surgery 112:130–139
29. Pogrebniak HW, Matthews WA et al (1990) Reactive oxygen species can amplify macrophage tumor necrosis factor production. Surg Forum 16:101–103
30. Yasumoto K, Inada Y (1986) Effect of coenzyme Q10 on endotoxin shock in dogs. Crit Care Med 14:570–574
31. Sugino K, Dohi K, Yamada K et al (1987) The role of lipid peroxidation in endotoxin induced hepatic damage and the protective effects of antioxidants. Surgery 101:746–752
32. Lelli JL, Drongowski RA, Gastman B et al (1993) Effects of coenzyme Q10 on the mediator cascade of sepsis. Circ Shock 39:178–187
33. Peavy PL, Fairchild EJ (1986) Evidence for lipid peroxidation in endotoxin-poisoned mice. Infect Immunol 52:613–616
34. Powell RJ, Machiedo GW, Rush BF et al (1991) Oxygen free radicals: effect on red cell deformability in sepsis. Crit Care Med 19:732–735
35. Peck MD, Alexander JW (1991) Survival in septic guinea pigs is influenced by vitamin E, but not by vitamin C in enteral diets. J Parent Ent Nutr 15:433–436
36. Nonaka A, Manabe T, Tobe T (1990) Effect of a new synthetic free radical scavenger, 2-octadecyl ascorbic acid, on the mortality in mouse endotoxemia. Life Sci 47:1933–1939

N-Acetylcysteine in Sepsis

C. Spies and K. Reinhart

Sepsis and Tissue Perfusion

Sepsis, septic shock and multiple organ dysfunction syndrome are characterized by progressive inadequate tissue perfusion and maldistribution of blood flow [1]. Endothelium-derived relaxing factor is considered to be important in maintaining nutrive blood flow [2]. Increased oxygen radicals known to be generated in large amounts during endotoxic shock and sepsis [3–8] inactivate nitric oxide or *S*-nitrocysteine, which account for the vasodilator action of endothelium-derived relaxing factor [9–12]. A constitutive nitric oxide synthase is present in endothelial cells [9], certain neurons [3, 14], endocardium [15], myocardium [16] and platelets [17, 18].

Clinical and experimental findings demonstrate that sepsis induces depletion of glutathione and endothelium-derived relaxing factor [8, 19–22] due to the increased oxygen radical load. Pacht and coworkers reported that the alveolar epithelial lining of patients with adult respiratory distress syndrome was deficient in total reduced glutathione [20]. Brigham and coworkers also showed a depletion of glutathione in patients with established acute respiratory distress syndrome [8]. Chin and coworkers found that endothelium-derived relaxing factor was inactivated by oxidized lipoproteins [19]. Myers and coworkers showed that endotoxin decreased endothelium-derived relaxing factor activity and nitric oxide production under both basal and bradykinin stimulated conditions after prolonged (i.e., 1 h coincubation followed by 1 h washout) exposure [11]. Free radicals, in particular the hydroxyl radical and hypochlorus acid, damage endothelial cells directly as a result of membrane lipid peroxidation [4]. As membrane lipid peroxidation occurs, mitochondrial membranes may also be damaged leading to impaired mitochondrial function and decreased ATP formation [23]. Remote indicators of oxyradical production include the consumption of common oxyradical scavenging compounds such as glutathione.

The hypothesis of an initial nitric oxide and glutathione lack in sepsis [8, 19–22] is supported by the fact that vascular damage is a prominent feature of this disease, and endothelial damage may be of particular importance [24]. Endotoxin induces widespread endothelial damage in vivo [25] and exposure of endothelial cells in culture to endotoxin [26], interferon-γ [26], or tumor necrosis factor-α [26] leads to cell death.

Vascular endothelial cells exhibit a diverse array of complex functions which include receptor-mediated endocytosis, eicosanoid metabolism, the expression of numerous species of plasmalemmal membrane receptors, vasomotor regulation through the nitric oxide system, the generation of reactive oxygen species, procoagulant activity, and connective tissue synthesis. Clearly, modulation of these pivotal endothelial cell functions by components of the hemodynamic environment will influence the initiation, progression and distribution of lesions.

Septic subjects react to the progression of the disease by induction of a second type of nitric oxide synthase that is not constitutively present. Endotoxin, interleukin-1 and tumor necrosis factor induce the expression of this inducible nitric oxide synthase [17, 18, 27–30]. It is expressed in a wide variety of cells after exposure to endotoxin or cytokines [31]. The list of cells capable of expressing inducible nitric oxide synthase include endothelial cells, vascular smooth muscle cells, macrophages, neutrophils, cardia myocytes, endocardial cells [31] and human hepatoytes [32]. Nitric oxide released from macrophages [33, 34] and neutrophils [35, 36] may contribute to host defense [37–39].

The speed of expression of this inducible nitric oxide synthase may vary between blood vessels and between species [40]. In the rat aorta significant expression is seen within 2 h of exposure to endotoxin [27]. It may also vary in patients with different diseases such as hypertension, congestive heart failure, diabetes mellitus, atherosclerosis, psychosocial stress, thrombosis or coagulopathies, which are known to induce to some extent endothelial dysfunction.

Antioxidants and Critical Care Resuscitation

The failure to address inflammatory host autoinjury as the paramount pathophysiology in sepsis has led to investigations in critical care resuscitation and the potential role of radical scavengers in the therapy of sepsis. Innumerable sources of oxyradical production exist such as eicosanoid metabolism [41, 42], ischemia/reperfusion syndrome [42–45], activated neutrophils and macrophages [4, 5, 46–49]. Ruptured cardiac myocytes in response to oxidative stress are capable of inducing peroxidative damage to membranes [50]. It has been emphasized that commonly used critical care resuscitative measures may represent key directives to alleviate oxyradical stress [51]. Maximizing oxygen consumption by increasing oxygen delivery and ensuring optimal microvasculature substrate delivery may be important in minimizing incomplete reduction of oxygen.

Supranormal values of cardiac index, oxygen delivery and consumption are often reported in critically ill patients and are considered as compensatory responses associated with a higher survival rate [52–55]. In some of these studies, it was essential that the goals were reached within a short time after onset of sepsis [53–55]. In a previous study of Hayes and coworkers [53] improved outcome was shown when increased oxygen delivery led to increased oxygen consumption in the first 24 h after admission to the intensive care unit. The lactate concentrations decreased significantly and only 1 out of 15 patients died (mortality rate: 7%). However, failure to improve oxygen consumption because of ineffective therapy or delays in the initiation of therapy was associated with a mortality rate of 16 out of 17 patients (94%).

Improvement of regional oxygenation and perfusion such as in the splanchnic region is also reported as an important determinant of outcome [56]. Mesenteric hypoperfusion is an important factor in alterations of permeability of the gut epithelium in endotoxicosis and sepsis [57–59]. The gastric intramucosal pH determined indirectly by back diffusion of carbon dioxide [60] correlates well with pH values measured directly with a needle electrode [61] and closely mirrors oxygen consumption [62]. A fall in gastric mucosal pH indicates impaired intestinal oxygenation and poor prognosis and is therefore used as a therapeutic index of tissue oxygenation in critically ill patients [56, 63].

These results indicate that it is important to improve tissue perfusion and oxygenation as early as possible after the onset of sepsis to reduce the risk of ischemia, reperfusion syndrome, vascular damage and multiple organ dysfunction syndrome.

Radical scavengers such as superoxide dismutase [64–67], α-tocopherol [23, 68–71], lazaroids [68], dimethyl sulfoxide [72], nitrones [73–76] and coenzyme Q10 [23, 77], administered before or at the onset of sepsis, were shown to improve survival rate in animal models of sepsis.

Pretreatment with coenzyme Q10 was found to decrease lactate production [77], preserve hemodynamic function [78], decrease pulmonary artery pressure and improve pulmonary compliance [77] in an animal model of sepsis. In a rat model of sepsis induced by cecal ligation/puncture, pretreatment with exogenous α-tocopherol preserved peripheral oxygen utilization as demonstrated by normal mixed venous oxygen saturations and arterial-venous oxygen content differences [79]. In addition, endotoxin-mediated decreases in erythrocyte deformability was prevented by pretreatment with α-tocopherol [79].

Regional improvement of tissue oxygenation is suggested in animal models of sepsis by the early treatment or pretreatment with scavengers. In the splanchnic region gastric mucosal pathology was attenuated [80], mesocecum microcirculatory derangements were prevented [74] and intestinal necrosis at autopsy was diminished [75]. Hepatic adenosine triphosphate content was preserved [23] and accumulation of thiobarituric acid reactive species was reduced [23]. Lung injury was attenuated [67, 81, 82]. The microvascular leakage was reduced [67, 83].

It should be appreciated that several cytokines commonly elevated in the setting of sepsis such as tumor necrosis factor-α, interleukin-1β and interferon-γ may induce the transcription and translation of a variety of oxyradical scavenger enzymes including superoxide dismutase and catalase [84]. Human serum catalase is reported to decrease endothelial cell injury from hydrogen peroxide [85]. Moreover, oxyradicals themselves such as hydrogen peroxide may enhance the transcription of the antioxidant elements of the organism such as the glutathione-*S*-transferase in response to the oxidant stress [86].

Nitrone treated septic animals demonstrated a significant reduction in peak levels of tumor necrosis factor and interferon-γ [75]. Pretreatment with coenzyme Q10 prevented spontaneous plasma peroxidation and blunted the increase in tumor necrosis factor and interleukin-6 [78].

N-Acetylcysteine

As protein sulfur amino acids are particularly susceptible to oxidant stress, it is not surprising that investigators have examined the use of exogenous sulfhydryl compounds such as *N*-acetylcysteine (NAC) as therapeutic interventions in sepsis-associated oxidant stress. NAC has antioxidant properties [8, 87, 88] and as a sulfhydryl donor may contribute to the regeneration of endothelium-derived relaxing factor and glutathione [8, 89, 90]. Reduced glutathione is essential for several enzymes, for example as a substrate for glutathione peroxidases which reduce radicals or transferases [91]. Interaction between antioxidants via a glutathione-dependent α-tocopherol free radical reductase is also indicated by cytosolic reduced glutathione and the membrane-bound α-tocopherol [92].

NAC enhances regeneration of endothelium-derived relaxing factor by replenishing tissue sulfhydryl groups or by increasing cysteine levels [11, 89]. Nitric oxide reacts readily with oxygen radicals [11, 12, 93] which are produced in large amounts during sepsis [8, 19–22]. Consumed nitric oxide can be restored by the glutathione cycle. If the endogenous scavenging mechanisms are being overwhelmed by oxygen radicals or the glutathione cycle is impaired by increased levels of oxidized glutathione disulfide, exogenous sulfhydryl compounds may have protective effects and facilitate regeneration of endothelium-derived relaxing factor as shown in other clinical settings such as nitrate tolerance [94–96] or normobaric hyperoxia [97, 98].

Like other inflammatory mediators, nitric oxide is reported to be both protective and damaging, depending on the amount produced, the site of synthesis and the response of the target tissues [40]. The hemodynamic environment can be influenced by substances which may act on the vasomotor regulation by promoting or inhibiting nitric oxide synthesis. The response to these agents will depend on the extent of dysfuncion or destruction of the endothelial cells. Dependent on the amount of nitric oxide synthesized in sepsis there are potential advantages and disadvantages in the treatment of sepsis with NAC.

Evidence for N-Acetylcysteine in Sepsis

There is increasing evidence that NAC has action pertinent to microcirculatory blood flow and tissue oxygenation. NAC has been shown to enhance whole body oxygen consumption via increased oxygen extraction in patients 18 h after the onset of fulminant liver failure [89]. It has been speculated that

NAC might also exert beneficial effects on impaired nutritive blood flow in patients with severe sepsis [89].

NAC is undergoing clinical trials to evaluate its usefulness in sepsis [112] and acute respiratory distress syndrome [113]. In a previous study [112] in maximum conventionally resuscitated septic patients we infused NAC over 90 min according to the standard regimen for acetaminophen induced liver failure. A subset of almost half the patients treated with NAC responded with a significant increase in whole body oxygen consumption, oxygen delivery, cardiac index and gastric intramucosal pH, and a decrease in venoarterial carbon dioxide gradient. The changes from baseline in whole body oxygen consumption, oxygen delivery and cardiac index after NAC infusion are shown in Fig. 1. Subsequently, these patients who responded to the NAC treatment had a much higher survival rate than the nonresponding patients. The fact that those parameters changed after optimized conventional therapy is suggestive of an effect on the extraction capability of tissues. The improvement of gastric intramucosal pH in our septic patients who responded to NAC treatment accompanied with increased oxygen consumption could reflect improved tissue oxygenation in the gut [114].

Recently there has been increasing attention to venous hypercarbia and increases in the carbon dioxide gradient between mixed venous and arterial blood in septic shock [115, 116]. Nonsurvivors had a significantly higher venoarterial carbon dioxide gradient than survivors [116]. The venoarterial carbon dioxide gradient in all of our patients, both responders and nonresponders to the NAC treatment, was at baseline in the range reported for the survivors in septic shock patients [116]. A further decrease in the venoarterial carbon dioxide gradient in patients who responded to the NAC treatment indicates that tissue perfusion further improved with the NAC treatment. Unfortunately, we could not find any characteristics to help predict which septic patients would be responders. The only difference we found was that the patients who responded to the NAC treatment were studied approximately 1 day earlier in their course of sepsis than the nonresponders.

Patients in septic shock have evidence of biventricular myocardial depression [117]. As has previously been seen in patients with fulminant liver failure [89] we found an increase in cardiac output, stroke volume index and left ventricular stroke work index as well as a decrease in systemic vascular resistance in a subset of almost half the septic shock patients treated with NAC [112]. Brigham and coworkers also found an increase in cardiac output and oxygen delivery in patients with established acute respiratory distress syndrome [8]. In an animal model of myocardial ischemia NAC was reported to improve myocardial contractility [119]. Another thiol drug, *N*-(2-mercaptopropionyl)glycine, has also been shown to improve recovery of myocardial contractile function infused prior to reperfusion [120]. The reason for the increases in stroke volume and left ventricular stroke work index during NAC infusion is unclear; NAC itself is not known to have a positive inotropic action [118], and the effect occurred only when the patients were critically ill [89, 112]. Thus it is possible that critically ill patients who responded to the

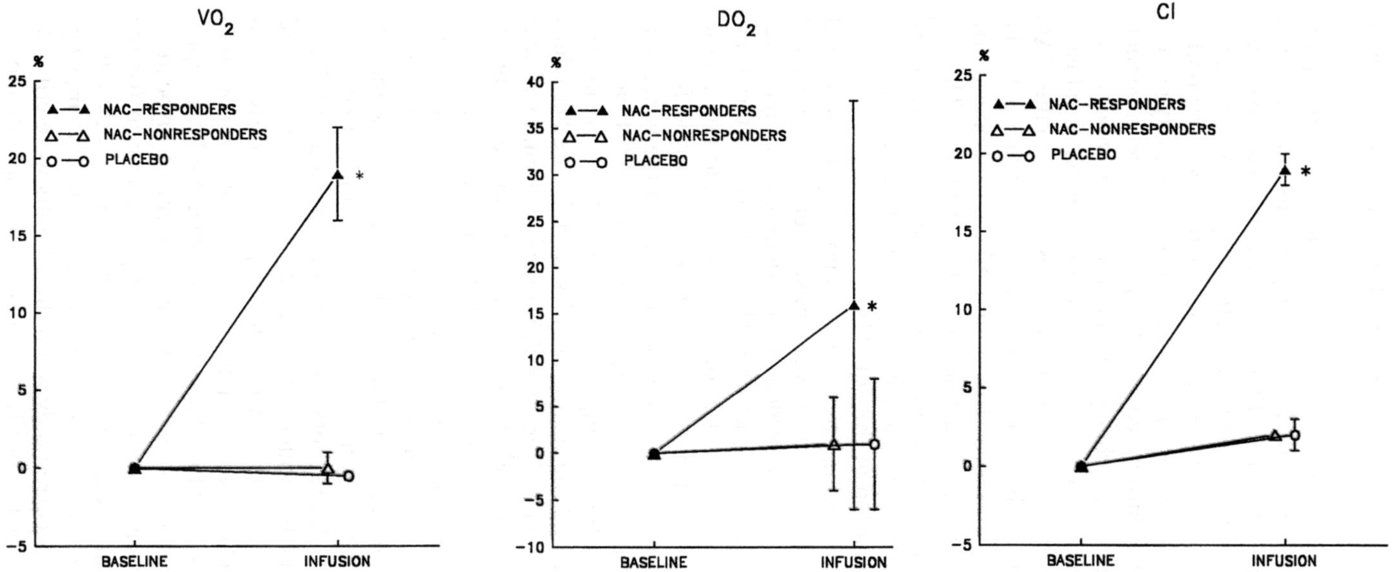

Fig. 1. Effects of *N*-acetylcysteine (*NAC*) infusion or placebo on whole body oxygen consumption ($\dot{V}O_2$), oxygen delivery (DO_2) and cardiac index (*CI*). Relative changes from baseline. *NAC-responders,* septic patients who responded to NAC treatment; *NAC-nonresponders,* those who did not respond to NAC treatment

NAC treatment had some combination of increased contractility, decreased afterload and microcirculatory or tissue effects.

In adult respiratory distress syndrome NAC acted as an anticoagulant and perhaps decreased pulmonary fibrin uptake [121]. However, no improvement could be demonstrated in the PaO_2/FiO_2 ratio in these patients [121]. Pulmonary compliance was higher in the NAC group in this study but this difference did not reach the chosen 5% level of significance [121]. Brigham and coworkers found in patients with established acute respiratory distress syndrome that NAC caused a more rapid clearing of radiological evidence of pulmonary edema than in the placebo group [8].

In animal studies the role of NAC in sepsis was investigated more intensively. NAC given early (1 h after induction of endotoxemia) to awake sheep attenuated the early phase rise in pulmonary artery pressure and the increase in pulmonary vascular resistance and prevented the decrease in cardiac output associated with endotoxemia [88]. These findings, supported by the marked attenuation of the endotoxin induced rise in thromboxane B_2 and 6-keto-prostaglandin-$F_{1\alpha}$, suggest that NAC interfered with the usual postendotoxin cascade of events [88]. NAC in vitro inhibited granulocyte aggregation and scavenged free radicals [88]. It reduced the increase in lung permeability and attenuated the alterations in lung mechanics, compliance and resistance to airflow [88]. NAC also markedly blunted both the early and late phase increase in thoracic lymph flow [88]. Histologic studies revealed electron microscopic evidence of endothelial cell damage 30 min postendotoxemia, although light microscopy did not reveal edema formation until 2 h later [122]. Thus it is possible that microvascular permeability increases early in response to endotoxemia and that NAC attenuated this pathological response. Further support for the ability of NAC to attenuate endotoxin induced permeability changes is found in the late (3–4 h) phase response, where a high relatively protein-rich lymph flow occurs, which has been associated with demonstrable nonhydrostatic pulmonary edema [123]. A related investigation using a porcine model of *E. coli* reported that NAC inhibited lipid peroxidation while limiting pulmonary albumin extravasation [124]. NAC has also been shown to be protective in prevention of hepatotoxicity secondary to lipopolysaccharides which probably involve oxygen radicals [125].

Other reduced sulfhydryl compounds in form of dimethyl sulfoxide and dimethylthiourea have been shown to act as scavengers and attenuate endotoxin induced respiratory and metabolic changes [72, 126–129].

NAC replenishes glutathione and nitric oxide. Replenishment of nitric oxide by NAC leads to reduced endothelial damage by inactivation of free oxygen radicals [11, 12]. It inhibits neutrophil superoxide anion production via a direct action on the NADPH oxidase [99]. Modulation of white blood cells [100], decreased platelet aggregation [17, 18, 101] and, hence, decreased sludge is shown. Vasodilation is reported [102] in vasoconstricted areas by increasing cyclic 3′,5′-guanosine monophosphate [40]. Due to the replenishment of nitric oxide by NAC shear stress, the transit time of cells and molecules may change [103–106]. Shear stress may modify both the endothelial expression and the synthesis of a number of proteins and bioactive compounds that determine important endothelial cell functions. At least two observations provide a potential link with endothelial thromboresistance, namely, increased synthesis of tissue plasminogen activator and its mRNA [107], and enhanced synthesis and secretion of prostacyclin [108, 109]. Recently it has also been shown that the postshear adherence of both monocytes and platelets to endothelial cells is greater on endothelial cells preexposed to low, relative to high, shear [110]. This effect is shear-time dependent, suggesting that the synthesis of mediating cytokines and cell adhesion molecules is likely. In baboons with septic shock there is widespread expression of endothelial leukocyte adhesion molecule 1 with strong histologic staining in the lung, liver, and kidneys. Endothelial leukocyte adhesion molecule 1 expression was evident in capillaries, venules, small veins, arterioles and arteries [111]. Neutrophil activation, measured by granulocyte elastase levels was much more pronounced in animals with septic shock than in those with traumatic hypovolemic shock [111]. Consistent with these findings are the higher levels of circulating tumor necrosis factor and other cytokines as well as lipopolysaccharides in sepsis [111]. NAC may reduce shear stress by acting as an anticoagulant [121], inhibiting granulocyte aggregation [88], decreasing pulmonary [88] and systemic vascular resistance [89, 112], increasing cardiac output [8, 89, 112, 119], preventing microvascular permeability increases [123, 124] and by acting on the vasomotor tone due to the replenishment of nitric oxide [11].

In septic animals nitric oxide is reported to promote protection from hepatic [130, 131], intestinal mucosal [132] and cardiac damage [133]. At least the constitutive nitric oxide-dependent vasodilator tone is vital for organ perfusion and survival during endotoxin shock [133]. Inhibition of nitric oxide synthesis resulted in increased hepatic damage during acute murine endotoxemia [130] and nitric oxide synthesis was found to play an important role in preserving intestinal mucosal integrity in rats [132]. As observed by Hollenberg and coworkers there are additional vasodilatory mechanisms, other than the release of endothelium-derived relaxing factor, involved in septic shock patients [134].

Evidence Against N-Acetylcysteine in Sepsis

The role of nitric oxide in sepsis, however, is still controversial. The benefit of nitric oxide promoting agents such as NAC in sepsis may be time-dependent. After the initiation of the cascade with an overshoot of nitric oxide by induction of an inducible nitric synthase no further benefit from the treatment may be expected. Nitric oxide released in large amounts from the inducible enzyme also stimulates guanylate cyclase, but has additional toxic effects which are independent from cyclic guanosine monophosphate [40]. Nitric oxide inhibits mitochondrial respiration and, hence, oxygen consumption in vitro [135]. It interacts with iron-sulfur centered enzymes [34, 136] and reacts with oxygen free radicals to form, for example, hydroxyl radicals [137, 138] and peroxynitrate [139]. However, the effects of nitric oxide on oxygen consumption in vivo are not known and changes in blood flow coupled with a direct effect on respiratory chain enzymes may lead to alterations in oxygen consumption that are only metabolic effects [140].

Clinical and experimental studies have been performed that directly implicate the overproduction of nitric oxide by an inducible nitric oxide synthase in the mediation of hypotension in septic shock [133, 141–144]. In patients with life threatening septic shock and severe refractory hypotension nonresponsive to fluid replacement and catecholamine management, treatment with the nitric oxide synthase inhibitor N^Gmonomethyl-L-arginine has been shown to produce dose-dependent increases in blood pressure [145]. Meyer and coworkers found reversal of the hyperdynamic response to continuous endotoxin administration by the inhibition of nitric oxide synthesis [146]. The finding of circulating methylated arginine analogues that are competitive inhibitors of nitric oxide synthase suggests the extensive of endogenous mechanisms to regulate nitric oxide synthesis found, e.g., in chronic renal failure [147]. Another endogenous vasoconstrictor which is elevated in sepsis is plasma endothelin [148, 149]. These findings suggest that the septic organism has to a certain extent automechanisms to compensate for the imbalance.

Biochemical evidence for increased production of nitric oxide in sepsis is provided by studies showing increased plasma concentrations of nitrite and nitrate, breakdown products of nitric oxide, in patients with septic shock [142]. In addition, plasma concentrations of arginine, the substrate for nitric oxide synthesis, are reduced in patients with sepsis, particularly in those patients who do not survive [150]. This finding is consistent with the increased activity of the L-arginine/nitric oxide pathway. However, another study has suggested that the reduced concentrations of arginine reflect a global reduction in plasma amino acid concentrations in sepsis [151].

Experimentally, after injection of endotoxin, plasma concentrations of nitrite and nitrate also increase [131] and nitrosohemoglobin, which results from the reaction of nitric oxide with deoxyhemoglobin, can be detected in the circulating blood [22, 152]. Nitrosohemoglobin appeared in rats 2–3 h after endotoxin infusion and increased to maximum after 6–8 h [22]. Nitrite and nitrate levels in human platelets which were stimulated by cytokines and endotoxin were over three times higher after 48 h than after 24 h [32].

One study showed endothelium-derived relaxing factor as a possible mediator of sepsis induced arteriolar dilation in skeletal muscle [143]. As reported by Finkel and coworkers in an isolated hamster papillary muscle model the negative inotropic effects of cytokines on the heart are also mediated by the overproduction of nitric oxide [153]. Induction of the nitric oxide synthase in the coronary circulation of the rabbit causes vasodilation and a reduced response to vasoconstrictors [154].

The cytotoxic effects of endotoxin, interferon-γ, and tumor necrosis factor-α in vitro are mediated in part by nitric oxide [26, 155]. In addition to damaging endothelial cells, nitric oxide increases vascular permeability [156, 157], although the mechanisms are not fully understood. Nitric oxide mediated damage to hepatocytes [135] and pancreatic islet cells [158, 159] has been demonstrated in vitro, and the recent observation that astrocytoma cells express inducible nitric oxide synthase after exposure to endotoxin [160] provides a mechanism whereby sepsis might lead to neurologic dysfunction.

In most of the studies in which treatment with NAC had no effect there were also no detrimental effects observed. NAC at high concentrations, however, can have cytotoxic effects upon sheep leukocytes as seen in both aggregation and enzyme release studies [88]. It is unlikely that such concentrations are achieved in vivo. Under normal conditions NAC may be excreted via the kidneys only slowly, while under conditions of oxidant stress, it is readily metabolized by cells via the glutathione reductase pathway and the metabolites are readily excreted via the kidneys [88]. Due to this metabolism there are some theoretical points of view whether thiol drugs really have a potential for attenuating tissue damage. Thiol drugs such as NAC or *N*-(2-mercatopropionyl)glycine have shown to be effective in inhibiting free radical production [50]. The thiyl radical formed when these thiols act as antioxidants can be removed by mutual annihilation (bimolecular termination) or, under aerobic conditions, can react with oxygen to form the thiyl peroxyradicals [161]. This latter species shows considerable reactivity [162] and may be involved in initiating deleterious modification of cellular constituents. The formation and subsequent reactions of this type of radical may be the reason for the relatively ineffective suppression of peroxidative degradation effected by *N*-(2-mercatopropionyl)glycine [50].

The only reproducible finding after NAC treatment was a moderate deterioration in gas exchange, but there was no alteration in lung mechanics [88]. The etiology might be reverse reflex hypoxic pulmonary vasoconstriction as a typical response to pulmonary vasodilators such as was observed with prostacyclin in critically ill patients [163].

Perspectives

A common and often lethal outcome of sepsis is the progression of the disease to multiple organ dysfunction syndrome. Depletion of endothelium-derived relaxing factor or of tissue sulfhydryl groups due to the consumption by reactive oxygen species may play a role very early in sepsis in the reduction of nutritive blood flow. Inadequate microcirculatory blood flow after the onset of sepsis might be at least partly reversible by the early use of the oxygen radical scavenger and sulfhydryl group donor NAC. In one of our studies NAC infusion improved whole body oxygen consumption, gastric intramucosal pH and venoarterial carbon dioxide gradient in almost half of the septic shock patients [112]. These NAC responders experienced a much higher survival rate than the nonresponders. During that early stage, treatment with oxyradical scavengers such as NAC may help to reduce the vascular damage and therefore limit the progression of sepsis to multiple organ dysfunction syndrome.

NAC enhances regeneration of nitric oxide, which is ubiquitous, and by this action contributes to the maintenance of an adequate nutritive blood flow in sepsis. Therefore, NAC may prevent the initially imbalanced supply/demand ratio of nitric oxide production and consumption with subsequent global imbalances in whole body oxygen consumption and delivery which may lead to ischemia in some regions. With the progression of sepsis the endothelial cells may provide a physiological response to improve tissue oxygenation by expression of an inducible nitric oxide synthase and the enhanced production of cytokines. During that stage the net nitric oxide production consumption ratio is increased and therefore hyporeactivity to vasoconstrictors may occur.

Despite the rapid expansion of studies exploring the nature of the interface between hemodynamic environment, on the one hand, and mediators and endothelial structure and function, on the other, there remain many important unsolved questions on the pathogenesis of sepsis. How might components of the hemodynamic environment influence macromolecular transcytosis? Does the hemodynamic environment regulate the synthesis of endothelium-derived relaxing factor or the generation of reactive oxygen species? By what mechanism does the hemodynamic environment modulate leukocyte or platelet adherence to the endothelium? The beneficial or harmful effects of nitric oxide synthase promoting or inhibiting agents are dose- and time-dependent [40, 112, 144] and there are many unsolved riddles on the exact role of these agents.

References

1. Members of the American College of Chest Physicians/Society of Critical Care Medicine, Consensus Conference Committee (1992) American College of Chest Physicians/Society of Critical Care Medicine Consensus Conference: definitions for sepsis and organ failure and guidelines for the use of innovative therapies in sepsis. Crit Care Med 20:864–874
2. Sun D, Messina EJ, Koller at al (1992) Endothelium-dependent dilation to L-arginine in isolated rat skeletal muscle arterioles. Am J Physiol 262:H1211–1216
3. Takeda Y, Shimada Y, Okada T et al (1986) Lipid peroxidation in experimental septic rats. Crit Care Med 14:719–723
4. Weiss SJ (1989) Tissue destruction by neutrophils. NEJM 320:365–375
5. Flohe L, Giertz H (1987) Endotoxins, arachodonic acid and superoxide formation. Rev Infect Dis 9:553–561
6. Byrne K, Schneider A, Carey D et al (1989) Enhanced rate of superoxide anion generation among circulating neutrophils following pseudomonas aeruginosa sepsis in the pig. Circ Shock 27:330–334
7. Keen RR, Stella L, Flanigan P et al (1991) Differential detection of plasma hydroperoxides in sepsis. Crit Care Med 19:1114–1119
8. Brigham KL (1991) Oxygen radicals – an important mediator of sepsis and septic shock. Klin Wochenschr 69:1004–1008

9. Palmer RMJ, Ferrige AG, Moncada S (1987) Nitric oxide release accounts for the biological activity of endothelial-derived relaxing factor. Nature 327:524–526
10. Ignarro LJ, Byrns RE, Buga GM et al (1987) Endothelium-derived relaxing factor from pulmonary artery and vein possesses pharmacologic and chemical properties identical to those of nitric oxide radical. Circ Res 61:866–879
11. Myers PR, Minor RL Jr, Guerra R Jr et al (1990) Vasorelaxant properties of the endothelium-derived relaxing factor more closely resemble S-nitrosocysteine than nitric oxide. Nature 345:161–163
12. Gryglewski RJ, Palmer RM, Moncada S (1986) Superoxide anion is involved in the breakdown of endothelium-derived vascular relaxing factor. Nature 320:454–456
13. Garthwaite J, Charles SL, Chess-Williams R (1988) Endothelium-derived relaxing factor release on activation of NMDA receptors suggests role as intracellular messenger in the brain. Nature 336:385–388
14. Bredt DS, Hwang PM, Glatt CE et al (1991) Cloned and expressed nitric oxide synthase structurally resembles cytochrom P-450 reductase. Nature 351:714–718
15. Schulz R, Smith JA, Lewis MJ et al (1991) Nitric oxide synthase in cultured endocardial cells of the pig, Br J Pharmacol 104:21–24
16. Schulz R, Nava E, Moncada S (1992) Induction and potential biological relevance of a Ca^{2+}-independent nitric oxide synthase in the myocardium. Br J Pharmacol 105:575–580
17. Radomski MW, Palmer RMJ, Moncada S (1990) Characterization of the L-arginine: nitric oxide pathway in human platelets. Br J Pharmacol 101:325–328
18. Radomski MW, Palmer RMJ, Moncada S (1987) Comparative pharmacology of endothelium-derived relaxing factor, nitric oxide and prostacyclin in platelets. Br J Pharmacol 92:181–187
19. Chin JH, Azhar S, Hoffmann BB (1992) Inactivation of endothelium derived relaxing factor by oxidized lipoproteins. J Clin Invest 89:10–18
20. Pacht ER, Timerman AP, Lykens MG et al (1991) Deficiency of alveolar fluid glutathione in patients with sepsis and the adult respiratory distress syndrome. Chest 100:1397–1403
21. Ishii Y, Partridge CA, DelVecchio PJ et al (1992) Tumor necrosis factor alpha-mediated decrease in glutathione increases the sensitivity of pulmonary vascular endothelial cell to H_2O_2. J Clin Invest 89:794–802
22. Westenberger U, Thanner S, Ruf HH et al (1990) Formation of free radicals and nitric oxide derivative of hemoglobin in rats during shock syndrome. Free Radic Res Commun 11:167–178
23. Sugino K, Dohl K, Yamada K et al (1987) The role of lipid peroxidation in endotoxin induced hepatic damage and the protective effects of antioxidants. Surgery 101:746–752
24. Kirkpatrick CJ, Klosterhalfen B, Hauptmann S (1992) The role of the endothelium in multiple organ failure. In: Vincent J-L (ed) Yearbook of intensive care and emergency medicine. Springer, Berlin Heidelberg New York, pp 14–25
25. Onda M, Toba M, Andoh T et al (1986) Ultrastructural studies of experimental endotoxin shock in the liver and spleen. Therapeutic of low-dose heparin on reticuloendothelial disturbances. Circ Shock 18:11–19
26. Palmer RMJ, Bridge L, Foxwell NA et al (1992) The role of nitirc oxide in endothelial cell damage and its inhibition by glucocorticoids. Br J Pharmacol 105:11–12
27. Rees DD, Cellek S, Palmer RMJ et al (1990) Dexamethasone prevents the induction by endotoxin of a nitric oxide synthase and the associated effects on the vascular tone: an insight into endotoxin shock. Biochem Biophys Res Commun 173:541–547
28. Busse R, Mulsch A (1990) Induction of nitric oxide synthase by cytokines in vascular smooth muscle, FEBS Lett 275:87–90
29. Fleming I, Gray GA, Schott C et al (1991) Inducible but not constitutive production of nitric oxide by vascular smooth muscle cells. Eur J Pharmacol 200:375–376
30. Vallance P, Palmer RMJ, Moncada S (1992) The role of induction of nitric oxide

synthesis in the altered response of jugular veins from endotoxaemic rats. Br J Pharmacol 106:459–463
31. Moncada S, Palmer RMJ, Higgs EA (1991) Nitric oxide: Physiology, pathophysiology and pharmacology. Pharmacol Rev 43:109–142
32. Nussler AK, DiSilvio M, Billar TR et al (1992) Stimulation of the nitirc oxide synthase pathway in human hepatocytes by cytokines and endotoxin. J Exp Med 176:261–264
33. Hibbs JB Jr, Vavrin Z, Taintor RR (1987) L-arginine is required for expression of the activated macrophage effector mechanism causing selective metabolic inhibition in target cells. J Immunol 138:550–565
34. Hibbs JB Jr, Taintor RR, Vavrin Z et al (1988) Nitric oxide: a cytotoxic activated macrophage effector molecule. Biochem Biophys Res Commun 157:87–94
35. McCall T, Boughton-Smith NK, Palmer RMJ et al (1989) Synthesis of nitric oxide from L-arginine by neutrophils. Biochem J 261:293–296
36. Rimele TJ, Sturm RJ, Adams LM et al (1988) Interaction of neutrophils with vascular smooth muscle: identification of a neutrophil-derived relaxing factor. J Pharmacol Exp Ther 245:102–111
37. Adams LB, Hibbs JB Jr, Tainter RR et al (1990) Microbiostatic effect of murine macrophages for Toxoplasma gondii: role of synthesis of inorganic nitrogen oxides from L-arginine. J Immunol 144:2725–2729
38. Liew FY, Millott S, Parkinson C et al (1990) Macrophage killing of Leishmania parasite in vivo is mediated by nitric oxide from L-arginine. J Immunol 144:4794–4797
39. Denis M (1991) Tumor necrosis factor and granulocyte macrophage-colony stimulating factor stimulate human macrophages to restrict growth of virulent Mycobacterium avium and to kill avirulent M. avium. Killing effector mechanism depends on the generation of reactive nitrogen intermediates. J Leukoc Biol 48:380–387
40. Vallance P, Moncada S (1993) Role of endogenous nitric oxide in septic shock. New Horizons 1:77–86
41. Paterson IS, Klausner JM, Goldman G et al (1989) Pulmonary edema after aneurysm surgery is modified by mannitol. Ann Surg 210:796–801
42. Schiller HJ, Reilly P, Bulkley GB (1993) Antiooxidant therapy. Crit Care Med 21:S92–S102
43. McCord JM (1985) Oxygen-free radicals in postischemic tissue injury. NEJM 312:159–163
44. Goldhaber JI, Weiss JN (1992) Oxygen free radicals and cardiac reperfusion abnormalities. Hypertension 20:118–127
45. Ambrosio G, Santoro G, Tritto I et al (1992) Effects of ischemia and reperfusion on cardiac tolerance to oxdative stress. Am J Physiol 262(31):H23–H30
46. Holman RG, Maier RV (1988) Superoxide production by neutrophils in a model of adult respiratory distress syndrome. Arch Surg 123:1491–1495
47. Nathan CF, Root RK (1977) Hydrogen peroxide release from mouse peritoneal macrophages. J Exp Med 146:1648–1653
48. Makino R, Tanaka T, Iizuka T et al (1986) Stoichometric conversion of oxygen to superoxide anion during the respiratory burst in neutrophils. J Biol Chem 261:11444–11447
49. Marshall PJ, Lands WEM (1986) In vitro formation of activators for prostaglandin synthesis by neutrophils and macrophages from humans and guinea pigs. J Lab Clin Med 108:525–530
50. Turner JJO, Rice-Evans CA, Davies MJ et al (1991) The formation of free radicals by cardiac myocytes under oxidative stress and the effects of electron-donating drugs. Biochem J 277:833–837
51. Youn Y-K, Lalonde C, Demling R (1991) Use of antioxidant therapy in shock and trauma. Circ Shock 35:245–249
52. Tuchschmidt J, Fried J, Astiz M et al (1992) Elevation of cardiac output and oxygen delivery improves outcome in sptic shock. Chest 102:16–20
53. Hayes MA, Yau EHS, Timmins AC et al (1993) Response of critically ill patients to

treatment aimed at achieving supranormal oxygen delivery and consumption. Relationship to outcome. Chest 103:886–895
54. Shoemaker WC (1993) A stitch in time saves lives. Chest 103:663–664
55. Shoemaker WC, Appel PL, Kram HB et al (1988) Prospective trial of supranormal values of survivors as therapeutic goals in high risk surgical patients. Chest 94:1176–1186
56. Gutierrez G, Palizas F, Doglio G, Wainsztein N et al (1992) Gastric intramucosal pH as a therapeutic index of tissue oxygenation in critically ill patients. Lancet 339:195–199
57. Fink MP (1993) Adequacy of gut oxygenation in endotoxemia and sepsis. Crit Care Med 21:S4–S8
58. Arndt H, Kubes P, Granger DN (1991) Involvement of neutrophils in ischemia-reperfusion injury of the small intestine. Klin Wochenschr 69:1056–1060
59. Siems W, Kowalewski J, Werner A et al (1989) Radical formation in the rat small intestine during and following ischemia. Free Radic Res Commun 7:347–353
60. Fiddian-Green RG, Baker S (1987) Predictive value of the stomach wall pH for complications after cardiac operations: comparison with other monitoring. Crit Care Med 5:153–156
61. Antonsson JB, Boyle CC, Kruithoff KL et al (1990) Validity of tonometric measures of gut intramural pH during endotoxemia and mesenteric occlusion in pigs. Am J Physiol 259:G519–G523
62. Grum CM, Fiddian-Green RG, Pittenger GL et al (1984) Adequacy of tissue oxygenation in intact dog intestine. J Appl Physiol 56(4):1065–1069
63. Doglio GR, Pusajo FJ, Egurrola MA et al (1991) Comparison between gastric intramucosal pH and pulmonary artery oxygen transport measurement on the intensive care unit. Crit Care Med 19:1037–1040
64. Kunimoto F, Morita T, Fujita T (1987) Inhibition of lipid peroxidation improves survival rate of endotoxemic rats. Circ Shock 21:15–22
65. Broner CW, Shenep JL, Stidham GL et al (1988) Effect of scavengers of oxygen-derived free radicals on mortality in endotoxin-challenged mice. Crit Care Med 16:848–854
66. Morgan RA, Manning PB, Coran AG et al (1988) Oxygen free radical during live E. coli septic shock in the dog. Circ Shock 25:319–323
67. Schneider J, Friderichs E, Heintze K et al (1990) Effects of the recombinant human superoxide dismutase on increased lung permeability and respiratory disorder in endotoxemic rats. Circ Shock 30:97–106
68. Powell RJ, Machiedo GW, Rush BJ et al (1991) Effect of oxygen-free radical scavengers on survival in sepsis. Am Surg 57:86–88
69. Peck MD, Alexander JW (1991) Survival in septic guinea pigs is influenced by vitamin E, but not by vitamin C in enteral diets. J Parenter Ent Nutr 15:433–436
70. Peavy PL, Fairchild EJ (1986) Evidence for lipid peroxidation in endotoxin-poisened mice. Infect Immunol 52:613–616
71. McKechnie K, Furman BL, Parrat JR (1986) Modification by oxygen free radical scavengers of the metabolic and cardiovascular effects of endotoxin infusion in conscious rats. Circ Shock 19:429–439
72. Brackett DJ, Lerner MR, Wilson MF (1991) Dimethyl sulfoxide antagonizes hypotensive, metabolic, and pathologic responses induced by endotoxin. Circ Shock 33:156–163
73. Hamburger SA, Mc Cay PB (1989) Endotoxin-induced mortality in rats is reduced by nitrones. Circ Shock 29:329–334
74. Novelli GP (1992) Oxygen radicals in experimental shock: effects of spin-trapping nitrones in ameliorating shock pathophysiology. Crit Care Med 20:499–507
75. Progrebniak HW, Merino J et al (1992) Spin trap salvage from endotoxemia: the role of cytokine down-regulation. Surgery 112:130–139
76. Progrebniak HW, Matthews WA et al (1990) Reactive oxygen species can amplify macrophage tumor necrosis factor production. Surg Forum 16:101–103

77. Yasumoto K, Inada Y (1986) Effect of coenzyme Q10 on endotoxin shock in dogs. Crit Care Med 14:570–574
78. Lelli JL, Drongowski RA, Gastman B et al (1993) Effects of coenzyme Q10 on the mediator cascade of sepsis. Circ Shock 39:178–187
79. Powell RJ, Machiedo GW, Rush BF et al (1991) Oxygen free radicals: effect on red cell deformability in sepsis. Crit Care Med 19:732–735
80. Arvidsson S, Fält K, Merklund S et al (1985) Role of free oxygen radicals in the development of gastrointestinal mucosal damage in Escheria coli sepsis. Circ Shock 16:383–393
81. Koyama S, Kobayshi T, Kubo K et al (1992) Recombinant human superoxide dismutase attenuates endotoxin-induced lung injury in awake sheep. ARRD 145:1404–1409
82. Brigham KL, Meyrick B, Berry LC et al (1987) Antioxidants protect cultured bovine lung endothelial cells from injury by endotoxin. J Appl Physiol 63:840–850
83. Matsuda T, Eccleston CA, Rubinstein et al (1991) Antioxidants attenuate endotoxin-induced microvascular leakage of macromolecules in vivo. J Appl Physiol 70:1483–1489
84. Harris CA, Derbin KS, Hunte-McDonugh B (1991) Manganese superoxide dismutase is induced by IFN-γ and tumor necrosis factor or IL-1. J Immunol 147:149–154
85. Leff JA, Oppegard MA, Tereda LS et al (1991) Human serum catalase decreased endothelial cell injury from hydrogen peroxide. J Appl Physiol 71(5):1903–1906
86. Rushmore TH, Morton MR, Pickett CB (1991) The antioxidant responsive element. J Biol Chem 266:11623–11639
87. Aruoma OI, Halliwell B, Hoey BM et al (1989) The antioxidant action of N-acetylcysteine: its reaction with hydrogen peroxide, hydroxyl radical, superoxide, and hypochlorous acid. J Free Radicals Biol Med 6:593–597
88. Bernard GR, Lucht WD, Niedermeyer ME et al (1984) Effect of N-acetylcysteine on the pulmonary response to endotoxin in the awake sheep and upon in vitro granulocyte function. J Clin Invest 73:1772–1784
89. Harrison PM, Wendon JA, Gimson AES et al (1991) Improvement by acetylcysteine of hemodynamics and oxygen transport in fulminant hepatic failure. NEJM 324:1852–1857
90. Suttorp N, Kästle S, Neuhof H (1991) Glutathione redox cycle is an important defense system of endothelial cells against chronic hyperoxia. Lung 196:203–214
91. Meister A (1992) On the antioxidant effects of ascorbic acid and glutathione. Biochem Pharmacol 44:1905–1915
92. Chow CK (1991) Vitamin E and oxidative stress. Free Radic Biol Med 11:215–232
93. Rubanyi GM, Vanhoutte PM (1986) Superoxide anions and hyperoxia inactivate endothelium-derived relaxing factor. Am J Physiol 250:H822–H827
94. Packer M, Lee WH, Kessler PD et al (1987) Prevention and reversal of nitrate tolerance in patients with congestive heart failure. NEJM 317:799–807
95. May DC, Popma JJ, Black WH et al (1987) In vivo induction and reversal of nitroglycerin tolerance in human coronary arteries. NEJM 317:805–809
96. Henry PJ, Horowitz JD, Louis WJ (1989) Determinants of in vitro nitroglycerine tolerance induction and reversal: influence of dose regimen, nitrate-free period, and sulfhydryl supplementation. J Cardiovasc Pharmacol 14:31–37
97. Patterson CE, Butler JA, Byrne FD et al (1985) Oxidant lung injury: interventions with sulfhydryl reagents. Lung 163:23–32
98. Spies CD, Hannemann L, Reinhart K et al (1992) N-Acetylcysteine (NAC) prevents decreased oxygen consumption during hyperoxia. Anesthesiology 77:A105
99. Clancy RM, Leszczynska-Piziak J, Abramson SB (1992) Nitric oxide, an endothelial cell relaxation factor inhibits neutrophil superoxide anion production via a direct action on the NADPH oxidase. J Clin Invest 90:1116–1121
100. Bath PMW, Hassal DG, Gladwin A-M et al (1991) Nitric oxide and prostacyclin: divergence of inhibitory effects on monocyte chemotaxis and adhesion to endothelium in vitro. Arterioscler Thromb 11:254–260

101. Mellion BT, Ignarro LJ, Ohlstein EH et al (1981) Evidence for the inhibitory role of guanosine 3′,5′monophosphate in ADP induced human platelet aggregation in the presence of nitric oxide and related vasodilators. Blood 57:946–955
102. Ignarro LJ, Kadowitz PJ (1985) The pharmacological and physiological role of cyclic GMP in vascular smooth muscle relaxation. Annu Rev Pharmacol Toxicol 24:171–191
103. Schwartz CJ, Valente AJ, Sprague EA, Kelley JL, Nerem RM (1991) The pathogenesis of atherosclerosis: an overview. Clin Cardiol 14:1–16
104. Schwartz CJ, Sprague EA (1992) Vascular endothelium and hemodynamic stress. Nutr Metab Cardiovasc Dis 2:99–100
105. Ku DN, Giddens DP, Zarins CK et al (1985) Pulsatile flow and atherosclerosis in the human carotid bifurcation. Positive correlation between plaque localization and low and oscillating shear stress. Arteriosclerosis 5:293–302
106. Asakura T, Karino T (1990) Flow patterns and spatial distribution of atherosclerotic lesions in human coronary arteries. Circ Res 66:1045–1066
107. Diamond SL, Eskin SG, McIntire LV (1989) Fluid flow stimulates tissue plasminogen activator secretion by cultured human endothelial cells. Science 243:1483–1485
108. Frangos JA, McIntire LV, Eskin SG et al (1985) Flow effects on prostacyclin production by cultured human endothelial cells. Science 227:1477–1479
109. Grabowski EF, Jaffe EA, Weksler BB (1985) Prostacyclin production by cultured endothelial cell monolayers exposed to step increases in shear stress. J Lab Clin Med 105:36–45
110. Cayatte AJ, Schwartz CJ, Nerem RM, Rozek MM, Sprague EA (1989) Decreased adherence of platelets and monocytes to preendothelialized porous polyester mesh exposed to prolonged elevated shear stress. In: Norman J (ed) Cardiovascular science and technology: basic and applied: I. Oxymoron, Louisville, Kentucky, pp 57–59
111. Redl H, Dinges HP, Schlag G et al (1991) Expression of endothelial leukocyte adhesion molecule-1 in septic but not traumatic/hypovolemic shock in the baboon. Am J Pathol 139:461–466
112. Spies C, Reinhart K et al (1993) Influence of N-Acetylcysteine on O_2 consumption and gastric intramucosal pH in septic patients. Crit Care Med 21:S183
113. Bernard GR, Swindell BB, Meredith MJ et al (1989) Glutathione repletion by N-acetylcysteine (NAC) in patients with the adult respiratory distress syndrome. ARRD 139:A221
114. Fiddian-Green RG (1993) Associations between intramucosal acidosis in the gut and organ failure. Crit Care Med 21:S103–S107
115. Mecher CE, Rackow EC, Astiz A et al (1990) Venous hypercarbia associated with severe sepsis and systemic hypoperfusion. Crit Care Med 18:585–589
116. Bakker J, Vincent JL, Gris P et al (1992) Veno-arterial carbon dioxide gradient in human septic shock. Chest 101:509–515
117. Parrillo JE, Parker MM, Natanson C et al (1990) Septic shock in humans. Advances in the understanding of pathogenesis, cardiovascular dysfunction and therapy. Ann Intern Med 113:227–242
118. Horowitz JD, Antman EM, Lorell BH et al (1983) Potentiation of the cardiovascular effects of nitroglycerin by N-acetylcysteine. Circulation 68:1247–1253
119. Forman MB, Puett DW, Cates CU et al (1988) Glutathione redox pathway and reperfusion injury: effect of N-acetylcysteine of infarct size and ventricular function. Circulation 78:202–213
120. Bolli R, Jeroudi MO, Patel BS et al (1989) Marked reduction of free radical generation and contractile dysfunction by antioxidant therapy begun at the time of reperfusion. Circ Res 65:607–622
121. Jepsen S, Herlevsen P, Knudsen P et al (1992) Antioxidant treatment with N-acetylcysteine during adult respiratory distress syndrome: a prospective, randomized, placebo-controlled study. Crit Care Med 20:918–923

122. Meyrick B, Brigham KL (1983) Acute effects of Escherichia coli endotoxin on the pulmonary microcirculation of anesthetized sheep: structure-function relationships. Lab Invest 48:458–470
123. Esbenshade AM, Newman JH, Lams PM et al (1982) Respiratory failure after endotoxin infusion in sheep: lung mechanics and lung fluid balance. L Appl Physiol 53:967–976
124. Groeneveld ABJ, deHollander W, Straub J et al (1990) Effects of N-acetylcysteine and terbutaline treatment on hemodynamics and regional albumin extravasation in porchine septic shock. Circ Shock 30:185–205
125. Ghezzi P, Saccardo B, Bianchi M (1989) Role of reactive oxygen intermediates in the hepatotoxicity of endotoxin. Immunopharmacology 12:241–244
126. Olson NC, Anderson DL, Grizzle MK (1987) Dimethyl thiourea attenuate endotoxin-induced acute respiratory failure in pigs. J Appl Physiol 63:2426–2432
127. Tate RM, Van Benthuysen KM, Shasby DM et al (1981) Dimethylurea, a hydroxyl radical scavenger, blocks oxygen radical-induced acute edematous lung injury in an isolated perfused lung. ARRD 123:243 (abstract)
128. Miller JS, Cormwell DG (1978) the role of cryoprotective agents as hydroxyl scavengers. Cryobiology 15:585–588
129. Ashwood-Smith MJ (1975) Current concepts concerning radioprotective and cryoprotective properties of dimethylsulfoxide in cellular systems. Ann NY Acad Sci 243:246–256
130. Harbrecht BG, Billiar TR, Stadler J et al (1992) Nitric oxide synthesis serves to reduce hepatic damage during acute murine endotoxemia. Crit Care Med 20:1568–1574
131. Billiar RT, Curran RD, Harbrecht BG et al (1990) Modulation of nitrogen oxide synthesis in vivo: N^G-methyl-L-arginine inhibits endotoxin-induced nitrite/nitrate biosynthesis while promoting hepatic damage. J Leukoc Biol 48:565–569
132. Hutcheson IR, Whittle BJR, Boughton-Smith NK (1990) Role of nitric oxide in maintaining vascular integrity in endotoxin-induced acute intestinal damage in the rat. Br J Pharmacol 101:815–820
133. Wright C, Rees D, Moncada S (1992) Protective and pathological roles of nitric oxide in endotoxin shock. Cardiovasc Res 26:48–57
134. Hollenberg SM, Cunnion RE, Parrillo JE (1992) Effect of septic on vascular smooth muscle: in vitro studies using rat aortic rings. Crit Care Med 20:993–998
135. Stadler J, Billiar TR, Curran RD et al (1991) Effect of exogenous and endogenous nitric oxide on mitochondrial respiration of rat hepatocytes. Am J Physiol 260:C910–916
136. Pellat C, Henry Y, Drapier J-C (1990) IFN-gamma-activated macrophages: detection by electron paramagnetic resonance of complexes between L-arginine derived nitric oxide and non-heme iron proteins. Biochem Biophys Res Commun 166:119–125
137. Beckman JS, Beckman TW, Chen J et al (1990) Apparent hydroxyl radical production by peroxynitrate: implications for endothelial injury from nitric oxide and superoxide. Proc Natl Acad Sci USA 87:1620–1624
138. Hogg N, Darley-Usmar D, Wilson MT et al (1992) Production of hydroxyl radicals from the simultaneous generation of superoxide and nitric oxide. Biochem J 281:419–424
139. Radi R, Beckman JS, Bush KM et al (1991) Peroxynitrate oxidation of sulfhydryls: the cytotoxic potential of superoxide and nitric oxide. J Biol Chem 266:4244–4250
140. Boyd O, Bennett ED (1992) Is oxygen consumption an important clinical target? In: Vincent J-L (ed) Yearbook of intensive care and emergency medicine. Springer, Berlin Heidelberg New York, pp 310–324
141. Kilbourn RG, Jubran A, Gross SS et al (1990) Reversal of endotoxin-mediated shock by N^G-methyl-L-arginine, an inhibitor of nitric oxide synthesis. Biochem Biophys Res Commun 172:1132–1138
142. Ochoa JB, Ukdekwu AO, Billiar TR et al (1991) Nitrogen oxide levels in patients after trauma and during sepsis. Ann Surg 214:621–626

143. Lübbe AS, Garrison RN, Cryer HM et al (1992) Endothelium-derived relaxing factor as a possible mediator of sepsis – induced arteriolar dilation in skeletal muscle. Am J Physiol 262:H880–H887
144. Nava E, Palmer RMJ, Moncada S (1991) Inhibition of nitric oxide synthesis in septic shock: how much is beneficial? Lancet 338:1555–1557
145. Petros A, Bennett D, Vallance P (1991) Effect of nitric oxide synthase inhibitors on hypotension in patients with septic shock. Lancet 338:1557–1558
146. Meyer J, Traber LD, Nelson S et al (1992) Reversal of hyperdynamic response to continuous endotoxin administration by inhibition of NO synthesis. J Appl Physiol 73(1):324–328
147. Vallance P, Leone A, Calver A et al (1992) Accumulation of an endogenous inhibitor of nitric oxide synthesis in chronic renal failure. Lancet 339:572–575
148. Voerman HJ, Stehouwer CDA, van Kamp GJ et al (1992) Plasma endothelin levels are increased during septic shock. Crit Care Med 20:1097–1101
149. Pittet J-F, Morel DR, Hemsen A et al (1991) Elevated plasma endothelin-1 concentrations are associated with the severity of illness in patients with sepsis. Ann Surg 213:261–264
150. Freund H, Atamian S, Holroyde J et al (1979) Plasma amino acids as predictors of the severity and outcome of sepsis. Ann Surg 190:571–576
151. Vente JP, von Meyenfeldt MF, van Eijk HMH et al (1989) Plasma amino acid profiles in sepsis and stress. Ann Surg 209:57–62
152. Wang Q, Jacobs J, DeLeo J et al (1991) Nitric oxide hemoglobin in mice and rats in endotoxin shock. Life Sci 49:55–60
153. Finkel MS, Oddis CV, Jacob TD et al (1992) Negative inotropic effects of cytokines on the heart mediated by nitric oxide. Science 257:387–389
154. Smith REA, Palmer RMJ, Moncada S (1991) Coronary vasodilation induced by endotoxin in the rabbit isolated perfused heart is nitric oxide – dependent and inhibited by dexamethasone. Br J Pharmacol 104:5–6
155. Estrada C, Gomez C, Martin C et al (1992) Nitric oxide mediates tumor necrosis factor-α cytotoxicity in endothelial cells. Biochem Biophys Res Commun 186:475–482
156. Cirino G, Cicala C, Sorrentino L et al (1991) Effect of bradykinin antagonist, N^G-monomethyl-L-arginine and L-N^G-nitro arginine on phospholipase A_2 induced edema in rat paw. Gen Pharmacol 22:801–804
157. Hughes SR, Williams TJ, Brain SD et al (1990) Evidence that endogenous nitric oxide modulates edema formation induced by substance P. Eur J Pharmacol 191:481–484
158. Kroncke K-D, Kolb-Bachofen V, Berschick B et al (1991) Activated macrophages kill pancreatic syngeneic islet cells via arginine-dependent nitric oxide generation. Biochem Biophys Res Commun 175:752–758
159. Bergmann L, Kroncke K-D, Suscheck C et al (1992) Cytotoxic action of IL-1b against pancreatic islet cells is mediated via nitric oxide formation and is inhibited by N^G-monomethyl-L-arginine. FEBS Lett 299:103–106
160. Salvemini D, Mollace V, Pistelli A et al (1992) Cultured astrocytoma cells generate a nitric oxide-like factor from endogenous L-arginine and glyceroltrinitrate: effect of E. coli lipopolysaccharide. Br J Pharmacol 106:931–936
161. Monig J, Asmus K-D, Forni LG et al (1987) Detection of thiyl radicals. Int Radiat Biol 52:589–602
162. Saez G, Thornalley PJ, Hill HAO (1982) The production of free radicals during the autooxidation of cysteine and their effect on isolated rat hepatocytes. Biochim Biophys Acta 719:24–31
163. Bihari D, Smithies M, Gimson A et al (1987) The effects of vasodilation with prostacyclin on oxygen delivery and uptake in critically ill patients. NEJM 317:397–403

Immunoaugmentation: A Contribution to Prophylaxis and Treatment of Sepsis?

E. Faist, A. Markewitz, R. Maier and S. Lang

Introduction

Trauma and the subsequent stress response have been associated with widely varied changes in host defense. A large body of information has been accumulated characterizing the various types of immune dysfunction following injury and suggests that major accidental, burn, or operative trauma causes substantial immunosuppression [1–4]. The deficit of immunocompetence together with an overwhelming nondiscriminant whole body inflammatory response explains the high susceptibility of the injured individual for developing sepsis with consecutive multiple organ dysfunction syndrome (MODS). We and others have demonstrated that the alterations of cell-mediated immunity (CMI) following trauma is mainly due to the disruption of intact monocyte (MØ)/T cell interaction [5, 6]. Within this phenomenon we see a shift of the cell ratio in the compartment of peripheral blood mononuclear cells (PBMCs) with a considerable increase of prostaglandin E_2 (PGE_2)-synthesizing MØs and a simultaneous decrease of functionally competent CD3+ and CD4+ lymphocytes. T cell dysfunction in states of profound mechanical stress is characterized by impaired synthesis of two crucial cytokines – interleukin-2 (IL-2) and γ-interferon (γ-IFN) [7, 8]. The inability to produce adequate amounts of IL-2 results in incomplete proliferative T cell responses to antigenic stimuli, while a lack of γ-IFN results in inefficient MØ antigen presentation. It has been demonstrated that both defects are keystones of suppressed CMI function following trauma with subsequent development of sepsis. The information derived from the dissection of down-regulatory mechanisms responsible for the development of injury-related immunoincompetence also provided incentive for the development of therapeutic regimens designed to prevent a major collapse of CMI.

The use of three classes of substances seemed to be most suitable for immunoprotection and/or immunorestoration:

1) Nonsteroidal anti-inflammatory drugs (NSAID), which block immunoreactive PGE_2, the common mediator in the malfunction of the MØ/T cell interactive network in states of trauma.

2) The synthetic thymomimetic substance thymopentin (TP-5) with its crucial characteristics – restoration of immunobalance, T cell activation and acceleration of T cell recruitment.
3) Human recombinant IL-2 (hrIL-2), the crucial cytokine for the development of adequate CMI.

We have conducted a number of clinical trials in recent years in order to scrutinize the immunoaugmenting potential of TP-5 and of the cyclooxygenase inhibitor indomethacin (Indo) in patients undergoing major surgery. A perioperative two-shot subcutaneous administration of 50 mg TP-5 in patients undergoing open heart surgery resulted in a restoration of the *in vitro* lymphocyte proliferative responses and in delayed type hypersensitivity (DTH) responses compared to a placebo treated control population. However, T cell receptor protection (CD3+, CD4+) and restoration of IL-2 synthesis could not be achieved with this treatment modality.

Conversely, postoperative administration of Indo in patients undergoing gastrectomy or reconstruction of the abdominal aorta resulted in an impressive protection of T cell receptor expression for the CD3+, CD4+, and IL-2 receptor+ subpopulations. This treatment also controlled overwhelming monocytosis. Furthermore, preservation of the preoperative *in vivo* immunoreactivity could be demonstrated. However, restoration of depressed IL-2 synthesis (DTH skin response) could not be achieved with Indo administration, which was in contrast to numerous *in vitro* experiments showing that Indo restores depressed IL-2 production [9].

Study Design

In view of the findings in these single agent studies, and based on the knowledge that trauma induced depression of CMI represents a multimechanistic phenomenon, the protocol for a combined agent therapeutic trial was designed. It was the objective of an extensive prospective randomized study to quantify, specify and compare the immunorestorative potential of a combined therapy with the cyclooxygenase inhibitor Indo and the thymomimetic substance TP-5 vs single drug administration of Indo following extracorporeal circulation (ECC) [10].

Experimental Protocol

For the prospectively randomized study 60 patients (45 men, 15 women) with an average age of 63±7 years were divided into three groups. All patients had acquired or congenital heart disease and had to undergo ECC surgery with coronary artery bypass grafting (CABG) or valve replacement. Group A patients (PA) ($n=20$) were given Indo (Confortid, Dumex, Denmark),

100 mg i.v., immediately after surgery (day 0) and three times 50 mg i.v. daily between postoperative days 1 and 5. Group B patients (PB) ($n=20$), besides Indo therapy, also received 50 mg of TP-5 (Timmunox, Cilag, FRG) subcutaneously, 2 h preoperatively, as well as 48 h and 96 h postoperatively. Group C patients (PC) ($n=20$) served as the control population, undergoing conventional ICU therapy postoperatively. Age, underlying disease, and quality of surgical procedure were highly comparable in all three groups. Immunologic screening of the patients was carried out twice preoperatively, immediately after admission and on the day of the operation (but calculated as one preoperative value) and on days 1, 3, 5 and 7 postoperatively.

The immune parameters studied *in vivo* and *in vitro* included the DTH skin response to recall antigens, PBMC phenotyping, specific and nonspecific induction of lymphoproliferative responses and the *in vitro* synthesis of IL-1β, IL-2, IL-6, and tumor necrosis factor-α (TNF-α). Additionally, for CMI serum markers, we evaluated the concentration of D-erythro-neopterin (NPT), a MØ metabolite and a very sensitive indicator of MØ activation, as well as the concentration of γ-IFN as a marker for T cell activation.

Results

In contrast to the findings in the control group, the *in vitro* IL-2 synthesis in cell cultures of PB on consecutive postoperative days did not show any suppression and the values were always on or above baseline level. To our knowledge, these findings represent the first report of a successful intervention to preserve adequate T cell capacity for IL-2 production in humans following trauma.

The serum levels of γ-IFN in the patient population treated with Indo/TB-5 continuously increased on consecutive postoperative days, with an average rise of +50% above baseline between days 3 and 7. The increased amount of γ-IFN released in PB provides evidence for the complex efficacy of T cell activation, triggered through that specific immunomodulatory treatment. γ-IFN serum levels in PA were within the baseline range on day 7 in contrast to an average reduction of 35% compared to preoperative levels in PC on day 7.

NPT rose much more rapidly in PC within the first 72 h post-trauma than in PB. By day 7 postoperatively, NPT concentrations were identical in all three patient groups. The analysis of the supernatants of lipopolysaccharide (LPS) stimulated PBMC cultures of PA, PB and PC for the proinflammatory cytokines IL-1, IL-6 and TNF-α revealed that the cardiopulmonary bypass procedures result in a substantial activation of the acute phase response. In PC we found an up-regulation of IL-6 synthesis while IL-1 and TNF-α production was substantially depressed during the first days post-trauma.

IL-1 and TNF-α synthesis was significantly higher in PB cultures than in these of PA and PC. Conversely IL-6 production in MØs and lymphocytes could be substantially reduced through combined therapy of TP-5 and Indo compared to single cyclooxygenase inhibition therapy or the untreated controls.

Discussion

In a study of Ertel et al. [11] it was demonstrated that administration of the cyclooxygenase inhibitor ibuprofen resulted in the restoration of adequate IL-1 and TNFα synthesis and, in parallel, in down-regulation of IL-6 synthesis. As previously stated, our investigation could corroborate the effect of PGE_2 counter-regulation in terms of IL-1 and TNF-α synthesis [12]. The entire body of information derived from this study provides us with striking evidence for the salutary mechanism of action induced by the Indo/TP-5 treatment. Simultaneous PGE_2 blockade, via Indo, and T cell activation, via TP-5, apparently represent an ideal strategy to provide protection for the successful development of an immune response for which several levels of control are necessary. Essential steps within the forward regulatory immune response pathway include: synthesis and release of IL-1 from MØs, intact MØ function, intact T cell receptor function, a sufficient number of functionally intact T helper cells, IL-2 synthesis and adequate IL-2 release, as well as IL-2 sensitive responder cells with intact capacity of IL-2 receptors. Moreover, MØ participation can only be sustained via γ-IFN production by activated T cells [13]. The down-regulation of CMI occurs mainly due to PGE_2, a regulatory mediator released from inhibitory MØ, which are present in large amounts following injury. One of the most prominent PGE_2 immunoregulatory activities consists of the regulation of IL-2 synthesis. Mediators such as PGE_2 that are associated with both specific and nonspecific immunosuppression have been demonstrated to impinge on the prostaglandin cAMP pathway, and it has been postulated that agents which interfere with these mechanisms may counteract the immunosuppressive influences. Thus, it has been recognized that an immunopharmacological attack on T cell disturbances in trauma should either contrasuppress the suppressor, PGE_2 by blocking cAMP, or it should have immunorestorative capacities in terms of promoting cGMP, as for example, thymomimetic substances like TP-5 do.

Based on these reflections it appears logical that a treatment regimen that combines blocking ideally with enhancing action should consist of a combination of immunopotentiating agents that complement each other functionally.

Indo/TP-5 therapy resulted in protection of all T cell functions tested, and it alleviated postoperative monocytosis and MØ overactivation. We found a convincing concurrence between the results of our long-term series of *in vitro* mechanistic studies and the findings derived from the simultaneous *in vivo* studies (administration of blocking and enhancing agents) in terms of protection of adequate MØ/T cell interaction following major operative trauma.

Finally, we conducted a clinical study including 40 patients with bronchial cancer undergoing elective surgery. The aim of this study was to evaluate the anti-infective effect of an immunomodulating treatment with subcutaneous low-dose hrIL-2 (Eurocetus, Frankfurt, FRG), with or without the addition of Indo. The treatment groups were comparable regarding age, tumor stage and the extent of surgery. (Patients with remote metastases were excluded). Immunological monitoring included testing of the DTH response and proliferation capacity as well as the determination of cytokine production. In the individual treatment groups, for dose determining reasons we investigated four different doses: 150000, 300000, 450000, 600000 IU hrIL-2 was administered to the patients daily between postoperative days 1 and 10. Patients receiving Indo were given a maximal dose of 3×50 mg i.v. between day 0 (110 mg) and day 6. This pilot study could demonstrate that serum neopterin levels, expressing the degree of CMI activation, were significantly elevated in hrIL-2 treated patients. The increment of serum neopterin concentrations was directly proportional to the corresponding hrIL-2 dose used. The addition of Indo seemed to alleviate the metabolic symptoms following hrIL-2 administration; however, when Indo treatment was discontinued on day 7, a number of patients immediately showed febrile peaks. Further studies are underway to obtain sufficient information about the immunomechanistics and clinical effects of preventive immunomodulation for surgical patients at risk.

Summary and Perspective

Major trauma with and without septic complications exerts a dramatic suppressive effect on CMI-specific and nonspecific inflammatory mechanisms. These abnormalities become strikingly evident when the synthesis patterns of T cell- and MØ-derived cytokines are analyzed. In a number of studies, we characterized the trauma-induced alteration of MØ/T cell interaction in injured humans by scrutinizing the ex vivo behavior of PBMCs in stimulated and unstimulated cell cultures. A major disruption of CMI responses is caused through an overrepresentation of suppressor-active MØs and inadequate T helper cells. The correlates for this observed phenomenon within the complex of cytokine regulation are manyfold. A major element of T cell dysfunction appears to be the severe deficit of IL-2 synthesis, which is most likely due to suppressive serum substances including prostaglandins causing defective transmembrane signaling and a massive elevation of intracellular cAMP.

Complement, endotoxin and antibody-antigen complexes cause a massive MØ activation and abnormal release of crucial cell products such as PGE_2, IL-1, IL-6, IL-8, TGFβ and TNFα. The monocyte/macrophage system is very sensitive to minimal changes in its environmental conditions. PGE_2 seems to be the major factor responsible for the overwhelming suppressor activity of the MØ, and it also functions as a major regulator within the cascade of proinflammatory cytokines. Cytokines are primarily regulated on a transcriptional or posttranscriptional level. First *in vivo* therapeutic trials, designed to counteract the trauma induced alteration of cytokine synthesis patterns and thus to alleviate the immune abnormalities which are responsible for the high susceptibility to infection, have been completed [14]. We saw a stunning concurrence between *in vitro* and *in vivo* cytokine regulation, a finding which could contribute to the design of an adequate therapeutic strategy to prevent malignant hyperinflammation and inefficient immune cell function in states of major trauma.

References

1. Hoyt DB, Ozkan AN (1991) Immunosuppression in trauma patients. Intensive Care Med 6:71–90
2. Mannick JA (1993) Trauma, sepsis and immune defects – an overview. In: Faist E, Meakins JL, Schildberg FW (eds) Host defense dysfunctions in trauma, shock and sepsis. Springer, Berlin Heidelberg New York (in press)
3. Ninnemann JL (1989) The immune consequences of trauma: an overview. In: Faist E, Ninnemann JL, Green D (eds) The immune consequences of trauma, shock and sepsis. Springer, Berlin Heidelberg New York, pp 3–8
4. Wood JJ, Rodrick ML, O'Mahony JB et al (1984) Inadequate interleukin 2 production: a fundamental immunological deficiency in patients with major burns. Ann Surg 200:287–292
5. Faist E, Ertel W, Mewes A et al (1989) Trauma-induced alterations of the lymphokine cascade. In: Faist E, Ninnemann JL, Green D (eds) The immune consequences of trauma, shock and sepsis. Springer, Berlin Heidelberg New York, pp 79–94
6. Miller-Granziano CL, Szabo G, Takayama T et al (1989) Alterations of monocyte function following major injury. In: Faist E, Ninnemann JL, Green D (eds) The immune consequences of trauma, shock and sepsis. Springer, Berlin Heidelberg New York, pp 95–108
7. Faist E, Mewes A, Baker CC et al (1987) Prostglandin E2 (PGE2)-dependent suppression of interleukin-2 (IL-2) production in patients with major trauma. J Trauma 27:837
8. Rodrick ML, Wood JJ, Grbic JT et al (1986) Defective IL-2 production in patients with severe burns and sepsis. Lymphokine Res 5:75
9. Faist E, Ertel W, Cohnert T et al (1990) Immunoprotective effects of cyclooxygenase inhibition in patients with major surgical trauma. J Trauma 30:8–18
10. Faist E, Markewitz A, Fuchs D et al (1991) Immunomodulatory therapy with thymopentin (TP-5) and indomethacin: successful restoration of interleukin-2 (IL-2) synthesis in patients undergoing major surgery. Ann Surg 214:264–275
11. Ertel W, Morrison MS, Meldrum DR et al (1993) Ibuprofen restores cellular immunity and decrease susceptibility to sepsis following hemorrhage. J Surg Res (in press)
12. Ertel W, Morrison MH, Ayala A et al (1991) Blockade of prostaglandin production increases cachectin synthesis and prevents depression of macrophage functions after hemorrhagic shock. Ann Surg 213:77–83
13. Polk HC, Galandiuk S, Sonnenfeld G et al (1993) The rationale for gamma interferon administration in trauma patients. In: Faist E, Meakins JL, Schildberg FW (eds) Host defense dysfunction in trauma, shock and sepsis. 2nd edn. Springer, Berlin Heidelberg New York (in press)
14. Browder W, Williams D, Pretus H et al (1990) Beneficial effect of enhanced macrophage function in the trauma patient. Ann Surg 211:605–613

What Is Certain in the Treatment with Immunoglobulins?

H. G. Kress

Introduction

Almost a century ago, in the time of von Behring, Ehrlich and Roux, the beneficial and in many cases live-saving concept of passive immunization with toxin- or pathogen-specific antisera was born and put into practice in Europe. The concept of passive immunotherapy and immunoprophylaxis against bacterial infections, although obviously efficacious, has been superseded by antimicrobial therapy with a continuously growing number of antibiotic agents. Interestingly enough, intramuscular immunoglobulins continue to be widely used in the prophylaxis and treatment of viral diseases such as measles, mumps, varicella, rubella and hepatitis.

During the last decades, although the use of appropriate antibiotics has remained the mainstay of sepsis treatment, their failure in reducing morbidity and mortality has again attracted attention to immunoglobulin therapy. The reevaluation of antibody treatment in critically ill patients as an at least theoretically promising adjunctive therapeutical approach has received renewed interest.

The objective of this article is to critically review our current knowledge of the use and efficacy of intravenous human standard immunoglobulin (IVIG) preparations for the prophylaxis and treatment of severe bacterial infections, with special reference to sepsis and septic shock.

Historical Background and Properties of Currently Available Human Immunoglobulin Preparations

The history of passive immunization dates back to the pioneering work at the end of the nineteenth century, when its concept, clinical efficacy and the quantitative dose–response relationship were established with antitoxin sera produced in animals [1, 2]. As early as 1907 the Italian Cenci used human convalescent sera for the prevention of measles and thus circumvented the problem of serum sickness resulting from heterologous plasma proteins.

During the 1930s lyophilized pooled adult sera were used, and Karelitz [3] demonstrated the protective effect of a globulin fraction prepared from the immune serum of healthy adults. In 1938 the antibody nature of the gamma globulin fraction was identified using the newly developed electrophoretic method [4]. Shortly thereafter, Cohn [5] established his fractionation method for the separation of plasma proteins (reduced ionic strength and pH in the presence of low alcohol concentration at low temperature), which readily became the basis of large scale immunoglobulin preparation. These conventional preparations (Cohns' fraction II) had to be given intramuscularly because the intravenous infusion resulted in severe anaphylactoid reactions.

It took another 20 years for the first IVIG to become commercially available (Gamma-Venin, Behringwerke, Marburg, Germany) [6]. This pepsin-treated preparation has been in clinical use for three decades and is still available in some countries. It consists mainly of $F(ab)_2$ fragments with a sedimentation coefficient of 5S, as the so-called Fc fragment (crystallizable antibody fragment), which is enzymaticly cleaved by the proteolytic digestion from the native 7S immunoglobulin molecule. The resulting antibody preparation has a considerably reduced biological half-life (<24 h) within the patient and is therefore unsuitable for replacement therapy in patients with antibody deficiency. It further lacks Fc functions such as activation of the classical complement pathway via C1q, Fc receptor-mediated opsonization and phagocytosis. Other enzymes such as plasmin have also been used for this purpose. Although this preparation was the real breakthrough in safe intravenous immunoglobulin therapy, fragmented products are now purely of historical interest and have been abandoned in favor of unfragmented 7S immunoglobulins with intact Fc functions. These became available in Europe in the mid-1960s and 1970s from various commercial producers [7–14].

Currently available 7S preparations consist of either intact unmodified or chemically modified immunoglobulins. Unmodified preparations are manufactured using cold alcohol fractionation, large-scale chromatography or hydrolase-polyethylene-glycol (PEG) fractionation procedures and show comparable IgG half-lives of 20–30 days. They also have low anaphylactoid reaction rates, show only traces of low-molecular weight material and no loss of biologic activity. Other methods of rendering purified IgG molecules safe for intravenous use are sulfonation, reduction and alkylation or stabilization with β-propiolactone [8, 11, 12]. Sulfonation splits the molecule reversibly and though reassembly occurs in the blood, Fc functions and half-life are slightly reduced compared with the native molecule. This is also more or less true for all modified IgG preparations that have been reported to show altered Fc functions or slightly diminished half-life [10, 15–17]. The clinical relevance of these changes is not very clear.

In the mid-1980s a β-propiolactone-stabilized IVIG preparation enriched for IgM (12%) and IgA (16%) was added to the spectrum of commercial standard immunoglobulins (Pentaglobin, Biotest, Dreieich, Germany). Mainly due to its IgM content this preparation showed high antibody titers against bacterial antigens and the lipid A component of endotoxin [18]. It proved superior to standard IVIG in mouse protection tests. Since the half-life of IgM is less than 3 days, only repeated or continuous infusions can provide measurable IgM replacement over a longer period of time. Experi-

What Is Certain in the Treatment with Immunoglobulins?

H. G. Kress

Introduction

Almost a century ago, in the time of von Behring, Ehrlich and Roux, the beneficial and in many cases live-saving concept of passive immunization with toxin- or pathogen-specific antisera was born and put into practice in Europe. The concept of passive immunotherapy and immunoprophylaxis against bacterial infections, although obviously efficacious, has been superseded by antimicrobial therapy with a continuously growing number of antibiotic agents. Interestingly enough, intramuscular immunoglobulins continue to be widely used in the prophylaxis and treatment of viral diseases such as measles, mumps, varicella, rubella and hepatitis.

During the last decades, although the use of appropriate antibiotics has remained the mainstay of sepsis treatment, their failure in reducing morbidity and mortality has again attracted attention to immunoglobulin therapy. The reevaluation of antibody treatment in critically ill patients as an at least theoretically promising adjunctive therapeutical approach has received renewed interest.

The objective of this article is to critically review our current knowledge of the use and efficacy of intravenous human standard immunoglobulin (IVIG) preparations for the prophylaxis and treatment of severe bacterial infections, with special reference to sepsis and septic shock.

Historical Background and Properties of Currently Available Human Immunoglobulin Preparations

The history of passive immunization dates back to the pioneering work at the end of the nineteenth century, when its concept, clinical efficacy and the quantitative dose–response relationship were established with antitoxin sera produced in animals [1, 2]. As early as 1907 the Italian Cenci used human convalescent sera for the prevention of measles and thus circumvented the problem of serum sickness resulting from heterologous plasma proteins.

During the 1930s lyophilized pooled adult sera were used, and Karelitz [3] demonstrated the protective effect of a globulin fraction prepared from the immune serum of healthy adults. In 1938 the antibody nature of the gamma

moted by the destruction of mechanical barriers (penetrating wounds, invasive diagnostic and therapeutic interventions) or poor tissue perfusion and ischemia. Under these circumstances compromised cellular (circulating neutrophils, fixed and circulating macrophages) and humoral defense mechanisms (complement, antibodies for opsonization) may become crucial factors deciding the outcome of sepsis in these patients [34, 35]. Enhanced proteolysis, consumption of pathogen-specific antibodies and external and internal protein loss can give rise to relative and absolute deficiencies in opsonic and neutralizing capacity of the circulating blood, which have been related to the presence of circulating endotoxin-like activity and poor clinical prognosis. Thus, deficiency in specific antibody appears to be one risk factor for developing disease.

On the basis of this pathophysiologic scenario theoretical arguments can be found for the use of IVIG as an adjunctive in the treatment of sepsis. Antibodies demonstrate neutralizing, binding and activating properties. Immunoglobulins of both IgG and IgM isotype facilitate phagocytosis and killing by neutrophils or macrophages with or without activation of the classical complement pathway [17, 36]. Consequently, effector cells such as neutrophils, macrophages and lymphocytes are stimulated by direct (Fc receptors, C3b receptors) or indirect mechanisms (chemotactic factors, mediators, cytokines). *In vitro* and animal experiments impressively demonstrated a synergism of IVIG with β-lactam antibiotics in the protective efficiency against various pathogens and toxins [37–39]. Furthermore, both standard and hyperimmune globulin have been extensively shown to provide functional antibacterial and antiviral antibodies for the prevention and treatment of bacterial and viral diseases in humans, especially in individuals suffering from primary immunodeficiency syndromes with defects of antibody formation [40–43].

Although sepsis and septic shock have traditionally been considered states of overall suppressed immunity, this is not completely true. Uncontrolled activation of the inflammatory response (whole body inflammation) is assumed to play a central role in the pathophysiology of the disease [44]. Potential immunomodulatory effects of IVIG have therefore attracted some attention to the idea that high-dose IVIG could eventually down-modulate activated inflammatory effector cells [45–49] and subsequently interrupt the vicious circle. Though the depression of the pathological expression of activation markers on endothelial cells and the down-regulation of activated immune cells and monocytes have been experimentally shown, their potential relevance to sepsis therapy remains highly speculative and unproven.

Elevated levels of circulating endotoxin antibodies (IgM or IgG) correlate with survival in patients with gram-negative infections. A study published nearly 20 years ago reported that bacteremic patients with elevated titers of anti-O antibody or anti-Re antibody had reduced mortality rates. Pollack and Young [50] also showed that elevated amounts of circulating anti-endotoxin IgG and IgM correlated significantly with decreased mortality rates from *Pseudomonas* sepsis.

Thus, the rationale for the administration of standard IVIG preparations in septic patients is to restore impaired defense mechanisms and to provide patients with specific antibodies to pathogens and toxins. Whereas the prophylactic and therapeutic use of IVIG in primary and secondary immunodeficiency states is an accepted clinical practice, its use as an adjunctive therapy in severe bacterial infections and sepsis is controversial and still considered to require further investigation.

Controlled, Randomized Clinical Studies

Accepted and well established indications for IVIG include replacement therapy in primary immunodeficiency syndromes and in secondary immunodeficiency resulting from hematological malignancies, radiotherapy or chemotherapy. Therapeutic effects have also been documented in children with acquired immune deficiency syndrome (AIDS), and in patients with immune thrombocytopenic purpura (ITP) or Kawasaki syndrome. In contrast, there appears to exist almost absolute uncertainty about the clinical usefulness of IVIG in the treatment of sepsis. Thus, the potential beneficial effects of IVIG administration in severe bacterial infections are still under debate. During the last two decades, various studies with small number of patients or anecdotal reports of beneficial effects of IVIG in sepsis have appeared in the literature, without establishing this new indication. Most of these studies did not include proper controls, nor did they furnish evidence that significant amounts of antibodies had been used. In addition, schedule and duration of treatment varied widely, as did underlying diseases and selection of patients, definition and stage of sepsis or critical supportive care measures.

Like any other pharmacological agent, IVIG preparations have to prove their protective and therapeutic efficacy not only in experimental animal studies but in the septic patient. The types of studies that are needed to definitely judge the value of IVIG in the treatment of sepsis are large, placebo-controlled, prospective and randomized trials in one or preferentially multiple centers, with patients included on the basis of clearly defined stages of disease and comparable supportive care regimens. At present only surprisingly few clinical trials fulfill these criteria.

Prophylaxis of Bacterial Infection and Sepsis

Much evidence exists demonstrating the efficiency of commercial IVIG products in preventing severe bacterial infections and sepsis in newborns and infants (Table 1). Due to the relative immaturity of their humoral and cellular immune systems including important antibacterial defense mechanisms such as opsonic antibodies, complement and polymorphonuclear leukocytes, newborns, especially if they are premature, are highly susceptible to bacterial infections and sepsis [51–55]. Therefore, nosocomial infection contributes

Table 1. Prophylactic efficacy of commercial IVIG preparations in neonates: controlled, randomized trials

Author	Patients	IVIG preparation	*n*	Protection infection rate	Mortality
Haque [53]	P/LBW	IgG	150	$p<0.005$	$p<0.001$
Chirico [52]	LBW	IgG	133	n.s.	n.s.
	(<1500 g)	IgG	83/133	$p<0.05$	$p<0.04$[a]
	(>1500 g)	IgG	50/133	n.s.	n.s.
Stabile [56]	P/LBW	IgG	96	n.s.	n.s.
Magny [55]	P/LBW	IgG	253	n.s.	n.s.
Baker [51]	P/LBW	IgG	588	$p<0.015$	—

IVIG, intravenous human immunoglobulin; P, preterm infant; LBW, low birth weight infants; *n*, number of patients; n.s., not significant.
[a] Only in a subgroup of patients.

substantially to morbidity and mortality in such infants, particularly in very low birth weight infants (<1500 g). Since the transplacental transport of maternal IgG occurs predominantly after 32 weeks gestation, and the infants' own IgG production does not begin before 24 weeks after birth, such premature babies suffer from severe hypogammaglobulinemia. These facts provide a strong rationale for immunoglobulin replacement.

Several controlled studies on the prophylaxis of neonatal bacterial infections with IVIG have been reported in the literature. In a prospective, randomized study from Saudi Arabia [53] including 150 preterm and low birth weight infants, a significant reduction of the infection rate (4% with IVIG vs 16% in the control group) and mortality were observed using one or two doses of 120 mg/kg of a β-propiolactone-stabilized standard 7S IVIG preparation (Intraglobin, Biotest, Dreieich, Germany). Interestingly, about 33% of the causative pathogens were *Salmonella* (*Escherichia coli* 50%, *Klebsiella* 17%, *Serratia* 8%), which can be explained by the specific situation in a developing country. Also, the incidence of neonatal sepsis reported in this study was much higher than that seen in developed parts of the world (22% vs 0.2%–14%). Similarly, Chirico et al. [52] reported a significant reduction in total infections (51% vs 77% in the control group), sepsis rate (5% vs 20%) and mortality rate (2% vs 15%) in 83 very low birth weight infants (<1500 g) by administration of 500 mg/kg/wk of native 7S IVIG (Sandoglobulin, Sandoz Ltd., Basel, Switzerland). However no significant effect was noted in 50 infants with birth weights above 1500 g randomly allocated to the IVIG or control group. Two other prospective, randomized prophylaxis studies from Italy [56] and France [55] using Italian and French IVIG preparations, respectively, did not demonstrate any significant differences in the infection rates of treated and control patients. Whether this discrepancy is due to differences in causative pathogens and/or specific antibody contents of the IVIG products remains unclear.

Recently the Multicenter Group for the Study of Immune Globulin in Neonates [51] presented a placebo-controlled prophylaxis study in 588 premature neonates weighing 500–1750 g at birth. This demonstrated a significant reduction in the risk of a first nosocomial infection (56 day period) in recipients of 500 mg/kg/day of an intact 7S IVIG preparation (Gammagard, Baxter Healthcare, Glendale, CA, USA). Smaller controlled prophylaxis studies in two US hospitals showed similar prophylactic efficacy [57, 58]. However, another study by Kinney et al. [59] was not conclusive. In conclusion, the majority of controlled prophylaxis studies with commercial 7S IVIG products suggest a significant protective effect at least in preterm infants with birth weights below 1500 g. Furthermore, doses of 500–700 mg/kg of IVIG have been administered to hundreds of human neonates without severe side effects. Thus, the prophylactic use of IVIG in these patients has proven safe and effective.

Adult patients suffering from hematological or other malignancies with secondary immunodeficiency syndromes (multiple myeloma, chronic lymphocytic leukemia, small cell carcinoma of the lung, malignant central nervous system tumors) developed significantly fewer infections under various prophylactic IVIG treatments than did respective control groups [28, 60–64]. As demonstrated by a randomized, double-blind, placebo-controlled multicenter study, patients at increased risk of bacterial infection were significantly protected by 500 mg/kg IVIG every 3 weeks over a 1 year period [28].

In surgical patients, only a few controlled trials have been published [65–70] (Table 2). In a pioneering, controlled, randomized trial [66] of 150 postoperative surgical patients the administration of a relatively low prophylactic dose (10 g on the first and second postoperative day) of a β-propiolactone-stabilized IVIG product (Intraglobin, Biotest, Dreieich, Germany) signifi-

Table 2. Controlled, randomized prophylaxis studies of IVIG administration in adult surgical patients

Author	Patients	IVIG preparation	IVIG dose	n	Protection
Duswald [66]	Surgery	IgG	2.5/10 g	150	$p<0.01^{b}$
Glinz [67]	Trauma	IgG	36 g	150	$p=0.01^{c}$
Kress [69]	Cardiac surgery[a]	IgG+ IgM	20 g	40	$p<0.01$
IVIG Group [70]	Surgery	IgG HIgG	1.6 g/kg 1.6 g/kg	109/329 108/329	$p=0.03/p=0.04^{c}$ n.s.

IVIG, intravenous human immunoglobulin; HIgG, hyperimmune IgG preparation; *n*, number of patients; n.s., not significant.

[a] Selected group of high-risk patients.

[b] Only in a subgroup of patients.

[c] Incidence of pneumonia.

cantly reduced the postoperative rate of local infections in patients with moderate infectious risk, but no significance was found with respect to urinary tract infections or pneumonia. Also no significant difference was found in the so-called high-risk group (contaminated and dirty operations). Not surprisingly, the "homeopathic" dose of 2.5 g IVIG did not provide any protection. As discussed by the authors, the incidence of systemic infectious symptoms was significantly lower in patients at moderate risk who had been treated with a 20 g dose of IVIG.

In 1985, the first randomized, double-blind study [67] on the prophylactic use of standard IVIG (Sandoglobulin, Sandoz Ltd., Basel, Switzerland) in 150 artificially ventilated multiple trauma patients was reported. The total dose of 36 g IVIG (12 g on days 0, 5 and 12 after admission to the ICU) resulted in a significantly reduced incidence of pneumonia (more than 30% reduction). No significant effects were observed in the mortality and sepsis rate. In an "at-risk" group of adult cardiopulmonary bypass patients, Kress et al. [68, 69] reported a significant reduction in the overall incidence and severity of early postoperative infections (2 week observation period) by the prophylactic postoperative infusion of 20 g of Pentaglobin (Biotest, Dreieich, Germany) which is an IgM- and IgA-enriched IVIG product. In this prospective, randomized, blinded, placebo-controlled study the state of preoperative cutaneous anergy identified the study group of patients at high-risk for postsurgical infection [71] who had otherwise been considered in optimum clinical condition for elective open-heart surgery.

Recently, a double-blind, placebo-controlled, clinical trial [70] investigated the prophylactic efficacy of two IVIG preparations, one of which was eightfold enriched in antibodies to the core lipopolysaccharide (LPS) of *Salmonella minnesota*. A total of 329 ICU patients at high risk of postsurgical infection received either standard 7S IVIG (Gammagard, Baxter Healthcare, Hyland Division, Glendale, CA, USA), hyperimmune IVIG; (identically manufactured and given in the same dose as standard IVIG, 400 mg/kg, maximum of four doses), or albumin as placebo. The prophylactic administration of standard IVIG significantly reduced the overall incidence of infections and pneumonia, especially due to gram-negative bacteria. In analogy to the results obtained with standard IVIG in traumatized patients [67], no effect on the rate of systemic infections, shock or mortality were observed under IVIG prophylaxis. Surprisingly, the hyperimmune IVIG preparation conferred no detectable protection. This study contrasts with a previous prophylaxis trial in surgical patients who had been effectively protected against gram-negative infections, sepsis and shock by the prophylactic administration of an antiserum to the core glycolipid of *E. coli* J5 endotoxin [65]. The reason for this discrepancy remains unclear, although it has been speculated that plasma components other than core-specific IgG may be the protective agents that are active in these preparations [72, 73].

In conclusion, there is strong evidence that various commercial IVIG products have prophylactic efficacy in both severely traumatized patients and in adult postsurgical patients at risk for the development of infections. However, sepsis rate and mortality obviously remain unchanged.

Adjunctive Treatment of Sepsis and Septic Shock

Relevant clinical studies are summarized in Table 3. In contrast to their well proven efficacy in the prophylaxis of infection in preterm, low birth weight infants, the definite role of standard IVIG preparations in the treatment of fully established neonatal sepsis has still to be determined by large placebo-controlled, double-blind, multicenter studies, because only limited data are presently available in the literature. Nonetheless, significant therapeutic effects of commercial IVIG products have been independently reported [74, 75]. Sidiropoulos et al. [75] studied the therapeutic effect of IVIG (Sandoglobulin, Sandoz Ltd., Basel, Switzerland) in neonates with sepsis confirmed by positive blood cultures. Only in premature infants weighing below 2500 g was the mortality significantly reduced by adjunctive IVIG therapy (six consecutive doses of 500 or 1000 mg/day). In the study by Haque et al. [74] using four doses of 250 mg/kg/day of a commercial IgM and IGM- and IGA-enriched IVIG-preparation (Pentaglobin, Biotest, Dreieich, Germany) and broad-spectrum antibiotic therapy, mortality was significantly reduced from 20% (controls, $n=30$) to 3.3% (IVIG, $n=30$). *E. coli* was the pathogen most frequently isolated, followed in decreasing frequency by *Klebsiella, Salmonella* and *Staphylococcus epidermitis.* Thus, these studies strongly suggest an adjunctive therapeutic efficacy of commercial IVIG preparations in neonatal

Table 3. Controlled, randomized studies of adjunctive IVIG therapy in sepsis and septic shock

Author	Patients	IVIG preparation	IVIG dose	n	Mortality
Sidiropoulos [75]	Neonates	IgG	6×0.5 g/day or 6×1 g/day	82	n.s. $p<0.04$[b]
Just [76]	Surgical	IgG+IgM	20 g	104	n.s. $p<0.01$[b]
Jesdinsky [77]	Peritonitis	IgG	70 g	288	n.s.
Haque [74]	Neonates	IgG+IgM	1 g/kg	60	$p<0.001$
Schedel [79]	Septic shock[a]	IgG+IgM	60 g	55	$p<0.01$
Dominioni [78]	Surgical ICU[a]	IgG	1 g/kg	62	$p<0.05$

IVIG, intravenous human immunoglobulin; n, number of patients; n.s., not significant.

[a] Selected group of high-risk patients.

[b] Only in a subgroup of patients.

sepsis. In analogy to the result of IVIG prophylaxis of neonatal infections, low birth weight infants appeared to benefit most from IVIG administration.

In adult patients, however, the varying results of clinical studies with commercial IVIG products do not allow a definite assessment of their potential beneficial effects as adjunctive therapeutical measure (Table 3). A randomized, controlled trial [76] was conducted with an IVIG preparation enriched in IgM and IgA (Pentaglobin, Biotest, Dreieich, Germany; four doses of 5 g in 36 h) in 104 surgical intensive care patients. At the first signs of infection, 50 patients received IVIG in addition to standard antibiotic treatment; control patients received antibiotics alone. Although the patients of the IVIG group recovered more rapidly from infections, overall mortality and mortality attributed to infections did not differ. Only in a subgroup of patients, preoperatively classified as "at high-risk," was the infectious mortality significantly lower in IVIG treated individuals. A randomized, controlled, multicenter trial in 288 patients suffering from diffuse fibrinopurulent peritonitis using an even higher dose of IVIG (70 g, Armour Pharmaceuticals, Eschwege, Germany) also failed to demonstrate any beneficial effects [77].

In contrast, two recently published prospective clinical studies reported unequivocally a significant reduction of mortality in septic patients treated with the respective commercial IVIG preparation [78, 79] (Table 3). The studies focused on different patient populations, surgical ICU vs clinical immunology ward. In the prospective, randomized, unblinded trial reported by Schedel et al. [79], 55 patients with septic shock and proven endotoxemia (>12.5 pg/ml) were either treated with or without additional administration of an IVIG product containing IgM and IgA (Pentaglobin, Biotest, Dreieich, Germany). The patients received a total of 1200 ml (60 g) during the first 3 days, starting with 30 g on day 1. IVIG treatment was started within 24 h after the onset of symptoms of septic shock. There were 38 patients who were referred from the medical division and only 17 patients were referred from the abdominal surgery division. The most frequent underlying diseases were neoplasms (19), chronic renal failure (7), chronic inflammatory bowel disease (6) and trauma or burns (6). During an observation period of under 6 weeks, death related to the septic process occurred in one (4%) of 27 IVIG patients, but nine (32%) of 28 control patients. Thus, in a preselected group of endotoxemic patients in the early phase of gram-negative septic shock, the administration of a relatively high dose (60 g) of IVIG was associated with significantly improved survival. Moreover, increased activity of circulating endotoxin and simultaneously decreased circulating anti-lipid A-specific IgG antibodies correlated with a fatal outcome,

In a randomized, double-blind, placebo-controlled, multicenter study, Dominioni et al. [78] investigated the therapeutic value of high dose IVIG administration (Sandoglobulin, Sandoz Ltd., Basel, Switzerland) vs placebo (albumin, $n=33$) in severely septic surgical and trauma ICU patients. The IVIG doses were 0.4 g/kg on day 0 and day 1, and 0.2 g/kg on day 5. Interestingly, in this trial a preselection based on a sepsis score of 20 or more (according to the grading system of Elebute and Stoner) was obligatory for enrollment of patients, in order to select patients with a high risk of mortality (>50%). As in the former study, a significantly reduced mortality was observed in the IVIG treated group (38% vs 67% in controls), even the mortality of septic shock was significantly lower (7% vs 33% in controls). Mortality from multiple organ failure (MOF) was unaffected (approximately 30% in both patient groups). There was a preponderance of gram-negative organisms isolated from the patients, but also gram-positive pathogens and *Candida* were found.

Thus, the two recent studies of Dominioni et al. [78] and Schedel et al. [79] proved for the first time the efficacy of commercial IVIG products in reducing mortality of patients with severe sepsis or septic shock. Both studies further demonstrated the safety and tolerance of even high dose IVIG treatment in these patients. The results of Schedel et al. [79] exclusively obtained in patients with gram-negative shock, and those of Dominioni et al. [78] in a more heterogeneous population strongly suggest that commercial preparations of polyvalent antibodies from pooled human sera are comparably effective in reducing mortality of severe gram-negative spesis, as previous studies have impressively demonstrated with polyvalent hyperimmune sera obtained from volunteers immunized with *E. coli* J5 [80]. However, taking into account the many disappointing results from other therapeutic trials with IVIG and the special selection criteria of the above mentioned studies, IVIG therapy cannot as yet be considered an established concept of adjunctive sepsis treatment.

Is There a Future for Immunoglobulin Therapy in Sepsis?

Only a few years ago, much hope focused on the potential beneficial effects of polyclonal and monoclonal pathogen-specific antibody preparations. So far, polyvalent IVIG preparations enriched with such pathogen-specific immunoglobulins have failed to prove their superior prophylactic and therapeutic efficacy against sepsis. After an enthusiastically celebrated first appearance, the hope raised in the "magic bullet" of monoclonal antibodies has been dampened by a rather unspectacular clinical reality. In spite of so many disappointing results reported from unsuccessful clinical trials with standard IVIG products, their prophylactic efficacy has been established in neonates and certain subgroups of adult postsurgical and trauma patients. In sepsis, their adjunctive therapeutic value still has to be substantially confirmed by large, well-controlled future studies. Nevertheless, in the days of monoclonal antibodies and cytokine receptor antagonists, the prophylactic and therapeutic potentials of standard IVIG products from pooled human sera remain interesting and promising. The present uncertainty reflects the inadequacy of our current insight into the nature and mechanisms of antibody-mediated protection against bacteria and their toxic products. Little is known about the correct indications, suitable administration schedules and optimum doses. Before their true therapeutic value can be determined, more investigational effort, more time and – last but not least – more money have to be invested. The promise of passive immunoprotection in sepsis still remains to be fulfilled.

References

1. Ehrlich P (1891) Experimentelle Untersuchungen über Immunität, I. über Ricin; II. über Abrin. Dtsch Med Wochenschr 17:976–979; 1218–1219
2. von Behring E, Kitasato (1890) Über das Zustandekommen der Diphtherie-Immunität und der Tetanus-Immunität bei Tieren. Dtsch Med Wochenschr 16:1113–1114
3. Karelitz S (1938) Prophylaxis against measles with the globulin fraction of immune adult serum. Am J Dis Child 55:768–775
4. Tiselius A, Kabat EA (1938) Electrophoresis of immune serum. Science 87:416–417
5. Cohn EJ, Luetscher JA Jr, Oncley JL et al (1940) Preparation and properties of serum and plasma proteins. J Am Chem Soc 62:3396–3400
6. Schultze HE, Schwick G (1962) Über neue Möglichkeiten intravenöser Gammaglobulin-Applikation. Dtsch Med Wochenschr 87; 1643–1650
7. Barandun S, Isliker H (1986) Development of immunoglobulin preparations for intravenous use. Vox Sang 51:157–160
8. Gronski P, Hofstaetter T, Kanzy EJ et al (1983) S-sulfonation: a reversible chemical modification of human immunoglobulins permitting intravenous application. I. Physiochemical and binding properties of S-sulfonated and reconstituted IgG. Vox Sang 45:144–154
9. Morell A (1986) Various immunoglobulin preparations for intravenous use. Vox Sang 51 [Suppl 2]:pp 44–49
10. Römer J, Morgenthaler JJ, Scherz R, Skvaril F (1982) Characterization of various immunoglobulin preparations for intravenous application. Vox Sang 42:62–73
11. Schroeder DD, Tankersley DL, Lundblad JL (1981) A new preparation of modified immune serum globulin (human) suitable for intravenous administration. Vox Sang 40:373–394
12. Stephan W (1969) Beseitigung der Komplementfixierung von Gammaglobulin durch chemische Modifizierung mit β-Propiolacton. Z Klin Chem Klin Biochem 7:282–286
13. Stephan W (1975) Undegraded human immunoglobulin for intravenous use. Vox Sang 28:422–437
14. Stephan W (1980) Intravenöse Immunglobuline. Proteinchemische und immunbiologische Charakterisierung der verschiedenen Präparatetypen. Arzneimittelforschung/Drug Res 30:116–117
15. Schreiber JR, Barrus VA, Siber GR (1985) Decreasd protective efficacy of reduced and alkylated human immune serum globulin in experimental infection with Haemophilus influenzae type b. Infect Immun 47:142–148
16. Stephan W, Dichtelmüller H (1984) Reduced efficacy of sulfitolysed intravenous immunoglobulin. Eur J Clin Microbiol 3:47
17. van Furth R, Leijh PCJ, Klein F (1984) Correlation between opsonic activity for various microorganisms and composition of gammaglobulin preparations for intravenous use. J Infect Dis 149:511–517
18. Stephan W, Dichtelmüller H, Schedel I (1985) Properties and efficacy of a human immunoglobulin M preparation for intravenous administration. Arzneimittelforschung/Drug Res 35:933–936
19. Berger D, Beger HG (1990) Adjuvant septic therapy with immunoglobulin – in vivo and in vitro studies. Intensive Care Med 16 [Suppl 1]:20
20. Garbett ND, Munro CS, Cole PJ (1989) Opsonic activity of a new intravenous immunoglobulin preparation: Pentaglobin compared with Sandoglobulin. Clin Exp Immunol 76:8–12

21. McCabe WR, DeMaria A Jr, Berberich H, Johns MA (1988) Immunization with rough mutants of Salmonella minnesota: protective activity of IgM and IgG antibody to the R 595 (Re chemotype) mutant. J Infect Dis 158:291–300
22. Collins MS, Roby RE (1984) Protective activity of an intravenous immune globulin (human) enriched in antibody against lipopolysaccharide antigens of Pseudomonas aeruginosa. Am J Med 76:168–174
23. Collins MS, Hector RF, Roby RE et al (1987) Prophylaxe gramnegativer und grampositiver Infektionen mit drei intravenösen Immunglobulin-Präparaten und Therapie der experimentellen polymikrobiellen Verbrennungssepsis mit intravenösem Pseudomonas-Immunglobulin G und Ciprofloxacin im Tiermodell. Infection 15 [Suppl 2]:51–59
24. Ferreira A, Garcia Rodriguez MC, Fontan G (1989) Follow-up of anti-IgA antibodies in primary immunodeficient patients treated with γ-globulin. Vox Sang 56:218–222
25. Winter PM, Manndorff P (1988) The frequency of IgA-deficiency in the Austrian population. Infusionstherapie 15:221–224
26. Björkander J, Cunningham-Rundles C, Lundin P et al (1988) Intravenous immunoglobulin prophylaxis causing liver damage in 16 of 77 patients with hypogammaglobulinemia or IgG subclass deficiency. Am J Med 84:107–111
27. Centers for Disease Control (1986) Safety of therapeutic immune globulin preparations with respect to transmission of human T-lymphotropic virus type III/lymphadenopathy-associated virus infection. MMWR 35:231–233
28. Cooperative Group for the Study of Immunoglobulin in Chronic Lymphocytic Leukemia (1988) Intravenous immunoglobulin for the prevention of infection in chronic lymphocytic leukemia: a randomized, controlled clinical trial. N Engl J Med 319:902–907
29. John TJ, Ninan GT, Rajagopalan MS et al (1979) Epidemic hepatitis B caused by commercial human immunoglobulin. Lancet 1:1074
30. Lever AML, Brown D, Webster ADB, Thomas HC (1984) Non-A, non-B hepatitis occurring in agammaglobulinaemic patients after intravenous immunoglobulin. Lancet 2:1062–1064
31. Ochs HD, Fischer SH, Virant FS et al (1985) Non-A, non-B hepatitis and intravenous immunnoglobulin. Lancet 1:404–405
32. Wells MA, Wittek AE, Epstein JS et al (1986) Inactivation and partition of human T-cell lymphotropic virus, type III, during ethanol fractionation of plasma. Transfusion 26:210–213
33. Yap PL (1988) Hepatitis transmission by blood products. J Hosp Infect 11 [Suppl A]:166–174
34. Alexander JW, Stinnett JD, Ogle CK et al (1979) A comparison of immunologic profiles and their influence on bacteremia in surgical patients with a high risk of infection. Surgery 86:94–104
35. Zimmerli W (1985) Impaired host defence mechanisms in intensive care unit patients. Intensive Care Med 11:174–178
36. Marodi L, Kalmar A, Szabo I (1989) Opsonic activity in serum from septic infants treated with intravenous immunoglobulin. Arch Dis Child 64:530–534
37. Dalhoff A (1984) Synergy between acylureidopenicillins and immunoglobulin G in experimental animals. Am J Med 76:91–100
38. Dalhoff A (1984) In vitro and in vivo effect of immunoglobulin G on the integrity of bacterial membranes. Infection 12:214–222
39. Offenbartel KS, Christensen P, Gullstrand P, Prellner K (1986) Synergism between gammaglobulin prophylaxis and penicillin treatment in experimental post-splenectomy sepsis in the rat. Int Arch Allery Appl Immunol 79:45–48
40. Cunningham-Rundles C, Siegal FP, Smithwick EM et al (1984) Efficacy of intravenous immunoglobulin in primary immunodeficiency disease. Ann Intern Med 101:435–439
41. Kark JD, Witztum E, Mazkin H et al (1984) The three-year incidence of non-B viral hepatitis morbidity in a controlled trial of pre-exposure immune serum globulin prophylaxis. Infection 12:251–255

42. Ohara H, Ebisawa I, Ohtani S (1986) Prophylactic efficacy of immune serum globulin against hepatitis A. Jpn J Exp Med 56:229–233
43. Sorenson RU, Polmar SH (1984) Efficacy and safety of high-dose intravenous immune globulin therapy for antibody deficiency syndromes. Am J Med 76 [Suppl 3A]:83–90
44. Glauser MP, Zanetti G, Baumgartner JD, Cohen J (1991) Septic shock: pathogenesis. Lancet 338:732–736
45. Dwyre JM (1992) Manipulating the immune system with immune globulin. N Engl J Med 326:107–116
46. Leung DYM, Burns JC, Newburger JW, Geha RS (1987) Reversal of lymphocyte activation in vivo in the Kawasaki syndrome by intravenous gamma globulin. J Clin Invest 79:468–472
47. Mannhalter JW, Eibl MM (1986) Polymeric IgG down modulates antigen presentation by human monocytes. In Eibl MM, Rosen FS (eds) Primary immunodeficiency diseases. Elsevier, Amsterdam, pp 281–286
48. Mannhalter JW, Ahmad R, Wolf HM, Eibl MM (1987) Effect of polymeric IgG on human monocyte functions. Int Arch Allergy Appl Immunol 82:159–167
49. Tsubakio T, Kurata Y, Katagiri S et al (1983) Alteration of T cell subsets and immunoglobulin synthesis in vitro during high dose γ-globulin therapy in patients with idiopathic thrombocytopenic purpura. Clin Exp Immunol 53:697–702
50. Pollack M, Young LS (1979) Protective activity of antibodies to exotoxin A and lipopolysaccharide at the onset of Pseudomonas aeruginosa septicemia in man. J Clin Invest 63:276–286
51. Baker CJ, Melish ME, Hall RT et al (1992) Intravenous immune globulin for the prevention of nosocomial infection in low-birth-weight neonates. N Engl J Med 327:213–219
52. Chirico G, Rondini G, Plebani A et al (1987) Intravenous gammaglobulin therapy for prophylaxis of infection in high risk neonates. J Pediatr 110:437–442
53. Haque KN, Zaidi MH, Haque SK et al (1986) Intravenous immunoglobulin for prevention of sepsis in preterm and low-birth-weight infants. Pediatr Infect Dis 5:622–625
54. Hill HR, Shigeoka AO, Gonzales LA, Christensen RD (1989) Intravenous immune globulin use in newborns. J Allergy Clin Immunol 84:617–624
55. Magny JF, Bremard-Oury C, Brault D et al (1991) Intravenous immunoglobulin therapy for prevention of infection in high risk premature infants: report of a multicenter, double-blind study. Pediatrics 88:437–443
56. Stabile A, Miceli Sopo S, Romanelli V et al (1988) Intravenous immunoglobulin for prophylaxis of neonatal sepsis in premature infants. Arch Dis Child 63:441–443
57. Bussel JB (1990) Intravenous gammaglobulin in the prophylaxis of late sepsis in very low-birth-weight infants: preliminary results of a randomized, double-blind, placebo-controlled trial. Rev Infect Dis 12 [Suppl 4]:S457–S462
58. Clapp DW, Kliegman RM, Baley JE et al (1989) Use of intravenously administered immune globulin to prevent nosocomial sepsis in low birth weight infants: report of a pilot study. J Pediatr 115:973–978
59. Kinney J, Mundorf L, Gleason C et al (1991) Efficacy and pharmakokinetics of intravenous immune globulin administration to high-risk neonates. Am J Dis Child 145:1233–1238
60. Besa EC (1984) Use of intravenous immunoglobulin in chronic lymphocytic leukemia. Am J Med 76 [Suppl 3A]:209–218
61. Gordon DS, Hearn EB, Spira TJ et al (1984) Phase I study of intravenous gamma globulin in multiple myeloma. Am J Med 76 [Suppl 3A] 111–116
62. Schedel I (1983) Intravenöse Immunglobulinsubstitution bei Patienten mit multiplem Myelom, Morbus Waldenström und chronischer lymphatischer Leukämie. In: Schmidt RE, Stroehmann I (eds) Immunglobuline – Grundlagen und klinische Anwendung. Karger, Basel, pp 52–58
63. Schmidt RE, Hartlapp JH, Niese D et al (1984) Reduction of infection frequency by intravenous gammaglobulins during intensive induction therapy for small cell carcinoma of the lung. Infection 12:167–170

64. Seybold JD, Bogdahn U, Seubert W, Krauseneck P (1991) 7S-Immunglobulin zur Infektprophylaxe bei Patienten mit malignen Hirntumoren unter zytostatischer Therapie, eine randomisierte prospektive Doppelblindstudie. Onkol Klin 3:38–48
65. Baumgartner JD, Glauser MP, McCutchan JA et al (1985) Prevention of gram-negative shock and death in surgical patients by prophylactic antibody to endotoxin core glycolipid. Lancet 2:59–63
66. Duswald KH, Müller K, Seifert J, Ring J (1980) Wirksamkeit von i. v. Gammaglobulin gegen bakterielle Infektionen chirurgischer Patienten – Ergebnisse einer kontrollierten, randomisierten klinischen Studie. Munch Med Wochenschr 122:832–836
67. Glinz W, Grob PJ, Nydegger UE et al (1985) Polyvalent immunoglobulins for prophylaxis of bacterial infections in patients following multiple trauma – a randomized, placebo-controlled study. Intensive Care Med 11:288–294
68. Kress HG, Scheidewig C, Engelhardt W et al (1989) Prediction and prevention, by immunological means, of septic complications after elective cardiac surgery. In: Schlag G, Redl H (eds) 2nd Vienna Shock Forum. Liss, New York, pp 1031–1035
69. Kress HG, Scheidewig C, Elert O (1990) Postoperative passive immunoprophylaxis prevents infections in "at-risk" patients after open-heart surgery. J Cardiothorac Anesth 4 [Suppl 3]:67
70. The Intravenous Immunoglobulin Collaborative Study Group (1992) Prophylactic intravenous administration of standard immune globulin as compared with core-lipopolysaccharide immune globulin in patients at high risk of postsurgical infection. N Engl J Med 327:234–240
71. Kress HG, Gehrsitz P, Elert O (1987) Predictive value of skin testing, neutrophil migration and C-reactive protein for postoperative infections in cardiopulmonary bypass patients. Acta Anaesthesiol Scand 31:397–404
72. Calandra T, Glauser M, Schellekens J, Verhoef J (1988) Treatment of gram-negative spetic shock with human IgG antibody to Escherichia coli J5: a prospective, double blind, randomized trial. J Infect Dis 158:312–319
73. Zanetti G, Glauser MP, Baumgartner JD (1991) Use of immunoglobulins in prevention and treatment of infection in critically ill patients: review and critique. Rev Infect Dis 13:985–992
74. Haque KN, Zaidi MH, Bakahim H (1988) IgM-enriched intravenous immunoglobulin therapy in neonatal sepsis. Am J Dis Child 142:1293–1296
75. Sidiropoulos D, Böhme U, von Muralt G et al (1981) Immunoglobulinsubstitution bei der Behandlung der neonatalen Sepsis. Schweiz Med Wochenschr 111:1649–1655
76. Just HM, Metzger M, Vogel W, Pelka RB (1986) Therapeutic effects of immunoglobulin in intensive care patients with severe infections. Klin Wochenschr 64:245–256
77. Jesdinsky HJ, Tempel G, Castrup HJ, Seifert J (1987) Cooperative group of additional immunoglobulin therapy in severe bacterial infections: results of a multicenter randomized controlled trial in cases of diffuse fibrinopurulent peritonitis. Klin Wochenschr 65:1132–1138
78. Dominioni L, Dionigi R, Zanello M et al (1991) Effects of high-dose IgG on survival of surgical patients with sepsis scores of 20 or greater. Arch Surg 126:236–240
79. Schedel I, Dreikhausen U, Nentwig B et al (1991) Treatment of gram-negative septic shock with an immunoglobulin preparation: a prospective, randomized clinical trial. Crit Care Med 19:1104–1113
80. Ziegler EJ, McCutchan JA, Fierer J et al (1982) Treatment of gram-negative bacteremia and shock with human antiserum to a mutant Escherichia coli. N Engl J Med 307:1225–1230

Arachidonic Acid Metabolism in Sepsis: What is the Role of Cyclooxygenase Inhibition?

G. R. Bernard

Introduction

Since the first report of Northover and Subramanian [1] in 1962 on the use of aspirin to prevent death due to endotoxin shock in mongrel dogs, there has been a near-continuous stream of investigations the results of which support the potential for cyclooxygenase inhibition in sepsis syndrome. Many of these studies are survival studies, i.e., intervention with cyclooxygenase inhibitors is intended to determine effects on mortality. It is clear from these data that treatment with inhibitors of cyclooxygenase improves survival, though the biochemical and physiological mechanisms responsible for this beneficial effect have not been well understood until recently [2–8]. With the discovery of arachidonic acid and its metabolites, which include prostaglandins, thromboxanes, and leukotrienes, interpretations of the physiologic effects of cyclooxygenase inhibition have been attributed to key metabolites of arachidonic acid [5, 6]. In the past 15 years data have become available linking abnormalities of prostaglandin metabolism with airway mechanics abnormalities, pulmonary hypertension and the associated hypoxemia, cardiovascular collapse, and multiple organ system failure [6–14].

There are now data to support the hypothesis that constrictor products of arachidonic acid, especially thromboxane A_2 (TxA_2), are produced in large quantities during human sepsis with or without shock [15]. These compounds are associated with and, on the basis of animal studies, are thought to be responsible for increased airflow resistance, decreased dynamic lung compliance, hypoxemia, and increased work of breathing [16, 17]. In addition, potent dilator prostaglandins, especially prostacyclin (PGI_2), are released into the circulation by vascular endothelium and act systemically to produce persistent systemic vasodilation and shock, thus contributing to progressive ischemic damage in the lung and other organs [12–14]. It is interesting to consider how constrictor and dilator effects of these metabolites can coexist in the same organism. This phenomenon may be explained by the fact that most active metabolites of arachidonate have extremely short half-lives, so that most effects occur in the immediate proximity of their production. It is also conceivable that differences in receptor concentrations in systemic versus pulmonary vascular beds may be important. In studies using whole animals it is difficult if not impossible to answer these kinds of mechanistic questions. In spite of these problems, studies of bronchodilator and pulmonary vasodilator effects of thromboxane inhibition resulting from use of either cyclooxygenase inhibitors or the more specific thromboxane receptor antagonists have been carried out in sheep [2, 14]. Cyclooxygenase inhibition has also been studied in those models where systemic vasodilation is the more prominent response to endotoxin, such as the primate and septic dog. In those experiments, cyclooxygenase inhibitors such as ibuprofen are associated with systemic vasoconstriction that results in restoration of blood pressure and improved survival [13]. In the latter studies, effects on blood pressure were noted even when ibuprofen was administered after endotoxin. Studies have also shown that TxA_2 and PGI_2, for example, can be produced in varying proportions from cells of different tissue beds. In this light, it has been shown that, when activated, macrophages from different species and different sites (e.g., pulmonary resident macrophages versus peritoneal resident macrophages) produce different arachidonic acid metabolites. Specifically, macrophages of pulmonary origin tend to produce more thromboxane and less prostacyclin than macrophages of peritoneal (systemic circulation) origin [18–20].

Because corticosteroids are often used in the therapy of the acute respiratory distress syndrome (ARDS) in humans, and because some studies have suggested that at least part of the mechanism of these drugs is related to inhibition of prostaglandin production, we and others examined the effect of methylprednisolone in septic patients and patients with ARDS caused chiefly by sepsis [21–24]. None of these trials were able to demonstrate a beneficial effect of corticosteroids on sepsis and related disorders.

It is now known that methylprednisolone, in concentrations generally found in patients receiving doses in the range of the ARDS study referred to above [24], does not substantially affect metabolism of arachidonic acid to thromboxane and prostacyclin. However, ibuprofen is capable of inhibiting cyclooxygenase at very low concentrations relative to the maximum achievable plasma levels in patients. The cyclooxygenase of mouse peritoneal macrophages is 95% inhibited by 30 μM (approximately 6 μg/ml) ibuprofen and 84% inhibited by 3 μM (approximately 0.6 μg/ml) ibuprofen [18].

The remainder of this paper will focus on the potential of ibuprofen rather than other cyclooxygenase inhibitors in sepsis because there is a very large body of information from animal models on this agent and human studies have been undertaken. It seems likely that cyclooxygenase inhibitors other than ibuprofen would achieve the same results based on what is known about the mechanism of action of this agent.

Basic Studies

As mentioned above, arachidonic acid metabolites may be produced in different proportions by macrophages of differing origin. Pulmonary macrophages harvested from mice and stimulated by zymosan have a response which is different from peritoneal macrophages in the relative proportions of PGI_2 and TxA_2 released. TxA_2 is the predominate product of pulmonary macrophages and no measurable PGI_2 is produced, whereas peritoneal macrophages produce some TxA_2 but 5- to 10-fold more PGI_2.

Several reports indicate that ibuprofen is capable of inhibiting leukocyte responses including aggregation, locomotion, enzyme release, and oxidative burst with the associated release of oxygen radicals [17, 18]. Ibuprofen has also been shown to slow the rate constant of the association of the chemotactic peptide FMLP, which mimics the effect of activated complement, with its receptor on the surface of the granulocyte (70% decrease at ibuprofen level of 125 μg/ml) while allowing dissociation of the peptide from the granulocyte to proceed uninhibited. Blockade of granulocyte surface receptors for inflammatory stimuli and the subsequent inhibition of chemotaxis and aggregation may be important in the clinical effects of ibuprofen that are seen at blood levels obtainable with oral therapy, i.e., between 60 and 250 μg/ml [19, 20].

Animal Studies

Data from animal studies have been used extensively to determine the potential for cyclooxygenase inhibition, because appropriate animal models of human disease offer a controlled situation in which to study sepsis pathophysiology. It is important to note that while most of these studies involve *"pretreatment"* with ibuprofen, we and others have been able to confirm similar effects when ibuprofen is administered as a *"post-treatment"*, that is, after the initiation of sepsis syndrome and in a time frame which might be considered to be within the realities of clinical medicine and clinical research.

Alterations in pulmonary hemodynamics are a major component of the whole animal response to the administration of a number of agents including endotoxin, glass beads, air emboli, and others, though not oleic acid [2]. The sheep model of endotoxin-induced ARDS has been particularly useful in studying and elucidating the mechanisms responsible for these changes. Infusion of *E. coli* endotoxin produces a consistent major increase in pulmonary artery pressure (PAP) and pulmonary vascular resistance (PVR) beginning approximately 30–45 min after infusion and persisting for at least 4–5 h. Tumor necrosis factor (TNF) produces a strikingly similar effect except that the response is nearly immediate, a finding compatible with the scenario that endotoxin activates macrophages to produce TNF, therefore, suggesting that the endotoxin-induced changes on the pulmonary vasculature are TNF-mediated. Regardless of the model of acute pulmonary hypertension, cyclooxygenase inhibitors have been capable of causing major attenuation and even total blockade of this response whether delivered prior to or following endotoxin administration [2, 16, 17]. Furthermore, some studies have suggested that the majority of TxA_2 produced after endotoxin originates in the lung and, possibly because of TxA_2's short half-life, does not cause significant systemic vasoconstriction [2].

Changes in dynamic compliance and airflow resistance are also well-documented responses to administration of endotoxin in the sheep model of ARDS. These changes are severe: a halving of dynamic compliance and a 5- to 10-fold increase in airflow resistance occurs within 30–45 min after endotoxin infusion and persists for at least 4–5 h [8, 15]. These changes are reversible by either nitroprusside, a nonspecific smooth muscle dilator, or ibuprofen, suggesting that some of these changes are due to bronchospasm rather than to pulmonary edema, airway secretions, or atelectasis [25]. The relative specificity of ibuprofen as an inhibitor of thromboxane production strongly suggests that thromboxane is the likely second messenger responsible for endotoxin-induced increases in airway resistance.

Although studies in the sheep endotoxin model show that pretreatment with ibuprofen and other cyclooxygenase inhibitors reduces pulmonary lymph flow, this effect appears to be due to a reduction in the early increase in hydrostatic pressure brought on by endotoxin. Studies by Gnidec et al. [26] in the sheep cecal ligation model have shown that ibuprofen given 24 h into the development of sepsis syndrome prevented the increase in lung lymph flow and lung water content. Ibuprofen has been shown to protect lung microvascular integrity in the canine oleic acid, sheep thrombin microembolism, rat endotoxin alveolitis, and smoke-induced pulmonary edema models [11, 27, 28].

Cyclooxygenase blockade appears to improve oxygenation in a number of models of abnormal gas exchange. In the ethchlorvynol-induced unilateral acute lung injury model in dogs, ibuprofen was shown to both prevent the development of hypoxemia if given as pretreatment and to restore oxygenation to control levels if given 60 min after injury [29]. In the canine lobar atelectasis model of hypoxemia, indomethacin restored pulmonary shunt to normal levels compared to controls [30]. In the sheep endotoxin model, pretreatment with ibuprofen prevented the development of hypoxemia after endotoxin [8].

The complexities of the multiple organ system failure (MOSF) seen in human sepsis have limited the elucidation of mechanisms through use of animal models. In spite of these difficulties some studies have demonstrated beneficial effects of cyclooxygenase inhibition on this phenomenon. Rats given infusions of live *E. coli* had significantly improved 24 h survival rates over control animals [31]. Newborn rats given group B streptococci (a model of neonatal sepsis) have shown significantly improved survival if given ibuprofen at the time of bacterial injection and a trend toward improved survival if treated as late as 4 h after bacterial injection. Investigations using the peritonitis and endotoxin models have shown that ibuprofen, whether given as pretreatment or several hours to 1 day after development of sepsis syndrome, is capable of improving systemic blood pressure, decreasing lactic acidosis, and restoring systemic vascular resistance [12, 13, 26]. There is even a suggestion that the massive resuscitation given patients in shock can activate the arachidonic acid cascade. This is supported by the finding that sheep (and humans) given very rapid infusions of concentrated albumin develop pulmonary hypertension and increased pulmonary artery wedge pressure (PAWP), which are blocked by pretreatment with ibuprofen. There is also evidence that some of the myocardial dysfunction occurring in sepsis is prostaglandin-related and may be reversible [14].

Of major concern when considering the use of ibuprofen for clinical studies is the fact that in certain clinical settings (not sepsis), ibuprofen has been shown to worsen preexisting renal failure. The concern in sepsis is that ibuprofen will aggravate the acutely ischemic kidney, possibly by inhibition of dilator prostaglandins, especially prostaglandin E_2 (PGE_2), resulting in decreased renal blood flow [32]. Studies in the canine sepsis model indicate that this renal vasoconstriction may be preventable by concomitant use of renal vasodilators such as low-dose dopamine without compromising the beneficial effects of ibuprofen [33]. It is possible that the effect of ibuprofen to reduce thromboxane in the circulation in sepsis might actually improve renal blood flow. This question will not be settled without adequate clinical study.

Human Data

Increasingly, data are becoming available with regard to the participation of prostaglandins in the pulmonary, cardiovascular, and other organ dysfunction of sepsis syndrome. Available data suggest that both thromboxane B_2 (TxB_2) (a stable metabolic of TxA_2) and 6-keto-prostaglandin $F_{1\alpha}$ (6-keto-$PGF_{1\alpha}$) a stable metabolite of PGI_2) are elevated in sepsis in humans [15] and that there is a positive correlation between plasma levels and mortality [31]. Only very recently have reliable techniques become readily available to study prostaglandin metabolism in man. The ability to measure metabolites indicative of *in vivo* prostaglandin production but which are not produced *ex vivo* in blood samples, and measurements of metabolites in urine, a fluid generally free of cells which can cause *ex vivo* production, constitute a major advance in this area [34].

At least one study has shown that abnormal lung mechanics are an important feature of ARDS as would be suggested by the animal models described above. Studies of gas exchange abnormalities in ARDS have focused on parenchymal alterations resulting from atelectasis, edema, and cellular infiltration, but the contribution of active airway dysfunction (bronchospasm) to ARDS has received little attention. Long-term survivors of ARDS appear to have increased bronchial reactivity, and data available from endotoxin-treated sheep demonstrate major airway mechanics changes prior to the development of significant pulmonary edema [2, 8, 17, 25]. If airway constriction is a major finding in sepsis, then the presence of dilator prostaglandins could produce hypoxemia by interfering with ventilation-perfusion matching and creation of shunt. Ibuprofen, through inhibition of vasodilating prostaglandins and airway-constricting thromboxane, could restore hypoxic vasoconstriction. Although no clinical studies exist to confirm or deny this line of reasoning, studies in patients with respiratory failure secondary to pneumonia have shown benefit to gas exchange through use of cyclooxygenase inhibition. Hanly et al. [35] studied ten such patients requiring mechanical ventilation and found an increase in PaO_2/FiO_2 from 128 ± 51 to 155 ± 53 mm Hg (mean $\pm$ SD) when patients were given indomethacin 1 mg/kg either orally or rectally ($p < 0.005$). This effect on oxygenation persisted for at least 2 h. In addition to potential benefits secondary to improved gas exchange, bronchodilation may lower peak and mean airway pressure, reduce the associated risk of barotrauma, prevent further parenchymal injury, and reduce the work of breathing [36].

If, as the animal studies would suggest, at least some of the pulmonary edema seen is a result of pulmonary hypertension secondary to venoconstriction, then it is possible that reduction in pulmonary microvascular pressure may benefit these patients. Further, if afterload on the right ventricle is reduced by lowering pulmonary vascular resistance, as is seen in the sheep endotoxin model, from often extremely high levels, then there would be the potential for improving cardiac output and oxygen delivery [37].

Studies in normal human volunteers given endotoxin clearly show that endotoxin causes release of TNF into the blood in measureable quantities. This release correlates with increased temperature, heart rate, as well as plasma ACTH and epinephrine levels. Although shock did not develop at these doses of endotoxin, pretreatment with orally administered ibuprofen blocked all symptoms and attenuated the fever, tachycardia, ACTH peak, and epinephrine peak even though TNF release was not blocked. Thus, the effects of low-dose endotoxin administration to humans appears to be largely mediated through the elaboration of TNF, which in turn produces physiologic responses through activation of the cyclooxygenase pathway [38].

Current Clinical Trials

We performed a second set of studies in order to characterize the airway mechanics abnormalities of patients with septic ARDS receiving mechanical ventilation both inclusive and exclusive of the effects of the endotracheal tube. Others have looked at effects of endotracheal tubes in non-ARDS patients, but no such studies are available in ARDS patients. We found that, even exclusive of the endotracheal tube resistance, patients with ARDS have airflow resistances more than five times those seen in other intubated patients, and that dynamic compliance (also grossly abnormal) correlates with PaO_2/PAO_2. Not surprising, but useful clinically, was the fact that peak airway pressure correlates with airflow resistance [35].

Finally, we conducted pilot studies of the effect of ibuprofen on patients with sepsis syndrome [15]. These studies were intended to determine if cyclooxygenase inhibition in humans (1) is possible, (2) results in clinically measureable positive results, and (3) is reasonably safe in the patient population under consideration here. Urinary concentrations of metabolites of thromboxane and prostacyclin in patients with well-defined sepsis syndrome undergoing a double-blind, placebo-controlled pilot study were measured. Previous investigators had shown that normal urinary concentrations of 2,3-dinor-6-keto-$PGF_{1\alpha}$ and 2,3-dinor-thromboxane B_2, the stable urinary metabolites of PGI_2 and TxA_2, were in the range of 0.15–0.20 ng/mg creatinine. At the time of study entry, patients with sepsis syndrome were shown to have markedly elevated values (prostacyclin metabolite concentration of 3.9 ± 2.0 ng/mg creatinine and thromboxane metabolite concentrations of 2.9 ± 0.7 ng/mg creatinine). These levels are 10- to 20-fold greater than normal, arguing for significant systemic platelet/macrophage activation and endothelial cell perturbation during sepsis syndrome. Values of both these metabolites remained significantly elevated for up to 5 days after enrollment in the study.

Ibuprofen-treated patients experienced a significant decrease in heart rate, body temperature, peak airway pressure, and minute ventilation. The ibuprofen-treated group experienced a significant decrease in urinary 2,3-dinor-6-keto-$PGF_{1\alpha}$ and 2,3-dinor-thromboxane B_2. There was a positive correlation between the thromboxane metabolite and peak airway and pulmonary artery pressures and an inverse correlation between the prostacyclin metabolite and mean systemic blood pressure. There also appeared to be a trend toward an increase in blood pressure, especially for those patients in shock at study entry, and more rapid resolution of pulmonary changes in ARDS blood gas criteria. The findings in this study were consistent with the hypothesis that both constrictor and dilator prostaglandins contribute to the pathophysiology in septic patients [15].

We found that urinary concentrations of the major metabolites of prostacyclin and thromboxane were markedly increased over those in normal subjects and that ibuprofen-treated patients experienced a marked decline in these levels. Abnormal physiology such as tachycardia, increased minute ventilation, high peak airway pressure and oxygenation, and hypotension tended to improve with therapy. No adverse effects of therapy were noted either with regard to bleeding abnormalities or impairment of renal function.

The pilot study indicated that ibuprofen was reasonably safe in sepsis and demonstrated potential efficacy. A larger, multicenter, randomized, placebo-controlled trial of intravenous ibuprofen delivered over 48 h to patients with sepsis sydnrome supported by the National Institutes of Helth, Division of Lung Diseases is currently underway. This larger study is designed to confirm the results of the pilot and to determine whether these beneficial effects seen in the preclinical and clinical work thus far will translate into improved survival of patients with sepsis syndrome.

References

1. Northover BJ, Subramanian G (1962) Analgesic-antipyretic drugs as antagonists of endotoxin shock in dogs. J Pathol Bacteriol 83:463–468
2. Brigham KL, Meyrick B (1986) State of the art: endotoxin and lung injury. Am Rev Respir Dis 133:913–927
3. Fletcher JR, Ramwell PW (1977) Modification, by aspirin and indomethacin, of the haemodynamic and prostaglandin releasing effects of E. coli endotoxin in the dog. Br J Pharmacol 61:175–181
4. Parratt JR, Sturgess RM (1975) E. coli endotoxin shock in the cat: treatment with indomethacin. Br J Pharmacol 53:485–488
5. Harris RH, Zmudka M, Maddox Y, Ramwell PW, Fletcher JR (1980) Relationships of TXB_2 and 6-Keto PGF_{1a} of the hemodynamic changes during baboon endotoxic shock. Adv Prostaglandin Thromboxane Leukotriene Res 7:843–849
6. Bowers RE, Ellis EF, Brigham KL, Oates JA (1979) Effects of prostaglandin cyclic endoperoxides on the lung circulation of sheep. J Clin Invest 63:131–137
7. Hinshaw LB, Solomon LA, Erdos EG, Reins DA, Gunter BJ (1967) Effects of acetylsalicylic acid on the canine response to endotoxin. J Pharmacol Exp Ther 157:665–671
8. Snapper JR, Hutchison AA, Ogletree ML, Brigham KL (1983) Effects of cyclooxygenase inhibitors on the alterations in lung mechanics caused by endotoxemia in the unanesthetized sheep, J Clin Invest 72:63–76
9. Mizus I, Michael J, Summer W, Gurtner G (1983) Acid aspiration induced pulmonary artery pressure rise is attenuated by hypoxia or ibuprofen. Crit Care Med 11:241 (abstract)
10. Perkowski SZ, Havill AM, Flynn JT, Gee MH (1983) Role of intrapulmonary release of eicosanoids and superoxide anion as mediators of pulmonary dysfunction and endothelial injury in sheep with intermittent complement activation. Circ Res 53:574–583
11. Perlman MB, Johnson A, Malik AB (1987) Ibuprofen prevents thrombin-induced lung vascular injury: mechanism of effect. Am J Physiol 252:H605–H614
12. Kopolovic R, Thraikill KM, Martin DT, Ambrose T, Vento M, Carey LC, Cloutier CT (1984) Effects of ibuprofen on a porcine model of acute respiratory failure. J Surg Res 36:300–305
13. Jacobs ER, Soulsby ME, Bone RC, Wilson FJ Jr, Hiller FC (1987) Ibuprofen in canine endotoxin shock. J Clin Invest 70:536–541
14. Soulsby ME, Jacobs ER, Perlmutter BH, Bone RC (1984) Protection of myocardial function during endotoxin shock by ibuprofen. Prostaglandins Leukotrienes Med 13:295–305
15. Bernard GR, Reines HD, Halushka PV et al (1991) Prostacyclin and thromboxane A_2 formation is increased in human sepsis syndrome: effects of cyclooxygenase inhibition. Am Rev Respir Dis 144:1095–1101
16. Wright PW, Bernard GR (1988) Effects of metaproterenol, atropine and ibuprofen on lung function during the late phase of endotoxemia in sheep. Am Rev Respir Dis 137:179
17. Wright PW, Bernard GR (1989) Mechanisms of the late hemodynamic and airway mechanics response to endotoxin in the awake sheep. Am Rev Respir Dis 140:672–678
18. Rouzer CA, Scott WA, Hamill AL, Cohn ZA (1982) Synthesis of leukotriene C and other arachidonic acid metabolites by mouse pulmonary macrophages. J Exp Med 155:720–733
19. Brown KA, Collins AJ (1977) Action of nonsteroidal, anti-inflammatory drugs on human and rat peripheral leucocyte migration in vitro. Ann Rheum Dis 36:239–243
20. Kaplan HB, Edelson HS, Korchak HM, Given WP, Abramson S, Weissmann G (1984) Effects of non-steroidal anti-inflammatory agents on human neutrophil functions in vitro and in vivo. Biochem Pharmacol 33:371–378

21. Bone RC, Fisher CJ, Clemmer TP et al (1987) A controlled clinical trial of high-dose methylprednisolone in the treatment of severe sepsis and septic shock. N Engl J Med 317:653–658
22. Luce JM, Montgomery AB, Marks JD et al (1988) Ineffectiveness of high-dose methylprednisolone in preventing parenchymal lung injury and improving mortality in patients with septic shock. Am Rev Respir Dis 138:62–68
23. The Veterans Administration Systemic Sepsis Cooperative Group (1987) The effects of high-dose glucocorticoid therapy on mortality in patients with clinical signs of systemic sepsis. N Engl J Med 317:659–665
24. Bernard GR, Luce JM, Sprung CL et al (1987) High-dose corticosteroids in patients with the adult respiratory distress syndrome. N Engl J Med 317:1565–1570
25. Wright P, Ishihara Y, Bernard GR (1988) Effects of nitroprusside on lung mechanics and hemodynamics after endotoxemia in awake sheep. J Appl Physiol 64:2026–2032
26. Gnidec AG, Sibbald W, Cheung H, Metz CA (1988) Ibuprofen ameliorates an increase in pulmonary microvascular fluid flux in a sheep model of surgically-induced peritonitis and permeability edema. J Appl Physiol 65:1024–1032
27. Rinaldo JE, Pennock B (1986) Effects of ibuprofen on endotoxin-induced alveolitis. Am J Med Sci 291:29–38
28. Shinozawa Y, Hales C, Jung W, Burke J (1986) Ibuprofen prevents synthetic smoke-induced pulmonary edema. Am Rev Respir Dis 134:1145–1148
29. Sprague RS, Stephanson AH, Dahms TE, Asner NG, Lonigro AJ (1987) Effects of ibuprofen on the hypoxemia of established ethchlorvynol-induced unilateral acute lung injury in anesthetized dogs. Chest 92:1088–1093
30. Garrett RC, Thomas HM III (1983) Meclofenamate uniformly decreases shunt fraction in dogs with lobar atelectasis. J Appl Physiol 540:284–289
31. Cook JA, Wise WC, Butler RR, Reines HD, Rambo W, Halushka PV (1984) The potential role of thromboxane and PGI_2 in endotoxic and septic shock. Am J Emerg Med 2:28–37
32. Passmore JC, Hartupee DA, Jackson BA (1987) Urinary and renal papillary solutes during cyclooxygenase inhibition with ibuprofen. J Lab Clin Med 110:807–812
33. Fink MP, Nelso R, Roethael R (1985) Low-dose dopamine preserves renal blood flow in endotoxin shocked dogs treated with ibuprofen. J Surg Res 38:582–591
34. FitzGerald GA, Pedersen AK, Patrono C (1983) Analysis of prostacyclin and thromboxane biosynthesis in cardiovascular disease. Circulation 67:1174–1177
35. Hanly PJ, Roberts D, Dobson K, Light RB (1987) Effect of indomethacin on arterial oxygenation in critically ill patients with severe bacterial pneumonia. Lancet i:351–354
36. Wright PW, Marini JJ, Bernard GR (1988) Increased airway resistance contributes to impaired lung mechanics in the ARDS. Am Rev Respir Dis 137:137
37. Hasselström LJ, Eliasen K, Mogensen T, Andersen JB (1985) Lowering pulmonary artery pressure in a patient with severe acute respiratory failure. Intensive Care Med 11:48–50
38. Michie HR, Manogue KR, Spriggs DR et al (1988) Detection of circulating tumor necrosis factor after endotoxin administration. N Engl J Med 318:1481–1486

Improvement of Monocyte Function – A New Therapeutic Approach?

W. D. Döcke, U. Syrbe, A. Meinecke, C. Platzer, A. Makki, K. Asadullah, C. Klug, H. Zuckermann, P. Reinke, H. Brunner, R. von Baehr and H. D. Volk

Introduction

Sepsis is a clinical syndrome that has become increasingly important in the last decades. Despite modern intensive care and antibiotic treatment, mortality of sepsis is high, ranging from 30%–40% in patients without shock and up to 70% in patients with septic shock [1]. Therefore, new therapeutic strategies are needed for this life threatening complication.

The role of the immune system in the pathogenesis of septic disease is ambivalent. It is well established that patients suffering from acquired immune deficiency (burn patients, polytrauma patients, patients undergoing major surgical procedures and transplant recipients) are predisposed to life threatening sepsis. Practically all late complications (morbidity and death) in surgical patients are due to infection [2]. Therefore, apart from appropriate surgical and antibiotic/antifungal therapy, reconstitution of that part of the immune system which is suppressed may be important for the clinical outcome of septic disease. However, uncontrolled immunostimulation (e.g., cytokines) may be harmful, as there is growing evidence that endogenous immune mediators (cytokines) play an important role in the imflammatory response against infectious agents [3].

When local infection develops into sepsis, a strong systemic reaction (whole body inflammation) occurs and cytokines, normally restricted to areas of local injury, can be detected systemically causing symptoms of septic shock [4]. One of these cytokines, tumor necrosis factor-α (TNF), is now regarded as a central mediator of the pathophysiological changes associated with bacteremia and sepsis syndrome [5]. Other cytokines such as interleukin-1 (IL-1) or the immunostimulatory cytokine interferon-γ (IFN-γ) act snyergistically with TNF in inducing septic shock in mice [6]. As a result, recent approaches using unspecific immunotherapy in septic disease are intended to neutralize the mediators of whole body inflammation or to inhibit their production. However, despite the promising results with anti-TNF monoclonal antibodies (anti-TNF) or interleukin-1 receptor antagonist (IL-1RA) in animal models of sepsis [7–10], several important aspects of pathophysiology should be kept in mind:

1. TNF and IL-1 have a short half-life in circulation and it should be difficult to start with the therapy on time.

2. Systemic treatment with anti-inflammatory mediators (IL-1RA or anti-TNF) may not be successful in cases with excessive compartmental inflammatory responses. So, anti-TNF treatment did not succeed in animal models of septic or sterile peritonitis [11, 12].
3. When considering the use of anti-TNF (or IL-1RA) therapies, the role of TNF (and IL-1) in anti-infectious defense must be taken into account. Experimental models of severe subacute gram-negative infection have shown a pattern of TNF release different from that after bolus inoculation. Anti-TNF failed to prevent death in these models or even increased mortality [12]. Moreover, anti-TNF may inhibit the closing off of infectious foci by decreasing the stimulatory action of TNF on fibrogenesis [13]. In agreement with this, anti-TNF enhanced the deleterious effects of cecal ligation and puncture in mice [14].

Most importantly, there are marked differences between almost all animal experiments and the clinical syndrome sepsis. While most experimental settings evaluate the benefit of anti-inflammatory therapy before or in the very early phase the onset of experimental sepsis, in the hospital the septic state may last weeks or even months. Many patients who survived the acute phase of septic shock because of modern intensive care died from multiple organ failure and persistent (opportunistic) infections weeks or even months later.

Recent strategies of unspecific immunotherapy have focused on the early period of whole body inflammation. Very little is known about the immune mechanisms that may be involved in the prolonged septic state and late death after the resolution of hyperacute septic shock. With this background, it may not be surprising that treatment with anti-inflammatory agents (anti-TNF, IL-1RA) seems to be successful in a subgroup of septic patients only [15].

Obviously, the development of strategies of immunotherapy for sepsis has to be paralleled by the development of diagnostic parameters in order to evaluate the individual patient's immune system. The state of the patient's immune system at the time of decision making should be the basis for the initiation of immunotherapy such as anti-inflammatory therapy or possible immunostimulatory therapy.

Monocytic cells probably have a pivotal role in mediating "physiological" and "harmful" anti-infectious responses. They can kill intracellular germs, release inflammatory mediators (cytokines, prostaglandins, complement), process and present antigens to specific T cells, remove and detoxify endotoxin. Therefore, in order to find relevant parameters for the present state of the immune system and for the individual prognosis of septic patients, we focussed our studies on the characterization of phenotype and function of monocytes in patients suffering from septic disease.

Inactivation of Monocytes in Septic Disease — Association with Fatal Outcome (Immunoparalysis)

Prognostic Value of Monocytic HLA-DR Expression for Clinical Management of Transplant Recipients

Transplant recipients suffering from septic disease. Sepsis is a life threatening complication of transplantation. The dilemma for transplant physicians in such a case results from the lack of objective parameters for the immunosuppressive management of these patients. Two alternate risks need to be minimized: death from septic disease or loss of graft due to uncontrolled reduction of immunosuppression.

Recently, we described the usefulness of an immune monitoring program as a guide for immunosuppression in allograft recipients with septic complications [16]. To judge from cytofluorometric analyses of mononuclear cells, HLA-DR antigen expression on monocytes seems to be a very helpful parameter for the clinical management of this life threatening complication in immunosuppressed patients. Monocytic HLA-DR expression was measured by dual monoclonal antibody staining and flow cytometry. Table 1 shows the uptdate of the above mentioned data. Septic transplant recipients were found to fall into two categories: those with extremely decreased expression of HLA-DR antigen on monocytes (45 of 77 patients) and patients with normal or marginally decreased HLA-DR antigen expression on monocytes (32 of 77 patients). The persistence of low HLA-DR antigen expression was associated with fatal outcome due to septic multiple organ failure (MOF). Reconstitution of diminished HLA-DR antigen expression after rapid tapering of immunosuppression was associated with a favorable outcome of sepsis. In septic patients with low HLA-DR expression on monocytes (<30%) who were continued on immunosuppression, mortality was >90%. Mortality was <10% in those with a low proportion of HLA-DR+monocytes whose immunosuppression was rapidly tapered.

While rapid tapering of immunosuppression in septic patients with normal or only marginally decreased HLA-DR antigen expression resulted in irre-

Table 1. Clinical outcome of transplant patients with septic disease. (From [61])

HLA-DR+ monocytes	Rapid tapering of immunosuppression	Patient survival	Graft survival
<30%	No	1/12 (8%)	—
<30%	Yes	30/33 (90%)*	29/30 (98%)
>30%	No	28/28 (100%)	28/28 (100%)
>30%	Yes	4/4 (100%)	0/4 (0%)

* $p<0.01$ (with respect to the above group); x^2 assay.

versible rejection, loss of graft has been observed in only one of 30 patients (liver graft recipient) in the group of patients with low HLA-DR antigen expression. Remarkably, patients in the last-mentioned group suffered significantly more frequently from opportunistic candida infections compared to the former group (40% vs 3%, $p<0.01$).

Monocytic MHC class II expression is known to have a central role in immunoregulation [17]. Our observations confirm that drastic reduction of monocytic MHC class II expression reflects a state of the immune system in which it is neither able to defend pathogens nor to reject allografts. Therefore, we termed this phenomenon immunoparalysis.

Iatrogenic oversuppression in transplant recipients. It is well established that HLA-class II antigen expression on monocytes/macrophages is regulated by different exogenous and endogenous mediators. T cell-derived cytokines such as interferon (IFN)-γ and granulocyte-macrophage colony-stimulating factor (GM-CSF) up-regulate HLA-class II antigen expression on monocytes [18–20]. Therefore, we wondered whether the loss of HLA-DR antigens on septic monocytes may result from a "cytokine lack syndrome" due to T cell-targeted immunosuppression. In fact, high-dose immunosuppressive regimens (i.e., prophylactic anti-T cell antisera (ATG) or anti-rejection therapy by ATG or methylprednisolone bolus) induced a temporary decrease of HLA-DR+monocytes. A drop of HLA-DR+monocytes to <30% (normal value: 85%–96%) following high-dose immunosuppression was associated with an increased risk for bacteremia/fungemia (Table 2). Therefore tapering of immunosuppression is indicated in such cases. Failing recovery of HLA-DR+monocytes after high-dose immunosuppression was often the first sign of septic complications.

Table 2. Association between drop in HLA-DR antigen expression on monocytes due to prophylactic high-dose immunosuppression and incidence of severe infections in transplant recipients. (From [61])

Infection	Incidence of systemic infections[a]	
	HLA-DR+monocytes <30% (1–2 days)	HLA-DR+moncytes >30%
Viremia	14/48 (29%)	8/43 (19%)
Bacteremia	15/48 (32%)	2/43 (5%)*
Fungemia	12/48 (25%)	2/43/(5%)*

* $p<0.01$.
[a] Follow-up 4 weeks after transplantation.

Prognostic Value of Monocytic HLA-DR Expression for Clinical Outcome in Surgical Patients with Septic Complications

Next we were interested to know whether the phenomenon of decreased HLA-DR antigen expression on monocytes is restricted to septic patients who received immunosuppression. In summary, we examined more than 400 patients admitted to the intensive care unit (ICU) because of septic syndrome (polytrauma patients, burned patients, patients suffering from perforation of gastrointestinal tract or acute pancreatitis) during the last 5 years. Patients were followed up two to three times per week until release from the ICU or hospital (more than 3000 cytofluorometrical investigations).

As in septic transplant recipients, patients differed with respect to HLA-DR antigen expression on their blood monocytes (Fig. 1). Patients with fatal outcome showed a marked and persistent decrease of the proportion and the absolute number of HLA-DR+monocytes. We have never seen

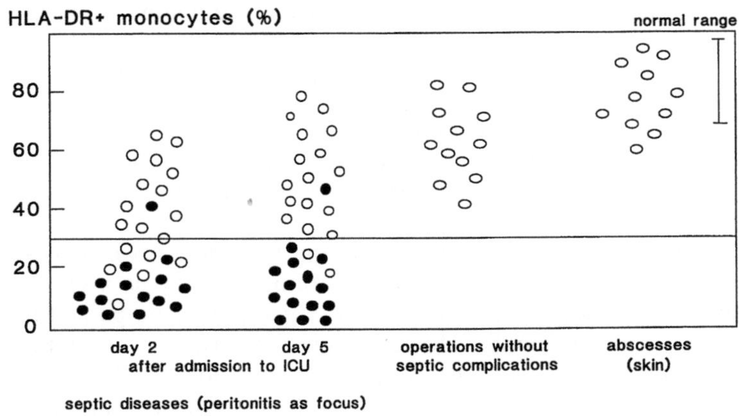

Fig. 1. Principal pattern of alterations in HLA-DR antigen expression on monocytes from surgical patients with and without septic complications.
Open circles, survivors; *closed circles,* nonsurvivors

Table 3. Predictive value of persistent decrease of HLA-DR antigen expression on monocytes for the clinical outcome of surgical patients with septic disease. (From [61])

HLA-DR+ monocytes <30%	Survival rate
Persistent for at least 5 days	12/98 (12%)
Not found or only short-term	131/149 (88%)*

* $p<0.01$; χ^2 assay.

a patient with low HLA-DR antigen expression whose condition would have allowed release from the ICU.

Using a sensitive cytofluorometer (FACS scan, EPICS profile), the critical cut-off seems to be 30% of HLA-DR+monocytes. The persistence of low HLA-DR antigen expression (<30%) for more than 3–4 days predicts fatal outcome in more than 85% of patients. In contrast to this, mortality in the group of patients with normal or moderately decreased HLA-DR antigen expression (>40%) was relatively low (12%) and was rarely associated with detectable bacteremia (mostly polytraumatic patients with septic syndrome). A summary of results from patients with follow up of more than 5 days is given in Table 3.

Septic patients (transplant patients or surgical patients) with a low proportion of HLA-DR+monocytes also showed decreased expression of another HLA-class II antigen, the HLA-DQ (1% vs 23%, $p<0.01$). In contrast to this, the expression of HLA-class I antigen on monocytes and lymphocytes was not diminished, nor was the expression of HLA-class II antigens on B-lymphocytes. The loss of HLA-class II antigen expression seems to be restricted to monocytes. However, the involvement of the specific immune system is indicated by a T cell-lymphopenia the degree of which is dependent on the duration of persistent immunoparalysis [16, 21–23].

A correlation between decreased monocytic MHC class II antigen expression (after severe trauma, burn and major elective surgery) and enhanced incidence of infectious complications and/or unfavorable clinical outcome was also described by other groups [24–27]. Ertel et al. [28] described a diminished MHC class II expression on peritoneal macrophages after hemorrhage in mice.

Based on our own and the above quoted findings we suggest that a diminished MHC class II expression on monocytes may be a sensitive sign of immunodepression induced by events which are accompanied by an excessive inflammatory response. However, the close correlation with fatal outcome especially in septic disease may result from the fact that temporary immunodepression in this situation leads to insufficient elimination of already present inducers (e.g., germs) of the inflammatory response. This results in further immunodepression. This vicious circle may lead to the persistence of immunodepression (immunoparalysis: HLA-DR expression <30% for more than 5 days) with commonly no spontaneous recovery and a fatal clinical outcome.

Functional Alterations Associated with Diminished Monocytic HLA-DR Expression in Fatal Septic Disease

Next we wondered whether the phenotypical changes of monocytes are associated with functional defects [29].

Diminished antigen presentation. Monocytes from septic patients with fatal outcome (HLA-DR+monocytes <30%) were not able to present tetanus toxoid or anti-CD 3 monoclonal antibody (mAb) to HLA-matched allogeneic lymphocytes from healthy donors. Nonetheless, lymphocytes from these patients showed an almost normal response in the presence of monocytes from healthy controls. Monocytes from septic patients with nearly normal HLA-DR antigen expression (>40%) could present both antigens.

Diminished capacity to form reactive oxygen species. Monocytes from septic patients with immunoparalysis (HLA-DR+monocytes <30%) showed also a diminished capacity to form reactive oxygen species (cytofluorometric assessment by dihydrorhodamine 123 [30] in response to tumor promoting activity (TPA) compared with healthy controls (132 ± 7 vs 96 ± 6 fluorescence channels (log scale), $p < 0.01$).

Altered lipopolysaccharide-induced cytokine production. Furthermore, we tested the spontaneous and lipopolysaccharide (LPS)-induced release of several cytokines (TNF, IL-1β, IL-6, IL-8) by monocytes in short-term cultures.

As shown in Fig. 2, monocytes from septic patients with low HLA-DR antigen expression showed a diminished capacity to release proinflammatory cytokines in response to LPS (and TPA, not shown) stimulation as compared to monocytes from septic patients with nearly normal HLA-DR antigen expression and from controls.

The value of these results for the in vivo situation has been confirmed by analysis of mRNA expression for TNF in freshly isolated mononuclear cells. TNF mRNA was only rarely detected by semiquantitative polymerase chain reaction (PCR) (for method see [31]) in cells from septic patients with immunoparalysis (HLA-DR+monocytes <30%). Meanwhile, it was even more frequently found in monocytes from septic patients without immunoparalysis than in monocytes from healthy donors (Table 4).

Statistical analysis confirmed a highly significant positive correlation between the percentage of HLA-DR+monocytes and the monocytic secretion of proinflammatory cytokines in ex vivo functional assays. Therefore the determination of monocytic HLA-DR expression can serve as handy parameter for monitoring the functional state of monocytes in septic disease.

Fig. 3 illustrates the prognostic value of persistent depression of monocytic cytokine production and HLA-DR expression in two cases. In the first case (Fig. 3a) the septic patient showed immunoparalysis with markedly depressed cytokine production and HLA-DR expression on days 12 and 13, a

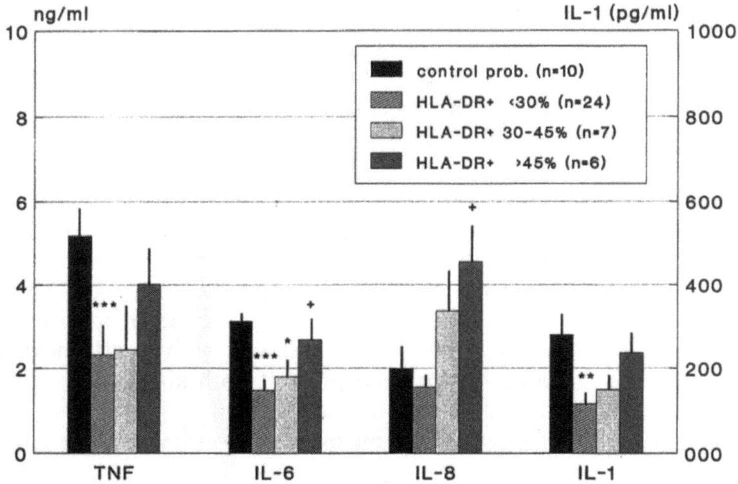

Fig. 2. Monocytes from septic patients with immunoparalysis have a diminished capacity to release inflammatory cytokines. Whole blood from septic patients and control donors was heparinized and suspended with RPMI (1:1). After short-term cultures (4 h) with 100 ng/ml lipopolysaccharide (LPS) cytokines were determined in supernatants by enzymoimmunoassays: tumor necrosis factor (*TNF*, Medgenix Diagnostics GmbH, Ratingen, FRG) and interleukin (IL)-1, IL-6, IL-8 (Biermann GmbH, Bad Nauheim, FRG). The readings were grouped according to the percentage of HLA-DR+monocytes in peripheral blood mononuclear cells of septic patients.
Mean values and standard error are given; * $p<0.05$, ** $p<0.01$, *** $p<0.001$ vs control group; $^{+}$ $p<0.05$ vs group with <30% HLA-DR+ monocytes; Student's *t* test for independent samples

temporary recovery, another drop of both parameters and finally a lasting recovery with normal HLA-DR expression and cytokine production. This patient survived. The second patient (Fig. 3b) showed persistent immunoparalysis and did not recover. Both parameters dropped even further and the patient died.

Munoz et al. [32] also described that monocytes from nonsurvivors with septic disease were marked by a persistently depressed capacity to produce cytokines. Mandi et al. [33] found a decrease of in vitro TNF production of leukocytes from septic patients with pancreatitis before fatal outcome.

In contrast to the diminished capacity of monocytes from septic patients with immunoparalysis to form proinflammatory cytokines, we observed a high spontaneous (not shown) and LPS-induced production of anti-inflammatory mediators (IL-1RA, soluble TNF receptor) in all septic patients, irrespective of existing immunoparalysis (Fig. 4).

Interestingly, unlike in whole blood cultures, we were not able to detect soluble TNF receptor (sTNF-R) after LPS stimulation in cultures of Ficoll Paque-separated mononuclear cells. These results indicate that the main source of sTNF-R in peripheral blood may be the granulocyte fraction.

Table 4. Detection of TNF mRNA in peripheral blood mononuclear cells of septic patients by competitive PCR[a]. (From [61])

Group	Detection of TNF mRNA	
	Yes	No
Healthy donors	8	8
Septic patients		
Immunoparalysis (HLA-DR+moncytes<30%)	2	16*
No immunoparalysis (HLA-DR+monocytes>45%)	26	4
Borderline group (HLA-DR+moncytes 30%–45%)	5	4

PCR, polymerase chain reaction; TNF, tumor necrosis factor; * $p<0.001$ (immunoparalysis vs no immunoparalysis); χ^2 assay.

[a] All cDNA samples to be compared were adjusted to contain equal amounts of input cDNA (competitive PCR between GAPDH cDNA and a control DNA). Equal band intensities of PCR products after the coamplification of equal amounts of GAPDH control fragment with the qualibrated cDNAs ensure that in the following PCRs with TNF-α specific primers identical amounts of cDNA were compared.

The even higher capacity to form anti-inflammatory cytokines may augment the deficiency of biological active inflammatory cytokines and anti-infectious defense in immunoparalytic septic patients.

Moreover, as it is known that during septic disease these anti-inflammatory mediators are enhanced in vivo [34–36], these results underline that the usefulness of therapy with IL-1RA or anti-TNF is rather doubtful in this situation.

In summary, these data on the inactivation of monocytes from septic patients with fatal outcome are in support of the concept of immunoparalysis as it is suggested for similar observations in septic transplant recipients.

Experimental Monocyte Inactivation

Inactivation of Monocytes by Phagocytic Stimuli in Vivo and In Vitro

Next we wondered what the cause of immunoparalysis might be. We found no correlation between the kind of bacteria detected in blood cultures and this phenomenon (gram-positive/gram-negative germs). Therefore, it does not seem to result from direct effects of specific bacterial toxins (e.g., LPS).

Only the detection of candida infection (antigen titer) was associated with the occurrence of immunoparalysis ($p<0.01$). This correlation may be ex-

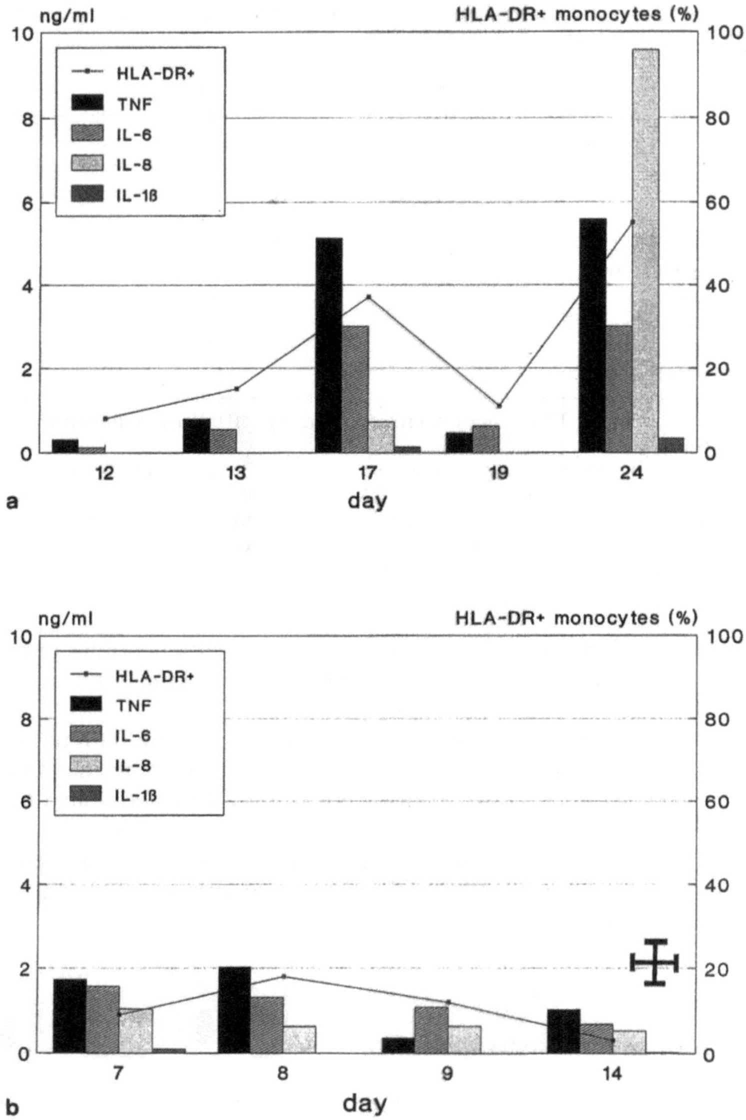

Fig. 3. a, b. Follow-up of monocytic HLA-DR expression and cytokine secretion capacity of two septic patients with immunoparalysis. **a** A septic patient with recovery of monocytic HLA-DR expression and cytokine secretion and good clinical outcome. **b** A septic patient with persistent depression of both parameters and fatal clinical outcome. Monocytic HLA-DR expression was cytofluorometrically monitored. Cytokine response to lipopolysaccharide (LPS; 100 ng/ml) was determined in supernatants of whole blood (1:1 with RPMI) short-term cultures (4 h) by enzymoimmunoassays (see Fig. 2).
TNF, tumor necrosis factor; IL, interleukin

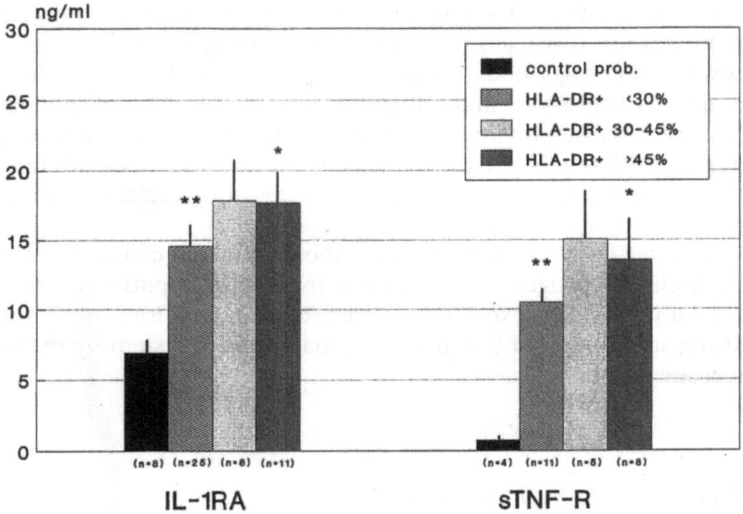

Fig. 4. White blood cells from septic patients with immunoparalysis have a normal or even enhanced capacity to release anti-inflammatory mediators. Whole blood from septic patients and control donors was heparinized and suspended in RPMI (1:1). After short-term cultures (4 h) with 100 ng/ml lipopolysaccharide (LPS), interleukin-1 receptor antagonist (*IL-1RA*) and soluble tumor necrosis factor receptor (*sTNF-R*) were determined in supernatants by enzymoimmunoassay (IL-1RA, Biermann GmbH, Bad Nauheim, FRG; sTNF-R, Medgenix Diagnostics GmbH, Ratingen, FRG). The readings were grouped according to the percentage of HLA-DR+monocytes in peripheral blood mononuclear cells of septic patients. Mean values and standard error are given; * $p<0.01$, ** $p<0.001$ vs control group; Student's *t* test for independent samples

plained by the fact that diminished immunological competence can result in the manifestation of opportunistic infections.

In order to confirm the hypothesis that an initial high-level inflammatory response can induce the phenomenon of immunoparalysis we tested the influence of inflammatory stimuli and sepsis mediators on the function of monocytic cells.

Living bacteria. In previous experiments we observed a significant reduction of the proliferative response of mouse spleen cells during infection with *Salmonella typhimurium* or *Listeria monocytogenes.* In order to find out whether this phenomenon was due to diminished antigen-presenting activity, separated lymphocytes and adherent spleen cells (monocytes/macrophages) from infected animals were cocultured with cells from untreated syngenetic mice. Our results indicated that the defect is located at the level of antigen-presenting monocytic cells.

Zymosan and fixed bacteria. Further experiments revealed that this phenomenon was not restricted to living bacteria. Injection of high-dose zymosan in Lewis rats (1 mg/g body weight, i.p.) also resulted in diminished MHC class II antigen expression and antigen-presenting function of monocytes.

Moreover, in previous experiments we observed a dose-dependent decrease of HLA-DR antigen expression on human monocytes in vitro induced by phagocytic stimuli (fixed bacteria, zymosan) resulting in diminished antigen-presenting function [37].

As a result, we assume that the most probable cause of the reduction of HLA-class II antigens on monocytes from surgical patients with septic immunoparalysis is the excessive release of inflammatory mediators following strong stimulation of the monocyte/macrophage system by bacteria, fungi or necrotic tissue.

High-Dose Tumor Necrosis Factor Simulates Phagocytosis-Mediated Effects

A key mediator in the pathogenesis of sepsis is TNF. However, we did not observe any association between the serum levels of total or free TNF and the clinical outcome of sepsis. Moreover, monocytes from patients with fatal outcome (immunoparalysis) did secrete lower amounts of TNF than monocytes from septic patients with favorable outcome (HLA-DR+monocytes >40%) as shown above. However, in follow-up studies of some patients we observed that the peak of serum TNF level was followed by immunoparalysis. Therefore, we wondered whether a short-term treatment with TNF would be able to simulate the inactivation of monocytic system in vivo.

Tumor necrosis factor induces loss of accessory activity of adherent spleen cells in mice. As shown in Fig. 5, mice treated with TNF for 2 weeks showed a diminished response of spleen cells to anti-CD3 mAb and concanavalin A (ConA). Coculture of spleen cells from these mice with mitomycin-treated whole spleen cells or an adherent spleen cell fraction restored the diminished proliferative response suggesting a defect of splenic antigen-presenting cells. Unlike in the human system, MHC class II antigen expression on murine splenic monocytes/macrophages was not diminished. Quite similar results were obtained by Gordon and Wofsy [38].

Inhibition of Interferon-γ production of human peripheral blood mononuclear cells by tumor necrosis factor. As monocytic inactivation may partly result from a deficiency of stimulatory cytokines (as is assumed by monocytic immunoparalysis in patients undergoing high-dose anti-rejection therapy) we investigated the in vitro influence of TNF on ConA-induced IFN-γ production of human mononuclear cells. As shown in Fig. 6, TNF inhibited IFN-γ release from mononuclear cells in a dose-dependent manner.

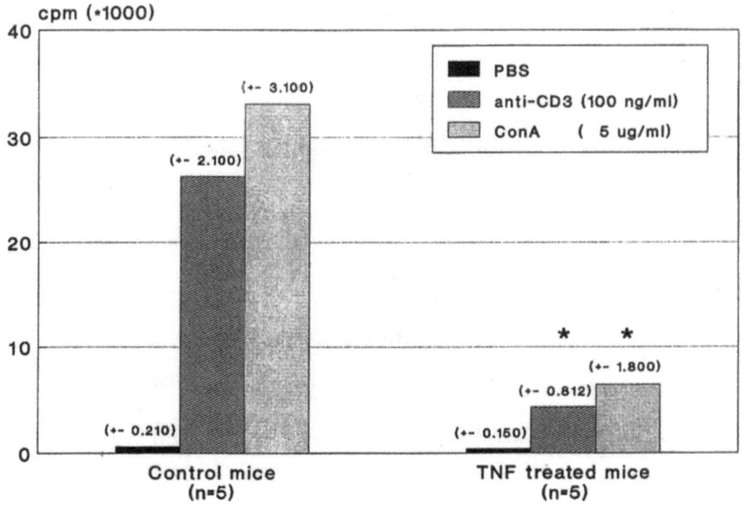

Fig. 5. Tumor necrosis factor (*TNF*) induces loss of accessory activity of adherent spleen cells in mice. Female Balb/c mice were injected six times with 2.5 μg recombinant human TNF (kindly provided by Dr. Haller, Bayer AG, Wuppertal, FRG) on alternate days. After killing the animals, spleen cells were prepared and resuspended (2×10^6/ml in RPMI supplemented with 10% heat-inactivated fetal calf serum and 5×10^{-5} *M* mercaptoethanol). Cells were cultured for 3 days with concanavalin A (ConA; 5 μg/ml) and rat anti-mouse CD3 monoclonal antibody (100 ng/ml) (Paesel Lorelei, FRG). Then, [^{3}H]thymidine incorporation after 8 h was measured by β-scintillation counter (Ionotech). *PBS,* phosphate-buffered saline. Mean values and, in parentheses, standard deviation are given; * $p < 0.01$ vs control group; Wilcoxon

Interleukin-10 Deactivates Monocytes

There seems to be obvious discrepancy between the fact that high-dose TNF is able to induce functional alteration as in immunoparalysis and the fact that in the state of immunoparalysis TNF production is markedly diminished. However, a long-lasting second messenger production which is induced by (even short-term) excessive levels of TNF and which in turn suppresses further production of inflammatory cytokines could be the solution to this problem.

Interleukin-10 (IL-10) is produced by monocytes in response to LPS in vitro and in vivo and IL-10 peak levels were preceded by TNF peak levels by several hours at least [39, 40]. IL-10 may act in an autoregulatory fashion in LPS-activated monocytes by suppressing monocytic synthesis of proinflammatory cytokines in response to LPS or IFN-γ [39, 41]. IL-10 is known to suppress monocytic MHC class II expression and, this way, to inhibit antigen-specific T cell proliferation [42]. Furthermore, it inhibits the IFN-γ production of lymphocytes via a monocyte-dependent mechanism [43].

We tested the influence of recombinant IL-10 on peripheral blood mono-

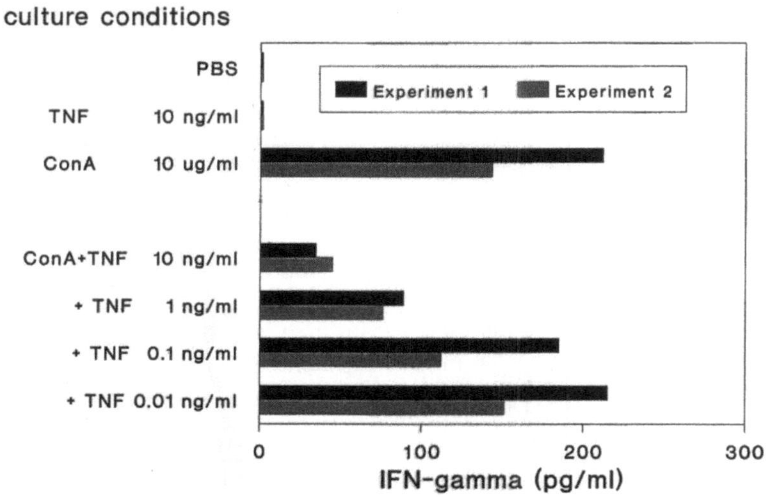

Fig. 6. Inhibition of interferon (*IFN*)-γ production of peripheral blood mononuclear cells (PBMNC) by tumor necrosis factor (*TNF*). Concanavalin A (*ConA*; 10 μg/ml)-induced IFN-γ secretion was determined by enzymoimmunoassay (Genzyme) in supernatants of human PBMNC (2×10^6/ml in RPMI supplemented with 10% fetal calf serum) short-term cultures (2 days) without or with addition of different doses of recombinant human TNF-α. Results of two independent experiments are given

nuclear cells from healthy donors and found a dose-dependent suppression of MHC class II expression on monocytes and on the proliferative response to anti-CD3 mAb.

Another interesting candidate for mediating immunosuppression in septic disease is transforming growth factor-β1 (TGF-β1) which is also produced by activated macrophages. TGF-β1 is known to depress monocytic cytokine production and MHC class II expression and to inhibit cytokine-induced macrophage activation [44–46].

Investigations whether TNF induces a monocytic IL-10 and/or TGF-β1 response in vitro are in progress in our laboratory.

Reconstitution of Monocyte Function and Phenotype – Evidence for Inhibitory Activity in Sepsis Plasma

After demonstrating that monocytes are inactivated in septic disease in vivo and that this can be reproduced using pertinent mediators of septic disease, we looked for possibilities to restore monocyte function and phenotype. Such approaches may be instrumental if a whole body inflammation leading to immunoparalysis could not be prevented.

T cell-derived cytokines such as IFN-γ and GM-CSF are known to augment monocyte function and to induce HLA class II expression on monocytes in vitro [20, 47, 48]. We wondered, if these cytokines are able to restore the diminished function and MHC class II antigen expression of monocytes from septic patients and in animals with monocytic inactivation.

In Vivo Reconstitution of MHC class II Expression on Monocytes of Zymosan-Treated Rats

In view of possible new therapeutic approaches it was interesting to examine the in vivo effect of IFN-γ on inactivated monocytes. IFN-γ administration to zymosan-treated rats normalized diminished MHC class II expression on monocytes in vivo [49].

In Vitro Reconstitution of Function and Phenotype of Monocytes from Septic Patients with Immunoparalysis – Inhibitory Activity in Sepsis Plasma

Next we tested if stimulatory T cell cytokines restore the phenotype and function of monocytes from septic patients with immunoparalysis ex vivo. Both cytokines, IFN-γ and GM-CSF, were able to normalize the diminished HLA-DR antigen expression on monocytes from such patients. Moreover, reconstitution of monocytic HLA-DR expression by IFN-γ was associated with normalization of accessory activity and cytokine production (not tested for GM-CSF).

However, both reconstitution of HLA-DR antigen expression and cytokine production (not tested for antigen-presenting activity) was almost completely inhibited by addition of plasma from septic patients with immunoparalysis instead of fetal calf serum or AB plasma from healthy donors (Fig. 7). Interestingly, 48 h culture with AB plasma alone already reconstituted diminished TNF secretion but not monocytic HLA-DR expression. We believe that there is a chronological dissociation of the reconstitution of TNF secretion capacity and HLA-DR expression of monocytes or that different amounts of stimulatory activity are required for the reconstitution. Therefore, monocytic expression of HLA-DR antigen may not reflect the functional state regarding cytokine production of monocytes in all cases.

We wondered whether this inhibition by sepsis plasma only occurs after presensitization of monocytes in septic patients. As shown in Fig. 8, sepsis plasma from patients with immunoparalyiss also prevented the IFN-γ-induced increase of HLA-DR expression and even supressed the cytokine secretion capacity of monocytes from healthy controls.

In conclusion, we suggest that the inhibitory activity in plasma from septic patients with immunoparalysis could be an independent pathogenic factor which participates in the inactivation of monocytes in the septic state.

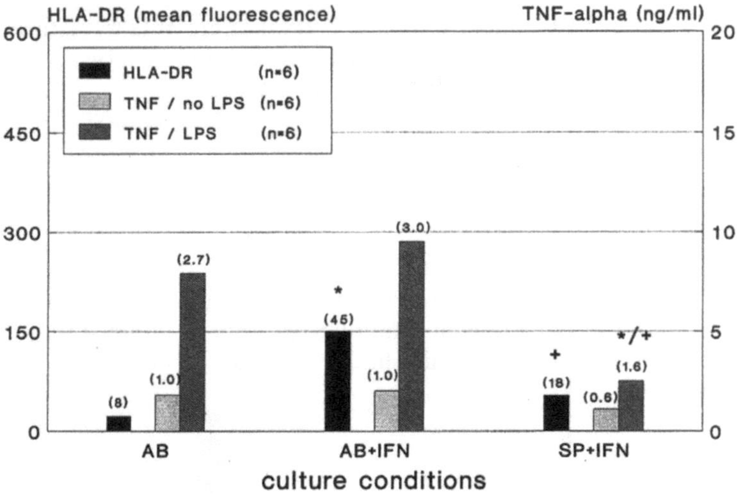

Fig. 7. Interferon (IFN)-γ restitutes diminished HLA-DR antigen expression and lipopolysaccharide (*LPS*)-induced tumor necrosis factor (*TNF*) secretion of monocytes from septic patients with immunoparalysis – evidence for inhibitory activity in sepsis plasma. Peripheral blood mononuclear cells from septic patients with immunoparalysis were cultured (48 h) with control AB plasma (*AB*, 20%) or sepsis plasma (*SP*, 20%) with or without IFN-γ (1 U/ml). Monocytic HLA-DR expression and LPS-induced TNF secretion were determined in short-term cultures (4 h) by flow cytometry and enzymoimmunoassay (Medgenix Diagnostics GmbH, Ratingen, FRG), respectively.
Mean values and, *in parentheses,* standard error are given; * $p<0.05$ vs AB culture without IFN-γ; $^{+}$ $p<0.05$ vs AB culture with IFN-γ; Wilcoxon test

Characterization of Inhibitory Activity in Sepsis Plasma

We examined if the inhibitory activity in sepsis plasma could be quantified by functional assays. By addition of different amounts of sepsis plasma we were able to demonstrate a dose-dependent inhibition of the IFN-γ-induced increase in HLA-DR expression on control monocytes in vitro (Fig. 9). Noticeable suppression was already found in cultures which were supplemented with only 5% of sepsis plasma. However, it was possible to overcome the inhibitory effects of sepsis plasma on control monocytes by adding different amounts of IFN-γ (Fig. 10). Therefore, we believe that there is a close functional association between the action of IFN-γ and the inhibitory activity in sepsis plasma.

Preliminary studies for identifying the inhibitory activity showed that the inhibitory factor(s) could not be neutralized neither by anti-endotoxin nor anti-TNF or by scavengers of reactive oxygen species or by protease inhibitors. The factor was found to be heat instable (>56°C) and not dialyzable (MW>6000).

Although we have not yet been able to fully characterize the inhibitory

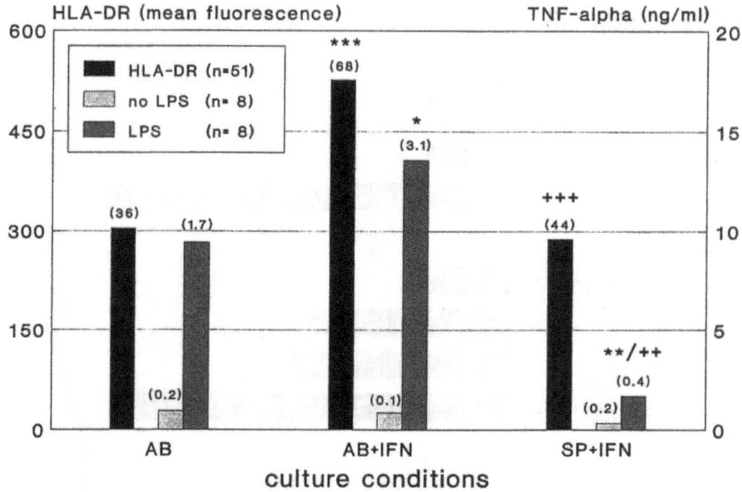

Fig. 8. Plasma from septic patients with immunoparalysis inhibits interferon (*IFN*)-γ-induced increase of HLA-DR expression and tumor necrosis factor (*TNF*) secretion of monocytes from healthy probands. Peripheral blood mononuclear cells from healthy donors were cultured (48 h) with control AB plasma (*AB*, 20%) or sepsis plasma (*SP*, 20%) with or without IFN-γ (1 U/ml). Monocytic HLA-DR expression and lipopolysaccharide (LPS-) induced TNF secretion were determined in short-term cultures (4 h) (see Fig. 7). Mean values and, *in parentheses*, standard error are given; * $p<0.05$, ** $p<0.01$, *** $p<0.001$ vs AB culture without IFN-γ; ++ $p<0.01$, +++ $p<0.001$ vs AB culture with IFN-γ; Wilcoxon test

activity until now, the functional definition of a prognostically relevant inhibitory factor in the plasma of septic patients ought to give rise to the development of new diagnostic and therapeutic approaches in septic disease.

Immunostimulatory Therapeutic Approaches in Septic Disease

Plasma Exchange Therapy in Septic Patients

In order to eliminate the inhibitory activity in sepsis plasma in vivo we started a clinical study with plasma exchange therapy in septic patients with immunoparalysis.

Patients who showed a monocytic HLA-DR expression lower than 30% for more than 3 days were included in the study. Plasma exchange (2–3 L/day, substitution by fresh frozen plasma) was commonly done in series of one per day over 3 consecutive days. If there was no clear recovery of monocytic HLA-DR expression after several days or again a drop to values below 30% HLA-DR+monocytes another series of plasma exchange therapy was started.

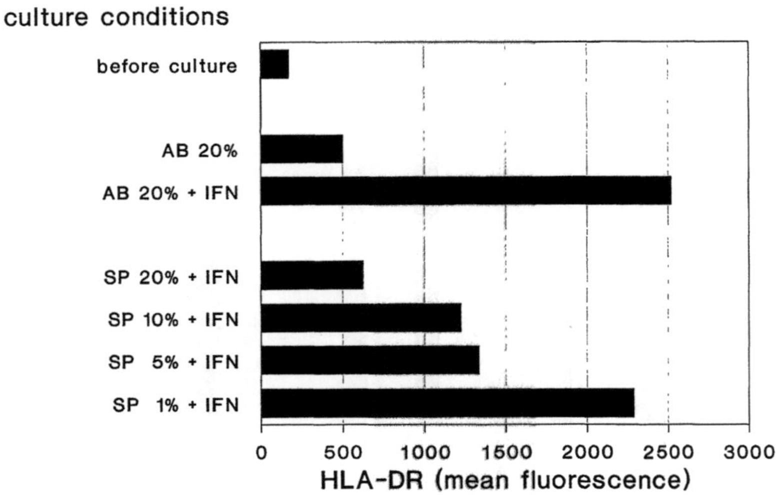

Fig. 9. Dose-dependent inhibition of interferon (*IFN*)-γ-induced increase of monocytic HLA-DR expression by sepsis plasma. Peripheral blood mononuclear cells from a healthy donor is cultured (48 h) with control AB plasma (*AB*) or different supplements of plasma from a septic patient with immunoparalysis (*SP*) with or without IFN-γ (1 U/ml). Monocytic HLA-DR expression is given as mean logarithmic fluorescence intensity in cytofluorometric determination

We observed four principal patterns of HLA-DR antigen expression and patient survival:

1. Lasting recovery of monocytic HLA-DR expression after one or more series of plasma exchange therapy and patient survival
2. No recovery of monocytic HLA-DR expression and fatal outcome of septic disease
3. Temporary recovery of monocytic HLA-DR expression followed by a drop and resistance to further series of plasmapheresis and eventually fatal outcome of septic disease
4. Lasting recovery of monocytic HLA-DR expression but fatal outcome mainly due to nonsepsis-related complications.

We never observed survival in a patient whose monocytic HLA-DR expression did not recover.

Although some patients did not or only temporarily respond to plasma exchange therapy our preliminary results show that this therapeutic approach significantly improved the prognosis of septic patients with immunoparalysis (Table 5). This finding agrees with the experience of other groups, who found a beneficial influence of plasma exchange therapy on the survival rates of septic patients [50, 51]. However, these immunodiagnostic parameters of monocytic activity (HLA-DR antigen expression and cytokine secre-

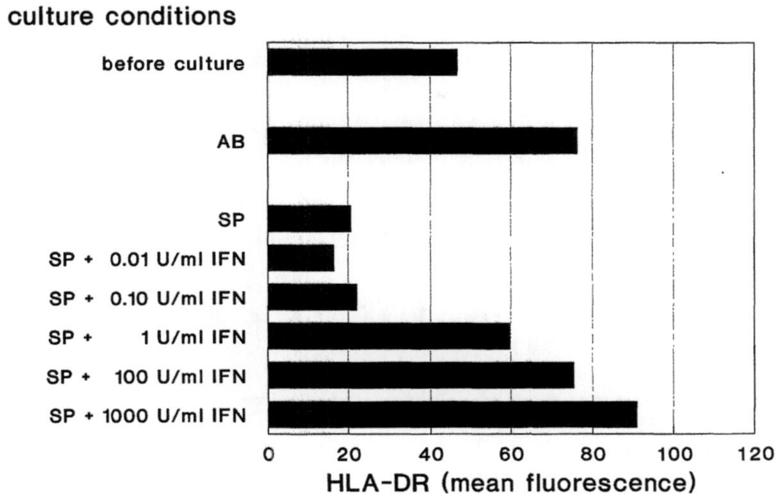

Fig. 10. Titration of the inhibitory activity in sepsis plasma with interferon (*IFN*)-γ. Peripheral blood mononuclear cells from a healthy donor was cultured (48 h) with control AB plasma (*AB*, 20%) or sepsis plasma (*SP*, 20%) and different concentrations of IFN-γ. Monocytic HLA-DR expression is given as mean logarithmic fluorescence intensity in cytofluorometric determination

Table 5. Influence of plasma exchange therapy on survival in septic patients with immunoparalysis (<30% HLA-DR+monocytes)

Immunoparalysis	Plasmapheresis	Survival rate
Yes	No	4/38 (11%)
Yes	Yes	15/31 (48%)*

* $p<0.01$; χ^2 assay.

tion capacity) can be used when deciding whether plasma exchange therapy is indicated and they are equally useful for the monitoring of the therapeutic success. Moreover, identification of the inhibitory factor(s) in sepsis plasma may encourage the search for new and more specific therapeutic approaches for preventing its production or for neutralizing or eliminating it.

Figures 11 and 12 show two cases of successful plasma exchange therapy in a septic patient with immunoparalysis. Figure 11 demonstrates the influence of plasma exchange on the functional capacity and HLA-DR expression of monocytes from a septic patient. First, plasma exchange therapy led to a recovery of monocytic HLA-DR expression but not of TNF formation capacity. HLA-DR expression dropped again (day 17). A second plasma exchange on day 17 led to lasting reconstitution of monocytic cytokine secretion capacity and MHC class II antigen expression.

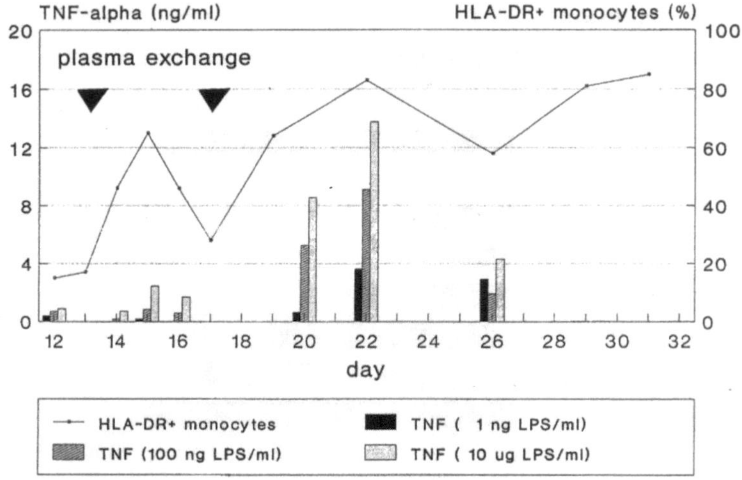

Fig. 11. Influence of plasma exchange therapy on HLA-DR expression and cytokine secretion capacity of monocytes from a septic patient with immunoparalysis. *Filled triangles* indicate the days on which the patient was treated by plasma exchange therapy. The *line* represents HLA-DR expression (in percent) on monocytes. The *columns* represent tumor necrosis factor (*TNF*) secretion in response to different lipopolysaccharide (*LPS*) concentrations in short-term cultures (4 h) of whole blood of the corresponding day

The influence of plasma exchange therapy on the inhibitory activity of plasma and the monocytic HLA-DR antigen expression of a patient with septic disease is illustrated in Fig. 12. Plasma exchange is followed by a noticeable decrease of inhibitory activity in the plasma and a recovery of HLA-DR antigen expression on the peripheral blood monocytes of the septic patient. Interestingly, following the first series of plasma exchange, sepsis plasma seems to contain stimulatory rather than inhibitory activity (day 18, not shown). The second series led to a lasting recovery of monocytic HLA-DR expression.

Although we found a fall in inhibitory plasma activity after plasmapheresis in all examined cases, in some cases this decrease was not associated with a recovery of the monocytic HLA-DR antigen expression and monocytic function. We suggest, that despite the elimination of inhibitory mediators by plasma exchange, stimulatory signals inducing a normalization of MHC class II antigen expression and monocyte function may be lacking in these patients. This hypothesis is supported by the fact that in sepsis-plasma-free cultures (control AB plasma) of peripheral blood mononuclear cells from some of the septic patients with immunoparalysis we found no spontaneous increase but rather a decrease of HLA-DR antigen expression and cytokine formation. This is in contrast to monocytes from healthy controls cultured under

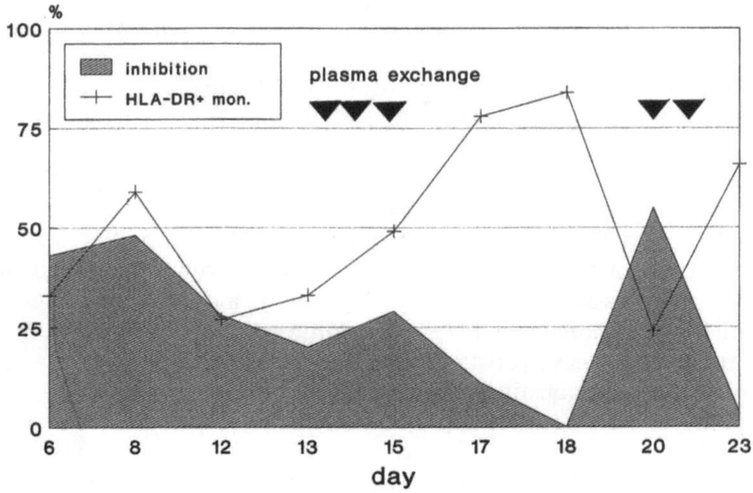

Fig. 12. Influence of plasma exchange therapy on the inhibitory activity of plasma from a septic patient with immunoparalysis. *Filled triangles* indicate the days on which the patient was treated by plasma exchange therapy. The *line* represents HLA-DR expression (in percent) on monocytes of the septic patient the plasma was obtained from. The *hatched area* represents the alterations of inhibitory activity in sepsis plasma. It was derived from the difference between HLA-DR expressions (in logarithmic fluorescence intensity) of monocytes which had been cultured with interferon-γ and either sepsis plasma (20%) from the respective day or control AB plasma (20%)

the same conditions, on which HLA-DR antigen expression increased in all cases.

In patients whose readings do not resume normal levels after elimination of inhibitory mediators, direct immunostimulation may be necessary.

Therapy with Immunostimulatory Cytokines in Septic Patients – A Critical Discussion

Candidates for immunostimulators could be agents which predominantly neutralize or suppress the formation of inhibitory mediators (e.g., anti IL-10) or which primarily act directly in a stimulatory way, e.g., IL-2, IFN-γ, GM-CSF.

Out of the second group, IFN-γ (and GM-CSF) may be the first candidate(s) for immunostimulatory therapy in the case of septic disease with severe monocyte inactivation.

It is well known that in severely injured patients there is depressed IFN-γ production [24, 52]. Septic complications may further enhance IFN-γ deficiency by TFN and IL-10 mediated mechanisms. Lack of sufficient amounts of IFN-γ may result in functional inactivation of monocytes and a diminished MHC class II antigen expression, as we could show in vitro [53].

However, our results demonstrate that IFN-γ is able to reconstitute the depressed cytokine production and MHC class II antigen expression of monocytes inactivated in experimental settings or of monocytes derived from septic patients with immunoparalysis. Moreover, it neutralized the inhibitory activity in plasma of septic patients.

Chomarat et al. [54] demonstrated that IFN-γ suppressed the monocytic production of IL-10, which, we suggest, is involved in monocytic inactivation after an excessive inflammatory response. It induces the production of TNF and IL-1 by monocytes [47, 55]. Additionally, IFN-γ inhibits the release of immunosuppressive prostaglandin E_2 [47]. Moreover, IFN-γ has been shown to be able to reconstitute the depressed cellular immunity by inhibiting the activity of T helper 2 cells [56]. Finally, IFN-γ up-regulates its own gene expression in lymphocytes [57, 58]. This way IFN-γ may be able to normalize the proportions of immunostimulatory and immunosuppressive mediators in the immunodepressive state of septic disease.

Nonetheless, as mentioned above, immunostimulatory therapy in septic disease may be dangereous in situations in which an excessive inflammatory response is present by amplifying cytokine (e.g., TNF and IL-1) effects leading to shock [6].

Despite all that, we were able to demonstrate that monocytes from septic patients with immunoparalysis were markedly depressed in their proinflammatory function. In these patients a relative deficiency of proinflammatory mediators exists. Therefore, we think that immunostimulatory therapy by IFN-γ (or GM-CSF) has to be initiated in septic patients with proven immunoparalysis only.

Clinical use of IFN-γ is established in the therapy of chronic granulomatous disease (CGD). Even though at least focal infection and inflammation may be present in this syndrome, no severe side effects were described. Only fever was observed more often [59].

Polk et al. [60] reported on a randomized clinical study with IFN-γ therapy after severe traumata. In this study, IFN-γ therapy resulted in a temporary recovery of diminished HLA-DR antigen expression on monocytes. However, IFN-γ was given early after injury (days 1–10) and its withdrawal resulted in a fast drop of monocytic HLA-DR expression to the same values as in the placebo group. There was no significant improvement of the survival rate. Although bacterial contamination was one of the entry criteria in this study, no inflammatory shock syndrome was reported as a consequence of IFN-γ therapy. Only fever was observed more often in the IFN-γ-treated group than in the placebo group (93% vs 83%). In fact, this higher incidence of fever may have resulted from an enhancement of the inflammatory response. However, in this study IFN-γ therapy was started early after the injury, i.e., in a phase during which an excessive inflammatory response was likely to be present. Monocytic inactivation (immunoparalysis), by contrast, was not an entry criteria in this study. The results show that IFN-γ therapy led to no significant improvement in clinical outcome. One reason for this could be the very formal design of the study, in which each patient was treated only the first 10 days after injury.

We think that here the same rule applies as for anti-inflammatory therapy: the success of any immunotherapeutic approach depends on the present situation of the immune system. Therefore, immunostimulatory therapy, e.g., with IFN-γ, in septic disease may be indicated but only in a state of lasting monocyte inactivation, because otherwise severe adverse effects have to be feared. In our experience, therapy has to be continued until functional recovery has been achieved. In order to carry this out, it is instrumental to have sufficient diagnostic means at hand, such as determination of monocytic HLA-class II expression and cytokine formation capacity. Moreover, in some patients an additional therapeutic approach for eliminating inhibitory mediators (e.g., plasma exchange therapy) may be necessary.

Summary

Monocytic inflammatory response is not generally enhanced in the septic state but may be severely depressed especially in the phase following acute septic shock when multiple organ failure and persistent (opportunistic) infections represent the main clinical problems.

In many of these patients we demonstrated a monocyte inactivation (diminished antigen-presenting capacity, formation of reactive oxygen species and of pro-inflammatory cytokines) which was associated with a diminished MHC class II antigen expression ($<30\%$ HLA-DR+) on monocytes. The persistence of monocytic inactivation for more than 5 days strongly correlated with a fatal outcome of septic disease.

High doses of inflammatory mediators (e.g., TNF) were able to induce similar monocytic alterations in vitro and in vivo. Therefore, we suggest, that an initial excessive inflammatory response (e.g., TNF) leads – via induction of immunosuppressive mediators (e.g., IL-10, TGF-β) – to a severe immunodepression, with monocyte inactivation the most crucial parameter (immunoparalysis) (Fig. 13). In contrast to this, an adequate initial inflammatory response will be limited by these mechanisms in a physiological feedback without leading to severe immunodepression.

Once monocyte inactivation has taken place in septic disease, immunostimulatory approaches (e.g., by IFN-γ or GM-CSF, which were shown to normalize monocytic function and phenotype in vitro) seem to be the adequate therapeutic measure while anti-inflammatory therapy (e.g., IL-1RA, anti-TNF) may be not effective.

If proven to be lasting, monocyte inactivation (immunoparalysis) is considered a “conditio sine qua non” for the initiation of immunostimulatory therapy, no severe adverse effects by IFN-γ-induced augmentation of TNF or

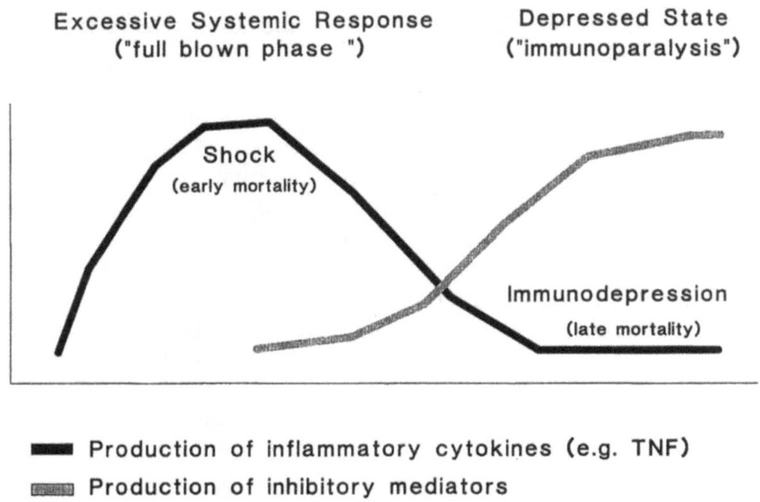

Fig. 13. Two phases of inadequate inflammatory response in whole body inflammation (hypothesis). Excessive systemic inflammatory response in the first phase may induce dysregulation of the immune system with dominating immunosuppressive and anti-inflammatory factors. Inhibitory mediators could be soluble tumor necrosis factor receptor (sTNF-R), interleukin (IL)-1 receptor antagonist (IL-1RA), soluble interferon-γ receptor, prostaglandin E_2 and cytokines (e.g., IL-10, transforming growth factor-β)

IL-1 response have to be feared. Functional recovery of monocytes should be regarded as an indicator of therapeutic success.

For assessing monocyte function, the determination of the monocytic cytokine formation capacity (in vitro) is very useful. However, in our experience, the cytofluorometrical measurement of HLA-DR antigen expression on blood monocytes ($<30\%$, the discrimination value for monocyte inactivation) was a valid substitute in almost all cases.

Since we demonstrated that in sepsis plasma an inhibitory activity exists which was able to induce monocyte inactivation and which counteracted the reconstitution of monocytic function and phenotype by IFN-γ, plasma exchange therapy was tested as a supplementary therapeutic tool in septic patients with immunoparalysis.

In fact, plasma exchange therapy did improve survival rates in septic patients with monocyte inactivation even without additional IFN-γ therapy.

Although it led to a decrease in inhibitory plasma activity in all cases, some patients showed no functional recovery and died. In these patients additional immunostimulatory therapy would seem to be instrumental.

References

1. Centers of Disease Control (1990) Increase in national hospital discharge survey rates for septicemia – United States. 1979–1987. JAMA 263:937–938
2. Meakins JL (1989) Prädisponierende Faktoren und körpereigene Abwehr bei Sepsis und septischem Schock. In: Reinhart K, Eyrich K (eds) Sepsis. Springer, Berlin Heidelberg New York
3. Heath AW (1990) Cytokines and infection. Current Opin Immunol 2/3:380–384
4. Glauser MP, Zanetti G, Baumgartner JD, Cohen J (1991) Septic shock: pathogenesis. Lancet 338:732–736
5. Spooner CE, Markowitz NP, Saravolatz LD (1992) The role of tumor necrosis factor in sepsis. Clin Immunol Immunopathol 62:11–17
6. Doherty GM, Lange JR, Langstein HN, Alexander HR, Buresh CM, Norton JA (1992) Evidence for IFN-gamma as a mediator of the lethality of endotoxin and tumor necrosis factor-alpha. J Immunol 149:1666–1670
7. Beutler B, Milsark IW, Cerami A (1985) Passive immunization against cachectin/tumor necrosis factor protects mice from lethal effect of endotoxin. Science 229:869–871
8. Tracey KJ, Fong Y, Hesse DG et al (1987) Anti-cachectin/TNF monoclonal antibodies prevent septic shock during lethal bacteraemia. Nature 330:662–664
9. Ohlsson K, Björk P, Bergenfeldt M, Hagemann R, Thompson RC (1990) Interleukin-1 receptor antagonist reduces mortality from endotoxin shock. Nature 348:550–552
10. Silva AT, Bayston KF, Cohen J (1990) Prophylactic and therapeutic effects of a monoclonal antibody to tumor necrosis factor-alpha in experimental gram-negative shock. J Infect Dis 162:421–427
11. Bagby GJ, Plessala KJ, Wilson LA, Thompson JJ, Nelson S (1991) Divergent efficacy of antibody to tumor necrosis factor-alpha in intravascular and peritonits models of sepsis. J Infect Dis 163:83–88
12. Zanetti G, Heumann D, Gérain J et al (1992) Cytokine production after intravenous or peritoneal gram-negative bacterial challenge in mice – comparative protective efficacy of antibodies to tumor necrosis factor-alpha and to lipopolysaccharide. J Immunol 148:1890–1897
13. Postlethwaite AE, Seyer JM (1990) Stimulation of fibroblast chemotaxis by human recombinant tumor necrosis factor-alpha (TNF-alpha) and a synthetic TNF-alpha 31–68 peptide. J Exp Med 172:1749–1756
14. Eskandari MK, Bolgos G, Miller C, Nguyen DT, DeForge LE, Remick DG (1992) Anti-tumor necrosis factor antibody therapy fails to prevent lethality after cecal ligation and puncture or endotoxemia. J Immunol 148:2724–2730
15. Spalding BJ (1993) In shocking Synergen, sepsis tallies third victim. Biotechnology 11:428–429
16. Volk HD, Reinke P, Falck P, Staffa G, Briedigkeit H, von Baehr R (1989) Diagnostic value of an immune monitoring program for the clinical management of immunosuppressed patients with septic complications. Clin Transplant 3:246–252
17. Janeway CA, Bottomly K, Babich J (1984) Quantitative variation in Ia antigen expression plays a central role in immune regulation. Immunol Today 5:99–105
18. Steeg PS, Johnson HM, Oppenheim JJ (1982) Regulation of murine macrophage Ia antigen expression by an immune IFN-like lymphokine: inhibitory effect of endotoxins. J Immunol 129:2402–2407
19. Gonwa TA, Frost JP, Karr RW (1986) All human monocytes have the capability of expressing HLA-DQ and HLA-DP molecules upon stimulation with interferon-gamma. J Immunol 137:519–524
20. Fischer HG, Frosch S, Reske K, Reske-Kunz AB (1988) Granulocyte macrophage colony-stimulating factor activates macrophages derived from bone marrow cultures to synthesis of MHC class II molecules and to augmented antigen presentation function. J Immunol 141:3082–3088
21. Volk HD, Lohmann T, Heym S et al (1990) Decrease of the proportion of HLA-

DR+monocytes as prognostic parameter for the clinical outcome of septic disease. In: Masihi KN, Lange W (eds) Immunotherapeutic prospects of infectious disease. Springer, Berlin Heidelberg New York, pp 298–301
22. Von Baehr R, Lohmann T, Heym S, Reinke P, Tausch W, Volk HD (1990) Immunparalyse bei Septikämien – Labordiagnostischer Nachweis und klinische Konsequenzen. Z Klin Med 45:1133–1137
23. Volk HD, Thieme M, Ruppe U et al (1993) Alterations in function and phenotype of monocytes from patients with septic disease: predictive value and new therapeutic strategies. In: Faist E, Meakins JL, Schildberg FW (eds) Host defense dysfunction in trauma, shock and sepsis. Springer, Berlin Heidelberg New York, pp 365–371
24. Livingston DH, Appel SH, Wellhausen SR, Sonnenfeld G, Polk HC (1988) Depressed interferon-γ production and monocyte HLA-DR expression after severe injury. Arch Surg 123:1309–1313
25. Cheadle WG, Hershman MJ, Wellhausen SR, Polk HC (1989) Role of monocytic HLA-DR expression following trauma in predicting clinical outcome. In: Faist E, Ninnemann J, Green D (eds) Immune consequences of trauma, shock, and sepsis. Springer, Berlin Heidelberg New York, pp 119–122
26. Gibbons RA, Martinez OM, Lim RC, Horn JK, Garovoy MR (1989) Reduction in HLA-DR, HLA-DQ and HLA-DP expression by Leu-M3+ cells from the peripheral blood of patients with thermal injury. Injury 19:263–266
27. Wakefield CH, Carey PD, Foulds S, Monson JRT, Guillou PJ (1993) Changes in major histocompatibility complex class II expression in monocytes and T cells of patients developing infection after surgery. Br J Surg 80:205–209
28. Ertel W, Morrison MH, Ayala A, Dean RE, Chaudry IH (1992) Interferon-gamma attenuates hemorrhage-induced suppression of macrophage and splenocyte functions and decreases susceptibility to sepsis. Surgery 111:177–187
29. Volk HD, Thieme M, Heym S et al (1991) Alterations in function and phenotype of monocytes from patients with septic disease – predictive value and new therapeutic strategies. Behring Inst Mitt 88:208–215
30. Rothe G, Oser A, Valet G (1988) Dihydrorhodamine 123: a new flow cytometric indicator for respiratory burst activity in neutrophil granulocytes. Naturwissenschaften 73:354–356
31. Platzer C, Richter G, Uberla K, Muller W, Blocker H, Diamantstein T, Blankenstein T (1992) Analysis of cytokine mRNA levels in interleukin-4-transgenic mice by quantitative polymerase chain reaction. Eur J Immunol 22:1179–1184
32. Munoz C, Carlet J, Fitting C, Misset B, Blériot JP, Cavaillon JM (1991) Dysregulation of in vitro cytokine production by monocytes during sepsis. J Clin Invest 88:1747–1754
33. Mandi Y, Farkas G, Karacsonyi S, Beladi I (1992) Tumor necrosis factor production in septic conditions following pancreatitis (preliminary report). Orv Hetil 26:211–214
34. Granowitz EV, Santos AA, Poutsiaka DD, Cannon JG, Wilmore DW, Wolff SM, Dinarello CA (1991) Production of interleukin-1-receptor antagonist during experimental endotoxaemia. Lancet 338:1423–1424
35. Fischer E, Van Zee KJ, Marano MA et al (1992) Interleukin-1 receptor antagonist circulates in experimental inflammation and in human disease. Blood 79:2196–2200
36. Van Zee KJ, Kohno T, Fischer E, Rock CS, Moldawer LL (1992) Tumor necrosis factor soluble receptors circulate during experimental and clinical inflammation and can protect against excessive tumor necrosis factor alpha in vitro and in vivo. Proc Natl Acad Sci USA 89:4845–4849
37. Gruner S, Volk HD, Falck P, von Baehr R (1986) The influence of phagocytic stimuli on the expression of HLA-DR antigens: role of reactive oxygen intermediates. Eur J Immunol 16:212–215
38. Gordon C, Wofsy D (1990) Effects of recombinant murine tumor necrosis factor-α on immune function. J Immunol 144:1753–1758
39. De Waal Malefyt R, Abrams J, Benett B, Figdor CG, de Vries JE (1991) Interleukin 10

(IL-10) inhibits cytokine synthesis by human monocytes: an autoregulatory role of IL-10 produced by monocytes. J Exp Med 174:1209
40. Durez P, Abramowicz D, Gérard C et al (1993) In vivo induction of interleukin 10 by anti-CD3 monoclonal antibody or bacterial lipopolysaccharide: differential modulation by cyclosporin A. J Exp Med 177:551–555
41. Howard M, Muchamuel T, Andrade S, Menon S (1993) Interleukin 10 protects mice from lethal endotoxemia. J Exp Med 177:1205–1208
42. De Waal Malefyt R, Haanen J, Spits H et al (1991) Interleukin 10 (IL-10) and viral IL-10 strongly reduce antigen-specific human T cell proliferation by diminishing the antigen-presenting capacity of monocytes via downregulation of class II major histocompatibility complex expression. J Exp Med 174:195
43. D'Andrea A, Aste-Amezaga M, Valiante NM, Ma X, Kubin M, Trinchieri G (1993) Interleukin 10 (IL-10) inhibits human lymphocyte interferon gamma-production by suppressing natural killer cell stimulatory factor/IL-12 synthesis in accessory cells. J Exp Med 178:1041–1048
44. Espenik T, Figari IS, Shalaby MR, Lewis GD, Shepard HM, Palladino MA Jr (1987) Inhibition of cytokine production by cyclosporin A and transforming growth factor β. J Exp Med 166:571
45. Czarniecki CW, Chiu HH, Wong GHW, McCabe SM, Palladino MA (1988) Transforming growth factor β modulates the expression of class II histocompatibility antigens on human cells. J Immunol 140:4217
46. Chandry D, Turner M, Abney A, Feldmann M (1989) Modulation of cytokine production by transforming growth factor β. J Immunol 142:4295
47. Boraschi D, Censini S, Tagliabue A (1984) Interferon-gamma reduces macrophage-suppressive activity by inhibiting prostaglandin E_2 release and inducing interleukin-1 production. J Immunol 133:764–768
48. Smith PD, Lamerson CL, Wong HL, Wahl LM, Wahl LM (1990) Granulocyte-macrophage colony-stimulating factor stimulates human monocyte accessory cell function. J Immunol 144:3829–3834
49. Volk HD, Lohmann T, Heym S et al (1992) Association between monocytic function and clinical outcome of sepsis. Microbiologist 3:20–26
50. McClelland P, Williams PS, Yaqoob M, Mostafa SM, Bone JM (1990) Multiple organ failure – a role for plasma exchange. Intensive Care Med 16:100–103
51. Pollack M (1992) Blood exchange and plasmapheresis in sepsis and septic shock. Clin Infect Dis 15:424–430
52. Faist E, Ertel W, Mewes A, Alkan S, Walz A, Strasser T (1989) Trauma-induced alterations of the lymphokine cascade. In: Faist E, Ninnemann J, Green D (eds) Immune consequences of trauma, shock, and sepsis. Springer, Berlin Heidelberg New York, pp 79–94
53. Volk HD, Waschke SR, Diezel W, Grunow R, von Baehr R, Fiebig H (1985) Decrease of HLA-DR antigen expression by human monocytes during cultivation in absence of exogenous or endogenous interferon. Immunol Lett 10:103–107
54. Chomarat P, Rissoan MC, Banchereau J, Miossec P (1993) Interferon-gamma inhibits interleukin-10 production by monocytes. J Exp Med 177:523–527
55. Philip R, Epstein LB (1986) Tumour necrosis factor as immunomodulator and mediator of monocyte cytotoxicity induced by itself, gamma-interferon and interleukin-1. Nature 323:86
56. Mosmann TR, Moore KW (1991) The role of IL-10 in cross-regulation of T_{H1} and T_{H2} responses. Immunol Today 12:A49
57. Hardy KJ, Sawada T (1989) Human interferon-gamma strongly up-regulates its own gene expression in peripheral blood lymphocytes. J Exp Med 170:1021
58. Cockfield SM, Ramassar V, Noujaim J, van der Meide PH, Halloran PF (1993) Regulation of IFN-gamma expression in vivo – IFN-gamma up-regulates expression of its mRNA in normal and lipopolysaccharide-stimulated mice. J Immunol 150:717–725
59. International Chronic Granulomatous Disease Cooperative Study Group (1991)A con-

trolled trial of interferon gamma to prevent infection in chronic granulomatous disease. N Engl J Med 324:509–516

60. Polk HC Jr, Cheadle WG, Livingston DH et al (1992) A randomized prospective clinical trial to determine the efficacy of interferon-gamma in severely injured patients. Am J Surg 163:191–196
61. Volk HD, Döcke WD, Syrbe U, Meinecke A, Klug C, Zuckermann H, Reinke P, Platzer C, Brunner H, Kox P, von Baehr (1994) Monocyte deactivation in fatal septic disease (submitted)

From Localized Angioedema to Generalized Capillary Leak Syndrome: Evidence for a Pivotal Role of C1-Inhibitor in Septic Shock-like Syndromes

B. Eisele and U. Delvos

Introduction

C1-inhibitor (C1-INH) is the only known inhibitor of the classical pathway of complement system and the most important inhibitor of factor XII-mediated contact activation. The genetic deficiency of C1-INH (hereditary angioedema) causes acute edema formation which is in most cases locally restricted to the upper extremities, neck, and face. Acute onset of an attack often results in life-threatening events such as laryngeal edema, which is resistant to treatment with corticosteroids.

When causal replacement therapy with C1-INH concentrate became available in the mid-1970s, admission of affected patients to intensive care units and life-saving resuscitation maneuvers declined in numbers considerably. The administration of the concentrate was found to be consistently effective in both preventing and resolving edema formation.

In the meantime evidence has been accumulated that the pathogenetic role of C1-INH is not restricted to the genetic defect. Rather, it appears to have a causative role in the regulation of the body's inflammatory response. Inflammation is a critical component of the normal healing process. If the organism fails to localize it, the inflammatory response becomes generalized and might progress to a septic shock-like syndrome with the clinical signs of generalized capillary leak syndrome and refractory hypotension. Under these circumstances the uncontrolled activation of complement and contact systems appears to play a causative role. As both systems are almost exclusively regulated by a single inhibitor, C1-INH, and as clinical signs of generalized capillary leakage resemble those of angioedema attack, C1-INH was given to patients who presented with capillary leak syndrome and/or refractory hypotension in the course of a systemic inflammatory response. In this paper the rationale behind and first results of treatment with C1-INH concentrate are reported.

Biology of C1-Inhibitor

Structure and Function

The C1-INH protein is a single-chain glycoprotein containing 478 aminoacid residues [1–3]. The molecular weight of the fully glycosylated molecule is 105 kD [2], of which the carbohydrate side chains comprise 26%–35% [2, 4]. C1-INH is a member of the serine protease inhibitor (serpin) "superfamily" which contains several plasma protease inhibitors, including α_1-protease inhibitor, antithrombin III, α_2-antiplasmin, and heparin cofactor II.

C1-INH inhibits its target proteases by binding to the reactive site. The inhibitor mimics the substrate and a covalently bound bimolecular complex with the respective protease is formed [5]. This complex formation results both in the masking of epitopes on the enzyme and in the generation of neoantigenic determinants on the inhibitor-protease complex [6].

Control of Complement and Contact Systems

The activation of the classical pathway of complement and of (bradykinin-forming) contact systems is regulated by C1-INH. C1-INH is the only known inhibitor in plasma of the first component of complement (C1) as well as of its two subcomponents C1r and C1s [7, 8]. Furthermore, it is able to inactivate kallikrein [9], plasmin [9], coagulation factors XIa and XIIa [10], and the enzymatically active fragments derived from factor XIIa (i.e., factor XIIf) [11]. However, only inhibition of activated C1-complex, kallikrein, and factors XIIa and XIIf appears to be physiologically relevant.

Besides the fact that C1-INH is the only known inhibitor of the classical path of complement system, kinetic data suggest that C1-INH accounts for more than 90% of the inactivation of both factor XIIa and factor XIIf [12] (Fig. 1).

As activated factor XII can activate the classical pathway of complement [13, 14], there are close interrelations between both systems. Activation of the complement and contact systems has very important physiological effects as it results in the formation of biologically active peptides. Complement activation products, such as the anaphylatoxins C3a, C4a, C5a, and the terminal complement complex (TCC), exhibit proinflammatory activities and have been shown to increase the permeability of endothelial cells [15]. Contact activation results inter alia in the formation of bradykinin, a nonapeptide cleaved from high-molecular-weight kininogen by kallikrein. Bradykinin has strong vasodilating properties, which are due to its capacity to induce the formation of nitric oxide (formerly endothelium-derived relaxing factor) in endothelial cells [16].

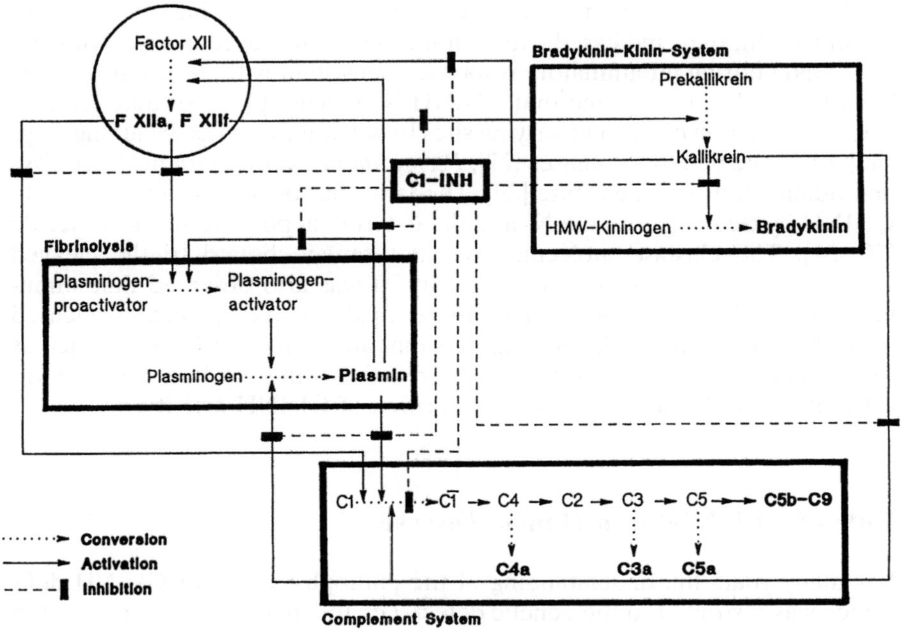

Fig. 1. The central role of C1-inhibitor (C1-INH) in the regulation of fibrinolysis and the complement (classical path) and bradykinin-kinin (contact) systems. C1-INH is the only known inhibitor of the classical pathway of the complement system and the major (>90%) inhibitor of factor XIIa and factor XIIf (fragments)

Production, Regulation, and Degradation

C1-INH is synthesized mainly by the liver [17], but also by skin fibroblasts, human umbilical vein endothelial cells [18], and human blood monocytes [19]. Due to their mobile nature, the synthesis of C1-INH by circulating monocytes seems to be important in the local regulation of inflammatory phenomena. Macrophages isolated from inflamed tissues produce larger amounts of complement components (including C1-INH) than do resident macrophages or monocytes [20]. In addition, the placenta is apparently capable of C1-INH synthesis [21] as well as megakaryocytes. Platelet alpha granules contain and secrete C1-INH during platelet activation [18].

Although our knowledge of the regulation of hepatic C1-INH synthesis is limited, a role for various cytokines and monokines in the stimulation of C1-INH synthesis has been established. Interferon-α, -β, and -γ (INF)- can stimulate de novo synthesis of C1-INH by human blood monocytes, INF-γ being the most potent [19, 22]. Recently, interleukin (IL)-6 was shown to increase the expression of C1-INH in HepG2 cells, and its activation was potentiated by IL-1 [23, 24]. IL-1 alone had no effect on C1-INH synthesis.

As IL-1 and IL-6 are important mediators of the acute phase response of inflammation, their increased expression leads to increased in vivo synthesis of C1-INH during inflammatory response. Consistent with this finding, it has been known for a long time that C1-INH is an acute phase protein [25].

C1-INH can be cleaved at varying sites by several proteases including trypsin [26], snake venom proteases [27], *Pseudomonas aeruginosa* protease [28], and human neutrophil elastase [29]. The latter has been shown to inactivate C1-INH by cleaving both the N- and the C-terminal portions of the molecule [30, 31]. The elastase molecule does not remain bound to the cleaved C1-INH but retains its enzymatic activity. It was also observed that stimulated neutrophils inactivate C1-INH more rapidly than do proteases released from the neutrophils [30]. This suggests that additional mechanisms, such as oxidation of amino acid residues in the reactive center by free oxygen radicals, may also play a role in the modification of C1-INH activity.

Role of C1-Inhibitor in Human Disease

For many years the understanding of the pathophysiology of C1-INH deficiency was restricted to the genetic defect, i.e., the inherited reduction in the production of functional active C1-INH protein (hereditary angioedema). Later on it was recognized that a reduction in functional C1-INH can be acquired due to anti-idiotype antibody in B-cell lymphoproliferative disorders or autoantibodies to C1-INH (acquired angioedema).

During recent years additional evidence has accumulated that the presence of an insufficient amount of functional C1-INH also plays a crucial role

Table 1. Characterization of C1-inhibitor (C1-INH) deficiency

I Hereditary deficiency
(mechanism: Genetic defects)
A Type I: Impaired synthesis of C1-INH
B Type II: Dysfunctional C1-INH

II Acquired deficiency
(mechanism: Antibody formation and/or uncontrolled triggering factors)
A Anti-idiotype antibody in lymphoproliferative diseases
B Autoantibody to C1-INH
C ACE inhibitors

III Relative deficiency
(mechanism: Increased demand not counterbalanced by increased production, i.e. capillary leak syndrome and (volume-) refractory hypotension in the course of systemic inflammatory response)
A Septic shock
B Interleukin-2 therapy
C Severe burns
D Bone marrow transplantation

in the pathogenesis of capillary leak syndrome (CLS) and (volume-)refractory hypotension during systemic inflammatory response syndrome (SIRS). As C1-INH belongs to the group of acute phase proteins, its production during SIRS is markedly increased, leading to enhanced antigenic levels of C1-INH. In this situation, increased production is accompanied by an increased turnover with target proteases (e.g., factors XIIa and XIIf, C1q, kallikrein) and cleavage by nontarget proteases (e.g., elastase). Patients with signs of CLS or (volume-)refractory hypotension in the course of SIRS present with a reduced functional index (activity/antigen) of C1-INH. In these patients functional C1-INH plasma levels may still be higher than in healthy persons, but they are markedly decreased compared to levels in patients with a similar underlying disease but without signs of CLS and/or (volume-)refractory hypotension. Consequently, it seems appropriate to characterize that condition as a "relative" C1-INH deficiency due to insufficient amounts of functional C1-INH despite increased production (Table 1).

Hereditary Angioedema

Clinical Manifestation

First described by Quincke [32] and Osler [33] more than 100 years ago as hereditary angio*neurotic* edema, the mode of inheritance of this condition was identified in 1917 as autosomal codominant, with equal sex and racial distribution [34]. The disease was defined biochemically in 1963, when Donaldson and Evans [35] demonstrated that patients with hereditary angioedema (HAE) lack the serum inhibitor of the first component of human complement. More recently, the detailed pathogenetic mechanisms of symptoms and phenotypic variants have been recognized [36–42].

On the basis of the apparent protein abnormality, two subtypes of HAE can be defined [43]. Type I, comprising about 85% of cases of HAE, is characterized by a reduced plasma level of functionally normal C1-INH. The underlying molecular event is the apparent lack of function of one C1-INH allele in the genome. Type II accounts for about 15% of HAE cases. It is characterized by the presence of normal or increased amounts of C1-INH, but the protein has markedly reduced functional activity [39, 44].

Both types of hereditary angioedema are characterized by recurrent, acute, local circumscribed edema of the skin or mucosa. The primary areas involved by edema are the extremities, face, larynx, and gastrointestinal tract. The edema is nonpitting and nonpruritic and is not painful except when there is gastrointestinal tract involvement, in which case patients present with acute, cramping abdominal pain. Frequently, this pain is associated with nausea and vomiting and can lead to emergency surgical intervention. The most serious, and potentially life-threatening manifestation of the disease is laryngeal edema. Prior to the institution of causal replacement therapy with C1-INH concentrate (Berinert P, Behringwerke AG, Germany), death from laryngeal edema commonly occurred. Genealogic data showed that more than 30% of relatives who had characteristic symptoms of HAE had died from laryngeal manifestation. Over the past decade, however, admission to intensive care units and life-saving resuscitation maneuvers (tracheostomy or intubation) have declined as administration of 500–1500 units of C1-INH concentrate has been shown to be consistently effective in reversing laryngeal and abdominal edema [36, 45] (Table 2).

Molecular Mechanism

A decrease in C1-INH functional acitivity is associated with angioedema attack. Since C1-INH is the only known inhibitor of the complement system (classical path) and the major inhibitor of factor XII-mediated contact activation, the mediators of those systems play an important role in the pathogenesis and mediation of the symptoms of angioedema.

C1-INH plasma deficiency allows autoactivation of the first component of complement with consumption of C4 and C2. Consequently, C4 levels are virtually undetectable during an attack, while C2 levels are substantially reduced [46]. Furthermore, levels of anaphylatoxins C3a and C4a are reported to be increased during attacks [41]. Uncontrolled activation of the contact system takes place leading to reductions in plasma levels of factor XII coupled with an increase in kallikrein activity and plasmin-α_2-antiplasmin complexes during attacks [47, 48]. These changes were demonstrated to be accompanied by decreased levels of prekallikrein (a substrate of activated factor XII and an indicator of bradykinin formation) and of high-molecular-weight kininogen (a substrate for kallikrein) [49]. Furthermore, induced blister fluids obtained from patients with HAE were found to contain activated kallikrein and decreased levels of prekallikrein and high-molecular-weight kininogen [50] (see Fig. 5). As a consequence, a kinin-like mediator and/or a C2-like derived split product are episodically released, resulting in edema of the subcutaneous or submucosal tissues.

Replacement therapy with C1-INH concentrate in patients with HAE is

Table 2. Treatment of attacks with C1-inhibitor (C1-INH) concentrate in patients with hereditary angioedema [36]

Site of edema	No. of patients	No. of infusions	C1-INH[a] (units)	Time until effective (min)
Abdominal	4	15	1000	60–120
Laryngeal	23	67	1000/1500	30–60

[a] One unit corresponds to the amount of C1-INH present in 1 ml normal human plasma.

followed by an increase in C4 [51] high-molecular-weight kininogen, and prekallikrein levels [40, 41] in parallel to rapid clinical improvement.

Acquired Angioedema

Immunologically Mediated Acquired Angioedema

Acquired angioedema (AAE) is characterized by symptoms identical to those of HAE but with onset after the fourth decade of life and in the absence of a family history of these symptoms. Two distinct forms are described. The first is caused by an associated disease (usually lymphoproliferative), while the second results from the presence of autoantibodies to C1-INH (autoimmune AAE). These autoantibodies may belong to all three major immunoglobulin classes. Apart from the biochemical characteristics of HAE (decrease in C1-INH, C2, and C4), the low plasma level of the C1 complex appears to be pathognomonic for the acquired form [44]. The demonstration of rapid in vivo turnover of C1 and C1-INH [52] and some experimental proofs of C1 activation and C1-INH depletion by the underlying lymphoproliferative or autoimmune disease [36, 53–55] led to the hypothesis that the cause of C1-INH deficiency should not be seen in C1-INH complexation but rather in marked C1 activation and subsequent consumption of the inhibitor. Recently an inactive C1-INH fragment (M 96000) in the plasma of patients with acquired C1-INH deficiency was found which is considered to be the result of cleavage of C1-INH (M 105000) by C1s [56].

In AAE, the leading pathogenetic mechanism seems not to be the reduced C1-INH functional activity favoring spontaneous autoactivation of the target proteases, but an overwhelming activation of proteases that is not counterbalanced by sufficient amounts of C1-INH. Consequently, effective treatment of AAE patients with normalization of C1-INH is not accompanied by substantial increases in the target proteases, as C1 complex and C4 invariably remain low [36].

The treatment of symptoms in AAE is identical to that in HAE, except that the amount of C1-INH concentrate needed in order to obtain regression of symptoms may be considerably higher (three to four times the dose required in HAE).

ACE-Inhibitor-Induced Acquired Angioedema

Angiotensin-converting enzyme (ACE) inhibitors have been in clinical use as antihypertensive agents since 1980. Reported side effects include cough, azotemia, hyperkalemia, hypotension, and angioedema. The incidence of angioedema associated with the use of ACE inhibitors ranges between 0.1% and 0.2% [57].

As ACE is partially responsible for the inactivation of bradykinin, the use of ACE inhibitors interferes with bradykinin degradation, thus potentiating its effects. As this protein is involved in the pathogenesis of angioedema attack, patients with hereditary and acquired angioedema are at a considerable risk of developing dramatic angioedema attacks during the course of treatment with ACE inhibitors, which may even result in severe hypotensive shock [58]. However, the occurrence of angioedema attacks seems not to be restricted to patients with genetic defects of C1-INH. There are numerous reports that C1-INH antigenic and functional plasma levels are not decreased during ACE-inhibitor-induced angioedema attacks [57, 59].

Caspritz [60] demonstrated that rat paw edema induced by the factor XII activator carrageenin and its potentiation by ACE inhibition could be totally blocked by infusion of C1-INH concentrate. Furthermore, Van der Starre et al. [61] reported that the kinin-mediated hypotension could be minimized by the administration of C1-INH concentrate. In consequence, C1-INH concentrate was administered in patients with ACE-inhibitor-induced angioedema as well, and was found to be effective [62] as it inhibited further progression of edema formation [63, 64].

Capillary Leak Syndrome

In 1960, Clarkson et al. [65] reported the case of a young woman who had several episodes of shock due to leakage of plasma from the circulation secondary to a sudden and striking increase in capillary permeability. No triggering event could be detected. Over the years more cases had been described but the pathophysiology of the syndrome remained unknown.

As one of the patients with spontaneous capillary leak [66] presented with post-partum angioedema of the vulva with rapid spread and subsequent involvement of almost the entire body, a decrease in C1-INH levels was accused as the causative factor. Thus, both antigenic and functional C1-INH plasma levels were measured in patients with spontaneously occurring systemic CLS but were found to be within the range seen in unaffected individuals [67, 68]. More detailed investigations revealed low complement proteins (C3, C4) and high complement activation products (C3a) despite normal C1-INH levels [69–71]. Furthermore, prekallikrein levels were found to be reduced to 50% of normal during attacks [72]. Both the clinical signs and the laboratory pattern resemble those seen in hereditary and acquired angioedema, except that C1-INH plasma levels are not decreased. Whether administration of C1-INH concentrate will be beneficial in patients with spontaneous CLS despite the fact that C1-INH plasma levels appear not to be decreased (as it is the case in ACE-inhibitor-induced angioedema), remains to be investigated. As spontaneous CLS is an extremely rare disease, no therapeutic intervention has yet been carried out.

Systemic Inflammatory Response

Generally, inflammation is regarded as the host response to injury (with or without exposure to bacteria and bacterial products) which aims at the removal of devitalized tissues, destruction of bacteria, and reestablishment of the integrity of host tissues. Inflammation is primarily a beneficial response to a particular stimulus rather than an essentially deleterious pathological process (Fig. 2).

In the late 1980s, a syndrome of multiple organ dysfunction seen in patients with sepsis, polytrauma, severe burns, pancreatitis, and other forms of cirtical illness was identified. This syndrome was associated with a high mortality [73] and was characterized by pulmonary, cardiovascular, hepatic, renal, gastrointestinal, and central nervous system dysfunction. An autopsy study in 35 polytraumatized patients revealed increased lung, heart, kidney, liver, and spleen organ weights, accumulation of polymorphonuclear leukocytes, and interstitial edema with no signs of circulatory overload [74]. In conclusion, it was hypothesized that multiple organ failure is the result of a generalized inflammatory reaction that produced deleterious effects on

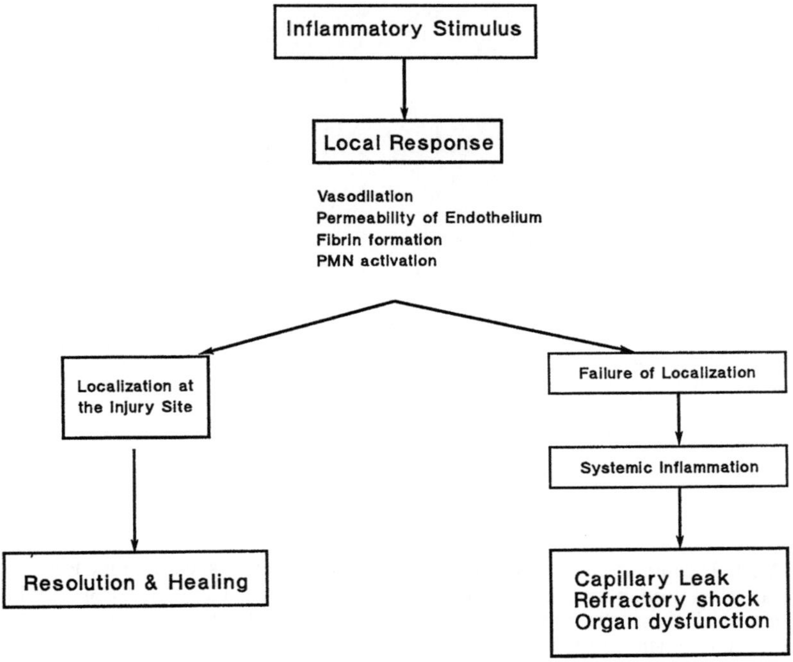

Fig. 2. Pathogenesis of organ injury. A failure of regulatory mechanisms to localize the inflammatory response may lead to systemic activation of cascade systems and bystander organ injury

bystander organs. Furthermore, it was recognized that although inflammation can be initiated by various events, the body's response to them is remarkably similar [75] (Fig. 3).

Following a triggering event, the host is immediately exposed to a number of proinflammatory substances. These mediators produce a specific response consisting of vasodilation, increased permeability, edema, thrombosis, and leukocyte emigration and activation. While these molecular mediators are locally confined in normal settings, their activity may beome deleterious during certain predisposing conditions like pancreatitis, long-bone injury with fat embolism, reperfusion injury, or mechanical, chemical, or thermal trau-

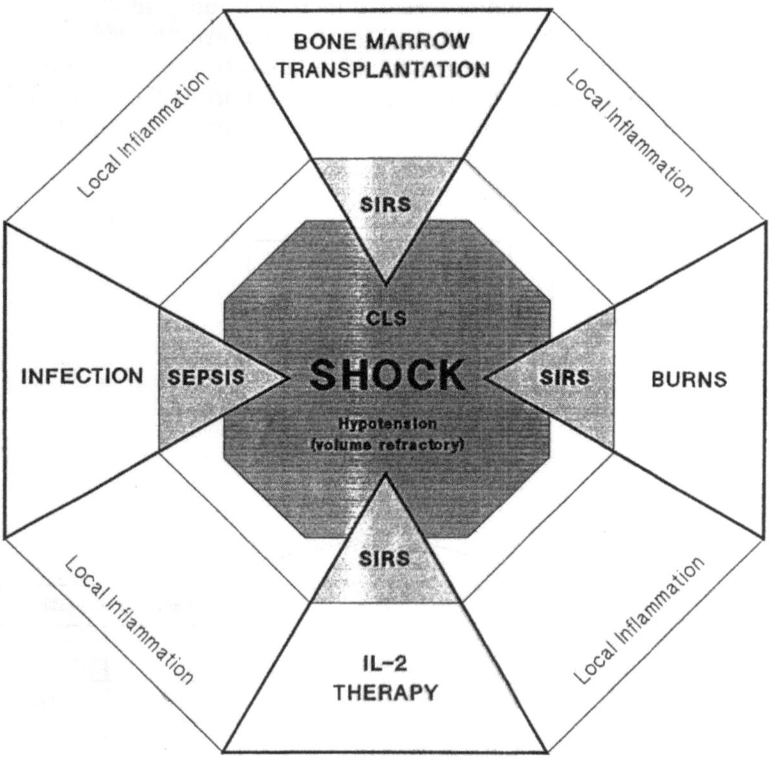

Fig. 3. Inflammation can be initiated by various events, such as infection, bone marrow transplantation, burns, and interleukin-2 (IL-2) therapy. The body's response to inflammation of all these etiologies is remarkably similar and includes vasodilation, increased permeability, edema formation, thrombosis, and leukocyte activation and emigration. When localization at the site of injury cannot be achieved, a systemic inflammatory response syndrome (SIRS) occurs. SIRS may exacerbate to its worst complication, shock with capillary leak syndrome (CLS) and volume-refractory hypotension. The unbalanced activation of complement and contact systems appears to be responsible for this catastrophic event

ma. An "all-out response" may occur [76], resulting in an exaggerated release of the mediators for which the term "systemic inflammatory response syndrome" (SIRS) was introduced.

Regulation of the Systemic Inflammatory Response

Development of a sound rationale for therapeutic intervention in SIRS requires two things: definition of regulatory mechanisms and, more important, recognition of the hierarchies between the biological systems involved.

For a long time it has been accepted that cytokines play an important role in the development of SIRS. Their plasma levels are elevated in clinical and experimental models of spesis [77–83]. Antibodies or other agents that neutralize the biological effects of cytokines in vivo have been shown to attenuate or even prevent the development of sepsis in animals [84–89]. Most interestingly, administration of cytokines to animals or humans induces a septic shock-like syndrome and leads to activation of neutrophils and of plasma cascade systems in a pattern similar to that seen after endotoxin challenge [81, 90–93]. This has been demonstrated for TNF, IL-1, and IL-2 [94–99]. However, most of the biological effects are not directly mediated by cytokines but are transmitted through cellular and humoral mediator systems [100, 101]. The complement and contact systems have both been implicated for more than 20 years in the development of the body's inflammatory response, but their role failed to be clearly defined (for review see [102, 103]). Now there is growing evidence that both systems are responsible for the induction of CLS and refractory shock in the course of SIRS.

The first evidence suggesting that the unbalanced activation of complement and contact systems represents the key factor in the pathogenesis of SIRS-related CLS was provided by Nürnberger et al. [104]. They reported on a premature baby who during the first days of life developed severe CLS. The symptoms were pericardial effusions, generalized edema, considerable weight gain, and consequent volume-refractory shock necessitating plasma transfusions and high-dose vasopressor medication. Laboratory analyses were consistent with an uncontrolled activation of the complement and cascade systems. C1-INH concentrate was administered at an initial dose of 300 U/kg body weight, followed by 100 U/kg body weight and 50 U/kg body weight during the subsequent days. Within 36 h dopamine infusion, which initially had been at a rate of more than 10 μg/kg per minute, could be stopped as the circulation stabilized. Within 6 days the edema completely resolved and body weight fell to the starting level. Although this successful administration of C1-INH concentrate was done as an uncontrolled, single-case intervention, the rapid stabilization of the patient's hemodynamic balance and the quick reduction of generalized edema provided the first suggestive evidence that the uncontrolled activation of complement and contact systems represents the final pathogenetic principle in the formation of SIRS-related CLS.

Septic Shock

Role of Complement and Contact Systems

Sepsis is synonymous to the systemic inflammatory response to invading microorganisms. Its clinical sequelae, however, result not from the pathogens but mainly from excessive triggering of endogenous mediator systems [86, 105–113]. When sepsis exacerbates to its worst complication, volume-refractory septic shock with concomitant signs of malperfusion, the complement and the contact systems come into play (Fig. 3). Both systems can be directly activated by gram-negative and gram-positive bacteria and their by-products (Fig. 5).

Levels of native complement factors are almost uniformly lowest in septic patients with (fatal) shock [114–116]. Activated complement factors C3a-desarg [77. 117], C3a activity [118], C4a-desarg [119], C5a-desarg [120], and TCC [118] are usually higher in patients with septic shock than in septic patients without shock. In patients with septic shock, a significant inverse correlation between initial plasma C5a activity and both systemic vascular resistance and mean arterial blood pressure has been found [96]. The anaphylatoxin C5a has hypotensive effects in various animal models [121–124] and decomplementation abolishes the hypotensive response to endotoxin [125]. In addition, direct effects of anaphylatoxin on the heart may contribute to hypotension. In a rabbit model, intracoronary administration of C3a causes tachycardia, impairment of atrioventricular conduction, left ventricular contractile failure, coronary vasoconstriction, and histamine release [126].

In primates, administration of a polyclonal antibody to C5a is able to partially attenuate the hypotensive response to live *E. coli* infusion [155]. In a rat endotoxin model, similar effects have been observed with F(ab')2 fragments of a polyclonal anti-C5a antibody [124]. Both studies show that neutralization of C5a does not completely prevent hypotension in sepsis, suggesting that other mechanisms are also involved.

Plasma levels of contact system proteins in patients with sepsis are low, in particular in those with shock [128–132] (see Fig. 5). Mean arterial pressure in 48 patients with sepsis (measured at the time of admission to the intensive care unit and at a time when the patients had not yet received significant vasopressor medication) significantly correlated with factor XII and prekallikrein levels as a parameter for bradykinin formation [133].

Recently, firm evidence for activation of the contact system in sepsis was provided by Pixley et al. [134], who demonstrated that infusion of a monoclonal antibody that blocks factor XII activity partially prevented the fall in blood pressure and significantly prolonged survival in septic baboons [134].

C1-INH: One Important Regulatory Principle of Systemic Inflammatory Response and Sepsis

As already stressed, C1-INH is the major inhibitor of the complement (classical path) and contact systems. Thus, C1-INH regulates the activity of two plasma cascade systems that are known for their vasodilating and vasopermeability-enhancing effects. C1-INH is therefore an important regulator of inflammatory reactions [135].

C1-INH is an acute-phase protein whose levels may increase up to twofold during uncomplicated infections and other inflammatory conditions. The increased synthesis of C1-INH under these conditions is most probably meant to protect the organism against the deleterious effects of (intravascular) activation of the complement and contact systems during acute-phase reactions [129]. Consequently, both functional and antigenic levels of C1-INH were increased during uncomplicated infections and sepsis [136]. If a patient presented with refractory shock, especially if the shock episode was fatal, functional plasma levels of C1-INH were not elevated in spite of its acute-phase properties. In addition, antigenic levels were higher than functional levels, indicating the presence of nonfunctional C1-INH. Probably, the nonfunctional C1-INH was due to increased degradation [136]. Neutrophil elastase, which is released by activated neutrophils, is most likely responsible for the catalytic inactivation of most serpins including C1-INH [29].

These findings led to the hypothesis that in the course of SIRS/sepsis increased degradation of C1-INH results in insufficient control of the complement and contact cascades, which enhances the activation of either system and contributes to the development of septic shock syndrome.

Therapeutic Intervention with C1-INH Concentrate

In a pilot study five patients with volume-refractory septic shock and signs of organ dysfunction (for eligibility criteria see [77, 119]) were treated with C1-INH concentrate for 5 days with a loading dose of 2000 U, followed by 1000 U every 12 h given as an intravenous infusion over 1 h. Before replacement therapy with C1-INH concentrate, all patients needed mechanical ventilatory support as well as volume substitution and therapy with vasopressor and positive inotropic drugs (dobutamine, dopamine, and/or norepinephrine) to maintain an adequate blood pressure.

In four patients replacement therapy with C1-INH concentrate resulted in an increase in plasma functional C1-INH levels and revealed signs of attenuated complement and contact systems activation (decrease in C3a and C5a levels, increase in prekallikrein and factor XII levels), which led to a substantial decrease in the amount of vasopressor medication needed.

In one patient who presented with liver cirrhosis as a concomitant disease there was almost no increase in plasma functional C1-INH levels during C1-INH replacement therapy. In this patient, the therapeutic intervention was not followed by attenuation of the unregulated activation of both complement and contact system, as indicated by unchanged levels of C3a and factor XII, and a further decrease in prekallikrein. Consequently, the hemodynamic situation worsened during the treatment period and the patient's need for vasopressor medication (dopamine and norepinephrine) increased further.

However, due to the variable recovery of C1-INH concentrate, which was attributed to proteolytic degradation by elastase and capillary leakage, the dosage regimen was changed during a subsequent dose-finding trial. The aim was to increase the dose of C1-INH during the first days of treatment in order to block unregulated complement and contact activation more efficiently, thereby preventing protein leakage through damaged endothelium and thus achieving a higher recovery of the drug (Fig. 4). Again, replacement therapy resulted in a quick (and loading-dose-related) restoration of plasma functional C1-INH levels followed by attenuation of complement and contact system activation. The overall results obtained (no toxic side effects, no sepsis-related mortality during the observation period, attenuation of complement and contact activation, and a possible beneficial effect on hypotension as reflected by a substantially decreased need for vasopressor medication) are very promising [135].

IL-2 Therapy

Role in Therapy

Studies by Rosenberg et al. [137, 138] have shown that administration of high doses of the cytokine IL-2 induces remissions in about 20% of patients with endstage cancer, in particular those with advanced renal cell carcinoma and melanoma. The administration of rIL-2, however, was found to be associated with serious dose-dependent side effects including fever, confusion, and hepatic and renal dysfunction. Even the formation of angioedema attacks in a patient with normal C1-INH activity was reported [90]. At higher doses, rIL-2 invariably induced a life-threatening CLS, characterized by vascular leakage and hypotension (Fig. 3). Hemodynamic studies have indicated that the circulatory changes induced by high doses of rIL-2 are similar to those seen in septic shock [94, 139]. The latter is not surprising as rIL-2 treatment not only induces the production of IL-1β and TNFα by peripheral blood mononuclear cells [140–142] but also activates other inflammatory mediators, such as neutrophils [90], complement [90, 92, 127], and contact (bradykinin-form-

→

Fig. 4. Different dosage regimens of C1-inhibitor (C1-INH) administered with the aim of arriving at a more efficient blocking of the unregulated complement and contact system activation. Treatment schedule 3 resulted in the most effective restoration of functional C1-INH plasma levels. This was followed by attenuation of complement and contact systems activation and, more importantly, by quick stabilization of the hemodynamics

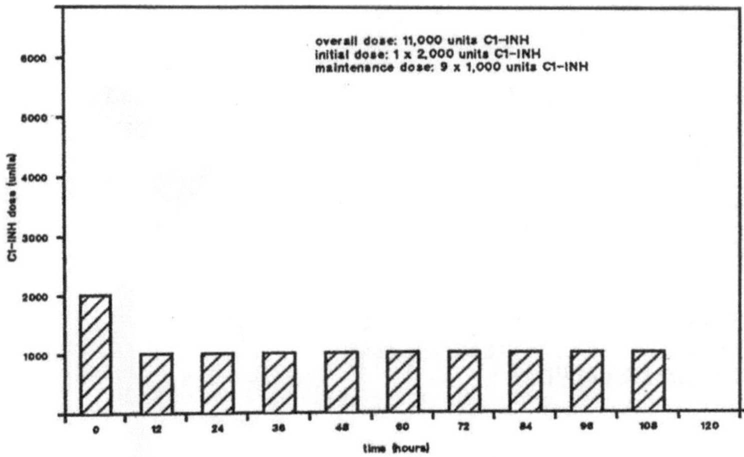

Treatment Schedule 1

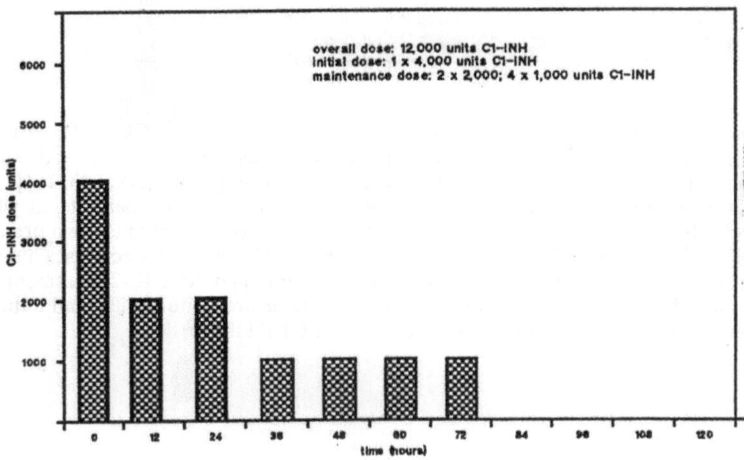

Treatment Schedule 2

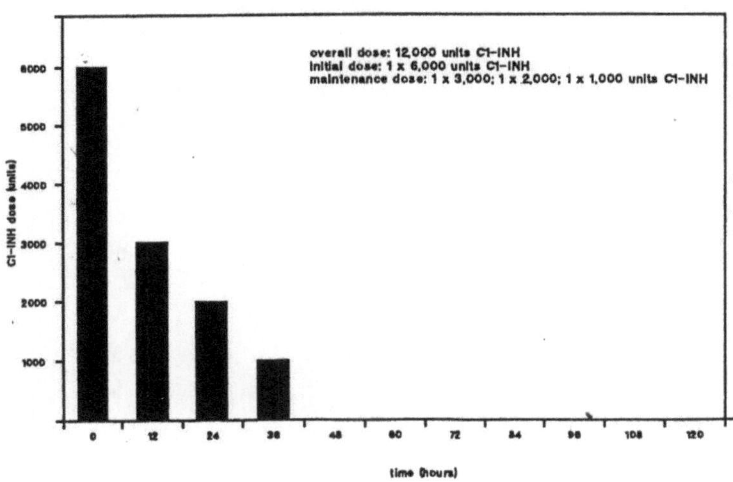

Treatment Schedule 3

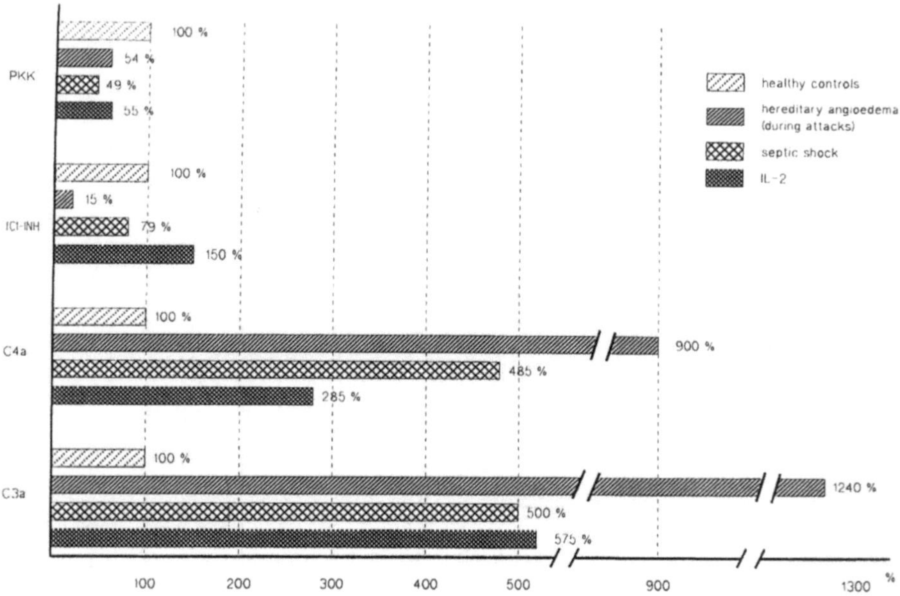

Fig. 5. Comparison of prekallikrein (PKK), functional C1-inhibitor (fC1-INH), C4a, and C3a levels between healthy controls and patients with angioedema attack, in septic shock, and after high-dose interleukin-2 (IL-2) treatment (taken from [40, 41, 119, 143, 154]). Results are given in percentage of normal levels except for IL-2-treated patients, in whom plasma levels after high-dose IL-2 treatment were compared to the patients' own pretreatment baseline. Despite the differences in plasma fC1-INH levels between patients with hereditary angioedema and those in septic shock or after high-dose IL-2 treatment, the laboratory patterns of the complement and contact systems are quite similar and indicates uncontrolled activation due to insufficient amounts of C1-inhibitor

ing) systems. In particular, levels of factor XII and prekallikrein markedly decrease during IL-2 therapy to yield levels comparable to those seen in severe sepsis and septic shock [143] (Fig. 5). These changes in contact system proteins correlate with the clinical signs and severity of CLS [143].

As patient populations with septic shock tend to be heterogeneous due to differences in the underlying diseases, the characteristics and number of infecting microorganisms, and the infectious focus, the results of intervention studies can be heavily influenced by unbalanced comorbidities. As toxic side effects (CLS and shock) of IL-2 therapy are generally considered as a human model for septic shock, attenuation of these side effects might not only reduce the mortality and morbidity of IL-2 therapy, but yield valuable information for the treatment of sepsis and septic shock in a more homogeneous patient population as well.

Therapeutic Intervention with C1-INH Concentrate

For the reasons just given, a trial was performed on the effect of the replacement therapy with C1-INH concentrate in the treatment of IL-2-induced septic shock-like syndrome [135]. Two groups of patients were treated exclusively with rIL-2 (Eurocetus, Amsterdam, The Netherlands). The first group (six patients) received rIL-2 at a fixed-dose regimen (18×10^6 U daily for 4 days), the second group (four patients) with escalating doses increasing by 18×10^6 U every 3rd day. A third group (six patients) received 72×10^6 U rIL-2 daily for 4 days together with C1-INH concentrate given at a dose of 2000 U initially, followed by 1000 U every 12 h for 4 days.

The C1-INH co-treated group was able to tolerate (at least) 2.7 times more rIL-2. These results suggested that C1-INH co-treatment was sufficient to reduce rIL-2 toxicity and rIL-2-induced complement and contact activation. Moreover, the effects of C1-INH replacement therapy observed in the rIL-2-treated patients were comparable to the effects seen in the C1-INH-treated patients with septic shock (i.e., attenuated complement activation, stabilized hemodynamic situation) [135]. In addition, the biochemical profile was favorable inasmuch as the degree of complement activation (C3a) plotted against the cumulative dose of rIL-2 given was less in the C1-INH co-treated group than in the other two groups [135].

Severe Burns

Host Response to Thermal Injury

The pathogenesis of circulatory shock in severe burn cases is currently acknowledged to be a continuous process comprising two different events. First a massive systemic inflammatory response is induced, and although it is initiated almost immediately, the systemic response progresses with time and peaks 5–7 days after injury [144, 145]. The initial burn injury activates the inflammatory mediator cascades, i.e., cytokines, complement and contact systems, and primes mononuclear cells. This response becomes more pronounced if any other subsequent triggering event occurs [146, 147]. With a second insult, e.g., when bacerial colonization of the wound progresses to severe infection, the production of inflammatory mediators increases. This further amplifies the process, leading to a vicious circle of inflammation resulting in hemodynamic instability and further tissue injury [148]. Early burn wound removal ameliorates the later response, indicating the importance of the wound in this process [149].

Again, the inflammatory response during the first stage is regarded as beneficial in that bacterial defenses are increased and devitalized tissues can be removed. However, it can result in a deleterious potentiation of autodestructive inflammation. As already seen in sepsis, also in severe burns IL-6 is also released very rapidly into the circulation and large increases in IL-6 correlate with mortality rates. Comparable to the situation in severe sepsis, IL-6 mediates the acute-phase response and thus increases the production of C1-INH, guaranteeing sufficient control of complement and contact activation. If the hemodynamic situation deteriorates, however, and a shock syndrome with CLS and volume-refractory hypotension occurs, functional active C1-INH appears to be insufficient (Fig. 3). In such patients the complement (classical path) and contact systems are markedly activated and the degree of activation correlates not only with the severity of the clinical situation but also with mortality rates [76, 150]. Thus, the administration of C1-INH concentrate appears as an appropriate therapeutic approach to reregulate the uncontrolled activation of complement and contact systems.

Therapeutic Intervention with C1-INH Concentrate

First clinical results obtained in a total of 12 burned patients with (volume-refractory) septic shock syndrome support this rationale. In almost all patients circulatory shock was successfully stopped and hemodynamics stabilized (personal communications from: F. Jostkleiglewe and K. A. Brandt; D. Kistler and R. Hettich; B. Stark, H. Horch, and G. Spilker).

As hemodynamic stabilization guarantees more rapid wound closure by early excision and grafting of the burn wound, and as rapid wound closure was found to improve mortality [151], the administration of C1-INH concentrate might already represent a promising therapeutic approach in managing severely burned patients. Whether this therapy is also sufficient to improve long-term survival in these patients will require a double-blind, placebo-controlled approach.

Bone Marrow Transplantation

Clinical Sequelae to Bone Marrow Transplantation

CLS is a frequent complication following bone marrow transplantation (BMT), with mortality rates up to 75% [72, 152]. The symptoms are the consequences of the loss of vascular fluids to extravascular spaces and resemble those commonly seen in the course of high-dose IL-2 treatment: generalized edema, weight gain, ascites, pleural or pericardial effusion, tachycardia, hypotension, and/or pre-renal failure (Fig. 3). Localized forms of CLS may also occur, e.g., lung edema or veno-occlusive disease, the latter being characterized as CLS of the liver [152].

Recently, it was demonstrated that the onset of CLS after BMT is accompanied by unregulated activation of the classical pathway of complement and decreasing functional levels of C1-INH, the latter due to reactions with target proteases. In patients with uneventful courses after BMT, i.e., those without development of CLS, complement proteins C3 and C4 as well as C1-INH increased during the first days after BMT and the complement activation product C4d remained almost unchanged. Those patients, however, who developed CLS after BMT exhibited a decrease in functional C1-INH levels coincident with the occurrence of CLS. This decrease in inhibitory capacity was accompanied by signs of strong complement activation, i.e., increase in C4d [152].

Therapeutic Intervention with C1-INH Concentrate

In view of the above findings, C1-INH concentrate was administered to four patients under an open protocol, primarily focusing on the question whether or not the administration of C1-INH resulted in a decrease of uncontrolled complement and contact activation. Seven doses of C1-INH concentrate were given: initial dose 60 U/kg, followed by 2 doses of 30 U/kg each and 4 doses of 15 U/kg each, every 12 h. After C1-INH administration, C4d levels decreased from 200% to 135% of baseline and prekallikrein levels (as a measure of bradykinin formation) increased from 60% to 75% of baseline. The amelioration of complement and contact activation was accompanied by a definite improvement of CLS in three-quarters of the patients. In one-quarter of the patients CLS improved but was recurrent, later necessitating a second but successful cycle of C1-INH replacement therapy [153].

The results of that pilot experience formed the basis for a controlled study in which patients are being randomly allocated to either standard therapy plus C1-INH concentrate or standard therapy without. The results of this study will shed light on whether amelioration of complement and contact activation results in reduced morbidity and mortality in patients with CLS after BMT.

Conclusions and Perspectives

Different predisposing conditions – extensive trauma, infection, pancreatitis – result in a remarkably similar inflammatory response. Although this inflammatory response primarily aims at the removal of devitalized tissues, destruction of bacteria, and reestablishment of the integrity of host tissues, it may potentially become unregulated and generalized and thereby produce effects deleterious to vital organs or the body as a whole. Cytokines play an important role in the development of the systemic inflammatory response. Most of their biological effects, however, are not directly mediated but exerted through other mediator systems. When the inflammatory response results in the formation of capillary leak syndrome and refractory hypotension, the unregulated activation of complement and contact systems appears to be the cause. Both systems are almost exclusively regulated by C1-INH. An unbalanced degradation of the inhibitor protein was found to be associated with the onset of capillary leakage in various conditions such as bone marrow transplantation, severe burns, and septic shock. Therapeutic intervention studies were initiated using high doses of C1-INH. Although tested in an uncontrolled fashion, first results are promising, as in most patients the administration of the drug was followed by a quick and marked improvement in hemodynamics. Whether the administration of C1-INH alone or in combination with other drugs is also sufficient to improve long-term survival has to be investigated in double-blind, placebo-controlled studies.

References

1. Bock SC, Skriver K, Nielsen E et al (1986) Human C1-inhibitor: primary structure, cDNA cloning and chromosomal localization. Biochemistry 25:4292–4301
2. Harrison RA (1983) Human C1-inhibitor: improved isolation and preliminary structural characterization. Biochemistry 22:5001
3. Nilsson T, Wiman B (1982) Purification and characterization of human C1-esterase inhibitor. Biochim Biophys 705:271
4. Perkins SJ, Smith KF, Amatayakul S et al (1990) Two-domain structure of the native and reactive centre cleaved forms of C1-inhibitor of human complement by neutron scattering. J Mol Biol 214:751–756
5. Laskowski M Jr, Kato I (1980) Protein inhibitors of proteinases. Ann Rev Biochem 49:593–626
6. Ziccardi RJ, Cooper NR (1978) Modulation of the antigenicity of C1r and C1s inactivator. J Immunol 121:2148–2152
7. Harpel PC, Cooper NR (1975) Studies on human plasma C1-inactivator enzyme interactions. I. Mechanisms of interaction with C1s, plasmin and trypsin. J Clin Invest 55:593–604
8. Ratnoff OD, Lepow IH (1957) Some properties of an esterase derived from preparations of the first component of complement. J Exp Med 106:327–343
9. Ratnoff OD, Pensky J, Ogston D, Naff GB (1969) The inhibition of plasmin, plasma kallikrein, plasma permeability factor, and the C1r subcomponent of the first component of complement by serum C1-esterase inhibitor. J Exp Med 129:315–331
10. Forbes CD, Pensky J. Ratnoff OD (1970) Inhibition of activated Hageman factor and

activated plasma thromboplastin antecedent by purified C1-inactivator. J Lab Clin Med 76:809–815
11. Schreiber AD, Kaplan AP, Austen KF (1973) Inhibition by C1-INH of Hageman factor fragment activation of coagulation, fibrinolysis, and kinin generation. J Clin Invest 52:1402–1409
12. De Agostini A, Lijnen HR, Pixley RA, Colman RW, Schapira M (1984) Inactivation of factor XII active fragment in normal plasma. J Clin Invest 73:1542–1549
13. Ghebrehiwet B, Siverberg M, Kaplan AP (1981) Activations of the classical pathway of complement by Hageman factor fragment. J Exp Med 153:665–676
14. Ghebrehiwet B, Randazzo BP, Dunn JT (1983) Mechanisms of activation of the classical pathway of complement by Hageman factor fragment. J Clin Invest 71:1450–1455
15. Bjork J, Hugli TE, Smedegård G (1985) Microvascular effects of anaphylatoxins C3a and C5a. J Immunol 134:1115–1119
16. Vane JR, Anggard EE, Botting RM (1990) Regulatory functions of the vascular endothelium. N Engl J Med 323:27–36
17. Johnson AM, Alper CA, Rosen RS, Craig JM (1971) C1-inhibitor: evidence for decreased hepatic synthesis in hereditary angioneurotic oedema. Science 173:553–554
18. Schmaier AH, Smith PM, Colman RW (1985) Platelet C1 inhibitor. A secreted alpha-granule protein. J Clin Invest 75:242–250
19. Lotz M, Zuraw BL (1987) Interferon gamma is a major regulator of C1-inhibitor synthesis by human blood monocytes. J Immunol 139:3382
20. Lappin D, Hamilton AO, Morrison L, Aref M, Whaley K (1986) Synthesis of complement components (C3, C2, B and C1-inhibitor) and lysozyme by human monocytes and macrophages. J Clin Lab Immunol 20:101–105
21. Gitlin D, Biasucci A (1969) Development of G, A, M, IC/IC, C1 esterase inhibitor, ceruloplasmin, transferrin, hemopexin, haptoglobin, fibrinogen, plasminogen, 1-antitrypsin, orosomucoid, lipoprotein, 2-macroglobulin, and prealbumin in the human conceptus. J Clin Invest 48:1433–1446
22. Heda GD, Mardente S, Weiner L, Schmaier AH (1990) Interferon gamma increases in vitro and in vivo expression of C1-inhibitor. Blood 75:2401
23. Falus A, Rokita H, Walcz E, Brozik M, Hidvegi T, Meretey K (1990) Hormonal regulation of complement biosynthesis in human cell lines. II. Upregulation of the biosynthesis of complement components C3, factor B and C1-inhibitor by interleukin-6 and interleukin-1 in human hepatoma cell line. Mol Immunol 27:197
24. Zuraw BL, Lotz M (1990) Regulation of the hepatic synthesis of C1-inhibitor by the hepatocyte stimulating factors interleukin-6 and interferon gamma. J Biol Chem 165:12664
25. Donaldson VH (1966) Serum inhibitor of C1-esterase in health and disease. J Lab Clin Med 68:369–382
26. Haupt H, Heimburger N, Kranz T, Schwick HG (1970) Ein Beitrag zur Isolierung und Charakterisierung des C1-Inaktivators aus Humanplasma. Eur J Biochem 17:254–261
27. Kress LF, Catanese J. Hirayama T (1983) Analysis of the effects of snake venom proteinases on the activity of human plasma C1-esterase inhibitor, α1-antichymotrypsin, and α2-antiplasmin. Biochim Biophys Acta 745:113–120
28. Catanese J, Kress LF (1984) Enzymatic inactivation of human plasma C1-inhibitor and 1-antichymotrypsin by Pseudomonas aeruginosa proteinase and elastase. Biochim Acta 789:37–43
29. Brower MS, Harpel PC (1982) Proteolytic cleavage and inactivation of α2-plasmin inhibitor and C1-inactivator by human polymorphonuclear leukocyte elastase. J Biol Chem 257:9849–9854
30. Pemberton PA, Harison RA, Lachmann PJ, Carrel RW (1989) The structural basis for neutrophil inactivation of C1-inhibitor. Biochem J 258:193–198
31. Reboul A, Prandini MH, Colomb MG (1987) Proteolysis and deglycosylation of human C1-inhibitor: effect on functional properties. Biochem J 244:117–119
32. Quincke H (1882) Über akutes umschriebenes Hautoedem. Monatsschr Prakt Dermatol 1:129–131

33. Osler W (1888) Hereditary angio-neurotic edema. Am J Med Sci 95:362–367
34. Crowder JR, Crowder TR (1917) Five generations of angioneurotic edema. Arch Intern Med 20:840–852
35. Donaldson VH, Evans RR (1963) A biochemical abnormality in hereditary angioneurotic edema: absence of serum inhibitor of C1-esterase. Am J Med 31:37–44
36. Agostoni A, Cicardi M (1992) Hereditary and acquired C1-inhibitor deficiency: biological and clinical characteristics in 235 patients. Medicine 71:206–215
37. Carreer FMJ (1992) The C1-inhibitor deficiency. A review. Eur J Clin Chem Clin Biochem 30:793–807
38. Colten HR (1987) Hereditary angioneurotic edema, 1887 to 1987. N Engl J Med 317:43–45
39. Davis AE (1988) C1-inhibitor and hereditary angioneurotic edema. Ann Rev Immunol 6:595–628
40. Kodama J, Uchida K, Yoshimura S, Katayama Y, Kushiro H, Yutani C et al (1984) Studies of four Japanese families with hereditary angioneurotic edema. Simultaneous activation of plasma protease systems and exogenous triggering stimuli. Blut 49:405–418
41. Sayama K, Shiraishi S, Miki Y (1985) Complement profile in a C1-inhibitor deficient family. Br J Dermatol 113:737–743
42. Widmer M, Späth P, Wüthrich B (1989) Hereditäres Angioödem (HAO): Substitutionstherapie mit C1-inhibitor Konzentrat zur Intervallbehandlung. Allergologie 12:432–439
43. Rosen FS; Charache P, Pensky J, Donaldson V (1965) Hereditary angioneurotic edema: two genetic variants. Science 148:957
44. Oltvai TN, Wong ECC, Atkinson JP, Tung KSK (1991) C1-Inhibitor deficiency: molecular and immunologic basis of hereditary and acquired angioedema. Lab Invest 65:381–388
45. Bork K, Kreuz W, Witzke G (1984) Hereditäres angioneurotisches Ödem. Dtsch Med Wochenschr 109:1331–1335
46. Huston DP, Bressler RB (1992) Urticaria and angioedema. Clin Allergy 76:805–840
47. Hentges F, Humbel R, Dicato M, Hemmer R, Kuntziger H (1986) Acquired C1-esterase inhibitor deficiency: case report with emphasis on complement and kallikrein activation during two patterns of clinical manifestations. J Allergy Clin Immunol 78:860–867
48. Nilsson T, Back O (1985) Elevated plasmin-α_2-antiplasmin complex levels in hereditary angioedema. Evidence for the in vivo efficiency of the intrinsic fibrinolytic pathway. Thromb Res 40:817–824
49. Schapira M, Silver LD, Scott CF, Schmaier AH, Prograis LJ Jr, Curd JG, Colman RW (1983) Prekallikrein activation and high-molecular weight kininogen consumption in hereditary angioedema. N Engl J Med 308:1050–1053
50. Curd JG, Prograis LJ Jr, Cochrane CG (1980) Detection of active kallikrein in induced blister fluids of hereditary angioedema patients. J Exp Med 152:742
51. Agostoni A (1989) Inherited C1-inhibitor deficiency. Complement Inflamm 6:112–118
52. Melamed J, Alper CA, Cicardi M, Rosen FS (1986) The metabolism of C1-inhibitor and C1q in patients with acquired C1-inhibitor deficiency. J Allergy Clin Immunol 77:322–326
53. Geha RS, Quinti I, Austen KF, Cicardi M, Sheffer A, Rosen FS (1985) Acquired C1-inhibitor deficiency associated with antiidiotypic antibody to monoclonal immunoglobulins. N Engl J Med 312:534–540
54. Hauptmann G, Petitjean F, Lang JM, Oberling F (1979) Acquired C1-inhibitor deficiency in a case of lymphosarcoma of the spleen. Reversal of complement abnormalities after splenectomy. Clin Exp Immunol 37:523–531
55. Schreiber AD, Zweiman B, Atkins P, Goldwein F, Pietra G, Atkinson B, Abdou NI (1976) Acquired angioedema with lymphoproliferative disorder: association of C1-inhibitor deficiency with cellular abnormality. Blood 48:567–580

56. Alsenz J, Bork K, Loos M (1987) Autoantibody-mediated acquired deficiency of C1-inhibitor. N Engl J Med 316:1360–1366
57. Chin HL, Buchan DA (1990) Severe angioedema after long-term use of an angiotensin-converting enzyme inhibitor (letter). Ann Intern Med 112:312–313
58. Agostoni A, Cicardi M (1991) Contraindications to the use of ACE-inhibitors in patients with C1-esterase inhibitor deficiency. Am J Med 90:278
59. Seidman MD, Lewandowski CA, Sarpa JR, Potesta E, Schweitzer VG (1990) Angioedema related to angiotensin-converting enzyme inhibitors. Otolaryngol Head Neck Surg 102:727–731
60. Caspritz G (1986) The blocking by human C1-inactivator of both carrageenin paw edema and its potentiation by the angiotensin converting enzyme-inhibitor ramipril. IRCS Med Sci 14:568–569
61. Van der Starre P, Sinclair D, Damen J. Brummelhuis H (1980) Inhibition of the hypotensive effect of plasma protein solutions by C1-esterase inhibitor. J Thorac Cardiovasc Surg 79:738–740
62. Wernze H (1988) Angioneurotisches Ödem unter ACE-Hemmern: Häufigkeit, klinische Charakteristik, Auslösemechamismen. Z Kardiol 77:61–64
63. (1991) Angioneurotische Ödeme und ACE-Hemmer. Bundesgesundheitsbl 7:353
64. Diehl KL, Wernze H (1992) Angioneurotisches Ödem durch Angiotensin-Konversionsenzym-Hemmer. Dtsch Med Wochenschr 117:727–732
65. Clarkson B, Thompson D, Horwith M, Luckey EH (1960) Cyclical edema and shock due to increased capillary permeability. Am J Med 29:193–216
66. Luke IW, Rubenstein E (1962) Fatal postpartum shock due to massive angioneurotic edema. Am J Obst Gynecol 83:322–327
67. George C, Regnier B, Le Gall JR, Gastinne H, Carlet J, Rain M (1978) Hypovolaemic shock with oedema due to increased capillary permeability. Intensive Care Med 4:159–163
68. Teelucksingh S, Padfield PL (1989) Systemic capillary leak syndrome. Lancet I:330–331
69. Cain JR, Bourgoignie JJ, Ahn YS, Schulz DR (1986) Systemic capillary leak syndrome (CLS): a rare cause of systemic edema. Kidney Int 29:181–186
70. Johansson BR, Löfdahl CG (1979) Ultrastructure of the microvessels in skeletal muscle in a case of systemic capillary leak syndrome. Acta Med Scand 206:413–416
71. Löfdahl CG, Sölvell L, Laurell AB, Johansson BR (1979) Systemic capillary leak syndrome with monoclonal IgG and complement alterations. Acta Med Scand 206:405–412
72. Atkinson JP, Waldmann TA, Stein SF et al (1977) Systemic capillary leak syndrome and monoclonal gamopathy. Medicine (Baltimore) 56:225–239
73. Knaus WA, Wagner DP (1989) Multiple systems organ failure: epidemiology and prognosis. Crit Care Clin 5:221
74. Nuytinck HKS, Offermans KK, Goris RJA (1987) Whole body inflammation in trauma patients, an autopsy study. First Vienna Shock Forum, Part A: pathophysiological role of mediators and mediator inhibitors in shock, pp 55–61
75. Williams JG, Maier RV (1992) The inflammatory response. Intensive Care Med 7:53–66
76. Bone RC (1992) Sepsis and multiple organ failure: consensus and controversy. In: Lamy M, Thijs LG (eds) Mediators of sepsis. Springer, Berlin Heidelberg New York pp 3–12
77. Hack CE, De Groot ER; Felt-Bersma RJF et al (1989) Increased plasma levels of interleukin-6 in sepsis. Blood 74:1704–1710
78. Hesse DG, Tracey KJ, Fong Y et al (1988) Cytokine appearance in human endotoxemia and primate bacteremia. Surg Gynecol Obstet 166:147–153
79. Martich GD, Danner RL, Ceska M. Suffredini AF (1991) Detection of IL-8 and TNF in normal humans after intravenous endotoxin: the effect of antiinflammatory agents. J Exp Med 173:1021–1024
80. Michie HR, Manogue KR, Spriggs DR et al (1988) Detection of circulating tumor necrosis factor after endotoxin administration. N Engl J Med 318:1481–1486

81. Van Deventer SJH, Büller HR, ten Cate JW, Aarden LA, Hack CE, Sturk A (1990) Experimental endotoxaemia in humans: analysis of cytokine release and coagulation, fibrinolytic, and complement pathway. Blood 76:2520–2526
82. Van Zee KJ, DeForge LE, Fischer E, Marano MA, Kenney JS, Remick DG Lowry SF, Moldawer LL (1991) IL-8 in septic shock, endotoxemia, and after IL-1 administration. J Immunol 146:3478–3482
83. Waage A, Brandtzaeg P, Halstensen A, Kierulf P, Espevik T (1989) The complex pattern of cytokines in serum from patients with meningococcal septic shock. Association between interleukin-6, interleukin-1 and fatal outcome. J Exp Med 169:333–338
84. Alexander HR, Doherty GM, Buresh CM, Venzon DJ, Norton JA (1991) A recombinant human receptor antagonist to IL-1 improves survival after lethal endotoxemia in mice. J Exp Med 173:1029–1032
85. Ashkenazi A, Marsters SA, Capon DJ et al (1991) Protection against endotoxic shock by tumor necrosis factor receptor immunoadhesion. Proc Natl Acad Sci USA 88:10535–10539
86. Beutler B, Milsark IW, Cerami A (1985) Passive immunization against cachectin/tumor necrosis factor protects mice from lethal effect of endotoxin. Science 229:869–871
87. Heremans H, Van Damme J, Dillen C, Dijkmans R, Billiau A (1990) Interferon gamma, a mediator of lethal lipopolysaccharide-induced Schwartzman-like shock reactions in mice. J Exp Med 171:1853–1869
88. Ohlsson K, Björk P, Bergenfeldt M, Hageman R, Thompson RC (1990) Interleukin-1 receptor antagonist reduces mortality from endotoxin shock. Nature 348:550–552
89. Starnes HF Jr, Pearce MK, Tewari A, Yim JH, Zou JC, Abrams JS (1990) Anti-IL-6 monoclonal antibodies protect against lethal Escherichia coli infection and lethal tumor necrosis factor-alpha challenge in mice. J Immunol 145:4185–4191
90. Baars JWS, Hack CE, Wagstaff J et al (1992) The activation of polymorphonuclear neutrophils and the complement system during immunotherapy with recombinant interleukin-2. Br J Cancer 65:96–101
91. Suffredini AF, Harpel P, Parillo JE (1989) Promotion and subsequent inhibition of plasminogen activator after administration of intravenous endotoxin to normal subjects. N Engl J Med 18:1165–1171
92. Thijs LG, Hack CE, Strack van Schijndel RJM et al (1990) Activation of the complement system during immunotherapy with recombinant interleukin-2: relation to the development of side effects. J Immunol 144:2419–2424
93. Vachino G, Gelfand JA, Atkins MB, Tamerius JD, Demchak P, Mier JW (1991) Complement activation in cancer patients undergoing immunotherapy with interleukin-2 (IL-2): binding of complement and C-reactive protein by IL-2-activated lymphocytes. Blood 78:2505–2513
94. Gaynor ER, Vitek L, Sticklin L et al (1988) The hemodynamic effects of treatment with interleukin-2 and lymphokine activated killer cells. Ann Intern Med 109:953–958
95. Natanson C, Eichenholz PW, Danner RL et al (1989) Endotoxin and tumor necrosis factor challenges in dogs simulate the cardiovascular profile of human septic shock. J Exp Med 169:823–832
96. Ognibene FP, Parker MM, Burch-Whitman C et al (1988) Neutrophil aggregating activity and septic shock in humans: neutrophil aggregation by C5a-like material occurs more frequently than complement component depletion and correlates with depression of systemic vascular resistance. Crit Care Med 3:103–111
97. Okusawa S, Dinarello CA, Yancey KB et al (1987) C5a induction of human interleukin 1. Synergistic effect with endotoxin or interferon-gamma. J Immunol 139:2635–2640
98. Okusawa S, Gelfland JA, Ikejima T, Connolly RJ, Dinarello CA (1988) Interleukin 1 induces a shock-like state in rabbits. J Clin Invest 81:1162–1172
99. Tracey KJ, Beutler B, Lowry SF et al (1986) Shock and tissue injury induced by human recombinant cachectin. Science 234:470–474
100. Piguet PF, Grau GE, Vassalli P (1990) Subcutaneous perfusion of tumor necrosis fac-

tor induces local proliferation of fibroblasts, capillaries, and epidermal cells, or massive tissue necrosis. Am J Pathol 136:103–110
101. Remick DG; Kunkel RG, Larric JW, Kunkel SL (1987) Acute in vivo effects of human recombinant tumor necrosis factor. Lab Invest 56:583–590
102. Colman RW (1992) The role of the kallikrein-kinin system in septic shock. In: Lamy M, Thijs LG (eds) Mediators in sepsis. Springer, Berlin Heidelberg New York, pp 99–112
103. Thijs LG, Hack CE (1992) Role of the complement cascade in severe sepsis. In: Lamy M, Thijs LG (eds) Mediators of sepsis. Springer, Berlin Heidelberg New York, pp 78–98
104. Nürnberger W, Göbel U, Stannigel H, Eisele B, Janssen A, Delvos U (1992) C1-inhibitor concentrate for sepsis-related capillary leak syndrome. Lancet 339:990
105. Beutler B, Cerami A (1987) Cachectin: more than a tumor necrosis factor. N Engl J Med 316:379–385
106. Bone RC (1991) The pathogenesis of sepsis. Ann Intern Med 115:457–469
107. Cohen J, Glauser MP (1991) Septic shock: treatment, Lancet 338:736–739
108. DeForge LE, Nguyen DT, Kunkel SL, Remick DG (1990) Regulation of the pathophysiology of tumor necrosis factor. J Lab Clin Med 116:429–438
109. Fong Y, Lowry SF (1990) Tumor necrosis factor in the pathophysiology of infection and sepsis. Clin Immunol Immunopathol 55:157–170
110. McCabe WR, Treadwell TL, De Maria A Jr (1983) Pathophysiology of bacteremia. Am J Med 75:7–18
111. Morrison DC, Ulevitch RJ (1978) The effects of bacterial endotoxins on host mediation systems. Am J Pathol 93:527–617
112. Parillo JE, Parker MM, Natanson C, Suffredini AF, Danner RL. Cunnion RE, Ognibene FP (1990) Septic shock in humans. Advances in the understanding of pathogenesis, cardiovascular dyscfunction, and therapy. Ann Intern Med 113:227–242
113. Parker MM, Parillo JE (1983) Septic shock. Hemodynamics and pathogenesis. JAMA 250:3324–3327
114. Fearon DT, Ruddy S, Schur PH, McCabe WR (1975) Activation of the properdin pathway of complement in patients with gram-negative bacteremia. N Engl J Med 292:937–940
115. Füst G, Petras G, Ujhelyi E (1976) Activation of the complement system during infections due to gram-negative bacteria. Clin Immunol Immunopathol 5:293–302
116. León C, Rodrigo MJ, Tomasa A et al (1982) Complement activation in septic shock due to gram-negative and gram-positive bacteria. Crit Care Med 10:308–310
117. Slotman GJ, Burchard KW, Williams JJ, D'Arezzo A, Yellin SA (1986) Interaction of prostaglandins, activated complement, and granulocytes in clinical sepsis and hypotension. Surgery 99:744–751
118. Brandtzaeg P, Mollnes TE, Kierulf P (1989) Complement activation and endotoxin levels in systemic meningococcal disease. J Infect Dis 16:58–65
119. Hack CE, Nuijens JH, Felt-Bersma RJF et al (1989) Elevated plasma levels of the anaphylatoxins C3a and C4a are associated with a fatal outcome in sepsis. Am J Med 86:20–26
120. Weinberg PF, Matthay MA, Webster RO, Roskos KV, Goldstein IM, Murray JF (1984) Biologically active products of complement and acute lung injury in patients with the sepsis syndrome. Am Rev Respir Dis 130:791–796
121. Bodammer G, Vogt W (1967) Actions of anaphylatoxin on circulation and respiration in the guinea pig. Int Arch Allergy 32:417–428
122. Lundberg C, Marceau F, Hugli TE (1987) C5a-induced hemodynamic and hematologic changes in the rabbit. Role of cyclooxygenase products and polymorphonuclear leukocytes. Am J Pathol 128:471–483
123. Pavel K, Piper PJ, Smedegård G (1979) Anaphylatoxin-induced shock and two patterns of anaphylactic shock: hemodynamics and mediators. Acta Physiol Scand 105:393–403

124. Smedegard G, Cui L, Hugli TE (1989) Endotoxin-induced shock in the rat. A role for C5a. Am J Pathol 135:489–497
125. Garner R, Chater BV, Brown DL (1974) The role of complement in endotoxin shock and disseminated intravascular coagulation. Experimental observations in the dog. Br J Haematol 28:393–401
126. Hachfeld del Balzo U, Levi R, Polley MJ (1985) Cardiac dysfunction caused by purified human C3a anaphylatoxin. Proc Natl Acad Sci 82:886–890
127. Thijs LG, Hack CE, Strack van Schijndel RJM et al (1989) Complement activation and high-dose of interleukin-2. Lancet II:395
128. Colman RW, Edelman R, Scott CF, Gilman RM (1978) Plasma kallikrein activation and inhibition during typhoid fever. J Clin Invest 61:287–296
129. Kalter ES; Daha MR, ten Cate JW, Verhoef J, Bouma BN (1985) Activation and inhibition of Hageman factor-dependent pathways and the complement system in uncomplicated bacteremia or bacterial shock. J Infect Dis 151:1019–1027
130. Mason JM, Kleeberg V, Dolan P, Colman RW (1970) Plasma kallikrein and Hageman factor in gram-negative bacteremia. Ann Intern Med 73:545–551
131. Nuijens JH, Huijbregts CC, Eerenberg-Belmer AJ et al (1988) Quantification of plasma factor XIIa-C1-inhibitor and kallikrein-C1-inhibitor complexes in sepsis. Blood 72:1841–1848
132. Robinson JA, Kloduycky ML, Lock HH, Racic MR, Gunner RM (1975) Endotoxin prekallikrein, complement and systemic vascular resistance sequential measurements in man. Am J Med 59:61–67
133. Hack CE, Nuijens JH, Strack van Schijndel RJM, Abink JJ, Eerenberg AJM, Thijs LG (1990) A model for the interplay of inflammatory mediators in sepsis – a study in 48 patients. Intensive Care Med 16:187–191
134. Pixley RA, De La Cadena R, Page JD et al (1993) The contact system contributes to hypotension but not disseminated intravascular coagulation in lethal bacteremia: in vivo use of a monoclonal antifactor XII antibody to block contact activation in baboons. J Clin Invest (in press)
135. Hack CE, Ogilvie AC, Eisele B, Eerenberg AJM, Wagstaff J, Thijs LG (1993) C1-inhibitor substitution therapy in septic shock and in the vascular leak syndrome induced by high doses of interleukin-2. Intensive Care Med 19:(in press)
136. Nuijens JH, Eerenberg-Belmer AJM, Huijbregts CCM et al (1989) Proteolytic inactivation of plasma C1-inhibitor in sepsis. J Clin Invest 84:443
137. Rosenberg SA, Lotze MT, Muul LM et al (1987) A progress report on the treatment of 157 patients with advanced cancer using lymphokine-activated killer cells and interleukin-2 or high-dose interleukin-2 alone. N Engl J Med 316:889–897
138. Rosenberg SA, Lotze MT, Mule JJ (1988) New approaches to the immunotherapy of cancer using interleukin-2. Ann Intern Med 108:853–864
139. Ognibene FP, Rosenberg SA, Lotze M, Skibber J, Parker MM, Shelhamer JH, Parillo JE (1988) Interleukin-2 administration causes reversible hemodynamic changes and left ventricular dysfunction similar to those seen in septic shock. Chest 94:750–754
140. Boccoli G, Masciulli R, Ruggeri EM et al (1990) Adaptive immunotherapy of human cancer: the cytokine cascade and monocyte activation following high-dose interleukin-2 bolus treatment. Cancer Res 50:5795–5800
141. Jablons DM, Mul' JJ, McIntosh JK et al (1989) IL-6/IFN-β-2 as a circulating hormone. Induction by cytokine administration in humans. J Immunol 142:1542–1547
142. Mier JW, Vachino G, Van der Meer JW et al (1988) Induction of circulating tumor necrosis factor (TNF alpha) as the mechanism for the febrile response to interleukin-2 (IL-2) in cancer patients. J Clin Immunol 8:426–436
143. Hack CE, Wagstaff J, Strack van Schijndel RJM, Eerenberg AJM, Pinedo HM, Thijs LG, Nuijens JH (1991) Studies on the contact system of coagulation during therapy with high doses of recombinant IL-2: implications for septic shock. Thromb Haemost 65:497–503
144. Nuytinck HKS, Offermans KK, Goris RJA (1988) Whole body inflammation in trauma patients. Arch Surg 123:1519

145. Oldham K, Guice K, Till G, Ward P (1988) Activation of complement by hydroxyl radical thermal injury. Surgery 104:272–277
146. Nerlich M, Flynn J, Demling R (1983) Effect of thermal injury on endotoxin induced lung injury. Surgery 92:289
147. Wilmore D, Orcutt T, Mason A (1975) Alterations in hypothalamic function following thermal injury. J Trauma 15:697
148. Youn YK, LaLonde C, Demling R (1992) The role of mediators in the response to thermal injury. World J Surg 16:30–36
149. Demling R, LaLonde C (1993) Early burn excision attenuates the post burn lung and systemic response to endotoxin. Surgery (in press)
150. Adam A, Damas J, Albert A, Ers P, Marichi J, Calay G, Laurent P (1986) Plasma prokallikrein and kininogens in burned patients. Thromb Res 41:537–543
151. Scott-Conner CEH, Meydrech E (1988) Quantitation of rate of wound closure and the prediction of death following major burns. Burns 14:373–378
152. Nürnberger W, Michelmann I, Petrik K et al (1993) Activity of C1-esterase inhibitor in patients with vascular leak syndrome after bone marrow transplantation. Ann Hematol 67:17–21
153. Nürnberger W, Petrik K, Kurre P, Lauermann G, Michelmann I, Burdach S, Göbel U (1993) Effect of C1-esterase inhibitor (C1-INH) on the activation of complement and contact system in capillary leakage syndrome (CLS) after bone marrow transplantation (BMT). Klin Paediatr 205:309
154. Martinez-Brotóns F, Oncins JR, Mestress J, Amargós V, Reynaldo C (1987) Plasma kallikrein-kinin system in patients with uncomplicated sepsis and septic shock – comparison with cardiogenic shock. Thromb Haemost 58:709–713
155. Stevens JH, O'Hanley P, Shapiro JM et al (1986) Effects of anti-C5a antibodies on the adult respiratory distress syndrome in septic primates. J Clin Invest 77:1818–1816

Potential for Gene Therapy in the Treatment of Sepsis

K. L. Brigham, A. E. Canonico, J. T. Conary, B. O. Meyrick and H. Schreier

Introduction

It now appears that much of the tissue injury which occurs in sepsis is a consequence of the inflammatory response run amok. This conclusion seemed first apparent when it became clear that the accumulation of neutrophils and their activation was intimately related to the pathogenesis of sepsis induced injury. The simple pathogenetic scheme initially cast neutrophils in the central role and implicated toxic products of neutrophils as the proximate mediators of cell injury. This concept provided several rationales for designing therapeutic interventions. These included interventions which might alter responses of neutrophils to activating stimuli and interventions which might inactivate either aggressive oxygen species or proteolytic enzymes released by activated neutrophils. As our understanding of the inflammatory process has progressed, the complexity of that process has become more clear. It is now obvious that a host of factors including cytokines, cell adhesion molecules, lipid mediators, and biologically active factors derived from endothelial cells, epithelial cells, and other cells all play important roles in inflammation and that all of these factors network their effects to result in the inflammatory response. While greatly complicating perception of the pathogenetic process in sepsis, this complexity offers a large number of new possibilities for therapeutic intervention. Several such interventions are currently under intensive investigation in the laboratory and some have reached the level of clinical investigation. Both increased understanding of the pathogenesis of sepsis induced injury and the emergence of many new pharmacologic agents with specific effects on the inflammatory response hold promise that effective pharmacologic intervention will be identified.

However, the need for novel new approaches to therapy is not diminished by the progress that has been made. With the explosion of the technology for manipulating nucleic acids and the development of strategies for *in vivo* delivery of functioning foreign DNA, the possibility of a new category of interventions which could be effective clinically is raised.

Gene Therapy and Gene Therapeutics

The characteristics of the molecular mechanisms for generating proteins in cells make manipulation of these processes attractive as a therapeutic tool. Through a process called transcription, DNA sequences encoding specific proteins generate messenger RNA which then commands the cellular protein synthetic machinery to generate the specific protein encoded in the gene. The specificity of this process is absolute. Therefore, if DNA could be introduced into cells in a functioning form, the cell could be directed to produce virtually any protein of interest.

Most of the focus in developing gene therapy as a clinical tool has been on diseases which are a consequence of a genetic abnormality. The concept here is simple. If it were possible to introduce into cells which lack a functioning specific gene, the normal gene, then the phenotypic consequence of the genetic abnormality could be corrected. Clinical trials using this approach are currently underway. For defects in genes encoding proteins which are secreted and have their effects extracellularly, it may not even be necessary to introduce the normal gene into the cells where it is deficient. In other circumstances, for example cystic fibrosis, the deficient protein is an integral membrane protein and therefore will presumably have to be placed into every defective cell in order to correct abnormal functioning of that cell. Clinical trials in humans are currently underway using gene therapy in both of these circumstances.

These concepts need not be limited to diseases which are a consequence of a genetic abnormality. For several years, molecular biologists have effectively introduced functioning foreign DNA into cells in culture in a manner in which the transgene is transiently expressed (transfection). If it were possible to increase expression of a gene encoding a protein which protects cells from sepsis related injury during the period the cell was at risk for injury, it would not be necessary to have prolonged expression of the introduced gene. In fact, that might not be desirable since the safety of such interventions might be dramatically enhanced by assuring transient functioning of the foreign DNA. This concept – the use of DNA in a form which assures that it does not integrate into the host genome and that the transgene is expressed only transiently – has been called transient gene therapy or gene therapeutics. The concept is, essentially, similar to other concepts in pharmacology. The only difference is that here the drug is DNA.

Over the past 5 years in the Center for Lung Research at Vanderbilt, we have attempted to use the concept of gene therapeutics to develop effective delivery systems for foreign DNA to the lungs and to design DNA constructs which will function *in vivo* transiently.

Expression of Reporter Genes

The gene delivery system which we have used most extensively involves the use of commercially available cationic liposomes (Lipofectin). These cationic liposomes, when incubated with DNA which is negatively charged, will form *DNA-liposome complexes* by charge-charge interaction (lipofection). This process occurs on simple incubation at room temperature. In a variety of cultured cell types, these *DNA-liposome complexes* traverse cell membranes and are relatively nontoxic.

To determine whether this process would effectively deliver foreign DNA to lung cells, we conducted studies in cultured bovine pulmonary artery endothelial cells. Using the commercially available cationic liposomes and a DNA construct in the form of a plasmid which contained the gene encoding a prokaryotic protein, chloramphenicol acetyltransferase (CAT), we were able to demonstrate the generation of the transgene product [1]. CAT activity could be demonstrated in bovine pulmonary artery endothelial cell cultures following exposure of the culture to *liposome-DNA complexes* overnight. Expression was seen as early as 1 day following transfection and expression persisted for at least a week.

Since the technique of lipofection appeared to be an effective way to deliver DNA to lung cells in culture, we wondered whether this might also work in intact animals. We reasoned that the lungs might be especially vulnerable to this approach because of their anatomic location. Material can be delivered to the lungs exclusively by aerosol or intra-airway administration, and even intravenous administration will result in exposure of the large lung microvascular bed to the injected substance as the first microvascular bed traversed. Using a plasmid DNA construct containing the coding region for CAT driven by a Rous sarcoma virus (RSV) promotor region, we injected mice with *liposome-DNA complexes* either intravenously through a tail vein or transtracheally. Animals were killed at different times following adminis-

Table 1. Chloramphenicol acetyltransferase (CAT) activity in lungs, liver and kidneys 72 h following DNA-liposome injection into mice. (From [2])

Route	CA (%) per h per μg protein $\times 10^{-2}$		
	Lungs	Liver	Kidneys
Intravenous			
30 μg DNA per mouse	24.5	0	0
15 μg DNA per mouse	10.1	0	0
Intratracheal			
30 μg DNA per mouse	35.7	0	0
Intraperitoneal			
30 μg DNA per mouse	0	0	0

CA, chloramphenicol acetylation

tration of the DNA and CAT activity was measured in the lungs, liver, and kidneys. We demonstrated expression of the transgene in the lungs following intravenous injection with a time course similar to that which we had seen in pulmonary endothelial cells in culture [2]. Transgene expression was apparent by 1 day following injection, expression peaked at day 3 and continued for as long as 5 days. As shown in Table 1, transgene expression in these studies appeared specific for the lungs.

Regardless of the route of administration, we could find no activity of the transgene product in either liver or kidneys. With intravenous injection of *DNA-liposome complexes*, transgene expression appeared to be related to the dose of DNA administered. Intratracheal administration appeared to result in greater transgene expression in the lungs than following intravenous injection. As expected, intraperitoneal injection of *DNA-liposome complexes* resulted in no detection of transgene activity in any organ studied.

In subsequent studies, we used a construct containing the gene encoding human growth hormone as a reporter gene. Human growth hormone is a protein which is, unlike CAT secreted. Radioimmunoassays are available which are specific for the human protein. Following intravenous injection of *liposome-DNA complexes,* we could show transgene expression. This was done by removing organs from mice following intravenous injection of *DNA-liposome complexes,* mincing the organs, and carrying them in organ culture for 24 h. Human growth hormone was then measured in the supernatant from the organ cultures [3]. We found generation of human growth hormone by the lungs from injected animals as early as 24 h following injection, with considerable decrease in activity by a week. As with the earlier studies, we found no transgene expression in liver or kidneys.

These studies demonstrate the phenomenonlogy. That is, it is possible using cationic liposomes to deliver functioning foreign genes to the lungs by either intravenous or intra-airway administration of *liposome-DNA complexes.*

In Vivo Expression of Relevant Transgenes

Genes encoding several proteins which might protect organs against injury in sepsis have been cloned. One such gene is α1-antitrypsin. If the generation of proteolytic enzymes by inflammatory cells in proximity to parenchymal cells of critical organs is an important part of the pathogenesis, endowing cells at risk with the capacity for generating increased amounts of an antiprotease might render them resistant to injury. The most abundant endogenous antiprotease is α1-antitrypsin. We have constructed an expression plasmid containing the cDNA for human α1-antitrypsin driven by a cytomegalovirus promotor. First, we determined whether, using cationic liposomes, this DNA construct would express the human antitrypsin protein in lung cells. In cultured bovine pulmonary artery endothelial cells, we were able to demonstrate by a variety of techniques that human α1-antitrypsin protein and message were expressed following lipofection [4]. Further, using this same construct, we showed in rabbits that intravenous injection of *DNA-liposome complexes* resulted in expression of the human transgene in the lungs. Using human-specific antibody, we demonstrated by western blotting that protein was produced; immunohistochemically, we were able to demonstrate the human protein in both airway epithelial cells and vascular endothelial cells; messenger RNA using a human specific probe was also detected [5]. In addition to demonstrating *in vivo* expression following intravenous injection, we also were able to demonstrate *in vivo* expression of the human α1-antitrypsin transgene in the lungs following aerosol administration of cationic *liposome-DNA complexes* [6]. We radiolabeled plasmids and injected them intravenously complexed to liposomes and then performed autoradiographic studies on sections of the lung in order to determine the location of the plasmid and to estimate the efficiency of delivery [7]. Following intravenous injection, we found localization of the radiolabeled plasmids in endothelial cells, particularly at the bifurcation of vessels, and in peripheral lung cells presumed to be endothelium although precise location could not be determined at the light microscopic level. We estimate that approximately 10% of the endothelial cells which could be visualized contained radiolabeled plasmid in these studies. Thus, it is possible to deliver a functioning human α1-antitrypsin gene to the lungs of animals using a liposome delivery technology. In these studies, organ specificity of transgene expression was less obvious than in the studies conducted using reporter gene constructs. We found evidence of gene expression in the liver following intravenous injection of *DNA-liposomes.* Some activity was also found in the liver even following aerosol administration of the *DNA-liposome complexes.* Thus, although relatively specific organ targeting of exogenously delivered DNA can be achieved in the lungs by choosing the route of administration, the material is not limited to the lungs even with administration in the airways.

There is abundant evidence that the generation of aggressive oxygen species is an important part of the mechanism of cell and organ injury which occurs in sepsis. This may be a consequence of the inflammatory response or may be a direct effect of bacterial endotoxin. Based on that pathogenetic information, it might be therapeutic to increase the generation of antioxidant enzymes in cells at risk to injury in sepsis. One such enzyme is superoxide dismutase (SOD). We made a DNA construct consisting of the gene encoding human manganous superoxide dismutase (MnSOD) driven by a cytomegalovirus promotor. Using cationic liposomes, we transfected this construct into cultured bovine pulmonary artery endothelial cells [8]. In these transfected cells, we were able to demonstrate increased message for MnSOD, increased generation of immunoreactive MnSOD protein (western blot) and increased SOD activity. To our surprise, these cells producing increased amounts of the antioxidant enzyme were not resistant to the direct effects of gram-negative bacterial endotoxin. It is of course possible that increased amounts of SOD simply result in increased generation of hydrogen peroxide and that a therapeutic benefit would be observed if increased amounts of catalase and other antioxidant enzymes were also achieved. We continue to pursue these studies in both cultured cell preparations and in intact animals.

Gene Transfer as Therapy in an Experimental Animal

The studies summarized so far clearly demonstrate the feasibility of using cationic liposomes as a delivery technology for achieving *in vivo* expression of transgenes in intact animals. Whether this is likely to prove applicable in the clinical setting will depend upon demonstration of both safety and efficacy. We have approached the efficacy issue initially by determining whether or not it was possible to alter responses of the lungs to endotoxin by transfecting animals *in vivo* with a DNA construct which hyperexpressed the gene encoding a protein which might render the lungs resistant to injury.

Initially, we have worked with the gene encoding prostaglandin synthase (PGG/H synthase). These studies were conducted in rabbits. We made a plasmid expression vector containing the cDNA for PGG/H synthase driven by a cytomegalovirus promotor. In cultured bovine pulmonary artery endothelial cells, we showed that lipofection with this construct resulted in increased generation of prostaglandin E_2 (PGE_2) and prostacyclin. Since both PGE_2 and prostacyclin have anti-inflammatory properties and since PGE_2 given exogenously has been shown to protect the lungs against damage due to endotoxin, we reasoned that if we could hyperexpress the PGG/H synthase gene predominantly in endothelial cells this might render the lungs resistant to endotoxin damage [9]. We first set about to determine whether we could cause increased generation of PGE_2 and prostacyclin in the lungs of intact animals using this approach. In rabbits, we infused intravenously liposome-DNA complexes [10]. At different times following injection, we killed animals and removed the lungs, carried lung minces in organ culture for 24 h, and measured PGE_2 and prostacyclin metabolites in the supernatant from these cultures. We showed a marked increase in generation of these two prostanoids in the lungs of transfected animals when compared to animals transfected with the empty plasmid vector. Further, using polymerase chain reaction (PCR), we could demonstrate specific messenger RNA for PGG/H synthase. Although the necessity to use PCR to demonstrate message implies fairly low level expression of the transgene, in this case we reasoned that a physiologic effect might still be seen because of the amplification resulting from the generation of prostacyclin and PGE_2, a process catalyzed by the transgene product. In order to determine whether this was the case, we transfected rabbits by intravenous injection of *DNA-liposome complexes* and 24 h later made an *in situ* blood perfused lung preparation in these same animals. We have thoroughly characterized the response of this preparation to the addition of endotoxin to the perfusate. Control animals included animals treated exactly as the experimental group except that the DNA construct given did not contain the DNA encoding PGG/H synthase

[11]. We found that animals transfected with the PGG/H synthase gene were resistance to the effects of adding endotoxin to the perfusate [11, 12]. This resitance was reflected in a marked reduction in the pulmonary hypertensive response and in the accumulation of lung water over approximately 2 h of perfusion following endotoxin.

This method of *in vivo* delivery of DNA also appears to be safe. We approached this evaluation by injecting *DNA-liposome complexes* intravenously into rabbits and in separate groups of animals delivery the same complexes by aerosol. *DNA-liposome complexes* were administered weekly for 4 weeks and animals were killed at weekly intervals in order to examine structural effects of this intervention. We found no toxic effects of the procedure. Lung mechanics did not change during the 4 week period, arterial blood gases remained constant, and post-mortem examination showed no difference between control animals and animals receiving *DNA-liposome complexes* [13].

We are encouraged to think that this approach to the *in vivo* delivery of potentially protective foreign genes to intact animals may be both safe and efficacious [14, 15].

Summary

The rapidly developing techniques of molecular biology provide, now, a unique potential for identifying new categories of therapies which could be effective in sepsis. Genes encoding several proteins which might be protective against sepsis induced injury have been cloned and are available. The technology for manipulating DNA and producing constructs which will hyperexpress these genes is available. Also, there are now emerging techniques for delivering these DNA constructs into organs of intact animals. Studies currently underway in humans aimed at determining efficacy and safety in patients with diseases which are a consequence of a genetic abnormality will pave the way for the application of these techniques in more acute diseases. The emergence of the category of therapies called gene therapeutics may be particularly applicable to patients with sepsis and organ failure. Studies already completed at a preclinical level demonstrate that functioning foreign genes can be delivered *in vivo* to the lungs and other organs and that, at least in the lungs, this technology can be used to protect the lungs against endotoxin induced injury. This will undoubtedly be a fruitful area for continued study and holds promise clinically for developing novel therapies for the treatment of sepsis induced injury.

Acknowledgements. This work was supported by the following: NIH, National Heart, Lung and Blood Institute Grants: HL 19153 (SCOR in Pulmonary Vascular Diseases); HL 07123 (NRSA Institutional Training Grant in Multidisciplinary Respiratory Diseases); R01 HL 34208. Also, grants from the John W. Cooke and Laura W. Cooke Foundation; the Bernard Werthan, Sr.

Foundation; and the Harry H. and Martha W. Straus Foundation. Dr. Brigham holds the Joe and Morris Werthan Chair for Investigative Medicine.

References

1. Brigham KL, Meyrick B, Christman B, Berry LC Jr, King G (1989) Expression of a prokaryotic gene in cultured lung endothelial cells following lipofection with a plasmid vector. Am J Respir Cell Mol Biol 1:95–100
2. Brigham KL, Meyrick B, Christman B, Magnuson M, King G, Berry LC Jr (1989) Rapid communication: In vivo transfection of murine lungs with a functioning prokaryotic gene using a liposome vehicle. Am J Med Sci 298:278–281
3. Brigham KL, Meyrick B, Christman B, Conary J, King G, Berry LC Jr, Magnuson M (1993) Expression of human growth hormone fusion genes in cultured lung endothelial cells and in the lungs of mice. Am J Respir Cell Mol Biol 8 (2):209–213
4. Canonico AE, Conary JT, Christman BW, Meyrick BO, Brigham KL (1991) In vitro transient gene expression of human α1 antitrypsin in bovine pulmonary artery endothelial cells. FASEB J 5:A6702
5. Canonico AE, Conary JT, Christman BW, Meyrick BO, Brigham KL (1991) Expression of a CMV promoter driven human alpha-1 antitrypsin gene in cultured lung endothelial cells and in the lungs of rabbits. Clin Res 39 (2):219A
6. Canonico AE, Conary JT, Meyrick BO, Brigham KL (1992) In vivo expression of a CMV promoter driven human alpha-1 antitrypsin (alpha-1AT) gene after intravenous or airway administration of DNA/liposome complex. Am Rev Respir Dis 145 (4):A200
7. Canonico AE, Conary JT, Meyrick BO, Brigham KL (1993) Cationic liposome mediated in vivo transfer of human alpha-1 antitrypsin gene to lungs of rabbits. Am J Respir Cell Mol Biol (submitted)
8. Branch M, Berry LC, Conary J, Yoshioka T, Brigham KL, Meyrick B (1993) Response of bovine pulmonary artery endothelial cells (BPAEC) to endotoxin following transfection of the human manganous superoxide dismutase (MnSOD) cDNA. Am Rev Respir Dis 147 (4):A206
9. Conary JT, Brown DL, Shepherd VE, Christman BW, King G, Brigham KL (1992) Expression of a CMV promoter driven ovine prostaglandin G/H synthase gene in cultured lung endothelial cells. Am Rev Respir Dis 145 (4):A839
10. Conary JT, Canonico AE, Parker RE, Christman BW, King G, Brigham KL (1992) Expression of a CMV promoter driven ovine prostaglandin G/H synthase gene in the lungs of rabbits. Am Rev Respir Dis 145 (4):A850
11. Conary JT, Parker RE, Christman BW, Faulks RD, King G, Brigham KL (1993) Alteration of the endotoxin response by expression of a CMV promoter driven ovine prostaglandin G/H synthase gene in the lungs of rabbits. Am Rev Respir Dis 147 (4):A546
12. Conary JT, Parker RE, Christman BW, Faulks RD, King G, Brigham KL (1993) Protection of rabbit lungs from endotoxin injury by in vivo hyperexpression of the prostaglandin G/H synthase gene. J Clin Invest (submitted)
13. Plitman JD, Canonico AE, Conary JT, Meyrick BO, Brigham KL (1992) The effects of inhaled and intravenous DNA/liposomes on lung function and histology in the rabbit. Am Rev Respir Dis 145 (4):A371
14. Brigham KL, Schreier H (1993) Cationic liposomes and DNA delivery. J Liposome Res 3 (1):31–49
15. Brigham KL, Canonico AE, Conary JT (1992) Mediator gene expression in sepsis: implications for therapy. In: Lamy M, Thijs LG (eds) Update in intensive care and emergency medicine, vol 16: mediators of sepsis. Springer, Berlin Heidelberg New York, pp 393–405

VII. Specific Therapeutic Aspects

Step-by-Step Treatment of Acute Respiratory Distress Syndrome

K. Lewandowski, R. Rossaint and K. J. Falke

Introduction

Acute respiratory distress syndrome (ARDS) is characterized by pulmonary edema due to injury of the capillary alveolar membranes and increased pulmonary artery pressure. It is further distinguished by severe hypoxemia, nonresponsive to common methods of support for respiratory failure. Hypoxemia is caused by intrapulmonary right-left shunting due to persistent perfusion of nonventilated alveoli. Another characteristic is the low thoracopulmonary compliance [1, 2]. The lesions in ARDS lungs are not homogeneously distributed. As has been shown by computer tomographic studies, the lesions are often found in dependent lung regions [3]. Gattinoni et al. [4] hypothesized that the inhomogeneous ARDS lung is a mixture of three different zones: healthy (H), recruitable (R) and diseased (D). Gas exchange is accomplished only in zones H and R. Based on this assumption, in adult patients with ARDS, the remaining healthy "baby" lung (zone H plus zone R), which is 20%–30% of a normal adult lung, must provide the body's whole oxygen demand. Additionally, ARDS is characterized not only by a low compliance, but also by high airway and tissue resistance [5–7].

Since first described in 1967 [8], the syndrome has been associated with a high mortality. Multicenter trials from Europe and the USA continue to report a mortality in excess of 50% [9, 10].

Recently, knowledge about the incidence of ARDS has been updated: Whereas in 1979 the National Heart, Lung, and Blood Institute (NHLBI) estimated that in the USA 150000 patients per year suffered from ARDS, reflecting an incidence of 75 per 100000/year [11]; latest studies suggest that this figure is a gross overestimation. Using a computerized search strategy employing ICD-9 codes, Earle et al. [12] found that only 21000 cases annually (10.5 per 100000/year) are to be expected in the USA. Thomsen et al. [13] determined the incidence of the syndrome in Utah, USA, to be 5.3–7.1 per 100000/year. Our own group established the incidence of ARDS in Berlin, Germany, a metropolis with 3440401 inhabitants, to be 3.0 per 100000/year [14]. Similar figures were derived from a retrospective study in a British health district: 4.5 per 100000/year [15]. An incidence of 1.5–3.5 per 100000/year was reported for the island of Gran Canaria, Spain, by Villar and Slutsky [16]. We recommend that citation of an incidence of 75 per 100000/year (or 150000 cases per year) in the USA from the 1979 task force [11] be abandoned.

Advanced treatment of ARDS currently consists of (1) ventilatory techniques aiming at reestablishment of impaired gas exchange such as pressure-controlled mechanical ventilation (pcCMV) [17–22], positive end-expiratory pressure (PEEP) [23], and permissive hypercapnea [24]; (2) adjunctive supportive measures which seek to improve ventilation-perfusion mismatch and reduce the extent of the pulmonary edema, such as positioning maneuvers [25] and dehydration [26–29]; (3) pharmacological interventions such as IV administration of vasodilators [30] and inhaling nitric oxide [31]; (4) establishment of artificial lungs for maintenance of adequate oxygenation and gas exchange until the lungs recover sufficiently to resume ventilatory function with only moderate mechanical support, e.g., extracorporeal membrane oxygenation (ECMO), extracorporeal CO_2 removal ($ECCO_2R$) [32–34] and intravascular oxygenator (IVOX) [35]. Each of these treatments has shown its clinical efficacy in certain populations of ARDS patients.

One could hypothesize that combined administration of all these measures would be the best treatment for all ARDS patients. However, a therapeutic option that is beneficial in a given patient could result in further deterioration, or even death, in another. No data exist substantiating the view that a combination of the cited therapeutic measures is superior to administration of selected options in a defined patient population.

Challenged by this lack of information, in 1989, we began to develop a step-by-step approach which amalgamated the most promising of the above mentioned therapeutic measures into an algorithm for treatment of severe ARDS. The objective here is to present our 4 year experience with the algorithm and evaluate its potential to reduce ARDS mortality rates. Furthermore we shall elucidate the question if the results of our approach need verification by a randomized controlled trial (RCT).

Application of the Algorithm

After inclusion and exclusion criteria for advanced treatment have been checked (Table 1), patients are transferred to our intensive care unit. Immediately after arrival, a Swan-Ganz catheter, a multilumen catheter, and a femoral artery catheter for measurement of extravascular lung water (EVLW) and arterial blood pressure are inserted. A chest X-ray and – if the patient's condition is stable – a computerized tomography with special emphasis on the lungs (high resolution CT) are obtained.

We then proceed with treatment according to the algorithm (Fig. 1). In patients meeting fast entry criteria (Table 2), venovenous extracorporeal membrane oxygenation (vv-ECMO) with heparin-coated internal surfaces (Carmeda, Sweden) is immediately instituted. Advanced conservative measures without vv-ECMO (Table 3) are administered to those patients not fulfilling fast entry criteria. If the combined administration of these measures

Table 1. Inclusion and exclusion criteria for advanced treatment of ARDS

Inclusion criteria
Typical findings of severe ARDS [8]
Presence of a severe persisting and progressive defect of arterial oxygenation for at least 48 h, requiring mechanical ventilation with $FiO_2 \geq 0.6$ and PEEP ≥ 10 cm H_2O leading to a $PaO_2 < 80$ mm Hg
Exclusion criteria
Extremely poor prognosis due to underlying disease, e.g., malignancy, unresolvable surgical problems
Immunosuppression
Irreversible damage of the central nervous system
Severe chronic pulmonary disease
Cardiogenic pulmonary edema (PCPW ≥ 18 mm Hg)

ARDS, acute respiratory distress syndrome; FiO_2, fraction inspired oxygen; PEEP, positive end-expiratory pressure; PaO_2, arterial oxygen tension; PCWP, pulmonary capillary wedge pressure.

does not prove to be successful, i.e., slow entry criteria (Table 2) are fulfilled within a time span of 24–120 h – assessed without nitric oxide (NO) inhalation – vv-ECMO is established.

Results

Since April 1989, 82 patients with severe ARDS have been transferred to our intensive care unit (ICU) for advanced treatment including vv-ECMO. The expected mortality rate in these patients was estimated to be 70%. We derive this figure from the European Collaborative ARDS Study evaluating patients fulfilling entry criteria for "group B" (arterial oxygen tension (PaO_2) < 75 mm Hg at a fraction of inspired oxygen (FiO_2) ≥ 0.5 plus PEEP = 5 cm H_2O) [9]. The distribution of patients based upon their etiology, survival rates and mode of treatment is shown in Table 4. Table 5 gives the number of patients treated and their survival rates according to their treatment groups. All of the survivors were discharged from the hospital without need for any further respiratory support.

Discussion

The main results presented in this chapter are: (1) Of the 50 patients who received advanced treatment without vv-ECMO, 44 (88%) survived. (2) Of the 23 patients who met slow entry criteria and received vv-ECMO, 14 (61%) survived. (3) Of the nine patients who met fast entry criteria and received vv-ECMO, three (33%) survived.

These results can be explained in only two ways: either our advanced treat-

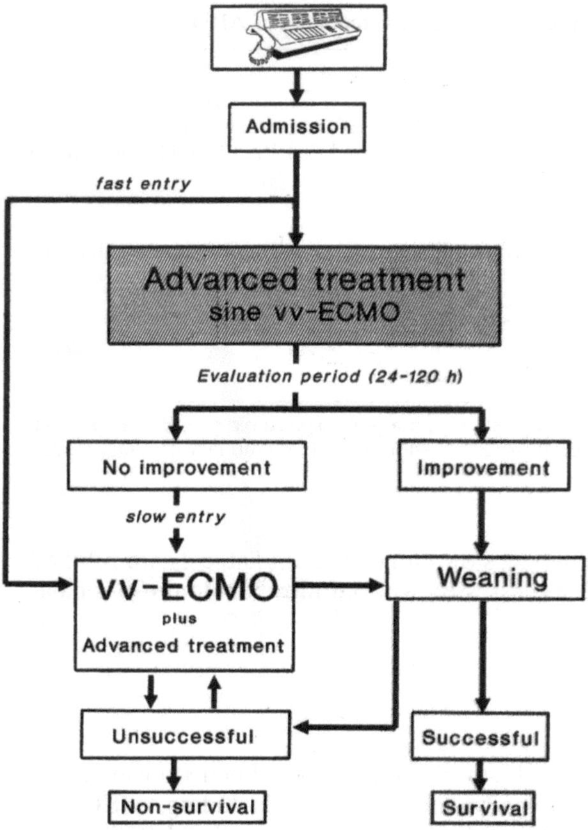

Fig. 1. Algorithm for treatment of severe acute respiratory distress syndrome (*ARDS*). *vv-ECMO,* venovenous extracorporeal membrane oxygenation

ment regimens (both with and without vv-ECMO) incorporate major therapeutic benefits, and/or the patients differ from those of other studies because of the selection process.

Our mortality figures are markedly below those reported by other major studies [9, 10, 37]. There is a selection process due to our inclusion criteria for advanced treatment. We can offer our advanced treatment only to patients reported to our ICU. We assume that there is a selection process prior to the first consultation with our ICU. Elderly patients, or those with severe underlying diseases, etc., are probably not reported to us. However, we had to refuse patients fulfilling inclusion criteria for advanced treatment because our ICU is capable of establishing a maximum of two ECMO circuits. However, our study population consisted of 82 patients who fulfilled the "classic" ARDS criteria and had a severely impaired gas exchange as reflected by our inclusion criteria for advanced treatment. Their overall mortality rate was

Table 2. Inclusion criteria for venovenous extracorporeal membrane oxygenation (vv-ECMO)

Fast entry criteria	
	$PaO_2/FiO_2 < 50$ mm Hg at $PEEP \geq 10$ cm H_2O for >2 h
Slow entry criteria	
After 24–120 h of maximal therapy the following criteria must be fulfilled:	
	$PaO_2/FiO_2 < 150$ mm Hg at $PEEP \geq 10$ cm H_2O
	$\dot{Q}_S/\dot{Q}_T \geq 30\%$ measured at $FiO_2 = 1.0$
	$EVLW \geq 15$ ml/kg body weight (method of Lewis et al. [36])
	Total respiratory compliance ≤ 30 ml/cm H_2O and/or recurrent pneumothoraces with bronchopleural fistula

PaO_2, arterial oxygen tension; FiO_2, fraction inspired oxygen; PEEP, positive end-expiratory pressure; Q_S/Q_T, intrapulmonary right-left shunt; EVLW, extravascular lung water.

only 26%. An unselected ARDS patient population (presence of an appropriate clinical setting and bilateral pulmonary infiltrates on chest roentgenogram, absence of a cardiac condition or chronic pulmonary disease) with similar impaired gas exchange was enrolled in the European Collaborative ARDS Study [9]. Mortality rate in 403 patients who fulfilled entry criteria for group B, i.e., $PaO_2 < 75$ mm Hg at $FiO_2 \geq 0.5$ plus $PEEP = 5$ cm H_2O, was 69%. A multicenter registry of patients with ARDS, defined as $PaO_2/FiO_2 \leq 250$, presence of an appropriate clinical setting and bilateral pulmonary infiltrates on chest roentgenogram, absence of chronic pulmonary disease, carcinoma or *Pneumocystis carinii* infection, determined to overall mortality rate to be 53% [10]. As our inclusion criteria referring the gas exchange criteria are similar to those of the above mentioned studies, we assume that our improved survival rates can, at least in part, be explained by applying our step-by-step procedure.

Many clinicians, however, would insist that our refined concept technique must be evaluated against standard treatment with a RCT. Until some sort of statistically sound comparative analysis is carried out, doubts about the benefits, costs, and ethics of our concept that includes vv-ECMO will persist. Multiple methodological, organizational and ethical problems would focus on the question whether vv-ECMO should be established when a combination of other therapeutic measures has failed to improve the patient's condition.

VV-ECMO is a technique for providing prolonged cardiopulmonary bypass to patients with potentially reversible pulmonary failure. Obviously, this technique cannot "heal" associated organ dysfunctions compromising the patient's prognosis in terms of survival. VV-ECMO could be described as a "one organ therapy". When initially developed in the 1950s, cardiopulmonary bypass could sustain patients for no more than several hours during surgical procedures. The development of membrane oxygenation, in the 1960s, however, made prolonged cardiopulmonary bypass a possibility. Following

Table 3. Therapeutic measures for treatment of ARDS

pcCMV	Respirator setting (Servo-ventilator 900 C): Pressure controlled mode, PIP: 30–35 cm H_2O FiO_2: aim at PaO_2 55–60 mm Hg Respirator rate: 12–16/min I/E ratio: Initial: 1:1, 2:1 if no improvement in oxygenation is achieved (consider "auto-PEEP," reduce PEEP accordingly)
PEEP	Determination of "best PEEP" (analysis of pressure-volume curves, results of lung CT) Avoid baro- and volutrauma
Permissive hypercapnea	Reduce PIP (30–35 cm H_2O), V_T (5–6 ml/kg body weight) Allow $PaCO_2$ to rise (70–80 mm Hg) pH_{art} not below 7.28
Positional maneuvers	Lateral position when asymmetric distribution of lung lesions is present Prone position in all ARDS patients for a a test period If $PaO_2\uparrow$, $\dot{Q}_S/\dot{Q}_T\downarrow$, positional maneuvers should be performed 2×/day for 4 h
Reduction of pulmonary edema Fluid restriction Pharmacologic dehydration Hemofiltration	Therapeutic goals: Hemoglobin level 14–15 g% PCWP < 10 mm Hg Central venous pressure 5–8 mm Hg Colloid osmotic pressure 25–29 mm Hg Urine output/h: 1 ml/kg body weight Assure success: Decrease of X-ray signs of pulmonary edema $PaO_2\uparrow$, $\dot{Q}_S/\dot{Q}_T\downarrow$, $SaO_2\uparrow$, EVLW ↓
Special ventilatory measures	Indication for differential lung ventilation: Asymmetric distribution of lung lesions Bronchopleural fistula with large air leak flow Indication for high frequency jet ventilation: Bronchopleural fistula with large air leak flow and sufficient compliance
vv-ECMO	Indication for vv-ECMO (see Table 2) Use of heparin-coated ECMO circuit Only minimal systemic anticoagulation required: ACT 130–150 s Extracorporal blood flow is adjusted so as to reduce respirator FiO_2 to 0.5 Respirator setting during vv-ECMO: PIP: 30–35 cm H_2O, "best PEEP", respirator frequency: 6–8/min, I/E-ratio: 1:1
IVOX	Oxygenator device implanted in the vena cava O_2/CO_2 transfer up to 142 cm^3/min Size of membrane surface: 0.21–0.52 cm^2 Systemic anticoagulation required (ACT ≈ 180 s)
NO	NO selectively improves perfusion in ventilated lung areas (dosage: 0.1–20 ppm) Significant improvement of oxygenation

ARDS, acute respiratory distress syndrome; PcCMV, pressure-controlled mechanical ventilation; PIP, peak inspiratory pressure; FiO_2, fraction inspired oxygen; PAO_2, arterial oxygen tension; I/E ratio, ratio of inspiration to exspiration; PEEP, positive end-expiratory pressure; V_T, tidal volume; $PACO_2$, arterial carbon dioxide tension; pH_{art}, arterial pH; $\dot{Q}_S\dot{Q}_T$, intropulmonary right-left shunt; PCWP, pulmonary capillary wedge pressure; SaO_2, arterial oxygen saturation; EVLW, extravascular lung water; vv-ECMO, venovenous extracorporeal membrane oxygenation; ACT, activated clotting time; IVOX, intravascular oxygenator: NO nitric oxide

Table 4. Etiology of ARDS in 82 patients according to mode of treatment and outcome

Etiology	Advanced treatment			
	Without vv-ECMO		With vv-ECMO	
	n	*s*	*n*	*s*
Polytrauma	23	22	9	6
Pneumonia	11	9	11	3
Aspiration	3	3	7	5
Sepsis	6	4	3	1
Major thoracic surgery	—	—	2	2
Pancreatitis	2	1	—	—
Intoxication	2	2	—	—
Burns	2	2	—	—
Fat embolism	1	1	—	—
Total	50	44	32	17

ARDS, acute respiratory distress syndrome; vv-ECMO, venovenous extracorporeal membrane oxygenation; *n*, number of patients treated; *s*, number of survivors.

Table 5. Treatment of ARDS: outcome study period april 1989–june 1993. Mean age of the patients was 31 ± 12 years

	Patients (*n*)	Survivors (*n*)	Survival rate (%)
Advanced treatment (without vv-ECMO)	50	44	88
vv-ECMO fast entry	9	3	33
vv-ECMO slow entry	23	14	61
Total	82	61	74

ARDS, acute respiratory distress syndrome; vv-ECMO, venovenous extracorporeal membrane oxygenation; *n*, number of patients treated.

reports of several successes with this new technology, the NHLBI sponsored a multi-institutional RCT comparing ECMO against standard therapy in adults with acute respiratory failure. Few patients survived in either treatment group, and interest in ECMO waned [38]. Refined concepts and development of surface-heparinized ECMO circuitry led to a "comeback" of the technique, especially in Europe. Survival rates of up to 61% were achieved [32]. Again, there was the necessity to test the refined ECMO technique against "advanced standard treatment" with a RCT. In 1992 Clemmer et al. [39] conducted such a RCT in a pulmonary intensive care unit of the University of Salt Lake City. The purpose of their study was to compare pressure-controlled inverse ratio ventilation (pcIRV) followed by extracorporeal CO_2-removal with low frequency positive pressure ventilation (LFPPV-

$ECCO_2R$) with continuous positive pressure ventilation (CPPV) in patients with ARDS. They found that survival was not significantly different in both groups, although overall survival rate had improved significantly when compared with historical experience (US-ECMO-Study [38]). With regard to this study, vv-ECMO should consequently be abolished. However, the continuous success of ECMO in Europe, reflected by a 46% survival rate (330 ARDS patients treated in six European centers, as of December 31, 1992) and the undoubted potential of the method to improve impaired gas exchange, make it an unrenounceable component in an advanced concept for treatment of severe ARDS. As a RCT to demonstrate its superiority over standard treatment is very unlikely to be established in the near future, we advocate the use of prospective observational studies, as proposed by Truog [40], to further elucidate the efficacy of the clinical application of ECMO.

Conclusion

Out of the 82 patients treated according to the proposed algorithm 61 (74%) survived. Therapeutic measures included in our algorithm are pressure-limited ventilation with PEEP and permissive hypercapnea, positioning maneuvers, special forms of ventilatory support, reduction of pulmonary edema, administration of inhaled agents to modify acute hypoxic pulmonary pressure response and establishment of extracorporeal gas exchange. Each of these treatments has shown its effectiveness in ameliorating at least one of the pathophysiologic manifestations of ARDS. This study demonstrates that a substantial proportion of patients with severe ARDS who did not respond to advanced supportive measures could be successfully treated with vv-ECMO. Improved survival rates of 70%–80% can be aspired to in the treatment of severe ARDS.

References

1. Murray JF, Matthay MA, Luce JM, Flick MR (1988) An expanded definition of the adult respiratory distress syndrome. Am Rev Respir Dis 138:720–723
2. Petty TL (1988) ARDS: refinement of concept and redefinition. Am Rev Respir Dis 138:724
3. Gattinoni L, Pelosi P, Vitale G, Pesenti A, D'Andrea L, Mascheroni D (1991) Body position changes redistribute lung computed-tomographic density in patients with acute respiratory failure. Anesthesiology 74:15–23
4. Gattinoni L, Pesenti A, Marcolin R et al (1992) Extracorporeal support in acute respiratory failure. In: Artigas A, Lemaire F, Suter PM, Zapol WM (eds) Adult respiratory distress syndrome. Churchill Livingstone, Edingburgh, pp 469–475
5. Broseghini C, Brandolese R, Poggi R, Polese G, Manzin E, Milic-Emili J, Rossi A (1988) Respiratory mechanics during the first day of mechanical ventilation in patients with pulmonary edema and chronic airway obstruction. Am Rev Respir Dis 138:355–361

6. Wright PE, Bernard GR (1989) The role of airflow resistance in patients with the adult respiratory distress syndrome. Am Rev Respir Dis 139:1169–1174
7. Eissa NT, Ranieri VM, Corbeil C, Chasse M, Robatto FM, Braidy J, Milic-Emili J (1991) Analysis of behavior of the respiratory system in ARDS patients: effects of flow, volume, and time. J Appl Physiol 70:2719–2729
8. Ashbaugh DG, Bigelow DB, Petty TL, Levine BE (1967) Acute respiratory distress in adults. Lancet 2:319–323
9. Artigas A, Carlet J, Le Gall JR, Chastang CL, Blanch L, Fernández R (1991) Clinical presentation, prognostic factors, and outcome of ARDS in the European Collaborative Study (1985–1987): a preliminary report. In: Zapol WM, Lemaire F (eds) Adult respiratory distress syndrome. Dekker, New York, pp 37–59
10. Sloane PJ, Gee MH, Gottlieb JE et al (1992) A multicenter registry of patients with acute respiratory distress syndrome. Am Rev Respir Dis 146:419–426
11. National Heart, Lung and Blood Institute Division of Lung disease (1979) Extracorporeal support for respiratory insufficiency. A collaborative study in response to RFP-NHLI-73-20
12. Earle LA, Grimm AM, Hopkins LE, Gottlieb JE (1993) Identifying patients with adult respiratory distress syndrome by utilizing a search strategy employing ICD-9 codes. Am Rev Respir Dis 147 [Suppl]:A348
13. Thomsen GE, Morris AH, Danino D, Ellsworth J, Wallace CJ (1993) Incidence of the adult respiratory distress syndrome in Utah. Am Rev Respir Dis 147 [Suppl]:A347
14. Lewandowski K, Metz J, Preiß H, Deutschmann C, Kuhlen R, Artigas A, Falke KJ (1993) Incidence, severity and mortality of acute respiratory failure in Berlin/Germany: a prospective multicenter trial in 72 intensive care units. Am Rev Respir Dis 147 [Suppl]:349A
15. Webster NR, Cohen AT, Nunn JF (1988) Adult respiratoy distress syndrome – how many cases in the UK? Anaesthesia 43:923–926
16. Villar J, Slutsky AS (1989) The incidence of the adult respiratory distress syndrome. Am Rev Respir Dis 140:814–816
17. Abraham E, Yoshihara G (1989) Cardiorespiratory effects of pressure controlled inverse ratio ventilation in severe respiratory failure. Chest 96:1356–1359
18. Andersen JB (1986) Changing ventilatory strategy may alter outcome in catastrophic lung disease. Intensive Care Med 12 [Suppl]:200A
19. Gurevitch MJ, Van Dyke J, Young ES, Jackson K (1986) Improved oxygenation and lower peak airway pressure in severe adult respiratory distress syndrome. Treatment with inverse ratio ventilation. Chest 89:211–214
20. Reynolds EOR (1971) Effect of alterations in mechanical ventilator settings on pulmonary gas exchange in hyaline membrane disease. Arch Dis Child 46:152–159
21. Lachmann B, Jonson B, Lindroth M, Robertson B (1982) Modes of artificial ventilation in severe respiratory distress syndrome. Lung function and morphology in rabbits after washout of alveolar surfactant. Crit Care Med 10:724–732
22. Tharratt RS, Allen RP, Albertson TE (1988) Pressure controlled inverse ratio ventilation. Chest 94:755–762
23. Falke KJ, Pontoppidan H, Kumar K, Leith DE, Geffin B, Laver MB (1972) Ventilation with endexpiratory pressure in acute lung disease. J Clin Invest 51:2315–2323
24. Hickling KG, Henderson SJ, Jackson R (1990) Low mortality associated with low volume pressure limited ventilation with permissive hypercapnea in severe adult respiratory distress syndrome. Intensive Care Med 16:372–377
25. Langer M, Mascheroni D, Marcolin R, Gattinoni L (1988) The prone position in ARDS patients. A clinical study. Chest 94:103–107
26. Sturm JA (1985) Traumatischer Schock und die Lunge. Gefäßschädigung und Volumentherapeutika im Experiment. In: Bergmann H, Brückner JB, Gemperle M, Henschel WF, Mayrhofer O, Meßmer K, Peter K (eds) Anästhesiologie und Intensivmedizin. Springer, Berlin Heidelberg New York, pp 1–118
27. Eisenberg PR, Hansbrough JR, Anderson D, Schuster DP (1987) A prospective study

of lung water measurement during patient management in an intensive care unit. Am Rev Respir Dis 136:662–668
28. Bone RC (1978) Treatment of adult respiratory distress syndrome with diuretics, dialysis, and positive end-expiratory pressure. Crit Care Med 6:136–139
29. Mitchell JP, Schuller B, Calandrino FS, Schuster DP (1992) Improved outcome based on fluid management in critically ill patients requiring pulmonary artery catheterization. Am Rev Respir Dis 145:990–998
30. Radermacher P, Santak B, Becker H, Falke KJ (1989) Prostaglandin E_1 and nitroglycerin reduce pulmonary capillary pressure but worsen ventilation-perfusion distributions in patients with adult respiratory distress syndrome. Anesthesiology 70:601–606
31. Rossaint R, Falke KJ, Lopez F, Slama K, Pison U, Zapol WM (1993) Inhaled nitric oxide for the adult respiratory distress syndrome. N Engl J Med 328:399–405
32. Lewandowski K, Rossaint R, Slama K, Falke KJ, Weidemann H (1993) Reduced mortality rates in severe adult respiratory distress syndrome. Chest 103:1309–1310
33. Gattinoni L, Pesenti A, Mascheroni D et al (1986) Low-frequency positive pressure ventilation with extracorporeal CO_2-removal in severe acute respiratory failure. JAMA 256:881–886
34. Morris AH, Menlove RL, Orme JF, Clemmer TP, Wallace CJ, Beck E (1989) A protocol-controlled trial of a new 3-step therapy including $ECCO_2R$ for adults with ARDS. In: Gille JP (ed) Neonatal and adult respiratory failure. Editions Scientifiques Elsevier, Paris, pp 137–148
35. Mortensen JD (1992) Intravascular oxygenator: a new alternative method for augmenting blood gas transfer in patients with acute respiratory failure. Artif Organs 16:75–82
36. Lewis FR, Ellings VB, Hill SL, Christensen JM (1982) The measurement of extravascular lung water by thermal-green indicator dilution. NY Acad Sci 384:394–410
37. Suchyta MR, Clemmer TP, Elliott CG, Orme JF, Weaver LK (1992) The adult respiratory distress syndrome. A report of survival and modifying factors. Chest 101:1074–1079
38. Zapol WM, Snider MT, Hill JD et al (1979) Extracorporeal membrane oxygenation in severe acute respiratory failure. A randomized prospective study. JAMA 242:2193–2196
39. Clemmer T, Morris A, Suchyta M, Wallace CJ, Orme J, Menlove R, Weaver L (1992) Extracorporeal support does not improve ARDS survival. Crit Care Med 20 [Suppl]:61A
40. Truog RD (1992) Randomized controlled trials: lessons from ECMO. Clin Res 40:519–527

Perfluorocarbons as an Alternative Respiratory Medium

A. S. Tütüncü and B. Lachmann

Introduction

Acute respiratory failure (ARF) represents one of the major problems in intensive care units because of its complex pathogenesis and high rates of morbidity and mortality [1, 2]. Since the clinical problems are similar regardless of the etiology of the lung injury, the therapeutic goal in ARF is to support patients until alveolocapillary membrane integrity is reestablished. Therefore, the main critical factors in clinical management of ARF are supply of adequate arterial and tissue oxygenation and treatment of the primary disorder. Different ventilatory support techniques have been introduced in respiratory failure to maintain adequate gas exchange in the lung with the least possible barotrauma and circulatory impairment.

Mechanical ventilation with high inflation pressures is associated with an increased incidence of barotrauma. Based on extensive evidence accumulated from animal studies showing that high tidal volumes and high peak inspiratory pressures can induce or even worsen acute lung injury [3–5], different ventilatory techniques have been investigated during the last 10 years. Hickling et al. demonstrated that mortality could be significantly reduced in patients with severe respiratory distress syndrome (RDS) by limiting peak inspiratory pressure (reducing tidal volume) and disregarding hypercapnia [6]. Other investigators have shown improved oxygenation with decreased airway pressures using pressure-controlled inverse ratio ventilation [7, 8]. High frequency jet ventilation has been proposed to achieve effective gas exchange using low tidal volumes at high respiratory rates [9, 10]. Extracorporeal membrane oxygenation (ECMO) and apneic oxygenation with extracorporeal CO_2 elimination have been administered in severe cases as nonconventional ventilatory support techniques where other ventilatory forms have failed to improve gas exchange. Although ECMO has resulted in clinical failure [11], it appears to be a promising technique in reducing mortality rates in patients with RDS [12]. The reestablishment of the functional integrity of the damaged surfactant in RDS in adults by exogenous surfactant replacement has been limited to few case reports [13, 14] because of nonavailability of surfactant in the required amounts and the high cost for adults.

Although more than two decades of clinical and laboratory research on RDS have passed, survival rates have remained virtually unchanged [2]. In clinical conditions, the diversity of the disorders associated with RDS has made it difficult to define the optimal ventilatory strategy. However, no controlled studies have demonstrated the superiority of one technique over other forms of ventilatory support. For these reasons, there has always been a search for ways to improve the clinical management of RDS.

As an alternative means of respiratory support, perfluorocarbon (PFC) liquids have been investigated extensively in liquid ventilation studies in animals, and this concept has led recently to the use of this new technique in preterm human neonates with severe RDS in whom conventional therapies have failed [15]. Although the technique of liquid ventilation has evolved since it was introduced first by Clark and Gollan [16], the search for a simpler means of PFC administration has given rise to a new method combining conventional gas ventilation and liquid ventilation, namely partial liquid ventilation [17–19]. In this new technique, PFC is given intratracheally while mechanical ventilation at conventional ventilator settings is superimposed on partly PFC-filled lungs.

This review summarizes the literature on liquid ventilation and partial liquid ventilation and describes the rationale behind partial liquid ventilation and, finally, the limitations and implications of partial liquid ventilation for future clinical application.

Liquid Ventilation

Perfluorocarbons

The most important physical properties of PFC liquids which make them suitable for ventilatory purposes are their remarkably low surface tension and extraordinary ability to dissolve oxygen (O_2) and carbon dioxide (CO_2) (Table 1).

PFC liquids are relatively simple organic compounds in which all hydrogen atoms have been replaced by fluorine; in addition, these chemicals also include compounds in which other halogen atoms such as bromine and iodine are present. These colorless, clear and odorless liquids are insoluble in aqueous media and they must first be emulsified before intravenous admin-

Table 1. Physical properties of some PFC liquids

	Perflubron	FC-77	RM-101
Density (g/ml)	1.92	1.75	1.77
Vapor pressure (mm Hg at 37°C)	10.5	75	64
Surface tension (dynes/cm)	18	14	15
O_2 solubility (ml/100 ml)	53	56	52
CO_2 solubility (ml/100 ml)	210	198	160

PFC, perfluorocarbon.

istration. Perfluorocarbons are very stable, chemically and biologically inert liquids due to the strong bond between carbon and fluorine atoms and cannot be metabolized in biological systems. PFC liquids are primarily eliminated by expiration from the lungs and, possibly, to a very minor degree via transpiration through the skin [20]. When administered into the lungs, systemic absorption and distribution of PFC to the other tissues in small amounts have been demonstrated and measurements in expired gases have documented a rapid elimination of PFC through the lung [21, 22]. The physicochemical properties of PFC liquids are described in detail elsewhere [23].

Biomedical Applications of Perfluorocarbons

As an oxygen carrier, PFC liquid is employed in various areas, either intravenously in emulsified form or intratracheally in neat (unemulsified) form. Since the first successful trial of Clark and Gollan on liquid breathing with PFC [16], liquid ventilation has been intensively investigated to support pulmonary gas exchange both in healthy and diseased lungs. PFC liquid breathing was administered also in other respiratory environment studies such as during deep diving and exposure to hyperbaric pressure [24].

The liquid ventilation technique has been employed as a controlled method to induce hypothermia. Studies have proven this technique to offer potential as a new approach for induced hypothermia in combining the higher heat capacity of PFC liquids and the lungs as an effective heat exchanger [25, 26].

Recent studies have indicated the feasibility of PFC liquids as a vehicle for pulmonary administration of drugs [27, 28]. The large exchange surface of the lung and the ability of PFC liquids to distribute easily through the lung make it a promising alternative route for delivery of agents.

PFC liquids have been used clinically as radiological contrast agent for bronchography and alveolography [29]. In addition, PFC liquids are ideal substances as a contrast agent for computer tomography, magnetic resonance imaging and ultrasound technology [30].

PFC emulsions are an effective oxygen carrier to tissues and, thus, have formed a related area of interest for research as a red cell substitute [31, 32]. In addition, emulsified PFC liquids have also been employed for improving tissue oxygenation in ischemic organs [33, 34].

Liquid Ventilation Technique

The use of saline as a respiratory medium to investigate the pulmonary structure and function relationship, particularly the study of tissue and alveolar surface active forces [35–37], has formed the basis for the evolution of the liquid breathing concept from the saline-filled lung to ventilation with inert liquids.

As in the studies with saline-filled lung early liquid breathing studies with PFC were performed by total body immersion of spontaneously breathing animals into the oxygenated liquid [16, 38], or manually regulated gravity-assisted insufflation of animals with oxygenated PFC [39–43]. However, while adequate oxygenation could be provided, ventilation with PFC liquid did not improve CO_2 elimination and acidosis in these systems.

The inherent problem of effective CO_2 elimination related to diffusional and flow limitations associated with the high density and viscosity of the PFC liquid was avoided by employing the demand-regulated and mechanically assisted breathing systems [44–48]. Development of a modified liquid ventilator enabled the liquid ventilation technique to be successfully used in subsequent studies, even in animals with ineffective gas exchange. In this technique, extracorporeally oxygenated, warmed PFC liquid is instilled into the animal's lung at a volume equivalent to functional residual capacity volume. After degassing the lungs with postural and thoracic manipulations, the animal is connected to the liquid breathing system, and tidal liquid volumes are delivered at a frequency depending on the animal's demands while exhaled liquid is purged of CO_2 and oxygenated extracorporeally between the breaths.

Liquid Ventilation in Healthy Animals

In 1966, Clark and Gollan were the first to introduce successful PFC liquid ventilation in mice [16]. They demonstrated that, unlike animals breathing other liquids (e.g., silicone oil), animals breathing PFC liquid for several hours survived the trial and were easily reconverted to gas breathing. This work was a major advance in the field of liquid breathing offering an alternative means of respiratory medium. The longest reported liquid ventilation trial was performed in dogs and lasted only 8 h [39]. In various studies with liquid ventilation, pulmonary gas exchange, respiratory mechanics, cardiovascular dynamics (such as cardiac output, organ blood flow) and alveolar surface tension characteristics of healthy animal lungs were investigated. Moreover, in addition to the early changes in lung functions after liquid ventilation, the morphologic, histologic and biochemical changes have been documented in these animals in long-term follow-up studies.

PFC liquid ventilation has been demonstrated to maintain adequate oxygenation in healthy animals [40–43, 49–52]. Although at satisfactory levels, paO_2 was consistently lower in all the studies during liquid ventilation when compared to the control levels. A commonly reported issue in these experiments is the observation of increases in $paCO_2$ and development of acidosis during liquid breathing [40–43]. The difficulty in effective elimination of CO_2 has been ascribed to the considerably high viscosity and density of the PFC liquid together with the low CO_2 diffusion coefficient [24]. Koen et al. have further explored and provided alternative ventilatory strategies to overcome this problem [47]. The changes in arterial pH were assumed to be related to changes in $paCO_2$ in some studies [39, 41]. However, with the development of liquid breathing systems effectively eliminating CO_2, acidosis was suggested to be a distinct metabolic disturbance secondary to hyperlactatemia associated with redistribution of blood flow [50]. In a recent study, ineffective intravascular volume status was emphasized as being responsible for the metabolic acidosis [52].

Liquid ventilation usually requires high airway pressures compared to gas ventilation. Considerably high (60–100 mm Hg) peak airway pressures have been reported in isolated lung preparations during liquid ventilation [50, 53]. In a study further investigating this issue, Curtis et al. have shown that real alveolar pressures are overestimated at proximal airway pressures but mean airway pressures can be used to reflect the alveolar pressures during liquid ventilation [51].

Several researchers have reported successful reconversion to gas breathing following liquid ventilation [39–43, 49, 51, 52]. However, a temporary impairment has been commonly observed in arterial oxygenation on returning to gas breathing [39–43, 51, 52] which took several days to return to preliquid breathing levels. This effect was attributed to residual PFC liquid remaining in the lung that was believed to cause a diffusion defect, low ventilation/perfusion areas or decreased alveolar pO_2 [40, 42, 52]. Similar to changes in arterial oxygenation, reversible changes in respiratory mechanics (decrease in respiratory system compliance and increase in airway resistance) have been documented after liquid ventilation [41, 42, 45]. Furthermore, both increased [51] or unchanged airway pressures [39] have been reported after reconversion to gas breathing.

The effect of liquid ventilation on pulmonary surfactant and its surface tension properties was subjected to both *in vivo* and *in vitro* studies more than 20 years ago. One study has revealed that surfactant was not removed from the lung and the surface tension-surface area characteristics of surfactant were not altered either after liquid ventilation or lung lavage with PFC [54]. In another study, demonstrating no changes in surfactant quantity after liquid breathing, the pressure-volume relationships of isolated healthy lungs as an indirect measure of surfactant function showed a transient increase in surface active properties of surfactant [55].

Great interest centers on the effects of liquid ventilation on lung morphology and histology. In various studies in different adult animals, hyperemia and an inflammatory reaction with macrophage infiltration were observed in the lungs only shortly after liquid ventilation [38, 40], and these were suggested to correlate with the changes in blood gases [40]. However, the alveolar structures appeared to be histologically normal within a few days, except that of residual vacuolated macrophages [40, 49, 56], and remained normal for several months [40, 42, 49, 56] and even 3 years after liquid ventilation [21, 43]. Additionally, in a morphologic study on newborn rabbits, electron microscopic data revealed that the ultrastructure of the lung remained unimpaired after liquid ventilation [57].

The limited hematologic and biochemical studies suggested that no permanent deleterious effect was produced after liquid ventilation [21, 56]. Despite the presence of residual PFC in all tissues, only minor changes in serum alkaline phosphatase, cholesterol, glutamic oxalacetic transaminase, glutamic pyruvate transaminase and white blood cell counts were detected, but they all returned to normal in less than 1 week following liquid ventilation.

Long-term follow-up studies have been conducted in adult animals to study the uptake, distribution and elimination of PFC liquids after various periods of liquid ventilation application. The longest reported follow-up studies, showing no adverse clinical effects, lasted approximately 3 years following 1 h liquid ventilation [21, 43]. Residual PFC was detected by gas chromatography in small amounts in all tissues, indicating systemic distribution; it was approximately 1000 times higher in the lungs and pulmonary lymph nodes than in the other tissues and, furthermore, fat contained a higher concentration of PFC than other tissues. Most importantly, residual PFC was not associated with any evidence of adverse reaction in any of the tissues. In other long-term studies, similar results have been reported and the elimination rate of PFC from lung tissue was found to be of an exponential character and dependent on vapor pressure of PFC; the higher the vapor pressure, the faster the elimination rate [21, 56, 58]. Additionally, the absence of excess inorganic fluoride ions in urine supported that PFC liquids are not metabolized in biologic systems [59]. The exact mechanisms for uptake, distribution and elimination of PFC warrants further investigation while some factors such as organ blood flow, tissue lipid composition, vapor pressure of PFC, and ventilation/perfusion matching in the lung are considered to play a role.

Liquid Ventilation in Animals with Acute Respiratory Failure

To date, there are only a few reports of respiratory support with liquid ventilation in adult animals with acute respiratory failure while much of the interest has focused on preterm animals with surfactant deficiency.

The elevated surface tension at the alveolar air-liquid interface contributes to the development of pulmonary pathology (i.e., atelectasis, intrapulmonary shunting and decreased compliance) due to either surfactant deficiency as in infant RDS, or surfactant dysfunction as in adult RDS. With the hypothesis that PFC liquid would eliminate the surface forces in the surfactant deficient lung and promote alveolar stability and, thus, improve lung mechanics, Shaffer et al. employed PFC liquid ventilation in premature animals which were subject to high alveolar surface tension and structural immaturity [60]. In this and subsequent studies, Shaffer et al. showed that in comparison to gas ventilation, liquid ventilation provided better pulmonary gas exchange in preterm animals [61, 62]. Moreover, these studies demonstrated that liquid-ventilated animals were successfully reconverted to gas ventilation, and gas exchange and lung mechanics parameters were improved compared to the initial gas ventilation: paO_2 and respiratory compliance increased, and alveolar-arterial O_2 difference and inflation pressures decreased.

Liquid ventilation was also applied to preterm animals with respiratory failure upon delivery, before initiating gas ventilation [63–65]. These studies demonstrated that liquid ventilation initiated immediately after birth provided effective pulmonary gas exchange while improving respiratory compliance and supporting cardiovascular stability.

The effect of short-term lung lavage with PFC liquid has been investigated in preterm animals and no significant changes were demonstrated in gas exchange and lung mechanics in contrast to liquid ventilation [66].

Histologic findings indicated that liquid ventilation was less harmful to the pulmonary structures when compared to gas ventilation in which hyaline membranes and epithelial necrosis were present [65, 67, 68]. In morphometric analysis, more homogeneously expanded and intact gas exchange units were documented in liquid-ventilated lungs in contrast to the gas-ventilated lungs [65, 69].

In an adult animal model of respiratory failure, liquid ventilation with gravity-assisted technique improved pulmonary gas exchange significantly and arterial oxygenation remained higher than in the only mechanically ventilated group even after liquid ventilation was terminated [70]. In an oleic acid model of lung injury in adult animals, short periods of whole lung lavage with oxygenated PFC liquid resulted in improvements in pulmonary gas exchange and respiratory system compliance while control animals showed deterioration [71]. These beneficial effects of lung lavage with PFC were believed to result from washing out the edema fluid and replacement of the edema fluid in the lung by the PFC with a low surface tension and high solubility for respiratory gases.

In view of the histologic and clinical data, the possible mechanisms by which liquid ventilation provided an effective therapeutic modality for treatment of respiratory failure were suggested as [65, 72]: elimination of increased alveolar surface tension in liquid filled-lung, improved alveolar stability and recruitment, even distribution of pulmonary blood flow in liquid-filled lung, improved ventilation-perfusion matching resulting in decreased intrapulmonary shunting.

Clinical Investigations of Liquid Ventilation

The first human trial of PFC liquid ventilation was reported by Greenspan et al. [15]. Short periods of liquid ventilation were administered by gravity-assisted technique to three premature infants with severe respiratory failure who were considered to be clinically at the terminal stage. Although the infants eventually died of their underlying disease, marked improvements in both arterial oxygenation and respiratory compliance were observed after liquid ventilation. Since the clinical condition of the infants was not improved with other treatment modalities, these results were considered promising for future applications of this technique at an earlier stage of pulmonary dysfunction.

In parallel to animal experiments with liquid ventilation, histologic analysis of the liquid-ventilated infant lungs demonstrated uniform, well expanded lung units when compared to conventionally ventilated infants [73]. Moreover, other organs were histologically similar to those of controls.

To study the uptake, distribution, and elimination of the PFC, expired gas samples, arterial blood and various tissues were analyzed by gas chromatography in infants following liquid ventilation and were compared with controls [74]. The results indicated that PFC was rapidly eliminated by vaporization through the lungs (PFC concentration in the expired gas was within control range in 8 h), and systemic absorption and distribution of PFC to the blood and other tissues occurred while deposition was in small amounts at 2.5 months following liquid ventilation. From the limited data, it was speculated that uptake, distribution and elimination of PFC could be related to lipid composition of the tissues, perfusion of the organs, and ventilation–perfusion matching in the lung.

Potential Problems and Future Implications of Liquid Ventilation

The progress of the liquid ventilation concept from laboratory experiments for studying pulmonary physiology to human trials to restore respiratory function is overwhelming. Based on the encouraging results of animal experiments and the limited data from clinical investigational trial liquid ventilation application has to be explored extensively in areas other than the infant RDS, such as the adult RDS, aspiration syndromes, pulmonary lavage in alveolar proteinosis and cystic fibrosis as potential therapeutic considerations in clinical conditions as stated elsewhere [75]. For this purpose, a better understanding of liquid ventilation is warranted with respect to safety and efficacy in clinical practice. More importantly, before large clinical trials are undertaken, PFC liquids and liquid ventilation have to be proven safe for administration for prolonged periods, and advantages over conventional therapeutic modalities have to be documented.

Although the principle of liquid ventilation is simple, the technology necessary to perform it is not encouraging. To employ liquid ventilation, there are extra technical requirements including an extracorporeal membrane oxygenator and a modified liquid ventilator. Moreover, one needs high volumes of PFC as a priming volume in liquid ventilation. At present, this complex and relatively expensive equipment has prevented liquid ventilation technique from becoming commonly and practically applied in clinical conditions. To overcome such problems, a new PFC administration technique has been explored in recent years as an alternative means of respiratory support. This new technique of partial liquid ventilation combines conventional mechanical gas ventilation and intratracheal PFC administration. In partial liquid ventilation, PFC liquid is administered into the lungs and mechanical gas ventilation is superimposed at conventional ventilator settings without necessitating an extracorporeal oxygenator and liquid ventilator.

Partial Liquid Ventilation

The search for a simpler PFC application technique to support pulmonary gas exchange has raised the concept of partial liquid ventilation, in that conventional mechanical ventilation is combined with intratracheal PFC administration.

Partial Liquid Ventilation in Healthy Animals

Recently, Fuhrman et al. published the first report on this new technique in healthy piglets, demonstrating effective oxygenation and ventilation [17]. After filling the lungs to the functional residual capacity volume with a PFC liquid which was fully saturated with oxygen, animals were volume-controlled ventilated for 1 h and these were compared to control animals subjected to the same ventilatory parameters with respect to gas exchange and respiratory mechanics.

In their study, arterial oxygenation was maintained about 400 mm Hg and average $paCO_2$ was 40 mm Hg, reflecting ventilation-perfusion matching during this technique which they named as "perfluorcarbon-associated gas exchange." More importantly, the adequate gas exchange was achieved at tidal volumes and airway pressures comparable with mechanically gas ventilated animals, suggesting that the presence of PFC did not alter the mechanical function of the lung.

For the possible mechanism of action for gas exchange during partial liquid ventilation in healthy animals, the authors speculated that filling the functional residual capacity volume of the lung with PFC maintained a respiratory medium for continuous gas exchange by allowing formation of air bubbles with the superimposed tidal gas volumes. The low surface tension of PFC, as they speculated, would serve as a suitable environment for in vivo bubble oxygenation and, thus, gas diffusion from PFC to alveolar vessels would provide an effective gas exchange during partial liquid ventilation.

Partial Liquid Ventilation in Acute Respiratory Failure

Based on the observations that preterm animals could be converted to mechanical gas ventilation following liquid ventilation with favorable effects of residual PFC on gas exchange and lung mechanics, experiments were performed to investigate the effects of intratracheal PFC administration in combination with conventional mechanical ventilation on pulmonary gas exchange in an animal model of RDS.

The first report on the effects of partial liquid ventilation in adult animals with acute respiratory failure was introduced by Tütüncü et al. [18]. After inducing RDS by repeated lung lavage with saline, PFC liquid was administered intratracheally in increasing doses (3–15 ml/kg) while animals were mechanically ventilated with volume-controlled ventilation and positive end-expiratory pressure. In contrast to isovolumic saline-treated animals, PaO_2 improved with PFC administration in a dose-dependent manner and $PaCO_2$ was maintained considerably lower. The improvement in PaO_2 with 15 ml/kg of PFC reached a level at which almost no intrapulmonary shunt occurred. The PFC doses tested were below the functional residual capacity volume (18 ml/kg) of the tested animals. Another interesting observation was that the inflation pressures were decreased to the same extent independent of the PFC dose and, thus, respiratory compliance was improved within the range of 20%–23% at all the PFC doses. Moreover, hemodynamic stability was not impaired during this type of respiratory support.

In another study from the same group [19], intratracheal PFC administration at functional residual capacity volume was tested in animals with acute respiratory failure and the effects of 3 h partial liquid ventilation on lung functions and lung histology were compared to conventional gas ventilation and saline controls. With this technique, pulmonary gas exchange was improved and maintained stable throughout the observation period in RDS-induced adult animals (mean PaO_2 was above 400 mm Hg and mean $PaCO_2$ was below 45 mm Hg). However, the same ventilatory conditions (tidal volume and positive end-expiratory pressure) resulted in persistent hypoxia and hypercarbia in conventionally ventilated animals and saline-treated animals. The administration of PFC provided lung inflation at lower airway pressures (an average of 23% less than in the untreated animals), and respiratory compliance consequently improved; these effects persisted throughout the study period. Additionally, there were marked decreases in respiratory resistance at inspiration.

Histologic data from the same study supported the clinical data and revealed that alveolar structures were well preserved with partial liquid ventilation, preventing alveolar distension and rupture. In both above-mentioned studies, metabolic acidosis was observed in PFC-treated animals despite the well preserved hemodynamic status, and was ascribed to changes in regional organ blood flow during mechanical ventilation with positive end-expiratory pressure.

These studies provided important data on the mechanisms by which PFC enhances gas exchange in the diseased lung, either during partial liquid ventilation or during gas ventilation following liquid ventilation. Moreover, the data provided physiologic implications with regard to the dissociation between the gas exchange and lung mechanics parameters during partial liquid ventilation. The dose-dependent improvement of gas exchange supported that large doses of PFC, approaching the normal functional capacity of the animal, are required to correct hypoxia as fully as possible. However, respiratory system compliance and airway pressures can be improved even with a small dose of PFC (3 ml/kg) and further doses do not make significant changes in the lung mechanics properties of lung-lavaged animals.

The responsible mechanism for the improvement in gas exchange during partial liquid ventilation was suggested to be mainly due to the filling of the alveoli with PFC liquid so that the more PFC applied, the more collapsed alveoli could be opened up and prevented from end-expiratory collapse. Thus, the lung volume participating in effective gas exchange would increase in parallel with the increasing PFC doses, thereby eliminating intrapulmonary shunt. The high solubility of O_2 and CO_2 in PFC would also contribute to the continuous pulmonary gas exchange in this system. This mechanism of action for PFC was confirmed by the well maintained PaO_2 for several hours, as well as by the histologic findings.

By contrast, the remarkably low surface tension of PFC liquid accounted for the changes in the mechanical behavior of the respiratory system independent of the PFC dose during partial liquid ventilation. The changes in respiratory mechanics suggested that, following administration of even a low dose of PFC (3 ml/kg), a thin film of PFC with a low surface tension is formed due to evaporation and covers the lung units in the whole lung. This hypothetical film of PFC reduces the elevated surface tension at the alveolar air-liquid interface in the diseased lung. Therefore, the reduction of surface tension by PFC facilitates easy lung expansion (improves respiratory compliance) during partial liquid ventilation. It follows that once the surface tension is reduced to the level of acting PFC, additional PFC doses would not cause further changes in the mechanical behavior of the lung.

These studies demonstrated the feasibility of partial liquid ventilation in improving pulmonary gas exchange and respiratory mechanics in animals with RDS and, in this regard, this new type of ventilatory support proved to offer advantages over conventional mechanical ventilation in the short term. Considering the remarkable reductions in airway pressures during partial liquid ventilation while identical ventilation parameters induced barotrauma during conventional ventilation, this new technique appears to be an alternative modality to minimize or prevent the progress of lung injury. Moreover, the data support the importance of a low surface tension at the air-liquid interface in the lung. Furthermore, as stated elsewhere [76], this technique holds major advantages compared with total liquid ventilation such as requirement of less PFC and ease of administration without necessitating extra technology (extracorporeal oxygenator, modified liquid ventilator).

Future Investigations and Implications of Partial Liquid Ventilation

Consideration of another ventilatory support modality for clinical use in critical care requires documentation of an advantage compared with available techniques. The advantage should be evident in one or more of the following areas: safety, expense, ease of operation, or therapeutic outcome.

At present, partial liquid ventilation is confined to only a few animal experiments and the available data are limited to short-term (3 h) effects on pulmonary gas exchange, respiratory mechanics and hemodynamic variables. In addition to long-term administration, efficacy in other models of acute respiratory failure has to be investigated as an alternative treatment modality. With respect to its safety and tissue toxicity, further studies are required, although the limited data on tissue toxicity have proven PFC to be safe both in animal studies with liquid ventilation [21] and in clinical trials as a contrast agent [77].

Another point for further investigation is the development of metabolic acidosis and hemodynamic compromise. Since PFC liquids are dense liquids, the effects of intratracheal PFC administration on cardiopulmonary interaction needs to be investigated as a contributory factor for altered organ blood flow and occurrence of lactic acidosis, although intravascular fluid volume plays an important role in maintaining adequate oxygen supply during liquid ventilation [52].

All types of mechanical ventilation modalities are means of supportive treatment until the primary disorder is cured. When the long-term administration of partial liquid ventilation is considered, repetitive doses of PFC will be inevitably required due to evaporation. In this respect, cost effectivity of this type of ventilatory support needs to be further investigated and compared with other treatment modalities, although this point makes partial liquid ventilation advantageous over liquid ventilation.

References

1. Rinaldo JE, Rogers RM (1982) Adult respiratory distress syndrome: changing concepts of lung injury and repair. N Engl J Med 306:900–909
2. Shale DJ (1987) The adult respiratory distress syndrome-20 years on. Thorax 42:642–645
3. Kolobow T, Morett MP, Fumagali R, Mascheroni D, Prato P, Chen V, Joris M (1987) Severe impairment in lung function induced by high peak airway pressure during mechanical ventilation. An experimental study. Am Rev Respir Dis 135:312–315
4. Sandhar BK, Niblett DJ, Argiras EP, Dunhill MS, Sykes MK (1988) Effects of positive end-expiratory pressure on hyaline membrane formation in a rabbit model of the neonatal respiratory distress syndrome. Intensive Care Med 14:538–546
5. Lachmann B, Jonson B, Lindroth M, Robertson B (1982) Modes of artificial ventilation in severe respiratory distress syndrome. Lung function and morphology in rabbits after wash-out of alveolar surfactant. Crit Care Med 10:724–732
6. Hickling KG, Henderson SJ, Jackson R (1990) Low mortality associated with low volume pressure limited ventilation with permissive hypercapnia in severe adult respiratory distress syndrome. Intensive Care Med 16:372–377
7. Anderson JB (1986) Changing ventilatory strategy may alter outcome in catastrophic lung disease. Intensive Care Med 12 [Suppl]:200A
8. Tharratt RS, Allen RP, Albertson TE (1988) Pressure controlled inverse ratio ventilation in severe adult respiratory failure. Chest 94:755–762

9. Sjöstrand U (1980) High-frequency positive-pressure ventilation (HFPPV): a review. Crit Care Med 8:345–364
10. Nielsen JB, Sjöstrand UH, Edgren EL, Lichtwarck-Aschoff M, Svensson BA (1991) An experimental study of different ventilatory modes in piglets in severe respiratory distress induced by surfactant depletion. Intensive Care Med 17:225–233
11. Zapol WM, Snider MT, Hill JD et al (1979) Extracorporeal membrane oxygenation in severe acute respiratory failure. A randomized prospective study. JAMA 242:2193–2196
12. Gattinoni L, Pesenti A, Mascheroni D et al (1986) Low frequency positive-pressure ventilation with extracorporeal CO_2 removal in severe acute respiratory failure. JAMA 256:881–886
13. Lachmann B (1987) The role of pulmonary surfactant in the pathogenesis and therapy of ARDS. In: Vincent JL (ed) Update in intensive care and emergency medicine. Springer, Berlin Heidelberg New York, pp 123–134
14. Lewis JF, Jobe AL (1993) Surfactant and the adult respiratory distress syndrome. Am Rev Respir Dis 147:218–233
15. Greenspan JS, Wolfson MR, Rubenstein SD, Shaffer TH (1990) Liquid ventilation of human preterm neonates. J Pediatr 117:106–111
16. Clark LC, Gollan F (1966) Survival of mammals breathing organic liquids equilibrated with oxygen at atmosphere pressure. Science 152:1755–1756
17. Fuhrmann BP, Paczan PR, DeFrancisis M (1991) Perfluorocarbon-associated gas exchange. Crit Care Med 19:712–722
18. Tütüncü AS, Faithfull NS, Lachmann B (1993) Intratracheal perfluorocarbon administration combined with mechanical ventilation in experimental respiratory distress syndrome: dose-dependent improvement of gas exchange. Crit Care Med 21:962–969
19. Tütüncü AS, Faithfull NS, Lachmann B (1993) Comparison of ventilatory support with intratracheal perfluorocarbon administration and conventional mechanical ventilation in animals with acute respiratory failure. Am Rev Respir Dis 148:785–792
20. Faithfull NS (1992) Artificial oxygen carrying substitutes. Adv Exp Med Biol 317:55–72
21. Calderwood HW, Ruiz BC, Tham MK, Modell JH, Hood CI (1975) Residual levels and biochemical changes after ventilation with perfluorinated liquid. J Appl Physiol 139:603–607
22. Wolfson MR, Clark LC, Hoffman RE, Davis SL, Greenspan JS, Rubenstein TH, Shaffer TH (1990) Liquid ventilation of neonates: uptake, distribution, and elimination of the liquid. Pediatr Res 27:37A
23. Sargent JW, Seffl RJ (1970) Properties of perfluorinated liquid. Fed Proc 29:1699–1703
24. Shaffer TH (1987) A brief review: liquid ventilation. Undersea Biomed Res 14:169–176
25. Forman DL, Bhutani VK, Tran N, Shaffer TH (1986) A new approach to induced hypothermia. J Surg Res 40:36–42
26. Shaffer TH, Forman DL, Wolfson MR (1984) The physiological effects of ventilation with liquid fluorocarbon at controlled temperatures. Undersea Biomed Res 11:287–298
27. Wolfson MR, Greenspan JS, Shaffer TH (1991) Pulmonary administration of vasoactive drugs (PAD) by perfluorocarbon liquid ventilation. Pediatr Res 29:336A
28. Zelinka MA, Wolfson MR, Calligaro S, Rubenstein SD, Greenspan JS, Shaffer TH (1991) Direct administration of gentamicin during liquid ventilation of the lamb: comparison of lung and serum levels to IV administration. Pediatr Res 29:290A
29. Liu MS, Long DM (1976) Biological disposition of perfluoroctylbromide: tracheal administration in alveolography and broncography. Invest Radiol 11:479–485
30. Mattrey RF (1989) Perfluoroctylbromide: a new contrast agent for CT, sonography and MR imaging. AJR 152:247–252
31. Mitsuno T, Ohyanagi H, Naito R (1982) Clinical studies of a perfluorochemical whole blood substitute (Fluosol-DA). Ann Surg 195:60–69
32. Tremper KK, Friedman AE, Levine EM, Lapin R, Camarillo D (1982) The pre-operative treatment of severely anemic patients with a perfluorochemical oxygen-transport fluid. N Engl J Med 307:277–283

33. Ricci JL, Sloviter HA, Ziegler MM (1985) Intestinal ischemia: reduction of mortality utilizing intraluminal perfluorochemical. Am J Surg 149:84–90
34. Forman MB, Gingham S, Kopelman HA, Wehr C, Sandler MP, Kolodgie F, Vaughn WK, Frieslinger GC, Virmani R (1985) Reduction of infarct size with intracoronary perfluorochemical in a canine preparation of reperfusion. Circulation 71:1060–1068
35. Neergard D Von (1929) Neue Auffassungen über einen Grundbegriff der Atemmechanik. Die Retraktionskraft der Lunge, abhängig von der Oberflächenspannung in den Alveolen. Gesammte Exp Med 66:373–394
36. Clements JA, Tierney DF (1965) Alveolar stability associated with altered surface tension. In: Fenn WO, Rahn H (eds) Handbook of physiology, section 3: respiration. American Physiological Society, Washington DC, pp 1565–1583
37. West JB, Dollery CT, Matthews CME, Zardini P (1965) Distribution of blood and ventilation in saline-filled lung. J Appl Physiol 20:1107–1117
38. Patel MJ, Syanto P, Yates B, Long DM (1970) Survival and histopathologic changes in lungs of hamsters following synthetic liquid breathing. Fed Proc 29:1740–1745
39. Modell JH, Newby EJ, Ruiz BC (1970) Long term survival of dogs after breathing oxygenated fluorocarbon liquid. Fed Proc 29:1731–1736
40. Modell JH, Hood CI, Kuck EJ, Ruiz BC (1971) Oxygenation by ventilation with fluorocarbon liquid (FX-80). Anesthesiology 34:312–320
41. Saga S, Modell JH, Calderwood HW, Lucas AJ, Tham MK, Swensson EW (1973) Pulmonary function after ventilation with fluorocarbon liquid P12-F (Caroxin-F). J Appl Physiol 34:160–164
42. Tuazon JG, Modell JH, Hood CI, Swensson EH (1973) Pulmonary function after ventilation with fluorocarbon liquid (Caroxin-D). Anesthesiology 38:134–140
43. Modell JH, Calderwood HW, Ruiz BC, Tham MK, Hood CI (1976) Liquid ventilation of primates. Chest 69:79–81
44. Moskowitz GD (1970) A mechanical respirator for control of liquid breathing. Fed Proc 29:1751–1752
45. Shaffer TH, Moskowitz GD (1974) Demand controlled liquid ventilation of the lungs. J Appl Physiol 36:208–213
46. Harris DG, Coggin RR, Roby J, Feezor M, Turner G, Bennett PB (1983) Liquid ventilation in dogs: an apparatus for normobaric and hyperbaric studies. J Appl Physiol 54:1141–1148
47. Koen PA, Wolfson MR, Shaffer TH (1988) Fluorocarbon ventilation: maximal expiratory flows and CO_2 elimination. Pediatr Res 24:291–296
48. Wolfson MR, Tran N, Bhutani V, Shaffer TH (1988) A new experimental approach for the study of cardiopulmonary physiology during early development. J Appl Physiol 65:1436–1443
49. Matthews WH, Balzer RH, Shelburne JD, Pratt PC, Kylstra JA (1978) Steady-state gas exchange in normothermic, anesthetized, liquid-ventilated dogs. Undersea Biomed Res 5:341–354
50. Lowe C, Tuma RF, Sivieri EM, Shaffer TH (1979) Liquid ventilation: cardiovascular adjustments with secondary hyperlactatemia and acidosis. J Appl Physiol 47:1051–1057
51. Curtis SE, Fuhrman BP, Howland DF (1990) Airway and alveolar pressures during perfluorocarbon breathing in infant lambs. J Appl Physiol 68:2322–2328
52. Curtis SE, Fuhrman BP, Howland DF, DeFrancisis M, Motoyama EK (1991) Cardiac output during liquid (perfluorocarbon) breathing in newborn piglets. Crit Care Med 19:225–230
53. Lowe CA, Shaffer TH (1981) Increased pulmonary vascular resistance during liquid ventilation. Undersea Biomed Res 8:229–238
54. Modell JH, Gollan F, Giammona ST, Parker D (1970) Effect of fluorocarbon liquid on surface tension properties of pulmonary surfactant. Chest 57:263–265
55. Ruefer R (1970) Surfactant and alveolar surface forces after breathing of an inert fluorinated liquid. Fed Proc 29:1813–1815
56. Calderwood HW, Modell JH, Rogow L, Tham MK, Hood CI (1973) Morphologic and

biochemical changes in dogs after ventilation with Caroxin-D fluorocarbon. Anesthesiology 39:488–495
57. Forman DL, Bhutani VK, Hilfer SR, Shaffer TH (1984) A fine structure study of the liquid-ventilated newborn rabbit lung. Fed Proc 43:647
58. Modell JH, Tham MK, Modell JH, Calderwood HW, Ruiz BC (1973) Distribution and retention of fluorocarbon in mice and dogs after injection or liquid ventilation. Toxicol Appl Pharmacol 26:86–92
59. Holaday DA, Fiserova-Bergerova V, Modell JH, Hood CI (1972) Uptake, distribution and excretion of fluorocarbon FX-80 (perfluorbertyl perfluorotetrahydrafuron) during liquid breathing in the dog. Anesthesiology 37:387–394
60. Shaffer TH, Rubenstein D, Moskowitz GD, Delivoria-Papadopoulos M (1976) Gaseous exchange and acid-base balance in premature lambs during liquid ventilation since birth. Pediatr Res 10:227–231
61. Shaffer TH, Douglas PR, Lowe CA, Bhutani VK (1983) The effects of liquid ventilation on cardiopulmonary function in preterm lambs. Pediatr Res 17:303–306
62. Shaffer TH, Lowe CA, Bhutani VK, Douglas PR (1984) Liquid ventilation: effects on pulmonary function in distressed meconium-stained lambs. Pediatr Res 18:47–52
63. Shaffer TH, Tran N, Bhutani VK, Sivieri EM (1983) Cardiopulmonary function in very preterm lambs during liquid ventilation. Pediatr Res 17:680–684
64. Wolfson MR, Tran N, Bhutani VK, Shaffer TH (1988) A new experimental approach for the study of cardiopulmonary physiology during early development. J Appl Physiol 65:1436–1443
65. Wolfson MR, Greenspan JS, Deoras KS, Rubenstein SD, Shaffer TH (1992) Comparison of gas and liquid ventilation: clinical, physiological, and histological correlates. J Appl Physiol 72:1024–1031
66. Shaffer TH, Ferguson JD, Koen PA, Moskowitz GD, Delivoria-Papadopoulos (1978) Pulmonary lavage in preterm lambs. Pediatr Res 12:695–698
67. Schwieler GH, Robertson B (1976) Liquid ventilation in immature newborn rabbits. Biol Neonate 29:343–353
68. Greenspan JS, Wolfson MR, Deoras KS, Rubenstein SD, Shaffer TH (1989) Minimal surface tension: clinical, physiologic, and histologic correlations in extremely premature lambs. Fed Proc 25:311A
69. Deoras KS, Wolfson MR, Greenspan JS, Shaffer TH (1989) Morphometric analysis of the ventilated immature lung: effect of minimizing surface tension. Physiologist 32:228
70. Calderwood HW, Modell JH, Ruiz BC, Brogdon JE, Hood CI (1973) Pulmonary lavage with liquid fluorocarbon in a model of pulmonary edema. Anesthesiology 38:141–144
71. Richman PS, Wolfson MR, Shaffer TH, Kelsen SG (1990) Lung lavage with oxygenated fluorocarbon improves gas exchange and lung compliance in cats with acute lung injury. Am Rev Respir Dis 141:A773
72. Wolfson MR, Shaffer TH (1990) Liquid ventilation during early development: theory, physiologic processes and application. J Dev Physiol 13:1–12
73. Deoras KS, Coppola D, Wolfson MR, Greenspan JS, Rubenstein SD, Shaffer TH (1990) Liquid ventilation of neonates: tissue histology and morphometry. Pediatr Res 27:29A
74. Wolfson MR, Clark LC, Hoffmann RE, Davis SL, Greenspan JS, Rubenstein SD, Shaffer TH (1990) Liquid ventilation of neonates: uptake, distribution, and elimination of the liquid. Pediatr Res 27:37A
75. Fuhrman BP (1990) Perfluorcarbon liquid ventilation: the first human trial. J Pediatr 117:73–74
76. Curtis S (1991) Perfluorcarbon-associated gas exchange: a hybrid approach to mechanical ventilation. Crit Care Med 19:600–601
77. Mattrey RF, Long DC (1988) Potential role of PFOB in diagnostic imaging. Invest Radiol 23[Suppl]:S298–S301

Subject Index

Springer-Verlag and the Environment

We at Springer-Verlag firmly believe that an international science publisher has a special obligation to the environment, and our corporate policies consistently reflect this conviction.

We also expect our business partners – paper mills, printers, packaging manufacturers, etc. – to commit themselves to using environmentally friendly materials and production processes.

The paper in this book is made from low- or no-chlorine pulp and is acid free, in conformance with international standards for paper permanency.

MIX
Papier aus verantwortungsvollen Quellen
Paper from responsible sources
FSC® C105338

If you have any concerns about our products,
you can contact us on
ProductSafety@springernature.com

In case Publisher is established outside the EU,
the EU authorized representative is:
Springer Nature Customer Service Center GmbH
Europaplatz 3, 69115 Heidelberg, Germany

Printed by Libri Plureos GmbH
in Hamburg, Germany